THE CHARACTER OF CONSCIOUSNESS

PHILOSOPHY OF MIND

Series Editor: David J. Chalmers, Australian National University

THE CHARACTER OF CONSCIOUSNESS

DAVID J. CHALMERS

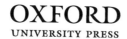

OXFORD
UNIVERSITY PRESS

2010

OXFORD
UNIVERSITY PRESS

Oxford University Press, Inc., publishes works that further
Oxford University's objective of excellence
in research, scholarship, and education.

Oxford   New York
Auckland   Cape Town   Dar es Salaam   Hong Kong   Karachi
Kuala Lumpur   Madrid   Melbourne   Mexico City   Nairobi
New Delhi   Shanghai   Taipei   Toronto

With offices in
Argentina   Austria   Brazil   Chile   Czech Republic   France   Greece
Guatemala   Hungary   Italy   Japan   Poland   Portugal   Singapore
South Korea   Switzerland   Thailand   Turkey   Ukraine   Vietnam

Copyright © 2010 by Oxford University Press, Inc.

Published by Oxford University Press, Inc.
198 Madison Avenue, New York, New York 10016

www.oup.com

Library of Congress Cataloging-in-Publication Data
Chalmers, David John, 1966–
The character of consciousness / David J. Chalmers.
p. cm. — (Philosophy of mind series)
ISBN 978-0-19-531110-5; 978-0-19-531111-2 (pbk.)
1. Consciousness. I. Title.
B808.9.C48 2009
126—dc22   2009038337

3 5 7 9 8 6 4 2

Printed in the United States of America
on acid-free paper

ACKNOWLEDGMENTS

I am grateful to far too many people to mention for discussion of the many topics in this book. Some but not all of them are acknowledged below for their help with individual chapters.

The chapters in this book were written over a period of just over a decade at four institutions: Washington University, University of California Santa Cruz, the University of Arizona, and the Australian National University. I am grateful to Andy Clark, David Hoy, Chris Maloney, and Frank Jackson for creating the conditions that made all of these institutions terrific places to work. I am also grateful to the Australian Research Council for a Federation Fellowship, which made much of this work possible.

A number of the chapters of this book were influenced by the extraordinary Summer Institute on Consciousness and Intentionality at UC Santa Cruz in 2002, sponsored by the National Endowment for the Humanities. I am grateful to the NEH, to my codirector, David Hoy, and to the participants in that institute for a remarkable intellectual experience.

I am also grateful to my coauthors, Tim Bayne and Frank Jackson, for their permission to include coauthored material in this book; to Karen Downing and Máire Ní Mhórdha for their help in preparing the manuscript; to Ole Koksvik and Brian Rabern for proof-reading and preparing the index respectively; to Berit Brogaard, Uriah Kriegel, and Susanna Siegel for their comments on the introduction; and to Robert Miller and Peter Ohlin at Oxford University Press for all their help with the process and for their patience.

As always, I am grateful to my (three) parents for their love and support. This book is dedicated to them.

Chapter 1 is drawn from *Journal of Consciousness Studies* 2: 200–19, 1995. This material was first presented at the 1994 "Toward a Science of Consciousness" conference in Tucson and was subsequently presented at conferences in Mexico City, Montreal, and Philadelphia and in talks at Caltech, Ohio State, UC San Francisco, UC Santa Cruz, and Yale. Thanks to Francis Crick, Peggy DesAutels, Matthew Elton, Liane Gabora, Stuart Hameroff, Christof Koch, Paul Rhodes, Gregg Rosenberg, and Sharon Wahl for their comments. The afterword draws on "Moving Forward on the Problem of Consciousness," published in *Journal of Consciousness Studies* 4 (1997): 3–46.

Chapter 2 is drawn from M. Gazzaniga, ed., *The Cognitive Neurosciences III* (MIT Press, 2004). It was first presented at a conference at King's College, London, in 1999 and subsequently at conferences in Amsterdam, Paris, Rio de Janeiro, Taipei, Tokyo, and Zaragoza, and in talks at Arizona, the Central Intelligence Agency, Cornell, CSU Long Beach, Mississippi, Montana, Northwestern, Prague, Queensland, Starlab (Brussels), Victoria, and Virginia. For commentaries in London and Paris, thanks to Scott Sturgeon and Jean Michel Roy. For comments on the written version, thanks to Christof Koch.

Chapter 3 is drawn from T. Metzinger, ed., *Neural Correlates of Consciousness: Empirical and Conceptual Issues* (MIT Press, 2000). It was first presented at the 1998 Association for the Scientific Study of Consciousness (ASSC) conference on "Neural Correlates of Consciousness" in Bremen, and subsequently in talks at the Australian National University (ANU), Arizona, Delaware, and the Ludwig Maximilian University in Munich. For comments, my thanks go to Stephen Engel, Christof Koch, Thomas Metzinger, and Alva Noë.

Chapter 4 is drawn from S. Hameroff, A. Kaszniak, and A. Scott, eds., *Toward a Science of Consciousness II: The Second Tucson Discussions and Debates* (MIT Press, 1998). It was first presented at the 1996 Tucson consciousness conference (this chapter is based on a transcript of that talk) and subsequently in talks at ANU, Berkeley, and Stanford.

Chapter 5 is drawn from S. Stich and F. Warfield, eds., *The Blackwell Guide to the Philosophy of Mind* (Blackwell, 2003) and from D. J. Chalmers, ed., *Philosophy of Mind: Classical and Contemporary Readings* (Oxford University Press, 2002). Thanks to Farid Masrour for comments.

A much-abridged version of chapter 6 appears in B. McLaughlin, A. Beckermann, and S. Walter, eds. *The Oxford Handbook of Philosophy of Mind* (Oxford University Press, 2009). Some of the material in this chapter is drawn from "Materialism and the Metaphysics of Modality" (*Philosophy and Phenomenological Research* 59: 473–93, 1999); "Does Conceivability Entail Possibility?" in T. S. Gendler and J. Hawthorne, eds., *Conceivability and Possibility* (Oxford University Press, 2002); and "Imagination, Indexicality, and Intensions" (*Philosophy and Phenomenological Research* 68: 182–90, 2004). Earlier versions of this material were presented as "Modal Rationalism and the Mind-body Problem," starting in 1998, at conferences in Arkansas, Buffalo, Kirchberg, Santa Barbara, South Bend, and Sydney, and at colloquia at ANU, NYU, Princeton, Stanford, the University of London, and the University of Nevada, Reno. Thanks go to too many people to mention for discussion and especially to Torin Alter, Ned Block, Tamar Gendler, John Hawthorne, Chris Hill, David Lewis, Brian Loar, Tom Nagel, Susanna Siegel, Daniel Stoljar, and Steve Yablo.

Chapter 7 is drawn from the *Philosophical Review* 110 (2001): 315–61. Thanks to Ned Block and two *Philosophical Review* referees for comments.

Chapters 8 and 9 are drawn from "The Content and Epistemology of Phenomenal Belief," in Q. Smith and A. Jokic, eds., *Consciousness: New Philosophical Perspectives* (Oxford University Press, 2003). This material was first presented at ANU in 1997 and subsequently at Princeton, UC Santa Cruz, the APA (Pacific Division), Metaphysical Mayhem (Syracuse), and the World Congress of Philosophy (Boston) and in Antwerp, Arizona, Delaware, Fribourg, Miami, Munich, Sydney, and Utah. Thanks to Fred Dretske, Alvin Goldman, Delia Graff, John Hawthorne, Mark Johnston, Keith Lehrer, John Pollock, and Tim Williamson for feedback. Special thanks to Martine Nida-Rümelin, Susanna Siegel, and Daniel Stoljar for lengthy discussions.

Chapter 10 is drawn from T. Alter and S. Walter, eds., *Phenomenal Concepts and Phenomenal Knowledge: New Essays on Consciousness and Physicalism* (Oxford University Press, 2006). It was greatly influenced by a round-table discussion at the 2002 NEH Summer Institute on Consciousness and Intentionality, involving Kati Balog, Ned Block, John Hawthorne, Joe Levine, and Scott Sturgeon, among many others. I was also influenced by Levine's paper, "Phenomenal Concepts and the Materialist Constraint," which develops closely related considerations by different sorts of arguments. This chapter was first formally presented at a session on David Papineau's book *Thinking about Consciousness* at the 2003 Pacific APA and has also been presented at ANU, Arizona, Birkbeck College, Sydney, Texas A&M, Texas Tech, Victoria, and Wisconsin, as well as at workshops in Buenos Aires and Copenhagen. Thanks to all those present on those occasions for very useful reactions. For comments on the written version, thanks also to Torin Alter, Murat Aydede, Janet Levin, Adam Pautz, David Papineau, Susanna Siegel, Scott Sturgeon, Daniel Stoljar, and Michael Tye.

Chapter 11 is drawn from Brian Leiter, ed., *The Future for Philosophy* (Oxford University Press, 2004). It was presented, starting in 2001, at Brown, Cornell, MIT, Rutgers, and the 2002 NEH Summer Institute on Consciousness and Intentionality. I would like to thank the audiences on all of these occasions for discussion. Special thanks to all of the participants in the NEH Institute for many valuable conversations and to Torin Alter, Justin Fisher, Terry Horgan, Uriah Kriegel, Brian Leiter, David Pitt, Sydney Shoemaker, Susanna Siegel, Brad Thompson, Leora Weitzman, and Wayne Wright for comments on a draft. Brad Thompson's dissertation on phenomenal content explores many of the same issues as this chapter, and I had much valuable discussion with him. This chapter has been influenced by the work of others in various obvious ways, but it has been influenced by the work of Sydney Shoemaker and Charles Siewert in ways that may be deeper than the obvious.

Chapter 12 is drawn from T. S. Gendler and J. Hawthorne, eds., *Perceptual Experience* (Oxford University Press, 2006). I owe a special debt to George Bealer for suggesting the central metaphor of this chapter in a memorable conversation at O'Hare airport. In discussing whether perfect properties could be instantiated in any possible world, George said, "Maybe that's how it was in Eden." I also owe a debt to Brad Thompson, whose exploration of a Fregean approach to phenomenal content in his dissertation helped to spark the line of thinking here. Conversations with John Hawthorne and Mark Johnston about primitivist views also had a significant influence on the ideas here. I first presented this material at a conference on the ontology of color in Fribourg in 2003, and comments from all of the participants there, especially Alex Byrne, Larry Hardin, Barry Maund, and Martine Nida-Rümelin, were very helpful. This material has also been presented at Arizona, Nottingham, NYU, and Virginia, and at conferences in San Francisco, Santa Barbara, and Florence. For their commentaries at NYU and at the Santa Barbara and Florence conferences, I am grateful to Tom Nagel, Gideon Rosen, Susanna Siegel, and Aaron Zimmerman.

Chapter 13 was first published in the philosophy section of *The Matrix* website (thematrix.com) in 2003 and in C. Grau, ed., *Philosophers Explore the Matrix* (Oxford University Press, 2005). It was first presented at Davidson College and at the Metaphysical Mayhem conference in Syracuse in 2002 and subsequently at conferences in Adelaide, Barcelona, Colorado, Idaho, Oxford, and Tucson and in lectures at Arizona, ANU, Bates, British Columbia, Dartmouth, Harvard, Maui, Montana, Nevada (Las Vegas), New Mexico State, Queensland, Texas Tech, UCLA, Vermont, Victoria, and Wisconsin. Thanks to people on all of these occasions and many others for discussion.

Chapter 14 is drawn from A. Cleeremans, ed., *The Unity of Consciousness: Binding, Integration, Dissociation* (Oxford University Press, 2003). It was first presented at the 2000 ASSC conference on the unity of consciousness in Brussels and subsequently at conferences in Boulder and Skaneateles and in talks at Alabama, Arizona, Barcelona, Munich, Skovde, University College London, and Wake Forest. Thanks to audience members on all of those occasions for helpful comments. Special thanks to Barry Dainton, Bernie Kobes, Graham Macdonald, and Paul Studtmann.

The appendix is abridged from "Two-dimensional Semantics" in E. Lepore and B. Smith, eds., *The Oxford Handbook of the Philosophy of Language* (Oxford University Press, 2006). Thanks to Brendan Jackson, Bernhard Nickel, and Adam Pautz for comments.

CONTENTS

INTRODUCTION

What is consciousness? How can it be explained? Can there be a science of consciousness? What is the neural basis of consciousness? What is the place of consciousness in nature? Is consciousness physical or nonphysical? How do we know about consciousness? How do we think about consciousness? What are the contents of consciousness? How does consciousness relate to the external world? What is the unity of consciousness?

We can think of these questions as limning a few dimensions of the character of consciousness. Consciousness is an extraordinary and multi-faceted phenomenon whose character can be approached from many different directions. It has a phenomenological and a neurobiological character. It has a metaphysical and an epistemological character. It has a perceptual and a cognitive character. It has a unified and a differentiated character. And it has many further sorts of character.

We will not understand consciousness by studying its character on just one of these dimensions. Studying the phenomenology or the neurobiology of consciousness alone may tell us a great deal, as might studying the metaphysics or the epistemology. The perceptual and cognitive aspects of consciousness pose huge challenges in their own right. But ultimately we must approach consciousness from all of these directions.

In this book, I address all of these issues about the character of consciousness and a number of others. It is not the last word (or even my last word) on any of them. There are many aspects of the character of consciousness that it does not address at all. Still, I hope that it provides a unified picture of many aspects of consciousness that repays attention.

The chapters of this book were first written as separate articles, so one might think that the book is bound to be fragmented. I have tried to structure and rework it in such a way that it works as a whole, however. Later chapters build on ideas put forward in earlier chapters, and there are many common themes throughout. In principle one could read the book from start to finish as if following a narrative thread. The book is long enough that perhaps this is too much to expect, but there are also many subbooks within it, some of which I will explain. I have added afterwords to some of the chapters, as well as new footnotes (marked with an asterisk). I have shifted some of the material and cut out the more blatant acts of repetition, although occasional repetition has survived, in part to assist readers who may not be reading straight through.

The book is structured as follows. Chapter 1 introduces the problems of consciousness in an accessible way. Chapters 2–4 address the science of consciousness by developing a positive picture of how the science works in light of the problems. Chapters 5–7 address the metaphysics of consciousness, arguing in detail against materialist views and for a view on which consciousness is irreducible. Chapters 8–10 address thought about consciousness and the epistemology of consciousness, developing an account of the concepts we use to think about consciousness and the distinctive knowledge that we have of consciousness. Chapters 11–13 address perceptual consciousness and the way it represents the external world. Chapter 14 addresses the unity of consciousness. The appendix gives an outline of the two-dimensional framework that plays a central role in a number of the more technical chapters.

Although the book contains some technical material, it also contains much that is intended to be highly accessible. Chapters 1–4 and 13 were written with a general audience in mind, and chapters 5 and 14 should be accessible to a reasonably broad audience. Chapters 6–12 are more technical and are likely to appeal mainly to philosophers or to those who are willing to work hard. To someone without much background in philosophy, I suggest skipping these chapters on a first reading. If pressed for time, start with chapters 1, 2, and 13, which have perhaps the broadest appeal. Likewise, for those especially interested in the science of consciousness, chapters 1–4 are the places to start, with perhaps some material of interest in chapters 13 and 14.

There are also many paths through the book for philosophers. Those especially interested in the mind-body problem might focus on chapters 1, 5–7, and 10 (with some relevant material in 2, 8, and 9). Those interested in issues about language, content, and concepts might focus on chapters 6–8 and 11–13, as well as the appendix. Those interested in epistemology might focus first on chapters 9 and 13, with relevant material also in 2, 4, 6, and 7. Those interested in phenomenology might find material of interest in chapters 11, 12, and 14. I urge philosophers not to skip chapter 13: the topic might seem frivolous, but the philosophical issues go as deep as in any chapter in the book.

This book could be considered a sort of sequel to my earlier book on consciousness, *The Conscious Mind* (*TCM*). That book received far more attention than I could reasonably have expected, for which I am enormously grateful. At the same time, it is very far from a perfect work (most of it was written as my PhD dissertation after four years of studying philosophy), and there is much about it that I would change if I were writing it now. There are also many relevant issues that it simply does not address. I would like to think that in subsequent years, I have come to understand a number of important issues better than I did then. In this book, I aim to flesh out a picture of consciousness that is clearer, fuller, and more adequate than the picture in *The Conscious Mind*.

The picture in this book is largely consistent with the picture in *The Conscious Mind*. I have not had an enormous change of mind since then, though there are some medium-sized changes: for example, I am somewhat less sympathetic to epiphenomenalism than I was then and somewhat more sympathetic to drawing close connections between consciousness and intentionality. A few chapters present arguments along the same lines as those in that book. In particular, chapters 1 and 5–7 cover the same sort of ground as the early chapters of *TCM*, in what I hope is a better fashion. In some of those chapters I have also responded to various critics of *TCM*. The chapters in sections II and IV address issues regarding the science of consciousness and concepts of consciousness that are touched on far too briefly in *TCM*, while sections V and VI move in new directions that are not explored at all there (those who want to explore entirely different issues could start here). I have not presupposed any knowledge of the earlier book; this book can stand alone.

One regret concerning *The Conscious Mind* is that the book has become known especially for a negative thesis, the thesis that consciousness is not physical. Perhaps this was to be expected, but my central goal in studying consciousness has always been positive rather than negative: I would like to find a theory of consciousness that works. Negative arguments are just a step on the way. So while this book contains its share of negative arguments (mainly in section III and to some extent in chapters 1 and 10), I have tried to put more focus on the positive. Chapters 2–4 outline a positive picture of how the science of consciousness can proceed (and is proceeding) even once the distinctive problems of consciousness are fully recognized. The second halves of chapters 1 and 5 sketch speculative positive pictures of the metaphysics of consciousness; chapters 8 and 9 try to tell a positive story about phenomenal concepts and the epistemology of consciousness; and the chapters in sections V and VI develop a positive picture of perceptual consciousness, its relation to the external world, and the unity of consciousness.

It is worth noting that many elements of this positive picture can be accepted by those who are not convinced by the negative arguments. Apart from chapters 1, 4–6, and 10, most of this book is quite compatible with various sorts of materialism. At the same time, there is at least a nonreductive spirit to many aspects of the picture. One might think of the book as a whole as an attempt to articulate a reasonably unified, broadly nonreductive vision of the character of consciousness.

In the remainder of this introduction I introduce each of the chapters in more detail, sketching some context and some informal background. I have permitted myself a few more personal remarks than elsewhere in the book. Readers can read this material or not as they like. The material can also be read before or after reading the chapters themselves.

Chapter 1 introduces the distinction between the "hard problem" and the "easy problems" of consciousness. The easy problems are those of explaining cognitive and behavioral functions such as discrimination, integration, and verbal report. The hard problem is that of explaining conscious experience. Where the easy problems are concerned, it suffices to explain how a function is performed, and to do this it suffices to specify an appropriate neural or computational mechanism. But where the hard problem is concerned, explaining cognitive and behavioral functions always leaves a further open question: why is the performance of these functions accompanied by experience? Because of this, the standard reductive methods of neuroscience and cognitive science that work for the easy problems do not work for the hard problem. I argue that this problem applies to any reductive explanation. In principle, these can explain only structure and function, and explaining conscious experience requires more than explaining structure and function. If this is right, there can be no wholly reductive explanation of consciousness. I go on to sketch an alternative nonreductive approach in which consciousness is taken as fundamental, and I sketch the outlines of a speculative theory of that sort.

I first presented this material in a talk at the first Tucson conference on the science of consciousness in April 1994. Although there is nothing especially original about the idea that consciousness poses a hard problem, I was in the right place at the right time. At the conference, the talk received an overwhelming and entirely unexpected reaction. Shortly afterward, I was invited to write up versions of this material for both *Scientific American* and the *Journal of Consciousness Studies*. The latter journal published four special issues containing a keynote article by me, around twenty-five responses, and a response by me in turn, all of which were later collected into the 1997 book titled *Explaining Consciousness: The Hard Problem* (edited by Jonathan Shear). The chapter here is a version of the original article in that journal.

As an afterword to chapter 1, I have also included an excerpt from my lengthy reply to the responses, "Moving Forward on the Problem of Consciousness." That article is too long to include here in full (it is available online), and much of it covers ground that is covered elsewhere in this book. But I have included a response to Daniel Dennett, both here and in the afterword to chapter 2, as his brand of highly deflationary materialism (the "type-A" materialism of chapter 5) is not discussed at length elsewhere in the book. I know that the debate between the deflationary and inflationary views of consciousness is of interest to readers both inside and outside philosophy, where the argument between the likes of Dennett and the likes of me is sometimes cast as an ideological battle. I learned long ago that I am not much of an ideological crusader: I do not believe that the world will be a hugely better place if everyone accepts my views, and I am only occasionally inclined to rhetorical extremes. Still, I think that one has a responsibility to the views that one has put forward, and the back-and-forth can at least shed some light on the underlying issues. So I have done my best to indicate how I see the core issues here.

I am fond of the original article on the hard problem in part because it makes the case against reductive theories of consciousness without any technicalities or far-out philosophical thought experiments. I have no objection to technicalities and thought experiments, which play a central role in the arguments of *The Conscious Mind*, but I think that the argument here is just as effective. There is a sense in which the argument here, which turns on simple issues about explanation, is more fundamental than conceivability arguments involving zombies, epistemological arguments involving Mary in her black-and-white room, and the like. And certainly it works better for an audience outside philosophy. It is sometimes supposed that nonreductive arguments turn essentially on these thought experiments, but this is just wrong. In fact, in chapter 5 and elsewhere, I suggest that the thought experiments turn essentially on points about structure and function that are close to the central points in this chapter. I see the thought experiments as a useful technical device for making the arguments more formal and more analyzable (as well as more vivid), and as a result they have produced much interesting and useful philosophical literature. Still, many of the common responses to those thought experiments have no clear application as a response to the simple arguments here (the phenomenal concept strategy discussed in chapter 10 is an exception, among others). Although the material in this chapter has been very widely cited, I have seen many fewer serious replies to its line of argument than to the line in *The Conscious Mind*. I would certainly be interested to see more.

Sixteen years after that first Tucson conference, the science of consciousness has gone from strength to strength. But the state of play in the science of consciousness with respect to the hard problem is very much as it was. Almost everyone in the field recognizes that there is a hard problem of consciousness that poses special challenges (perhaps this is a sort of progress, although I think that most people recognized it all along). There have been many neurobiological and cognitive models of consciousness, but few of them have been offered as a solution to the hard problem, and when they have, hardly anyone has been convinced. Any associated claims about the hard problem are usually driven by bits of philosophy that are largely independent of the science and can be responded to straightforwardly. I have occasionally been invited to write critical reviews of this sort of work, but one bonus of the phraseology is that it generates a critique that writes itself: the work addresses the easy problems but not the hard problem, it provides a correlate of conscious experience but not an explanation, and so on. So I have not usually felt the need to go back over this ground.

That being said, positive nonreductive theories of consciousness have not had a much easier time of it. The speculative "theory" outlined in the second half of this chapter has certainly not gained widespread acceptance, and even I am inclined to be skeptical about the more speculative parts of it, such as the double-aspect theory of information. There have been a handful of attempts at nonreductive theories (the work of Stuart Hameroff and Gregg Rosenberg comes to mind), but not many, and none has attained much support. Perhaps it is too early in the science for positive theories that address the hard problem in a substantial and successful way. Still, I think it is worth trying.

In any case, the science of consciousness is thriving. Most of the work in the field does not try to solve the hard problem of consciousness but is none the worse for that. There are robust research programs in neurobiology (especially vision, but also emotion, bodily awareness, and other areas), psychology (especially conscious and unconscious processing in memory and learning, and the relationship between perception, attention, and consciousness), clinical neurology (especially on the vegetative state and other postcoma conditions), and other areas. These programs raise all sorts of fascinating philosophical issues, and in chapters 2–4 I address some of them.

Chapter 2 gives an overview of the science of consciousness and presents a picture of how it can work even in the absence of a solution to the hard problem. The central role of the science, as I see it, is to provide a bridge between third-person data about brain and behavior and first-person data about consciousness, where it is data of the latter sort that make the science of consciousness truly distinctive. I suggest that the science is essentially correlative rather than reductive—at least, the central parts of the science make claims about correlation without making claims about reduction. Science of this sort can still have great explanatory power, however, by articulating powerful general principles that connect the first-person and third-person domains. The science of consciousness is not yet at the point of having that power, but if one squints, one can see the possibility of a framework of that sort in the distance. After discussing the role of much of the present work in the field, the chapter ends with discussion of some obstacles and of where the science might eventually go. I have tried to sketch a framework for the science that can be embraced by reductionists and nonreductionists alike.

I have given talks corresponding to chapter 2 at numerous conferences and other venues, including a memorable occasion at the Central Intelligence Agency in Virginia in 2000. (The talk was advertised without my knowledge as "Consciousness at the Millennium: The Mind-machine Connection"; I think the audience did not get what it was expecting, at least until I mentioned the consciousness meter.) Dan Dennett was present on a couple of occasions and responded in a debate at Northwestern with a paper titled "The Fantasy of First-person Science." I have not responded to Dennett's paper in print anywhere, so I have added an afterword indicating the general lines of my response, as well as discussing some other central issues involving first-person data.

Chapters 3 and 4 address what is arguably the centerpiece of the resurgence of the science of consciousness: the search for neural correlates of consciousness, especially of visual consciousness. Chapter 3 addresses conceptual issues about what it is to be a neural correlate of consciousness. The question might seem straightforward initially, but it generates all sorts of interesting puzzles. Must there be one neural correlate of consciousness, or might there be many? How strong a correlation is required? Over what range of cases? The chapter addresses these questions and a number of others and puts forward a proposal for understanding the notion of a neural correlate of consciousness in a way that does justice to the way the notion is used in the field. I use this analysis to draw some conclusions for the methodology of the search for neural correlates of consciousness.

Chapter 4 focuses directly on the epistemology of the search. The key question is: how can we isolate the neural correlate of consciousness in the absence of a "consciousness meter," which measures consciousness directly? The obvious answer is that we rely on verbal reports and other behavioral indicators of consciousness. Importantly, the use of these indicators tacitly relies on pre-experimental principles that connect these behavioral indicators to consciousness. The use of these principles is unavoidable, and it has a number of interesting consequences for the science. After drawing out some of the key principles, I once again draw some conclusions that bear directly on the practical methodology of the scientific work in this area.

Of course, there are many important issues in the science of consciousness that I do not address in these chapters. There is much to be said about the science of unconscious processes, especially regarding the philosophical assumptions behind the principles used in this area to ascribe conscious and unconscious mental states to subjects. I have discussed that work in talks (e.g., "Implicit Philosophy in Implicit Cognition Research") but not yet in print. Likewise, there are very interesting philosophical issues concerning how to monitor consciousness in apparently unresponsive patients, such as those diagnosed with vegetative state; I have recently started some collaborative work with neurologists and neurobiologists on this topic. The relationship between consciousness and attention also raises all sorts of interesting issues that I hope to address in future work.

Chapters 5–7 focus on issues about materialism and dualism with regard to consciousness. The arguments of chapter 1 make a case for a view in which consciousness is irreducible and nonphysical, but much more needs to be said to flesh out these arguments, to answer objections, and to investigate the resulting views.

Chapter 5 provides an overview of the territory. It starts by presenting the central arguments against materialism, which involve establishing an epistemic gap between the physical and the phenomenal, and moves from there to an ontological gap. It then distinguishes between the three most important sorts of materialist opposition to these arguments: what I call type-A materialism (which denies the epistemic gap), type-B materialism (which accepts the epistemic gap but denies the ontological gap), and type-C materialism (which holds that there is a deep epistemic gap but one that will be closed in the limit). I make the case, in reasonable detail but without technicality, that each of these three views should be rejected. In the second half of the chapter I investigate the most important nonreductive views that result: type-D dualism (or interactionism), type-E dualism (or epiphenomenalism), and type-F monism (Russellian monism, or panprotopsychism). I discuss the pros and cons of each, suggesting that all three have significant attractions and that none has fatal flaws.

My own loyalties are fairly evenly spread among these three views, depending on the day of the week. I have often been told that I am an

epiphenomenalist, based on the sympathetic discussion of epiphenomenalism in *The Conscious Mind*. Sometimes that is taken to be sufficient
reason to reject the arguments of the book, as epiphenomenalism is widely
regarded as crazy. But even in *TCM* I was just as sympathetic to Russellian
monism (in both panpsychist and nonpanpsychist variants) as to epiphenomenalism, and Russellian monism involves a causal role for consciousness. In addition, I now think that the criticisms of interactionism there
were much too quick (for reasons discussed in the section on type-D
dualism here) and that there are no decisive reasons for rejecting that view.
In any case, the proper conclusion of the anti-materialist arguments is disjunctive. The choice among the three disjuncts rests on further and largely
independent considerations. As things stand, the choice is wide open. At
the end of the day, the choice will come down to which of the disjuncts
yields the most successful detailed theory, in light of a well-developed science of consciousness.

Chapter 6 is mainly devoted to the conceivability argument against
materialism, viewed through the lens of the two-dimensional semantic
framework. An argument of this sort was one of the centerpieces of *The
Conscious Mind* and has attracted many replies. At the same time, the two-
dimensional argument there was not as clearly formulated as it could have
been. Here I have tried to give the argument a really clear formulation and
to answer all of the central objections that have been raised against it. This
chapter is unavoidably technical, but I would like to think that this is a
case in which technicality has some rewards, not just in understanding issues about consciousness, but also in understanding the metaphysics and
epistemology of modality.

The key issue in this chapter is whether conceivability (of some sort)
entails metaphysical possibility (of some sort). The key opponent is the
type-B materialist, who denies the entailment. Many objections and putative counterexamples to the conceivability–possibility thesis have been
mooted: the chapter discusses fifteen or so putative counterexamples, along
with ten or so objections of other sorts to the conceivability argument. I
think that on close examination there are straightforward replies to most
of them. Some raise deeper issues: about the apriority of modal epistemology, for example, or about the connection between concepts, rationality, and modality. Late in the chapter I sketch a positive grounding for
the sort of modal rationalism that drives the conceivability argument. In an
afterword I bring the analysis to bear on some other central arguments
against materialism (the knowledge argument, Kripke's modal argument,
the property dualism argument, the argument from disembodiment, the
semantic stability argument), arguing that the issues underlying each are

closely related and that a two-dimensional analysis can shed useful light on each.

Chapter 7 (coauthored with Frank Jackson) addresses a related form of opposition to the anti-materialist arguments. Some type-B materialists allow that a unique epistemic gap exists between physics and consciousness: truths about consciousness are not deducible from physical truths, but truths about water, life, and other high-level phenomena are deducible from physical truths. Others argue that these epistemic gaps arise in many high-level domains. In a 1999 paper, Ned Block and Robert Stalnaker respond in the second way to arguments given by Jackson, by Joseph Levine, and by me, suggesting that truths about water, life, and heat are no more deducible from physical truths than are truths about consciousness. If so, the case of consciousness is nothing special, and unless one is prepared to accept that water is nonphysical, one should reject the argument that consciousness is nonphysical.

In response, Jackson and I argue that there are in fact a priori entailments from a nearly physical base to truths about water, life, and so on. The base needs to be expanded a little to allow indexicals, a "that's all" truth, and of course truths about consciousness. But from this base, other ordinary macroscopic truths can be deduced by a priori reasoning. The argument here turns on some general observations about concepts and conceptual analysis. One of the key points is that there can be a priori entailments even in the absence of definitions or explicit analyses, contrary to what Block and Stalnaker appear to assume. The issues here are largely conceptual and epistemological, but we draw consequences for the explanatory gap regarding consciousness.

Chapters 6 and 7 raise issues in metaphysics, epistemology, and the philosophy of language that go well beyond issues about consciousness. Much more needs to be said about these issues, and in recent work I have tried to say some of it. A forthcoming book is devoted to issues in the philosophy of language and content, arguing for a Fregean approach to meaning and an internalist approach to mental content, grounded largely in the two-dimensional semantic framework that is central to chapter 6. Another forthcoming book takes up some of the issues in chapter 7 through the lens of the "scrutability" thesis, arguing that there is a limited class of truths from which all truths are deducible. I suggest that this scrutability thesis can be used to vindicate some (not all) of the aims of Rudolf Carnap and other logical empiricists, and that it has many interesting consequences in epistemology, the philosophy of language, metaphilosophy, and metaphysics. For me, these works grew out of seeds in work on consciousness and then took on a life of their own. This seems to me to be a sign of the fertility of issues about consciousness for thinking about philosophy more generally, although perhaps it is just a sign of the way that every issue in philosophy is connected to every other.

Chapters 8 to 10 concern our thoughts and beliefs about consciousness, and the concepts we use to think about consciousness. These concepts are now known throughout philosophy as phenomenal concepts. Chapter 8 develops an account of the distinctive nature of phenomenal concepts, grounded in part in an analysis of the epistemological and conceptual observations that drive the arguments against materialism. I argue that phenomenal concepts behave in a way that is quite unlike most other concepts, involving a very strong sort of direct reference, on which the phenomenal qualities that are the referents of the concepts are also somehow present inside their sense. Here, the two-dimensional framework is again a useful tool in analyzing the phenomenon. The account in this chapter is in principle compatible with materialism, and in recent years some materialists have developed closely related accounts, but I think the account itself is fairly neutral (perhaps ultimately with some support for dualism, for reasons given toward the end of chapter 10). In any case, the issues concerning concepts and belief are of much interest in their own right.

Chapter 9 concerns our knowledge of consciousness. It was originally the second half of a long paper also containing chapter 8, and it builds on the central idea of that chapter. The special phenomenal concepts of chapter 8 lead to a distinctive class of "direct phenomenal beliefs," which I argue have many interesting epistemological properties. For a start, they support a sort of infallibility thesis: direct phenomenal beliefs cannot be false. This thesis can do only limited epistemological work, but analysis of these beliefs leads to a more substantial epistemological view that involves a central role for acquaintance. I use the framework to analyze two important issues in the epistemology of consciousness: epistemological arguments against nonreductive views of consciousness, as well as Wilfrid Sellars's arguments against the "given." I suggest that with the appropriate analysis in hand, both sorts of arguments can be defanged. (Among other things, I think that this analysis provides a better response to the "paradox of phenomenal judgment" than I gave in *The Conscious Mind.*)

These chapters are explicitly concerned just with beliefs about consciousness, but much of the material here has application to a much broader class of beliefs. For example, I think that some perceptual beliefs are closely related to direct phenomenal beliefs, such that consciousness pays a central role in their constitution. Moreover, these consciousness-based beliefs may play a distinctive role in perceptual epistemology. The role for consciousness may go further still. Chapter 8 concludes by drawing some speculative morals for the role of consciousness in grounding intentionality quite generally (a topic that I revisit in chapters 11 and 12). Chapter 9 ends with some morals about the general role of consciousness in epistemology.

Chapter 10 concerns a role for phenomenal concepts in the debate over materialism. As I noted earlier, many type-B materialists think that a unique epistemic gap exists between physical and phenomenal truths, one that does not arise in other domains. It is then incumbent on them to explain why there should be such a gap in a purely physical world. By far the most popular strategy is to argue that the gap results from the way we think about consciousness (rather than from the nature of consciousness itself) and in particular from the nature of phenomenal concepts. Many different accounts of phenomenal concepts have been offered for this purpose. In chapter 6 I argue against two such accounts individually. In chapter 10 I discuss the accounts as a class and argue that no such account can work. In particular, I argue that there is no account of phenomenal concepts such that the nature of the concepts is both explainable in physical terms and capable of explaining our epistemic situation regarding consciousness. And I argue that without doing these things, the account is toothless in explaining away the epistemic gap. Put differently, if an account of phenomenal concepts is substantial enough to explain our distinctive epistemic situation regarding consciousness, it will itself be as difficult to explain in physical terms as consciousness was. If I am right about this, it removes perhaps the most powerful sort of opposition to the arguments of chapters 1, 5, and 6.

Chapters 11–13 concern the contents of consciousness: in particular, the way that consciousness represents the external world. A central theme is the connection between consciousness and intentionality. Chapters 11 and 12 are concerned with the contents of perceptual experience. Chapter 13 is concerned with external-world representation in belief rather than in perception, but the themes are closely connected.

Chapter 11 focuses on representationalism, or intentionalism: roughly, the view that consciousness is essentially and wholly a matter of representing goings-on in the world. Representationalism has been a central view in recent philosophy of perception and philosophy of consciousness more generally. It is often put forward as a reductive thesis and is used in the interest of reducing consciousness to the physical. It is also often forward as a radically externalist thesis, on which consciousness is grounded in states outside the head. These commitments are quite inessential to representationalism per se, however, and representationalism is much more plausible when it is detached from them. In this chapter I argue for a distinctive sort of nonreductive, internalist representationalism, one that has most of the benefits of other sorts of representationalism along with relatively few of the costs.

The first half of chapter 11 surveys the territory. I clarify the nature of representationalism and argue for its plausibility. I survey varieties of representationalism, making the case for a nonreductive, internalist variety. The second half of the chapter develops an account of the contents of perceptual experience. If internalism is true, it appears that standard forms of environment-dependent content are ruled out and that one needs a sort of narrow (or internal) content instead. I bring in some ideas from the two-dimensional semantic framework to analyze the content of perception into two dimensions: Fregean content and Russellian content. Fregean content is narrow, while Russellian content is not. I argue that Fregean content is closely associated with the phenomenal character of experience. An afterword to the chapter spells out the application of the two-dimensional framework to perception in more depth.

Chapter 12 takes up the issue of the contents of experience where chapter 11 leaves off. I argue that the account of Fregean content in chapter 11 has some important inadequacies concerning its relation to phenomenology and leaves some crucial issues unexplained. I develop a further account involving what I call Edenic content: content that represents primitive properties (such as primitive redness or greenness), properties that are not instantiated in our world but that one can imagine might have been instantiated in the Garden of Eden. I bring this account to bear on many questions in the philosophy of perception, including questions about color constancy, spatial content, the representation of objects, and more.

I originally intended chapters 11 and 12 to be one long piece of work, but they are each long enough as they stand. Separating them might give the sense that I had a change of mind between the chapters, but that is not quite right: the Edenic view in chapter 12 extends the Fregean view in chapter 11 without rejecting it. When it comes to the metaphysics of consciousness, I think the Edenic story is more fundamental: fundamentally, consciousness may consist in the phenomenal representation of certain primitive properties. However, more than one sort of content is required for an adequate account of the many aspects of representation in experience. This reflects a general pluralism about mental and semantic content: one almost always needs contents of many different sorts to properly understand the complex phenomena of representation.

Chapters 11 and 12, along with chapters 8 and 9, can also be viewed as a contribution to what is now often called the "phenomenal intentionality" research program: the program of grounding intentionality in phenomenology.

Chapters 11 and 12 suggest that a distinctive sort of intentionality is inherent in perceptual experience. Chapters 8 and 9 suggest that phenomenology can play a constitutive role in determining the content of our beliefs, along with a corresponding epistemological role. These suggestions might well be taken much further. While I doubt that all of intentionality is fully determined by phenomenology, I think that intentionality cannot be properly understood without giving phenomenology a central role. I am at least attracted to a view in which all "narrow" intentionality is grounded in phenomenal intentionality along with functional and/or inferential roles and in which "wide" intentionality is grounded in turn in narrow intentionality plus the environment in the way suggested by the two-dimensional framework. I cannot claim to have made the case for a view as strong as that here, but I hope to develop it in future work.

Chapter 13 uses the movie *The Matrix* to address issues about our knowledge of the external world. On the face of it, the movie raises a version of Descartes' skeptical challenge. Just as I cannot know I am not the victim of a evil genius, I also cannot know I am not in a matrix. And if I am in a matrix, so the challenge goes, most of my beliefs are false: I am not really seeing a table in front of me, I do not really live in Australia, and so on. In this chapter, I argue that this thought, although initially compelling, is wrong. Even if I am in a matrix, there are still tables and cars, and most of my beliefs remain true. That is, the hypothesis that I am in a matrix is not a skeptical hypothesis, as traditionally thought. Instead, it is a sort of metaphysical hypothesis about the underlying nature of our world. If we are in a matrix, the physical world is more fundamentally a computational world, in which things are made of bits. This is an interesting new metaphysics, but it does not lead to skepticism. I argue that much the same applies to many traditional skeptical hypotheses, such as the evil demon hypothesis and the hypothesis that my life is a dream. This does not provide a complete victory over skepticism (some skeptical hypotheses survive), but it nevertheless helps in the project of vindicating knowledge of the external world.

The conclusion of the chapter is in some ways reminiscent of antiskeptical conclusions by philosophers as diverse as Berkeley and Putnam. However, I arrive at the conclusion by a quite different route, one that involves reflection on the possible character of physics, as well as on the possible character of the mind-body relation and of creation. Most people start off very dubious about the conclusion (just as I did), but my experience is that the arguments bring a surprising number of people around. I am not sure what to make of this, except perhaps that in this domain people's Cartesian intuitions run less deep than one might think.

On the face of it, chapter 13 might seem distant from chapters 11 and 12, with little explicit discussion of perception and consciousness. In fact the issues are deeply linked. If the arguments in this chapter are correct, the beliefs of a subject in a matrix are largely true. The same goes for perception: the perceptual experiences of a subject in a matrix are largely veridical. This picture coheres well with the Fregean picture developed in chapter 11, according to which perception represents properties that are the normal causes of certain sorts of perceptual experiences. This Fregean content does not require properties of a highly constrained sort, so if it turns out that that the relevant experiences are typically caused by certain computational properties, then these properties are represented by our experiences. This way, our experiences can be largely veridical, and our corresponding beliefs largely true.

Still, there is a persisting intuition that, if we are in a matrix, the world is not wholly as it seems. This intuition can be accommodated by bringing in ideas from chapter 12. If we are in a matrix, our experiences are not *perfectly veridical:* that would require our world to have primitive color properties, primitive spatiotemporal properties, and so on, as in Eden. But a moral of the Matrix chapter is that a matrix world is no better and no worse than a nonmatrix world in which quantum mechanics, relativity, and so on are true. In such a world, we have already fallen from Eden. Even in the world as revealed by contemporary science, it seems that our experiences are not perfectly veridical (their Edenic contents are not true): at best, they are imperfectly veridical (their ordinary Fregean and Russellian contents are true). But imperfect veridicality is good enough. And imperfect veridicality is something that the world of science shares with the world of the Matrix.

In effect, Eden and the Matrix can be seen as two poles in a familiar philosophical dichotomy. Eden is akin to the manifest image: the world exactly as it seems to us. The Matrix is (very loosely) akin to the scientific image: the messy and complicated real world of science with its many divergences from the manifest. But despite the mismatch between these images, we have grown used to the idea that the world of the scientific image is good enough to make our ordinary beliefs about the world true. The world does not vindicate them completely: a perfect match would require primitive solidity, primitive redness, and primitive squareness, and nothing in our world is really that way. So in a sense, our manifest image puts demands on the world that it does not meet. Still, the world of science vindicates our beliefs and experiences well enough by meeting the standard of imperfect veridicality. Perfect veridicality would require our world to be Eden, but imperfect veridicality can be satisfied even in a matrix.

These two poles call to mind another famous dichotomy. Eden corresponds at least loosely to Kant's phenomenal world: the world of things as they appear. The Matrix corresponds loosely to Kant's noumenal world: the world of things in themselves. We might think of Eden as a pure phenomenal world: if we were in Eden, nothing would have a hidden nature. But if we are in the Matrix, the world has a hidden nature that is not revealed to us in perception or even in ordinary science. Like the analogy with the scientific image, the analogy with the noumenal world is imperfect. The movie offers us an un-Kantian route to see the things in themselves: the red pill reveals their computational nature, which of course just raises the question of the noumena underlying the computers in turn. Still, through this lens, the film no longer seems to be an illustration of Cartesian deception. Rather, it is an illustration of Kantian (or perhaps Russellian) humility. Perception and even science do not reveal the entire intrinsic character of the world. Perhaps it was unreasonable ever to expect that they would. Still, even if perception and science are not perfect, in their imperfect ways they are adequate to their tasks all the same.

Reflection on the Matrix scenario is fertile in many other ways. Coming to grips with it requires getting to the bottom of some of the deepest issues in philosophy. These include not just issues in epistemology but also those in metaphysics (what is the nature of objects?), the philosophy of language (what determines the reference of our expressions?), the philosophy of mind (how do we make cognitive contact with the world?), the philosophy of perception (how do we represent space?), the philosophy of physics (what is the role of spatiotemporal concepts in theoretical physics?), the philosophy of computation (what does it take to implement a computation?), and even the philosophy of religion (what should we say about God if our world is the product of imperfect creators?) and ethics (is life in a matrix as meaningful as a life outside it?). I address a few of these issues in the chapter and in the philosophical notes that follow. I am sure that I have not gotten to the bottom of any of them. Still, because of the way that it opens a door to all of these issues in such a simple way, this chapter is my favorite in the book.

Chapter 14 (coauthored with Tim Bayne) addresses another Kantian topic: the unity of consciousness. It is hard to turn this fuzzy topic into clear philosophy, but in recent years a few people have tried. This is our attempt. We start with the question of what it is for two states of consciousness (experiencing red and hearing middle C, say) to be unified. We analyze a number of different notions of unity in search of one that undergirds a nontrivial but still plausible unity thesis holding that consciousness is necessarily unified. This leads to a notion of phenomenal unity, defined in terms of a sort of conjoint phenomenal character. We suggest that there is a prima facie case that consciousness is necessarily unified in this sense and that prima facie counterevidence from split-brain syndrome can be accommodated by making relevant distinctions. To get a better handle on unity, we introduce a quasi-mereological analysis and an analysis in terms of entailment between phenomenal states. We use these analyses to argue against certain representationalist and higher-order theories of consciousness on the grounds that they cannot vindicate the unity thesis. We end by speculating about why consciousness is unified, if indeed it is.

The end of the chapter suggests a certain holistic view of the metaphysics of consciousness, one in which local states of consciousness (experiencing red, hearing middle C) are grounded in total states of consciousness for a subject at a time. It is tempting to think that these states are the basic units of consciousness. If we combine this picture with the picture in chapter 12, a more detailed hypothesis in the metaphysics of consciousness suggests itself: consciousness consists in the unified phenomenal representation of an Edenic world. I do not know whether this hypothesis is correct, but it is at least aesthetically pleasing.

The appendix provides an introduction to the two-dimensional semantic framework that I use in a number of the more technical chapters. This framework provides a very useful tool for analyzing the relationship between modal and epistemological issues, as well as for modeling the content of linguistic expressions and mental states in a way that is sensitive to their cognitive and epistemological roles. After outlining the framework and some of its applications, I address a number of objections that various philosophers have put forward. I think that once the framework is understood correctly, there are straightforward replies to many of these objections, although of course some objections raise substantial issues, too. But readers can decide for themselves.

Part I

THE PROBLEMS OF CONSCIOUSNESS

1

FACING UP TO THE PROBLEM OF CONSCIOUSNESS

1. Introduction

Consciousness poses the most baffling problems in the science of the mind. There is nothing that we know more intimately than conscious experience, but there is nothing that is harder to explain. All sorts of mental phenomena have yielded to scientific investigation in recent years, but consciousness has stubbornly resisted. Many have tried to explain it, but the explanations always seem to fall short of the target. Some have been led to suppose that the problem is intractable and that no good explanation can be given.

To make progress on the problem of consciousness, we have to confront it directly. In this chapter I first isolate the truly hard part of the problem, separating it from more tractable parts and giving an account of why it is so difficult to explain. I critique some recent work that uses reductive methods to address consciousness and argue that these methods inevitably fail to come to grips with the hardest part of the problem. Once this failure is recognized, the door to further progress is opened. In the second half of the chapter I argue that, if we move to a new kind of nonreductive explanation, a naturalistic account of consciousness can be given.

2. The Easy Problems and the Hard Problem

There is not just one problem of consciousness. "Consciousness" is an ambiguous term that refers to many different phenomena. Each of these phenomena needs to be explained, but some are easier to explain than others. At the start, it is useful to divide the associated problems of consciousness into "hard" and "easy" problems. The easy problems of consciousness are those that seem directly susceptible to the standard methods of cognitive science, whereby a phenomenon is explained in terms of computational or neural mechanisms. The hard problems are those that seem to resist those methods.

The easy problems of consciousness include those of explaining the following phenomena:[1]

- the ability to discriminate, categorize, and react to environmental stimuli
- the integration of information by a cognitive system
- the reportability of mental states
- the ability of a system to access its own internal states
- the focus of attention
- the deliberate control of behavior
- the difference between wakefulness and sleep

All of these phenomena are associated with the notion of consciousness. For example, one sometimes says that a mental state is conscious when it is verbally reportable or when it is internally accessible. Sometimes a system is said to be conscious of some information when it has the ability to react on the basis of that information or, more strongly, when it attends to that information or when it can integrate that information and exploit it in the sophisticated control of behavior. We sometimes say that an action is conscious precisely when it is deliberate. Often we say that an organism is conscious as another way of saying that it is awake.

There is no real issue about whether *these* phenomena can be explained scientifically. All of them are straightforwardly vulnerable to explanation in terms of computational or neural mechanisms. To explain access and reportability, for example, we need only specify the mechanism by which information about internal states is retrieved and made available for verbal report. To explain the integration of information, we need only exhibit mechanisms by which information is brought together and exploited by later processes. For an account of sleep and wakefulness, an appropriate neurophysiological account of the processes responsible for

1. *This is an imperfect list, as most of the phenomena on the list have experiential aspects that raise the hard problem. There are distinctive sorts of experience involved in attention and voluntary control, for example. The list should be understood as calling attention to the functional rather than the experiential aspects of these phenomena. It should be noted that the easy problems are *not* characterized as the problems of intentionality.

organisms' contrasting behavior in those states will suffice. In each case, an appropriate cognitive or neurophysiological model can clearly do the explanatory work.

If these phenomena were all there was to consciousness, then consciousness would not be much of a problem. Although we do not yet have anything close to a complete explanation of these phenomena, we have a clear idea of how we might go about explaining them. This is why I call these problems the easy problems. Of course, "easy" is a relative term. Getting the details right will probably take a century or two of difficult empirical work. Still, there is every reason to believe that the methods of cognitive science and neuroscience will succeed.

The really hard problem of consciousness is the problem of *experience*. When we think and perceive, there is a whir of information processing, but there is also a subjective aspect. As Nagel (1974) has put it, there is *something it is like* to be a conscious organism. This subjective aspect is experience. When we see, for example, we *experience* visual sensations: the felt quality of redness, the experience of dark and light, the quality of depth in a visual field. Other experiences go along with perception in different modalities: the sound of a clarinet, the smell of mothballs. Then there are bodily sensations from pains to orgasms; mental images that are conjured up internally; the felt quality of emotion; and the experience of a stream of conscious thought. What unites all of these states is that there is something it is like to be in them. All of them are states of experience.

It is undeniable that some organisms are subjects of experience, but the question of why it is that these systems are subjects of experience is perplexing. Why is it that when our cognitive systems engage in visual and auditory information processing, we have visual or auditory experience: the quality of deep blue, the sensation of middle C? How can we explain why there is something it is like to entertain a mental image or to experience an emotion? It is widely agreed that experience arises from a physical basis, but we have no good explanation of why and how it so arises. Why should physical processing give rise to a rich inner life at all? It seems objectively unreasonable that it should, and yet it does.

If any problem qualifies as *the* problem of consciousness, it is this one. In this central sense of "consciousness," an organism is conscious if there is something it is like to be that organism, and a mental state is conscious if there is something it is like to be in that state. Sometimes terms such as "phenomenal consciousness" and "qualia" are also used here, but I find it more natural to speak of "conscious experience" or simply "experience." Another useful way to avoid confusion (used by, e.g., Newell 1990; Chalmers 1996) is to reserve the term "consciousness" for the phenomena of experience, using the less loaded term "awareness" for the more straight-forward phenomena described earlier. If such a convention were widely adopted communication would be much easier; as things stand, those who talk about "consciousness" are frequently talking past each other.

The ambiguity of the term "consciousness" is often exploited by both philosophers and scientists writing on the subject. It is common to see a paper on consciousness begin with an invocation of the mystery of consciousness, noting the strange intangibility and ineffability of subjectivity and worrying that so far we have no theory of the phenomenon. Here, the topic is clearly the hard problem—the problem of experience. In the second half of the paper, the tone becomes more optimistic, and the author's own theory of consciousness is outlined. Upon examination, this theory turns out to be a theory of one of the more straightforward phenomena—of reportability, of introspective access, or whatever. At the close, the author declares that consciousness has turned out to be tractable after all, but the reader is left feeling like the victim of a bait-and-switch. The hard problem remains untouched.

3. Functional Explanation

Why are the easy problems easy, and why is the hard problem hard? The easy problems are easy precisely because they concern the explanation of cognitive *abilities* and *functions*. To explain a cognitive function, we need only specify a mechanism that can perform the function. The methods of cognitive science are well suited for this sort of explanation and so are well suited to the easy problems of consciousness. By contrast, the hard problem is hard precisely because it is not a problem about the performance of functions. The problem persists even when the performance of all of the relevant functions is explained. (Here "function" is not used in the narrow teleological sense of something that a system is designed to do but in the broader sense of any causal role in the production of behavior that a system might perform.)

To explain reportability, for instance, is just to explain how a system could perform the function of producing reports on internal states. To explain internal access, we need to explain how a system could be appropriately affected by its internal states and use information about them in directing later processes. To explain integration and control, we need to explain how a system's central processes can bring information together and use them in the facilitation of various behaviors. These are all problems about the explanation of functions.

How do we explain the performance of a function? By specifying a *mechanism* that performs the function.[2] Here, neurophysiological and cognitive modeling are perfect for the task. If we want a detailed, low-level explanation, we can specify the neural mechanism that is responsible for the function. If we want a more abstract explanation, we can specify a mechanism in computational terms. Either way, a full and satisfying explanation will result. Once we have specified the neural or computational mechanism that performs the function of verbal report, for example, the bulk of our work in explaining reportability is over.

In a way, the point is trivial. It is a *conceptual* fact about these phenomena that their explanation involves only the explanation of various functions, as the phenomena are *functionally definable*. All it *means* for reportability to be instantiated in a system is that the system has the capacity for verbal reports of internal information. All it means for a system to be awake is for it to be appropriately receptive to information from the environment and for it to be able to use this information in directing behavior in an appropriate way. To see that this is a conceptual fact, note that someone who says, "You have explained the performance of the verbal report function, but you have not explained reportability," is making a trivial conceptual mistake about reportability. All it could *possibly* take to explain reportability is an explanation of how the relevant function is performed; the same goes for the other phenomena in question.

Throughout the higher-level sciences, reductive explanation works in just this way. To explain the gene, for instance, we needed to specify the mechanism that stores and transmits hereditary information from one generation to the next. It turns out that DNA performs this function; once we explain how the function is performed, we have explained the gene. To explain life, we ultimately need to explain how a system can reproduce, adapt to its environment, metabolize, and so on. All of these are questions about the performance of functions and so are well suited to reductive explanation. The same holds for most problems in cognitive science. To explain learning, we need to explain the way in which a system's behavioral capacities are modified in light of environmental information, and the way in which new information can be brought to bear in adapting a system's actions to its environment. If we show how a neural or computational mechanism does the job, we have explained learning. We can say the same

2. *It is sometimes suggested that arguments for the explanatory gap turn on an outmoded "deductive-nomological" model of explanation. So it is worth noting that this chapter invokes a model of explanation in terms of functions and mechanisms. This model is closely related to models that have become popular in the philosophy of science in the years since the paper on which this chapter is based was published.

for other cognitive phenomena, such as perception, memory, and language. Sometimes the relevant functions need to be characterized quite subtly, but it is clear that insofar as cognitive science explains these phenomena at all, it does so by explaining the performance of functions.

When it comes to conscious experience, this sort of explanation fails. What makes the hard problem hard and almost unique is that it goes *beyond* problems about the performance of functions. To see this, note that even when we have explained the performance of all the cognitive and behavioral functions in the vicinity of experience—perceptual discrimination, categorization, internal access, verbal report—a further unanswered question may remain: *why is the performance of these functions accompanied by experience?* A simple explanation of the functions leaves this question open.

There is no analogous further question in the explanation of genes or of life or of learning. If someone says, "I can see that you have explained how DNA stores and transmits hereditary information from one generation to the next, but you have not explained how it is a *gene*," then they are making a conceptual mistake. All it means to be a gene is to be an entity that performs the relevant storage and transmission function. But if someone says, "I can see that you have explained how information is discriminated, integrated, and reported, but you have not explained how it is *experienced*," they are not making a conceptual mistake. This is a nontrivial further question.

This further question is the key question in the problem of consciousness. Why doesn't all of this information processing go on "in the dark," free of any inner feel? Why is it that when electromagnetic waveforms impinge on a retina and are discriminated and categorized by a visual system, the discrimination and categorization are experienced as a sensation of vivid red? We know that conscious experience *does* arise when these functions are performed, but the very fact that it arises is the central mystery. There is an *explanatory gap* (a term due to Levine 1983) between the functions and experience, and we need an explanatory bridge to cross it. A mere account of the functions stays on one side of the gap, so the materials for the bridge must be found elsewhere.

This is not to say that experience has no function. Perhaps it will turn out to play an important cognitive role, but for any role it might play, there will be more to the explanation of experience than a simple explanation of the function. Perhaps it will even turn out that in the course of explaining a function, we will be led to the key insight that allows an explanation of experience. If this happens, though, the discovery will be an extra explanatory reward. There is no cognitive function such that we can say in advance that explanation of that function will automatically explain experience.

To explain experience, we need a new approach. The usual explanatory methods of cognitive science and neuroscience do not suffice. These methods have been developed precisely to explain the performance of cognitive functions, and they do a good job of it. Still, as these methods stand, they are equipped to explain *only* the performance of functions. When it comes to the hard problem, the standard approach has nothing to say.

4. Some Case Studies

In the last few years, a number of works have addressed the problems of consciousness within the framework of cognitive science and neuroscience. This might suggest that the foregoing analysis is faulty, but in fact a close examination of the relevant work only lends the analysis further support. When we investigate just which aspects of consciousness these studies are aimed at and which aspects they end up explaining, we find that the ultimate target of explanation is always one of the easy problems. I illustrate this with two representative examples.

The first is the "neurobiological theory of consciousness" outlined by Crick and Koch (1990; see also Crick 1994). This theory centers on certain 35–75 hertz neural oscillations in the cerebral cortex; Crick and Koch hypothesize that these oscillations are the basis of consciousness. This is partly because the oscillations seem to be correlated with awareness in a number of different modalities—within the visual and olfactory systems, for example—and also because they suggest a mechanism by which the *binding* of information might be achieved. Binding is the process whereby separately represented pieces of information about a single entity are brought together to be used by later processing, as when information about the color and shape of a perceived object is integrated from separate visual pathways. Following others (e.g., Eckhorn et al. 1988), Crick and Koch hypothesize that binding may be achieved by the synchronized oscillations of neuronal groups representing the relevant contents. When two pieces of information are to be bound together, the relevant neural groups will oscillate with the same frequency and phase.

The details of how this binding might be achieved are still poorly understood, but suppose that they can be worked out. What might the resulting theory explain? Clearly it might explain the binding of information, and perhaps it might yield a more general account of the integration of information in the brain. Crick and Koch also suggest that these oscillations activate the mechanisms of working memory, so that there may be an account of this and perhaps other forms of memory in the distance. The theory might eventually lead to a general account of how perceived information is bound and stored in memory for use by later processing.

Such a theory would be valuable, but it would tell us nothing about why the relevant contents are experienced. Crick and Koch suggest that these oscillations are the neural *correlates* of experience. This claim is arguable—does not binding also take place in the processing of unconscious information?—but even if it is accepted, the *explanatory* question remains: why do the oscillations give rise to experience? The only basis for an explanatory connection is the role they play in binding and storage, but the question of why binding and storage should themselves be accompanied by experience is never addressed. If we do not know why binding and storage should give rise to experience, telling a story about the oscillations cannot help us. Conversely, if we *knew* why binding and storage gave rise to experience, the neurophysiological details would be just the icing on the cake. Crick and Koch's theory gains its purchase by *assuming* a connection between binding and experience and so can do nothing to explain that link.

I do not think that Crick and Koch are ultimately claiming to address the hard problem, although some have interpreted them that way. A published interview with Koch gives a clear statement of the limitations on the theory's ambitions:

> Well, let's first forget about the really difficult aspects, like subjective feelings, for they may not have a scientific solution. The subjective state of play, of pain, of pleasure, of seeing blue, of smelling a rose—there seems to be a huge jump between the materialistic level, of explaining molecules and neurons, and the subjective level. Let's focus on things that are easier to study—like visual awareness. You're now talking to me, but you're not looking at me, you're looking at the cappuccino, and so you are aware of it. You can say, "It's a cup and there's some liquid in it." If I give it to you, you'll move your arm and you'll take it—you'll respond in a meaningful manner. That's what I call awareness. (What Is Consciousness? *Discover* [November 1992], 96.)

The second example is an approach at the level of cognitive psychology. This is Bernard Baars's global workspace theory of consciousness, presented in his book *A Cognitive Theory of Consciousness*. According to this theory, the contents of consciousness are contained in a *global workspace*, a central processor used to mediate communication between a host of specialized nonconscious processors. When these specialized processors need to broadcast information to the rest of the system, they do so by sending this information to the workspace, which acts as a kind of communal blackboard for the rest of the system, accessible to all the other processors.

Baars uses this model to address many aspects of human cognition and to explain a number of contrasts between conscious and unconscious cognitive functioning. Ultimately, however, it is a theory of *cognitive accessibility* that explains how it is that certain information contents are widely accessible within a system, as well as a theory of informational integration and reportability. The theory shows promise as a theory of awareness, the functional correlate of conscious experience, but an explanation of experience itself is not on offer.

One might suppose that, according to this theory, the contents of experience are precisely the contents of the workspace. However, even if this is so, nothing internal to the theory *explains* why the information within the global workspace is experienced. The best the theory can do is to say that the information is experienced because it is *globally accessible*. But now the question arises in a different form: why should global accessibility give rise to conscious experience? As always, this bridging question is unanswered.

Almost all of the work taking a cognitive or neuroscientific approach to consciousness in recent years could be subjected to a similar critique. The "neural Darwinism" model of Edelman (1989), for instance, addresses questions about perceptual awareness and the self-concept but says nothing about why there should also be experience. The "multiple drafts" model of Dennett (1991) is largely directed at explaining the reportability of certain mental contents. The "intermediate level" theory of Jackendoff (1988) provides an account of some computational processes that underlie consciousness, but Jackendoff stresses that the question of how these "project" into conscious experience remains mysterious.

Researchers using these methods are often inexplicit about their attitudes to the problem of conscious experience, although sometimes they take a clear stand. Even among those who are clear about it, attitudes differ widely. In relating this sort of work to the problem of experience, a number of different strategies are available. It would be useful if these strategic choices were more often made explicit.

The first strategy is simply to *explain something else*. Some researchers are explicit that the problem of experience is too difficult for now and perhaps even outside the domain of science altogether. These researchers instead choose to address one of the more tractable problems such as reportability or the concept of the self. Although I have called these problems the "easy" problems, they are among the most interesting unsolved problems in cognitive science, so this work is certainly worthwhile. The worst that can be said of this choice is that in the context of research on consciousness it is relatively unambitious, and the work can sometimes be misinterpreted.

The second choice is to take a harder line and *deny the phenomenon*. (Variations on this approach are taken by Allport 1988; Dennett 1991; Wilkes 1988.) According to this line, once we have explained the functions such as accessibility and reportability, there is no further phenomenon called "experience" to explain. Some explicitly deny the phenomenon, holding, for example, that what is not externally verifiable cannot be real. Others achieve the same effect by allowing that experience exists but only if we equate "experience" with something like the capacity to discriminate and report. These approaches lead to a simpler theory but are ultimately unsatisfactory. Experience is the most central and manifest aspect of our mental lives and indeed is perhaps the key explanandum in the science of the mind. Because of this status as an explanandum, experience cannot be discarded like the vital spirit when a new theory comes along. Rather, it is the central fact that any theory of consciousness must explain. A theory that denies the phenomenon "solves" the problem by ducking the question.

In a third option, some researchers *claim to be explaining experience* in the full sense. These researchers (unlike those mentioned above) wish to take experience very seriously; they lay out their functional model or theory and claim that it explains the full subjective quality of experience (e.g., Flohr 1992; Humphrey 1992). The relevant step in the explanation is typically passed over quickly, however, and usually ends up looking something like magic. After some details about information processing are given, experience suddenly enters the picture, but it is left obscure *how* these processes should suddenly give rise to experience. Perhaps it is simply taken for granted that it does, but then we have an incomplete explanation and a version of the fifth strategy below.

A fourth, more promising approach appeals to these methods to *explain the structure of experience*. For example, it is arguable that an account of the discriminations made by the visual system can account for the structural relations between different color experiences, as well as for the geometric structure of the visual field (see, e.g., Clark 1992; Hardin 1992). In general, certain facts about structures found in processing will correspond to and arguably explain facts about the structure of experience. This strategy is plausible but limited. At best, it takes the existence of experience for granted and accounts for some facts about its structure, providing a sort of nonreductive explanation of the structural aspects of experience (I say more on this later). This is useful for many purposes, but it tells us nothing about why there should be experience in the first place.

A fifth and reasonable strategy is to *isolate the substrate of experience*. After all, almost everyone allows that experience *arises* in one way or another from brain processes, and it makes sense to identify the sort of process from which it arises. Crick and Koch present their work as isolating the neural correlate of consciousness, for example, and Edelman (1989) and Jackendoff (1987) make related claims. Justification of these claims requires careful theoretical analysis, especially as experience is not directly observable in experimental contexts, but when applied judiciously this strategy can shed indirect light on the problem of experience. Nevertheless, the strategy is clearly incomplete. For a satisfactory theory, we need to know more than *which* processes give rise to experience; we also need an account of why and how. A full theory of consciousness must build an explanatory bridge.

5. The Extra Ingredient

We have seen that there are systematic reasons why the usual methods of cognitive science and neuroscience fail to account for conscious experience. These are simply the wrong sort of methods. Nothing that they give to us can yield an explanation. To account for conscious experience, we need an *extra ingredient* in the explanation. This makes for a challenge to those who are serious about the hard problem of consciousness: what is your extra ingredient, and why should *that* account for conscious experience?

There is no shortage of extra ingredients to be had. Some propose an injection of chaos and nonlinear dynamics. Some think that the key lies in nonalgorithmic processing. Some appeal to future discoveries in neurophysiology. Some suppose that the key to the mystery will lie at the level of quantum mechanics. It is easy to see why all of these suggestions are proposed. None of the old methods work, so the solution must lie with *something* new. Unfortunately, these suggestions all suffer from the same old problems.

Nonalgorithmic processing, for example, is suggested by Penrose (1989, 1994) because of the role it might play in the process of conscious mathematical insight. The arguments about mathematics are controversial, but even if they succeed and an account of nonalgorithmic processing in the human brain is given, it will still only be an account of the *functions* involved in mathematical reasoning and the like. For a nonalgorithmic process as much as an algorithmic process, the question is left unanswered: why should this process give rise to experience? In answering *this* question, there is no special role for nonalgorithmic processing.

The same goes for nonlinear and chaotic dynamics. These might provide a novel account of the dynamics of cognitive functioning, quite different from that given by standard methods in cognitive science. But from dynamics, one only gets more dynamics. The question about experience here is as mysterious as ever. The point is even clearer for new discoveries in neurophysiology. These discoveries may help us make significant progress in understanding brain function, but for any neural process we isolate, the same question will always arise. It is difficult to imagine what a proponent of new neurophysiology expects to happen over and above the explanation of further cognitive functions. It is not as if we will suddenly discover a phenomenal glow inside a neuron!

Perhaps the most popular "extra ingredient" of all is quantum mechanics (e.g., Hameroff 1994). The attractiveness of quantum theories of consciousness may stem from a law of minimization of mystery: consciousness is mysterious, and quantum mechanics is mysterious, so maybe the two mysteries have a common source. Nevertheless, quantum theories of consciousness suffer from the same difficulties as neural or computational theories. Quantum phenomena have some remarkable functional properties, such as nondeterminism and nonlocality. It is natural to speculate that these properties may play some role in the explanation of cognitive functions, such as random choice and the integration of information, and this hypothesis cannot be ruled out a priori. When it comes to the explanation of experience, however, quantum processes are in the same boat as any other. The question of why these processes should give rise to experience is entirely unanswered.[3]

(One special attraction of quantum theories is the fact that, according to some interpretations of quantum mechanics, consciousness plays an active role in "collapsing" the quantum wave function. Such interpretations are controversial, but in any case they offer no hope of *explaining* consciousness in terms of quantum processes. Rather, these theories *assume* the existence of consciousness and use it in the explanation of quantum processes. At best, these theories tell us something about a physical role that consciousness may play. They tell us nothing about why it arises.)

At the end of the day, the same criticism applies to *any* purely physical account of consciousness. For any physical process we specify there will be an unanswered question: why should this process give rise to experience? Given any such process, it is conceptually coherent that it could be instantiated in the absence of experience. It follows that no mere account of the physical process will tell us why experience arises. The emergence of experience goes beyond what can be derived from physical theory.

---

3. *In a reply to the paper on which this chapter is based, Hameroff and Penrose (1996) explicitly endorse the idea that experience is a fundamental element of nature.

Purely physical explanation is well suited to the explanation of physical *structures* by explaining macroscopic structures in terms of detailed micro-structural constituents. It also provides a satisfying explanation of the performance of *functions* by accounting for these functions in terms of the physical mechanisms that perform them. This is because once the internal details of the physical account are given, the structural and functional properties fall out as an automatic consequence. However, the structure and dynamics of physical processes yield only more structure and dynamics, so structures and functions are all we can expect these processes to explain. The facts about experience cannot be an automatic consequence of any physical account, as it is conceptually coherent that any given process could exist without experience. Experience may *arise* from the physical, but it is not *explained* by the physical.

The moral of all this is that *you can't explain conscious experience on the cheap*. It is a remarkable fact that reductive methods—methods that explain a high-level phenomenon wholly in terms of more basic physical processes—work well in so many domains. In a sense, one *can* explain most biological and cognitive phenomena on the cheap, in that these phenomena are seen as automatic consequences of more fundamental processes. It would be wonderful if reductive methods could explain experience, too; I hoped for a long time that they might. Unfortunately, there are systematic reasons why these methods must fail. Reductive methods are successful in most domains because what needs explaining in those domains are structures and functions, and these are the kinds of thing that a physical account can entail. When it comes to a problem over and above the explanation of structures and functions, these methods are impotent.

This might seem reminiscent of the vitalist claim that no physical account could explain life, but the cases are disanalogous. What drove vitalist skepticism was doubt about whether physical mechanisms could perform the many remarkable functions associated with life, such as complex adaptive behavior and reproduction. The conceptual claim that explanation of functions is what is needed was implicitly accepted, but, lacking detailed knowledge of biochemical mechanisms, the vitalists doubted whether any physical process could do the job and proposed the hypothesis of the vital spirit as an alternative explanation.[4] Once it turned out that physical processes could perform the relevant functions, vitalist doubts melted away.

---

4. *Garrett (2006) suggests that one vitalist, Nehemiah Grew, gave conceivability arguments closely related to those concerning consciousness. I think that on examination even Grew's view is consistent with the idea that the vital spirit is invoked to explain the functions. It is just that, once the vital spirit is invoked in this role, one can then imagine other, counterfactual systems in which it is absent.

With experience, on the other hand, physical explanation of the functions is not in question. The key is instead the *conceptual* point that the explanation of functions does not suffice for the explanation of experience. This basic conceptual point is not something that further neuroscientific investigation will affect. In a similar way, experience is disanalogous to the *élan vital*. The vital spirit was presented as an explanatory posit in order to explain the relevant functions and could therefore be discarded when those functions were explained without it. Experience is not an explanatory posit but an explanandum in its own right and so is not a candidate for this sort of elimination.

It is tempting to note that all sorts of puzzling phenomena have eventually turned out to be explainable in physical terms. But these were all problems about the observable behavior of physical objects and came down to problems in the explanation of structures and functions. Because of this, these phenomena have always been the kind of thing that a physical account *might* explain, even if at some points there have been good reasons to suspect that no such explanation would be forthcoming. The tempting induction from these cases fails in the case of consciousness, which is not a problem about physical structures and functions. The problem of consciousness is puzzling in an entirely different way. An analysis of the problem shows us that conscious experience is just not the kind of thing that a wholly reductive account could succeed in explaining.

6. Nonreductive Explanation

At this point some are tempted to give up, holding that we will never have a theory of conscious experience. McGinn (1989), for example, argues that the problem is too hard for our limited minds; we are "cognitively closed" with respect to the phenomenon. Others have argued that conscious experience lies outside the domain of scientific theory altogether.

I think this pessimism is premature. This is not the place to give up; it is the place where things get interesting. When simple methods of explanation are ruled out, we need to investigate the alternatives. Given that reductive explanation fails, *nonreductive* explanation is the natural choice.

Although a remarkable number of phenomena have turned out to be explicable wholly in terms of entities simpler than themselves, this is not universal. In physics, it occasionally happens that an entity has to be taken as *fundamental*. Fundamental entities are not explained in terms of anything simpler. Instead, one takes them as basic and gives a theory of how they relate to everything else in the world. For example, in the nineteenth century it turned out that electromagnetic processes could not be explained in terms of the wholly mechanical processes that previous physical theories appealed to, so Maxwell and others introduced electromagnetic charge and electromagnetic forces as new fundamental components of a physical theory. To explain electromagnetism, the ontology of physics had to be expanded. New basic properties and basic laws were needed to give a satisfactory account of the phenomena.

Other features that physical theory takes as fundamental include mass and space-time. No attempt is made to explain these features in terms of anything simpler. This does not rule out the possibility of a theory of mass or of space-time, however. There is an intricate theory of how these features interrelate and of the basic laws they enter into. This theory is used to explain many familiar higher-level phenomena concerning mass, space, and time.

I suggest that a theory of consciousness should take experience as fundamental. We know that a theory of consciousness requires the addition of *something* fundamental to our ontology, as everything in physical theory is compatible with the absence of consciousness. We might add some entirely new nonphysical feature from which experience can be derived, but it is hard to see what such a feature would be like. More likely, we will take experience itself as a fundamental feature of the world, alongside mass, charge, and space-time. If we take experience as fundamental, then we can go about the business of constructing a theory of experience.

Where there is a fundamental property, there are fundamental laws. A nonreductive theory of experience will add new principles to the basic laws of nature. These basic principles will ultimately carry the explanatory burden in a theory of consciousness. Just as we explain familiar high-level phenomena involving mass in terms of more basic principles involving mass and other entities, we might explain familiar phenomena involving experience in terms of more basic principles involving experience and other entities.

In particular, a nonreductive theory of experience will specify basic principles that tell us how experience depends on physical features of the world. These *psychophysical* principles will not interfere with physical laws, as it seems that physical laws already form a closed system. Rather, they will be a supplement to a physical theory. A physical theory gives a theory of physical processes, and a psychophysical theory tells us how those processes give rise to experience. We know that experience depends on physical processes, but we also know that this dependence cannot be derived from physical laws alone. The new basic principles postulated by a nonreductive theory give us the extra ingredient that we need to build an explanatory bridge.

Of course, by taking experience as fundamental, there is a sense in which this approach does not tell us why there is experience in the first place, but this is the same for any fundamental theory. Nothing in physics tells us why there is matter in the first place, but we do not count this against theories of matter. Certain features of the world need to be taken as fundamental by any scientific theory. A theory of matter can still explain all sorts of facts about matter by showing how they are consequences of the basic laws. The same goes for a theory of experience.

This position qualifies as a variety of dualism as it postulates basic properties over and above the properties invoked by physics. But it is an innocent version of dualism, entirely compatible with the scientific view of the world. Nothing in this approach contradicts anything in physical theory; we simply need to add further *bridging* principles to explain how experience arises from physical processes. There is nothing particularly spiritual or mystical about this theory—its overall shape is like that of a physical theory, with a few fundamental entities connected by fundamental laws. It expands the ontology slightly, to be sure, but Maxwell did the same thing. Indeed, the overall structure of this position is entirely naturalistic, allowing both that the universe ultimately comes down to a network of basic entities obeying simple laws and that there eventually may be a theory of consciousness cast in terms of such laws. If the position is to have a name, *naturalistic dualism* is a good choice.

If this view is right, then in some ways a theory of consciousness will have more in common with a theory in physics than a theory in biology. Biological theories involve no principles that are fundamental in this way, so biological theory has a certain complexity and messiness to it; but theories in physics, insofar as they deal with fundamental principles, aspire to simplicity and elegance. The fundamental laws of nature are part of the basic furniture of the world, and physical theories are telling us that this basic furniture is remarkably simple. If a theory of consciousness also involves fundamental principles, then we should expect the same. The principles of simplicity, elegance, and even beauty, which drive physicists' search for a fundamental theory, will also apply to a theory of consciousness.

(Some philosophers [the type-B materialists of chapter 5] argue that even though there is a *conceptual* gap between physical processes and experience, there need be no metaphysical gap, so that experience might in a certain sense still be physical. I argue against this view in chapters 5–7 and chapter 10. Still, if what I have said so far is correct, this position must at least concede an *explanatory* gap between physical processes and experience. For example, the principles connecting the physical and the experiential will not be derivable from the laws of physics, so such principles must be taken as *explanatorily* fundamental. So even on this sort of view, the explanatory structure of a theory of consciousness will be much as I have described.)

7. Outline of a Theory of Consciousness

It is not too soon to begin work on a theory. We are already in a position to understand certain key facts about the relationship between physical processes and experience and about the regularities that connect them. Once reductive explanation is set aside, we can lay those facts on the table so that they can play their proper role as the initial pieces in a nonreductive theory of consciousness and as constraints on the basic laws that constitute an ultimate theory.

There is an obvious problem that plagues the development of a theory of consciousness, and that is the paucity of objective data. Conscious experience is not directly observable in an experimental context, so we cannot generate data about the relationship between physical processes and experience at will. Nevertheless, we all have access to a rich source of data in our own case. Many important regularities between experience and processing can be inferred from considerations about one's own experience. There are also good indirect sources of data from observable cases, as when one relies on the verbal report of a subject as an indication of experience. These methods have their limitations, but we have more than enough data to get a theory off the ground.

Philosophical analysis is also useful in getting value for money out of the data we have. This sort of analysis can yield a number of principles relating consciousness and cognition, thereby strongly constraining the shape of an ultimate theory. The method of thought experimentation can also yield significant rewards, as we will see. Finally, the fact that we are searching for a *fundamental* theory means that we can appeal to nonempirical constraints such as simplicity and homogeneity in developing a theory. We must seek to systematize the information we have, to extend it as far as possible by careful analysis, and then to make the inference to the simplest possible theory that explains the data while remaining a plausible candidate to be part of the fundamental furniture of the world.

Such theories will always retain an element of speculation that is not present in other scientific theories because of the impossibility of conclusive intersubjective experimental tests. Still, we can certainly construct theories that are compatible with the data that we have and evaluate them in comparison to each other. Even in the absence of intersubjective observation, there are numerous criteria available for the evaluation of such theories: simplicity, internal coherence, coherence with theories in other domains, the ability to reproduce the properties of experience that are familiar from our own case, and even an overall fit with the dictates of common sense. Perhaps there will be significant indeterminacies remaining even when all of these constraints are applied, but we can at least develop plausible candidates. Only when candidate theories have been developed will we be able to evaluate them.

A nonreductive theory of consciousness will consist in a number of *psychophysical principles*, principles that connect the properties of physical processes to the properties of experience. We can think of these principles as encapsulating the way in which experience arises from the physical. Ultimately, these principles should tell us what sort of physical systems will have associated experiences, and for the systems that do, they should tell us what sort of physical properties are relevant to the emergence of experience and just what sort of experience we should expect any given physical system to yield. This is a tall order, but there is no reason we should not get started.

In what follows, I present my own candidates for the psychophysical principles that might go into a theory of consciousness. The first two of these are *nonbasic principles*—systematic connections between processing and experience at a relatively high level. These principles can play a significant role in developing and constraining a theory of consciousness, but they are not cast at a sufficiently fundamental level to qualify as truly basic laws. The final principle is my candidate for a *basic principle*, which might form the cornerstone of a fundamental theory of consciousness. This final principle is particularly speculative, but it is the kind of speculation that is required if we are ever to have a satisfying theory of consciousness. I can present these principles only briefly here; I argue for them at much greater length in *The Conscious Mind*.[5]

1. The Principle of Structural Coherence

This is a principle of coherence between the *structure of consciousness* and the *structure of awareness*. Recall that "awareness" was used earlier to refer to the various functional phenomena that are associated with consciousness. I am now using it to refer to a somewhat more specific process in the cognitive underpinnings of experience. In particular, the contents of awareness

---

5. *The three elements that follow are developed in chapters 6–8 of *The Conscious Mind*. Readers should feel free to skip or skim this material, which is not essential to the narrative of the remainder of this book.

are to be understood as those information contents that are accessible to central systems and brought to bear in a widespread way in the control of behavior. Briefly put, we can think of awareness as *direct availability for global control.* To a first approximation, the contents of awareness are the contents that are directly accessible and potentially reportable, at least in a language-using system.[6]

Awareness is a purely functional notion, but it is nevertheless intimately linked to conscious experience. In familiar cases, wherever we find consciousness, we find awareness. Wherever there is conscious experience, there is some corresponding information in the cognitive system that is available in the control of behavior and available for verbal report. Conversely, it seems that whenever information is available for report and for global control, there is a corresponding conscious experience. Thus, there is a direct correspondence between consciousness and awareness.

The correspondence can be taken further. It is a central fact about experience that it has a complex structure. The visual field has a complex geometry, for instance. There are also relations of similarity and difference between experiences, as well as relations in things such as relative intensity. Every subject's experience can be at least partly characterized and decomposed in terms of these structural properties: similarity and difference relations, perceived location, relative intensity, geometric structure, and so on. It is also a central fact that, to each of these structural features, there is a corresponding feature in the information-processing structure of awareness.

Take color experiences as an example. For every distinction between color experiences, there is a corresponding distinction in processing. The different phenomenal colors that we experience form a complex three-dimensional space, varying in hue, saturation, and intensity. The properties of this space can be recovered from information-processing considerations. Examination of the visual systems shows that waveforms of light are discriminated and analyzed along three different axes, and it is this three-dimensional information that is relevant to later processing. The three-dimensional structure of phenomenal color space therefore corresponds directly to the three-dimensional structure of visual awareness. This is precisely what we would expect. After all, every experienced color distinction corresponds to some reportable information and therefore to a distinction that is represented in the structure of processing.

6. *Awareness is closely related to Ned Block's "access consciousness" (1995). In effect, this principle suggests a certain coherence between the structure of phenomenal consciousness and the structure of access consciousness. This point is developed in a commentary on Block (Chalmers 1997a). The connection between availability and experience is also explored in chapter 4.

In a more straightforward way, the geometric structure of the visual field is directly reflected in a structure that can be recovered from visual processing. Every geometric relation corresponds to something that can be reported and is therefore cognitively represented. If we were given only the story about information processing in an agent's visual and cognitive system, we could not *directly* observe that agent's visual experiences, but we could nevertheless infer those experiences' structural properties.

In general, any information that is consciously experienced will also be cognitively represented. The fine-grained structure of the visual field will correspond to some fine-grained structure in visual processing. The same goes for experiences in other modalities and even for nonsensory experiences. Internal mental images have geometric properties that are represented in processing. Even emotions have structural properties, such as relative intensity, that correspond directly to a structural property of processing: where there is greater intensity, we find a greater effect on later processes. In general, precisely because the structural properties of experience are accessible and reportable, those properties will be directly represented in the structure of awareness.

It is this isomorphism between the structures of consciousness and awareness that constitutes the principle of structural coherence. This principle reflects the central fact that even though cognitive processes do not conceptually entail facts about conscious experience, consciousness and cognition do not float free of one another but cohere in an intimate way.

This principle has its limits. It allows us to recover structural properties of experience from information-processing properties, but not all properties of experience are structural properties. There are properties of experience, such as the intrinsic nature of a sensation of red, that cannot be fully captured in a structural description. The very intelligibility of inverted spectrum scenarios, where experiences of red and green are inverted but all structural properties remain the same, show that structural properties constrain experience without exhausting it. Nevertheless, the very fact that we feel compelled to leave structural properties unaltered when we imagine experiences inverted between functionally identical systems shows how central the principle of structural coherence is to our conception of our mental lives. It is not a *logically* necessary principle, as after all we can imagine all of the information processing occurring without any experience at all, but it is nevertheless a strong and familiar constraint on the psychophysical connection.

The principle of structural coherence allows for a very useful kind of indirect explanation of experience in terms of physical processes. For example, we can use facts about the neural processing of visual information to indirectly explain the structure of color space. The facts about neural processing can entail and explain the structure of awareness; if we take the coherence principle for granted, the structure of experience will also be explained. Empirical investigation might even lead us to better understand the structure of awareness within a bat, shedding indirect light on Nagel's vexing question of what it is like to be a bat. This principle provides a natural interpretation of much existing work on the explanation of consciousness (e.g., Clark 1992 and Hardin 1992 on colors and Akins 1993 on bats), although it is often appealed to inexplicitly. It is so familiar that it is taken for granted by almost everybody and is a central plank in the cognitive explanation of consciousness.

The coherence between consciousness and awareness also allows a natural interpretation of work in neuroscience directed at isolating the neural correlate of consciousness. This interpretation is developed further in chapter 4.

2. The Principle of Organizational Invariance

This principle states that any two systems with the same fine-grained *functional organization* will have qualitatively identical experiences. If the causal patterns of neural organization were duplicated in silicon, for example, with a silicon chip for every neuron and the same patterns of interaction, then the same experiences would arise. According to this principle, what matters for the emergence of experience is not the specific physical makeup of a system but the abstract pattern of causal interaction between its components. This principle is controversial, of course. Some (e.g., Searle 1980) have thought that consciousness is tied to a specific biology, so that a silicon isomorph of a human need not be conscious. I believe that the principle can be given significant support by the analysis of thought experiments, however.

Very briefly: suppose (for the purposes of a reductio ad absurdum) that the principle is false and that there could be two functionally isomorphic systems with different experiences. Perhaps only one of the systems is conscious, or perhaps both are conscious, but they have different experiences. For the purposes of illustration, let us say that one system is made of neurons and the other of silicon and that one experiences red where the other experiences blue. The two systems have the same organization, so we can imagine gradually transforming one into the other, perhaps replacing neurons one at a time by silicon chips with the same local function. We thus gain a spectrum of intermediate cases, each with the same organization but with slightly different physical makeup and slightly different experiences.

Along this spectrum, there must be two systems, A and B, between which we replace less than one-tenth of the system but whose experiences differ. These two systems are physically identical, except that a small neural circuit in A has been replaced by a silicon circuit in B.

The key step in the thought experiment is to take the relevant neural circuit in A and install alongside it a causally isomorphic silicon circuit, with a switch between the two. What happens when we flip the switch? By hypothesis, the system's conscious experiences will change—from red to blue, say. This follows from the fact that the system after the change is essentially a version of B, whereas before the change it is just A.

Given the assumptions, however, there is no way for the system to *notice* the changes. Its causal organization stays constant, so that all of its functional states and behavioral dispositions stay fixed. As far as the system is concerned, nothing unusual has happened. There is no room for the thought, "Hmm! Something strange just happened!" In general, the structure of any such thought must be reflected in processing, but the structure of processing remains constant here. If there were to be such a thought, it must float entirely free of the system and would be utterly impotent to affect later processing. (If it affected later processing, the systems would be functionally distinct, contrary to the hypothesis). We might even flip the switch a number of times, so that experiences of red and blue dance back and forth before the system's "inner eye." According to the hypothesis, the system can never notice these "dancing qualia."

This I take to be a reductio of the original assumption.[7] It is a central fact about experience, very familiar from our own case, that whenever experiences change significantly and we are paying attention, we can notice the change; if this were not the case, we would be led to the skeptical possibility that our experiences are dancing before our eyes all the time. This hypothesis has the same status as the possibility that the world was created five minutes ago: perhaps it is logically coherent, but it is not plausible. Given the extremely plausible assumption that changes in experience correspond to changes in processing, we are led to the conclusion that the original hypothesis is impossible and that any two functionally isomorphic

7. *I still find this hypothesis very odd, but I am now inclined to think that it is something less than a reductio. Work on change blindness has gotten us used to the idea that large changes in consciousness can go unnoticed. Admittedly, these changes are outside attention, and unnoticed changes in the contents of attention would be much stranger, but it is perhaps not so strange as to be ruled out in all circumstances. Russellian monism (see chapter 5) also provides a natural model in which such changes could occur. In *The Conscious Mind* I suggested that this "dancing qualia" argument was somewhat stronger than the "fading qualia" argument given there; I would now reverse that judgment.

systems must have the same sort of experiences. To put it in technical terms, the philosophical hypotheses of "absent qualia" and "inverted qualia," while logically possible, are empirically and nomologically impossible.

(Some may worry that a silicon isomorph of a neural system might be impossible for technical reasons. That question is open. The invariance principle says only that *if* an isomorph is possible, then it will have the same sort of conscious experience.)

There is more to be said here, but this gives the basic flavor. Once again, this thought experiment draws on familiar facts about the coherence between consciousness and cognitive processing to yield a strong conclusion about the relation between physical structure and experience. If the argument goes through, we know that the only physical properties directly relevant to the emergence of experience are *organizational* properties. This acts as a further strong constraint on a theory of consciousness.

3. The Double-Aspect Theory of Information

The two preceding principles are *nonbasic* principles. They involve high-level notions such as "awareness" and "organization" and therefore lie at the wrong level to constitute the fundamental laws in a theory of consciousness. Nevertheless, they act as strong constraints. What is further needed are *basic* principles that fit these constraints and that might ultimately explain them.

The basic principle that I suggest centrally involves the notion of *information*. I understand information in more or less the sense of Shannon (1948). Where there is information, there are *information states* embedded in an *information space*. An information space has a basic structure of *difference* relations between its elements, characterizing the ways in which different elements in a space are similar or different, possibly in complex ways. An information space is an abstract object, but following Shannon we can see information as *physically embodied* when there is a space of distinct physical states, the differences between which can be transmitted down some causal pathway. The transmittable states can be seen as themselves constituting an information space. To borrow a phrase from Bateson (1972), physical information is a *difference that makes a difference*.

The double-aspect principle stems from the observation that there is a direct isomorphism between certain physically embodied information spaces and certain *phenomenal* (or experiential) information spaces. From the same sort of observations that went into the principle of structural coherence, we can note that the differences between phenomenal states have a structure that corresponds directly to the differences embedded in physical processes; in particular, to those differences that make a difference down certain causal pathways implicated in global availability and control. That is, we can find the *same* abstract information space embedded in physical processing and in conscious experience.

This leads to a natural hypothesis: that information (or at least some information) has two basic aspects, a physical aspect and a phenomenal aspect. This has the status of a basic principle that might underlie and explain the emergence of experience from the physical. Experience arises by virtue of its status as one aspect of information, when the other aspect is found embodied in physical processing.

This principle is lent support by a number of considerations, which I can outline only briefly here. First, consideration of the sort of physical changes that correspond to changes in conscious experience suggests that such changes are always relevant by virtue of their role in constituting *informational changes*—differences within an abstract space of states that are divided up precisely according to their causal differences along certain pathways. Second, if the principle of organizational invariance is to hold, then we need to find some fundamental *organizational* property for experience to be linked to, and information is an organizational property par excellence. Third, this principle offers some hope of explaining the principle of structural coherence in terms of the structure present within information spaces. Fourth, analysis of the cognitive explanation of our *judgments* and *claims* about conscious experience— judgments that are functionally explainable but nevertheless deeply tied to experience itself—suggests that explanation centrally involves the information states embedded in cognitive processing. It follows that a theory based on information allows a deep coherence between the explanation of experience and the explanation of our judgments and claims about it.

Wheeler (1990) has suggested that information is fundamental to the physics of the universe. According to this "it from bit" doctrine, the laws of physics can be cast in terms of information, postulating different states that give rise to different effects without actually saying what those states *are*. It is only their position in an information space that counts. If so, then information is a natural candidate to also play a role in a fundamental theory of consciousness. We are led to a conception of the world in which information is truly fundamental and in which it has two basic aspects, one that corresponds to the physical and one that corresponds to the phenomenal features of the world.

Of course, the double-aspect principle is extremely speculative and also underdetermined, leaving a number of key questions unanswered. An obvious question is whether *all* information has a phenomenal aspect. One possibility is that we need a further constraint on the fundamental theory, indicating just what *sort* of information has a phenomenal aspect. The other possibility is that there is no such constraint. If not, then experience is much more widespread than we might have believed, as information is everywhere. This is counterintuitive at first, but on reflection the position gains a certain plausibility and elegance. Where there is simple information processing, there is simple experience, and where there is complex information processing, there is complex experience. A mouse has a simpler information-processing structure than a human and has correspondingly simpler experience; might a thermostat, a maximally simple information-processing structure, have maximally simple experience? Indeed, if experience is truly a fundamental property, it would be surprising for it to arise only every now and then; most fundamental properties are more evenly spread. In any case, this is very much an open question, but I think that the position is not as implausible as it is often thought to be.

Once a fundamental link between information and experience is on the table, the door is opened to some grander metaphysical speculation concerning the nature of the world. For example, it is often noted that physics characterizes its basic entities only *extrinsically*, in terms of their relations to other entities, which are themselves characterized extrinsically, and so on. The intrinsic nature of physical entities is left aside. Some argue that no such intrinsic properties exist, but then one is left with a world that is pure causal flux (a pure flow of information) with no properties for the causation to relate. If one allows that intrinsic properties exist, a natural speculation, given the preceding, is that the intrinsic properties of the physical—the properties that causation ultimately relates—are themselves phenomenal properties.[8] We might say that phenomenal properties are the internal aspect of information. This could answer a concern about the causal relevance of experience—a natural worry, given a picture in which the physical domain is causally closed and in which experience is supplementary to the physical. The informational view allows us to understand how experience might have a subtle kind of causal relevance in virtue of its status as the intrinsic nature of the physical. This metaphysical speculation is probably best ignored for the purposes of developing a scientific theory, but in addressing some philosophical issues it is quite suggestive.

8. *See the discussion of type-F monism in chapter 5 and of Russellian monism in chapter 6 for much more on this theme.

8. Conclusion

The theory I have presented is speculative, but it is a candidate theory. I suspect that the principles of structural coherence and organizational invariance will be planks in any satisfactory theory of consciousness; the status of the double-aspect theory of information is less certain. Indeed, right now it is more of an idea than a theory. To have any hope of eventual explanatory success, it will have to be specified more fully and fleshed out into a more powerful form. Still, reflection on just what is plausible and implausible about it and on where it works and where it fails can only lead to a better theory.

Most existing theories of consciousness either deny the phenomenon, explain something else, or elevate the problem to an eternal mystery. I hope to have shown that it is possible to make progress on the problem even while taking it seriously. To make further progress we will need further investigation, more refined theories, and more careful analysis. The hard problem is a hard problem, but there is no reason to believe that it will remain permanently unsolved.[9]

Afterword: From "Moving Forward on the Problem of Consciousness"

There are two quite different ways in which a materialist might respond to the challenge in this chapter. One sort of response denies that on reflection there is a "hard problem" distinct from the "easy" problems or at least holds that solving the easy problems (perhaps along with some philosophical reflection) suffices to solve the hard problem. Another accepts that there is a distinctive phenomenon that generates a distinctive hard problem that goes beyond the easy problems but argues that it can be accommodated within a materialist framework all the same. To a first approximation, the first sort of view corresponds to what I call type-A materialism in

---

9. Further reading. The problems of consciousness have been widely discussed in the recent philosophical literature. For some conceptual clarification of the various problems of consciousness, see Block (1995), Nelkin (1993), and Tye (1995). Those who have stressed the difficulties of explaining experience in physical terms include Hodgson (1991), Jackson (1982), Levine (1983), Lockwood (1989), McGinn (1989), Nagel (1974), Seager (1991), Searle (1991), Strawson (1994), and Velmans (1991), among others. Those who take a reductive approach include Churchland (1995), Clark (1992), Dennett (1991), Dretske (1995), Kirk (1994), Rosenthal (1997), and Tye (1995). There have not been many attempts to build detailed nonreductive theories in the literature, but see Hodgson (1991) and Lockwood (1989) for some thoughts in that direction. Two excellent collections of articles on consciousness are Block, Flanagan, and Güzeldere (1997) and Metzinger (1995).

chapter 5, while the second sort corresponds to type-B and type-C materialism. The second sort of response is much more popular than the first, and I discuss it at some length in other chapters here (especially chapters 6 and 10). So in this afterword I take the opportunity to address the first sort of response, as put forward in articles responding to this chapter by Paul Churchland (1996) and Daniel Dennett (1996).

The type-A materialist, more precisely, denies that there is any phenomenon that needs explaining, over and above accounting for the various functions: once we have explained how the functions are performed, we have thereby explained everything. Sometimes type-A materialism is expressed by denying that consciousness exists; more often, it is expressed by claiming that consciousness may exist but only if the term "consciousness" is defined as something like "reportability" or some other functional capacity. Either way, it is asserted that there is no interesting fact about the mind in the vicinity that is conceptually distinct from the functional facts and that needs to be accommodated in our theories. Once we have explained how the functions are performed, that is that.

This is an extremely counterintuitive position. At first glance, it seems to simply deny a manifest fact about us. But it deserves to be taken seriously: After all, counterintuitive theories are not unknown in science and philosophy. On the other hand, to establish a counterintuitive position, strong arguments are needed. And to establish a position as counterintuitive as this, one might think that extraordinarily strong arguments are needed. So what arguments do its proponents provide?

A common strategy for a type-A materialist is to deflate the hard problem by using analogies to other domains, where talk of such a problem would be misguided. Thus, Dennett imagines a vitalist arguing about the hard problem of "life" or a neuroscientist arguing about the hard problem of "perception." Similarly, Paul Churchland imagines a nineteenth-century philosopher worrying about the hard problem of "light." In these cases, we are to suppose, someone might once have thought that more needed explaining than structure and function, but in each case, science has proved them wrong. So perhaps the argument about consciousness is no better.

This sort of argument cannot bear much weight, however. Pointing out that analogous arguments do not work in other domains is no news. The whole point of antireductionist arguments about consciousness is that there is a disanalogy between the problem of consciousness and problems in other domains. As for the claim that analogous arguments in such domains might once have been plausible, this strikes me as something of a convenient myth. In the other domains, it is more or less obvious that structure and function are what need explaining, at least once any experiential aspects are left aside, and one would be hard pressed to find a substantial body of people who ever argued otherwise.

When it comes to the problem of life, for example, it is just obvious that what needs explaining is structure and function. How does a living system self-organize? How does it adapt to its environment? How does it reproduce? Even the vitalists recognized this central point. Their driving question was always, "How could a mere physical system perform these complex functions?", not "Why are these functions accompanied by life?". It is no accident that Dennett's version of a vitalist is "imaginary." There is no distinct hard problem of life, and there never was one, even for vitalists.

In general, when faced with the challenge "explain X," we need to ask: what are the phenomena in the vicinity of X that need explaining, and how might we explain them? In the case of life, what cries out for explanation are phenomena such as reproduction, adaptation, metabolism, and self-sustenance: all complex functions. There is not even a plausible candidate for a further sort of property of life that needs explaining (leaving aside consciousness itself), and indeed there never was. In the case of consciousness, on the other hand, the manifest phenomena that need explaining are things such as discrimination, reportability, integration (the functions), *and experience*, so this analogy does not even get off the ground.

If someone were to claim that something has been left out by reductive explanations of light (Paul Churchland's example) or of heat (an example used by Patricia Churchland 1997), what something might they be referring to? The only phenomenon for which the suggestion would be even remotely plausible is our subjective experience of light and hotness. The molecular theory of heat does not explain the sensation of heat, and the electromagnetic theory of light does not explain what it is like to see, and understandably so. The physicists explaining heat and light have quite reasonably deferred the explanation of their experiential manifestations until the time when we have a reasonable theory of consciousness. One need not explain everything at once. With consciousness itself, however, subjective experience is precisely what is at issue, so we cannot defer the question in the same way. So once again, the analogy is no help to a reductionist.

Paul Churchland suggests that parallel antireductionist arguments could have been constructed for the phenomenon of "luminescence" and might have been found plausible at the time. I have my doubts about that plausibility, but in any case it is striking that his arguments about luminescence all depend on intuitions about the conscious experience of light. His hypothetical advocate of a "hard problem" about light appeals to light's "visibility" and the "visual point of view"; his advocate of a "knowledge argument" about light appeals to blind Mary, who has never had the experience of seeing; and the advocate of a "zombie" argument appeals to the conceivability of a universe physically just like ours but in which everything is dark. That the first two arguments trade on intuitions about experience is obvious, and even for the third, it is clear on a moment's reflection that the only way such a universe might make sense is as a universe in which the same electromagnetic transmission goes on but in which no one has the experience of seeing.

Churchland might insist that by "luminescence" he means something quite independent of experience, which physical accounts still do not explain, but then the obvious reply is that there is no good reason to believe in luminescence in the first place. Light's structural, functional, and experiential manifestations exhaust the phenomena that cry out for explanation and the phenomena in which we have any reason to believe. By contrast, conscious experience presents itself as a phenomenon to be explained and cannot be eliminated in the same way.

So, analogies do not help. To have any chance of making the case, a type-A materialist needs to argue that for consciousness, as for life, the functions are all that need explaining. Perhaps some strong, subtle, and substantive argument can be given, establishing that once we have explained the functions, we have automatically explained everything. If a sound argument could be given for this surprising conclusion, it would provide as valid a resolution of the hard problem as any.

Is there any compelling, non-question-begging argument for this conclusion? The key word, of course, is "non-question-begging." Often a proponent will simply assert that functions are all that need explaining or will argue in a way that subtly assumes this position at some point, but that is clearly unsatisfactory. Prima facie, there is very good reason to believe that the phenomena that a theory of consciousness must account for include not just discrimination, integration, report, and other such functions but also experience, and prima facie there is good reason to believe that the question of explaining experience is distinct from the questions about explaining the various functions. Such prima facie intuitions can be overturned, but to do so requires very solid and substantial argument. Otherwise, the problem is being "resolved" simply by placing one's head in the sand.

Such arguments are not easy to find. Dennett is the one of the few philosophers who has attempted to give them, and his arguments are typically not extensive. In his response to this chapter, he spends about a paragraph making the case. I take it that this paragraph bears the weight of his piece, once the trimmings are stripped away. So it is this paragraph that we should examine.

Dennett's argument here, interestingly enough, is an appeal to phenomenology. He examines his own phenomenology and tells us that he finds nothing other than functions that need explaining. The manifest phenomena that need explaining are his reactions and his abilities; nothing else even presents itself as needing to be explained.

This is daringly close to a simple denial—one is tempted to agree that it might be a good account of *Dennett's* phenomenology—and it raises immediate questions. For a start, it is far from obvious that even all of the items on Dennett's list—"feelings of foreboding," "fantasies," "delight and dismay"—are purely functional matters. To assert without argument that all that needs to be explained about such things are the associated functions seems to beg the crucial question at issue. And if we leave these controversial cases aside, Dennett's list seems to be a systematically incomplete list of what needs to be explained in explaining consciousness. One's "ability to be moved to tears" and "blithe disregard of perceptual details" are striking phenomena, but they are far from the most obvious phenomena that I (at least) find when I introspect. Much more obvious are the experience of emotion and the phenomenal visual field themselves, and nothing Dennett says gives us reason to believe that these do not need to be explained or that explaining the associated functions will explain them.

What might be going on here? Perhaps the key lies in what has elsewhere been described as the foundation of Dennett's philosophy: "third-person absolutism." If one takes the third-person perspective on oneself—viewing oneself from the outside, so to speak—these reactions and abilities are no doubt the main focus of what one sees. But the hard problem is about explaining the view from the first-person perspective. So to shift perspectives like this—even to shift to a third-person perspective on one's first-person perspective, which is one of Dennett's favorite moves—is again to assume that what needs explaining are functional matters such as reactions and reports and so is again to argue in a circle.

Dennett suggests "subtract the functions and nothing is left." Again, I can see no reason to accept this, but in any case the argument seems to have the wrong form. An analogy suggested by Gregg Rosenberg (in conversation) is useful here. Color has properties of hue, saturation, and brightness. It is plausible that if one "subtracts" hue from a color, nothing phenomenologically significant is left, but this certainly does not imply that color is nothing but hue. So even if Dennett could argue that function were somehow required for experience (in the same way that hue is required for color), this would fall a long way short of showing that function is all that has to be explained.

A slight flavor of noncircular argument is hinted at by Dennett's suggestion: "I wouldn't know what I was thinking about if I couldn't identify them by their functional differentia." This tantalizing sentence suggests various interpretations, but all of the reconstructions that I can find fall short of making the case. If the idea is that functional role is essential to the (superpersonal) process of identification, this falls short of establishing that functioning is essential to the experiences themselves, let alone that functioning is all there is to the experiences. If the idea is rather that function is all we have access to at the personal level, this seems false and seems to beg the question against the intuitive view that we have knowledge of intrinsic features of experience. But if Dennett can elaborate this into a substantial argument, that would be a very useful service.

In his paper Dennett challenges me to provide "independent" evidence (presumably behavioral or functional evidence) for the "postulation" of experience. But this is to miss the point. Conscious experience is not "postulated" to explain other phenomena in turn; rather, it is a phenomenon to be explained in its own right. And if it turns out that it cannot be explained in terms of more basic entities, then it must be taken as irreducible, just as happens with categories such as space and time. Again, Dennett's "challenge" presupposes that the only explananda that count are functions.

(Tangentially, I would be interested to see Dennett's version of the "independent" evidence that leads physicists to "introduce" the fundamental categories of space and time. It seems to me that the relevant evidence is spatiotemporal through and through, just as the evidence for experience is experiential through and through.)

Dennett might respond that I, equally, do not give arguments for the position that something more than functions needs to be explained. There would be some justice here: while I do argue at length for my conclusions, all of these arguments take the existence of consciousness for granted, where the relevant concept of consciousness is explicitly distinguished from functional concepts such as discrimination, integration, reaction, and report. Dennett presumably disputes this starting point: he thinks that the only sense in which people are conscious is a sense in which consciousness is defined as reportability, as a reactive disposition, or as some other functional concept.

But let us be clear on the dialectic. It is prima facie obvious to most people that there is a further phenomenon here. In informal surveys, the large majority of respondents (even at Tufts!) indicate that they think something more than functions needs explaining. Dennett himself—faced with the results of such a survey, perhaps intending to deflate it—has accepted that there is at least a prima facie case that something more than functions needs to be explained, and he has often stated how "radical" and "counterintuitive" his position is. So it is clear that the default assumption is that there is a further problem of explanation; to establish otherwise requires significant and substantial argument.

I would welcome such arguments in the ongoing attempt to clarify the lay of the land. The challenge for those such as Dennett is to make the nature of these arguments truly clear. I do not think it a worthless project—the hard problem is so hard that we should welcome all attempts at a resolution—but it is clear that anyone trying to make such an argument is facing an uphill battle.

Part II

THE SCIENCE OF CONSCIOUSNESS

2

HOW CAN WE CONSTRUCT A SCIENCE OF CONSCIOUSNESS?

In recent years there has been an explosion of scientific work on consciousness in cognitive neuroscience, psychology, and other fields. It has become possible to think that we are moving toward a genuine scientific understanding of conscious experience. But what is the science of consciousness all about, and what form should such a science take? This chapter gives an overview of the agenda.

1. First-Person Data and Third-Person Data

The task of a science of consciousness, as I see it, is to systematically integrate two key classes of data into a scientific framework: *third-person data*, or data about behavior and brain processes, and *first-person data*, or data about subjective experience. When a conscious system is observed from the third-person point of view, a range of specific behavioral and neural phenomena present themselves. When a conscious system is observed from the first-person point of view, a range of specific subjective phenomena present themselves. Both sorts of phenomena have the status of data for a science of consciousness.[1]

1. *What is a datum—a phenomenon, a proposition, a judgment, a record? The issue is to some extent verbal, but for present purposes it is best to take data to be observed states of affairs (in a broad enough sense of "observed"): for example, the state of affairs of a specific subject having a certain sort of experience (first-person data) or exhibiting a certain sort of behavior or having a certain sort of brain process (third-person data). Here, states of affairs should be individuated in a fine-grained way that is sensitive to the mode of presentation, as befits the epistemological role of data. So, for example, "The glass contains water" (observed by tasting) and "The glass contains H_2O" (observed by chemical test) may count as different data.

Third-person data concern the behavior and the brain processes of conscious systems. These behavioral and neurophysiological data provide the traditional material of interest for cognitive psychology and cognitive neuroscience. Where the science of consciousness is concerned, some particularly relevant third-person data are those concerning perceptual discrimination and those involving verbal reports. Direct measurements of brain processes also play a crucial role in cognitive neuroscience, of course.

First-person data concern the subjective experiences of conscious systems. It is a datum for each of us that such experiences exist: we can gather information about them both by attending to our own experiences and by monitoring subjective verbal reports about the experiences of others. These phenomenological data provide the distinctive subject for the science of consciousness. Some central sorts of first-person data include those having to do with the following:

- visual experiences (e.g., the experience of color and depth)
- other perceptual experiences (e.g., auditory and tactile experience)
- bodily experiences (e.g., pain and hunger)
- mental imagery (e.g., recalled visual images)
- emotional experience (e.g., happiness and anger)
- occurrent thought (e.g., the experience of reflecting and deciding)

Both third-person data and first-person data need explanation. An example is provided by the case of musical processing. If we observe someone listening to music, relevant third-person data include those concerning the nature of the auditory stimulus, its effects on the ear and the auditory cortex of the subject, various behavioral responses by the subject, and any verbal reports the subject might produce. All of these third-person data need explanation, but they are not all that needs explanation. As anyone who has listened to music knows, there is also a distinctive quality of subjective experience associated with listening to music. A science of music that explained the various third-person data just listed but that did not explain the first-person data of musical experience would be a seriously incomplete science of music. A complete science of musical experience must explain both sorts of phenomena, preferably within an integrated framework.

2. Explaining the Data

The problems of explaining third-person data associated with consciousness are among the "easy" problems of consciousness from the last chapter.

The problem of explaining first-person data is the hard problem. In chapter 1 we saw that, to explain third-person data, we need to explain the objective functioning of a system and can do so in principle by specifying a mechanism. When it comes to first-person data, however, this model breaks down. The reason is that first-person data—the data of subjective experience—are not data about objective functioning. Merely explaining the objective functions does not explain subjective experience.

The lesson is that *as data*, first-person data are irreducible to third-person data and vice versa. That is, third-person data alone provide an incomplete catalogue of the data that need explaining: if we explain only third-person data, we have not explained everything. Likewise, first-person data alone are incomplete. A satisfactory science of consciousness must admit both sorts of data and must build an explanatory connection between them.

What form might this connection take? A common position holds that, although there are two sorts of data, we can explain first-person data wholly in terms of material provided by third-person data. For example, many think that we might wholly explain the phenomena of subjective experience in terms of processes in the brain. This position is very attractive, but in chapter 1 I give reasons to be skeptical about it. Here I present a simple argument that encapsulates some reasons for doubt:

1. Third-person data are data about the objective structure and dynamics of physical systems.
2. (Low-level) structure and dynamics explain only facts about (high-level) structure and dynamics.
3. Explaining structure and dynamics does not suffice to explain the first-person data.

_____

4. First-person data cannot be wholly explained in terms of third-person data.

Premise 1 captures something about the character of third-person data: these data always concern certain physical structures and their dynamics. Premise 2 says that explanations in terms of processes of this sort only explain further processes of that sort. There can be big differences between the processes, as when simple low-level structure and dynamics give rise to highly complex high-level structure and dynamics (in complex systems theory, for example), but there is no escaping the structural/dynamical circle. Premise 3 encapsulates the points, discussed earlier, that explaining structure and dynamics is only to explain objective functions and that to explain objective functions does not suffice to explain first-person data about subjective experience. From these three premises, the conclusion, 4, follows.[2]

Of course, it does not follow that first-person data and third-person data have nothing to do with one another; there is obviously a systematic association between them. We have good reason to believe that subjective experiences are systematically correlated with brain processes and behavior. It remains plausible that whenever subjects have an appropriate sort of brain process, they will have an associated sort of subjective experience. We simply need to distinguish correlation from explanation. Even if first-person data cannot be wholly explained in terms of third-person data, the two sorts of data are still strongly correlated.

It follows that a science of consciousness remains entirely possible. It is just that we should expect this science to take a nonreductive form. A science of consciousness will not reduce first-person data to third-person data, but it will articulate the systematic connections between them. Where there is systematic covariation between two classes of data, we can expect systematic principles to underlie and explain the covariation. In the case of consciousness, we can expect systematic *bridging principles* to underlie and explain the covariation between third-person data and first-person data. A theory of consciousness will ultimately be a theory of these principles.

Of course, these foundational issues are controversial, and there are various alternative views. One class of views (e.g., Dennett 1991) holds that the only phenomena that need explaining are those that concern objective functioning. The most extreme version of this view says that there are no first-person data about consciousness at all. A less extreme version of this view says that all first-person data are equivalent to third-person data (e.g., about verbal reports), so that explaining these third-person data explains everything. Another class of views (e.g., P. S. Churchland 1997) accepts that that first-person data need further explanation but holds that they might be reductively explained by future neuroscience. One version of this view holds that future neuroscience could go beyond structure and dynamics in ways we cannot currently imagine. Another version holds that if we can find sufficient correlations between brain states and consciousness, that will qualify as a reductive explanation. I argue against views of this sort in chapter 5.

In this chapter I focus on constructive projects for a science of consciousness. I will sometimes presuppose the reasoning sketched earlier, but much of what I say has application even to alternative views.

---

2. *For more on this argument and on just what "structure and dynamics" comes to, see the section on type-C materialism in chapter 5.

3. Projects for a Science of Consciousness

If what I have said so far is correct, then a science of consciousness should take first-person data seriously and should proceed by studying the association between first-person data and third-person data without attempting a reduction. In fact, this is exactly what one finds in practice. The central work in the science of consciousness has always taken first-person data seriously. For example, much central work in psychophysics and perceptual psychology has been concerned with the first-person data of subjective perceptual experience. In research on unconscious perception, the first-person distinction between the presence and absence of subjective experience is crucial. In recent years, a growing body of research has focused on the correlations between first-person data about subjective experience and third-person data about brain processes and behavior.

In what follows I articulate what I see as some of the core projects for a science of consciousness, with illustrations drawn from existing research.

Project 1: Explain the Third-Person Data

One important project for a science of consciousness is that of explaining the third-person data in the vicinity: explaining the difference between functioning in sleep and wakefulness, for example, and explaining the voluntary control of behavior. This sort of project need not engage the difficult issues relating to first-person data, but it may still provide an important component of a final theory.

One example of this sort of project is that of explaining binding in terms of neural synchrony, as discussed in the last chapter. It is not yet clear whether this hypothesis is correct, but if it is correct, it will provide an important component in explaining the integration of perceptual information, which in turn is closely tied to questions about consciousness. Of course, explaining binding will not on its own explain the first-person data of consciousness, but it may help us to understand the associated processes in the brain.

Research on the "global workspace" hypothesis also falls into this class. Baars (1988) has postulated such as a workspace as a mechanism by which shared information can be made available to many different cognitive processes. More recently, other researchers (e.g., Dehaene and Changeux 2004) have investigated the potential neural basis for this mechanism and postulated a neuronal global workspace. If this hypothesis is correct, it will help to explain third-person data concerning access to information within the cognitive system, as well as data about the information made available to verbal report. Again, explaining these processes will not in itself explain the first-person data of consciousness, but it may well contribute to the project (project 4 later in this chapter) of finding neural correlates of consciousness.

Project 2: Contrast Conscious and Unconscious Processes

Many cognitive capacities can be exercised both consciously and unconsciously, that is, in the presence or absence of associated subjective experience. For example, the most familiar sort of perceptual processing is conscious, but there is also strong evidence of unconscious perceptual processing (Merikle and Daneman 2000). One finds a similar contrast in the case of memory, where the now common distinction between explicit and implicit memory (Schacter and Curran 2000) can equally be seen as a distinction between conscious and unconscious memory. *Explicit memory* is essentially memory associated with a subjective experience of the remembered information; *implicit memory* is essentially memory in the absence of such a subjective experience. The same goes for the distinction between explicit and implicit learning (Reber 1996), which is in effect a distinction between learning in the presence or absence of relevant subjective experience.

Conscious and unconscious processes provide pairs of processes that are similar in some respects from the third-person point of view (e.g., both involve registration of perceptual stimuli) but differ from the first-person point of view (one involves subjective experience of the stimulus; one does not). Of course, there are also differences from the third-person point of view. For a start, a researcher's evidence for conscious processes usually involves a verbal report of a relevant experience, and evidence for unconscious processes usually involves a verbal report of the absence of a relevant experience. There are also less obvious differences between the behavioral capacities that go along with conscious and unconscious processes, as well as between the associated neural processes. These differences make for the beginning of a link between the first-person and third-person domains.

For example, evidence suggests that, while unconscious perception of visually presented linguistic stimuli is possible, semantic processing of these stimuli seems limited to the level of the single word rather than complex expressions (see Greenwald 1992). By contrast, conscious perception allows for semantic processing of very complex expressions. Here, experimental results suggest a strong association between the presence or absence of subjective experience and the presence or absence of an associated functional capacity—a systematic link between first-person and third-person data. Many other links of the same sort can be found in the literature on unconscious perception, implicit memory, and implicit learning.

Likewise, there is evidence for distinct neural bases for conscious and unconscious processes in perception. Appealing to an extensive body of research on visuomotor processing, Milner and Goodale (1995; see also Goodale 2004) have hypothesized that the ventral stream of visual processing subserves conscious perception of visual stimuli for the purpose of the cognitive identification of stimuli, while the dorsal stream subserves unconscious processes involved in fine-grained motor capacities. If this hypothesis is correct, one can again draw a systematic link between a distinction in first-person data (presence or absence of conscious perception) and a distinction in third-person data (visual processing in the ventral or dorsal stream). A number of related proposals have been made in research on memory and learning.

Project 3: Investigate the Contents of Consciousness

Consciousness is not simply an on-off switch. Conscious experiences have a complex structure with complex contents. A conscious subject usually has a manifold of perceptual experiences, bodily sensations, emotional experiences, and conscious thoughts, among other things. Each of these elements may itself be complex. For example, a typical visual experience has an internal structure representing objects with many different colors and shapes in varying degrees of detail. We can think of all of this complexity as composing the contents of consciousness.

The contents of consciousness have been studied throughout the history of psychology. Weber's and Fechner's pioneering work in psychophysics concentrated on specific aspects of these contents, such as the subjective brightness associated with a visual experience, and correlated it with properties of the associated stimulus. This provided a basic link between first-person data about sensory experience and third-person data about external stimuli. Later work in psychophysics and gestalt psychology took an approach of the same general sort, investigating specific features of perceptual experience and analyzing how these covary with the properties of a stimulus.

This tradition continues in a significant body of contemporary research. For example, research on visual illusions often uses subjects' first-person reports (and even scientists' first-person experiences) to characterize the structure of perceptual experiences. Research on attention (Mack and Rock 1998; Treisman 2003) aims to characterize the structure of perceptual experience inside and outside the focus of attention. Other researchers investigate the contents of consciousness in the domains of mental imagery (Baars

1996), emotional experience (Kaszniak 1998), and stream of conscious thought (Pope 1978; Hurlburt 1990).

An important line of research investigates the contents of consciousness in abnormal subjects. For example, subjects with synesthesia have unusually rich sensory experiences. In a common version, letters and numbers trigger reports of extra color experiences, in addition to the standard perceived color of the stimulus. Recent research strongly suggests that these reports reflect the subjects' perceptual experiences and not just cognitive associations. For example, Ramachandran and Hubbard (2001) find that certain visual patterns produce a perceptual "pop-out" effect in synesthetic subjects that is not present in normal subjects. When first-person data about the experiences of abnormal subjects are combined with third-person data about brain abnormalities in those subjects, this yields a new source of information about the association between brain and conscious experience.

Project 4: Find the Neural Correlates of Consciousness

This leads us to what is perhaps the core project of current scientific research on consciousness: the search for neural correlates of consciousness (Metzinger 2000; Crick and Koch 2004). A neural correlate of consciousness (NCC) can be characterized as a minimal neural system that is directly associated with states of consciousness (see chapter 3 for much more on this). Presumably the brain as a whole is a neural system associated with states of consciousness, but not every part of the brain is associated equally with consciousness. The NCC project aims to isolate relatively limited parts of the brain (or relatively specific features of neural processing) that correlate directly with subjective experience.

It may be that there will be many different NCCs for different aspects of conscious experience. For example, it might be that one neural system is associated with being conscious as opposed to being unconscious (perhaps in the thalamus or brainstem; see e.g., Schiff 2004), while another neural system is associated with the specific contents of visual consciousness (perhaps in some part of the visual cortex), and other systems are associated with the contents of consciousness in different modalities. Any such proposal can be seen as articulating a link between third-person data on brain processes and first-person data on subjective experience.

In recent years, by far the greatest progress has been made in the study of NCCs for visual consciousness. Milner and Goodale's (1995) work on the ventral stream provides an example of this sort of research. Another example is the research of Nikos Logothetis and colleagues on binocular rivalry in monkeys (e.g., Logothetis 1998; Leopold, Maier, and Logothetis 2003). When different stimuli are presented to the left and the right eyes, subjects usually undergo alternating subjective experiences. Logothetis trained monkeys to signal such changes in their visual experience and correlated these changes with changes in underlying neural processes. The results indicate that changes in visual experience are only weakly correlated with changes in patterns of neural firing in the primary visual cortex: in this area, neural firing was more strongly correlated with the stimulus than with the experience. In contrast, changes in visual experience were strongly correlated with changes in patterns of neural firing in later visual areas, such as the inferior temporal cortex. These results tend to suggest that the inferior temporal cortex is a better candidate than the primary visual cortex as an NCC for visual consciousness.

Of course, no single experimental result can provide conclusive evidence concerning the location of an NCC, but much evidence concerning the location of NCCs for vision has accumulated in the last few years (Koch 2004), and one can expect much more to come. If successful, this project will provide some highly specific connections between brain processes and conscious experiences.

Project 5: Systematize the Connection

To date, links between first-person data and third-person data have been studied in a somewhat piecemeal fashion. Researchers isolate correlations between specific aspects of subjective experience and specific brain processes or behavioral capacities in a relatively unsystematic way. This is to be expected at the current stage of development. We can hope that as the science develops, however, more systematic links will be forthcoming. In particular, we can hope to develop principles of increasing generality that link a wide range of first-person data with a correspondingly wide range of third-person data. For example, there might eventually be an account of the neural correlates of visual consciousness that will not only tell us which neural systems are associated with visual consciousness but will also yield systematic principles that tell us how the specific content of a visual experience covaries with the character of neural processes in these systems.

A few principles of this sort have been suggested to date in limited domains. For example, Hobson (1997) has suggested a general principle linking certain levels of neurochemical activity with different states of consciousness in wakefulness, sleep, and dreaming. It is likely than any such proposals will be heavily revised as new evidence comes in, but one can expect that in the coming decades increasingly well-supported principles of this sort will emerge. The possibility of such principles holds out the tantalizing prospect that eventually we might use them to predict features of an organism's subjective experience based on knowledge of its neurophysiology.

Project 6: Infer Fundamental Principles

If the previous project succeeds, we will have general principles that connect third-person data and first-person data, but these general principles will not yet be fundamental. The principles might still be quite complex, and limited both to specific aspects of consciousness and to specific species. A science of consciousness consisting of wholly different principles for different aspects of consciousness and different species would not be entirely satisfactory. It is reasonable to hope that eventually some unity will be discovered behind this diversity. We should at least aim to maximize the generality and the simplicity of the relevant principles wherever possible. In the ideal situation, we might hope for principles that are maximally general in their scope, applying to any conscious system whatsoever and to all aspects of conscious experience. In addition, we might hope for principles that are relatively simple in their form in the way that the basic laws of physics appear to be simple.

It is unreasonable to expect that we will discover principles of this sort anytime soon, and it is an open question whether we will be able to discover them at all. Currently, we have little idea what form such principles might take (notwithstanding the speculation at the end of chapter 1). Still, if we can discover them, principles of this sort would be candidates for fundamental principles: the building blocks of a fundamental theory of consciousness. If what I said earlier is correct, then something about the connection between first-person data and third-person data must be taken as primitive, just as we take fundamental principles in physical theories as primitive. But we can at least hope that the primitive element in our theories will be as simple and as general as possible. If, eventually, we can formulate simple and general principles of this sort, based on an inference from accumulated first-person and third-person data, we could be said to have an adequate scientific theory of consciousness.

What would this entail about the relationship between physical processes and consciousness? The existence of such principles is compatible with different philosophical views. One might regard the principles as laws that connect two fundamentally different domains. One might regard them as laws that connect two aspects of the same thing. Or one might regard them as grounding an identification between properties of consciousness and physical properties. Such principles could also be combined with different views of the causal relation between physical processes and consciousness. These matters are all discussed further in chapter 5, but for many purposes, the science of consciousness can remain neutral on these philosophical questions. One can simply regard the principles as principles of correlation while staying neutral on their underlying causal and ontological status. This makes it possible to have a robust science of consciousness even without having a widely accepted solution to the philosophical mind/body problem.

4. Obstacles to a Science of Consciousness

The development of a science of consciousness as I have presented it thus far may sound remarkably straightforward. We simultaneously gather first-person data about subjective experience and third-person data about behavior and brain processes, isolate specific correlations between them, formulate general principles governing these correlations, and infer the underlying fundamental laws. But of course it is not as simple as this in practice. There are a number of serious obstacles to this research agenda. The most serious obstacles concern the availability of the relevant data in both the third-person and first-person domains. In what follows I discuss a few of these obstacles.

Obstacles Involving Third-Person Data

The third-person data relevant to the science of consciousness include both behavioral and neural data. The availability of behavioral data is reasonably straightforward: one is constrained only by the ingenuity of the experimenter and the limitations of experimental contexts. In practice, researchers have accumulated a rich body of behavioral data relevant to consciousness. In contrast, the availability of neural data is much more constrained by technological and ethical limitations, and the body of neural data that has been accumulated to date is correspondingly much more limited.

In practice, the most relevant neurophysiological data come from two or three sources: brain imaging via functional magnetic resonance imaging (fMRI) and positron emission tomography (PET) technology, single-cell recording through insertion of electrodes, and surface recording through electroencephalographs (EEG) and magnetoencephalography (MEG).

Each of these technologies is useful, but each has serious limitations for the science of consciousness. Both EEG and MEG have well-known limitations in spatial localization. Brain imaging through fMRI and PET is better in this regard, but these methods are still spatially quite coarse grained. Single-cell recording is spatially fine grained but is largely limited to experimentation on nonhuman animals.

These limitations apply to all areas of cognitive neuroscience, but they are particularly pressing for the science of consciousness because the science of consciousness relies on gathering third-person and first-person data simultaneously. By far the most straightforward method for gathering first-person data is verbal report, but verbal report is limited to human subjects. By far the most useful third-person data are data at the level of single neurons, where one can monitor representational content that correlates with the content of consciousness (e.g., when one monitors a neuron with a specific receptive field, as discussed in chapter 3), but these experiments are largely limited to nonhuman subjects. As a result, it is extremely difficult to discover strong associations between first-person data and corresponding neural data with current techniques.

There have been numerous ingenious attempts to circumvent these limitations. The best known include Logothetis's experiments on monkeys, in which the animals are trained extensively to provide a substitute for a verbal report of visual consciousness by pressing a bar. Research on blindsight in monkeys by Cowey and Stoerig (1995) has done something similar. Still, the very fact that researchers have to go to such great lengths in order to gather relevant neural data illustrates the problem. Others have performed neuron-level measurements on human surgical patients (e.g., Kreiman, Fried, and Koch 2002), but there are obvious practical limitations here. Many others (e.g., Rees 2004) have tried to get as much relevant information as they can from the limited resources of brain imaging and surface recording; nevertheless, fewer deep correlations have emerged from this sort of work than from neuron-level studies.

One can hope that this is a temporary limitation imposed by current technology. If a technology is eventually developed that allows for noninvasive monitoring of neuron-level processes in human subjects, we might expect a golden age for the science of consciousness to follow.

Obstacles Involving First-Person Data

Where the availability of first-person data is concerned, a number of related obstacles run quite deep. I discuss three of these here.

1. Privacy

The most obvious obstacle to the gathering of first-person data concerns the privacy of such data. In most areas of science, data are intersubjectively available: they are equally accessible to a wide range of observers. But in the case of consciousness, first-person data concerning subjective experiences are directly available only to the subject having those experiences. To others, these first-person data are only indirectly available, mediated by observation of the subject's behavior or brain processes. Things would be straightforward if we had a "consciousness meter" (discussed in the next chapter) that could be pointed at a subject and reveal his or her subjective experiences to all. But in the absence of a theory of consciousness, no such consciousness meter is available. This imposes a deep limitation on the science of consciousness, but it is not a paralyzing limitation. For a start, subjects have direct access to first-person data concerning their own conscious experiences. We could imagine that Robinson Crusoe on a desert island, equipped with the latest brain-imaging technology, could make considerable progress toward a science of consciousness by combining this technology with first-person observation. More practically, each of us has indirect access to first-person data concerning others' experiences by relying on behavioral indicators of these data.

In practice, by far the most common way of gathering data on the conscious experiences of other subjects is to rely on their verbal reports. Here, one does not treat the verbal reports just as third-person data (as a behaviorist might, limiting the datum to the fact that a subject made a certain noise). Rather, one treats the report as a report of first-person data that are available to the subject. Just as a scientist can accumulate third-person data by accepting reports of third-person data gathered by others (rather than simply treating those reports as noises), a scientist can also gather first-person data by accepting reports of first-person data gathered by others. This is the typical attitude that researchers adopt toward experimental subjects. If there is positive reason to believe that a subject's report might be unreliable, a researcher will suspend judgment about it. But in the absence of any such reason, researchers will take a subject's report of a conscious experience as good reason to believe that the subject is having a conscious experience of the sort that the subject is reporting.

In this way, researchers have access to a rich trove of first-person data that is made intersubjectively available. Of course, our access to these data depends on our making certain assumptions: in particular, the assumption that other subjects really are having conscious experiences and that by and large their verbal reports reflect these conscious experiences. We cannot directly test this assumption; instead, it serves as a sort of background

assumption for research in the field. But this situation is present throughout other areas of science. When physicists use perception to gather information about the external world, for example, they rely on the assumption
that the external world exists and that perception reflects the state of the
external world. They cannot directly test this assumption; instead, it serves
as a sort of background assumption for the whole field. Still, it seems a
reasonable assumption to make, and it makes the science of physics possible. The same goes for our assumptions about the conscious experiences
and verbal reports of others. These seem to be reasonable assumptions to
make, and they make the science of consciousness possible.

Of course, verbal reports have some limits. Some aspects of conscious
experience (e.g., the experience of music or of emotion) are very difficult
to describe; in these cases we may need to develop a more refined language.
What is more, verbal reports cannot be used at all in subjects without language, such as infants and nonhuman animals. In these cases, one needs
to rely on other behavioral indicators, as when Logothetis relies on a
monkey's bar pressing. These indicators require further assumptions. For
example, Logothetis's work requires both the assumption that monkeys are
conscious and the assumption that visual stimuli that the monkey can
exploit in the voluntary control of behavior are consciously perceived.

These assumptions appear reasonable to most people, but they go beyond
those required in the case of verbal report. The farther we move away from
the human case, the more questionable the required assumptions become.
For example, it would be very difficult to draw conclusions about consciousness from experiments on insects. Still, verbal reports in humans,
combined with behavioral indicators in primates, give researchers enough
access to first-person data to enable a serious body of ongoing research.

2. Methodology

A second obstacle is posed by the fact that our methods for gathering first-
person data are quite primitive compared with our methods for gathering
third-person data. The latter have been refined by years of scientific practice, but the former have not received nearly as much attention. Where
simple first-person data are concerned, this problem is not too pressing.
There is usually no great difficulty in determining whether one is having an
experience of a certain color in the center of one's visual field, for example.
Where more subtle aspects of subjective experience are concerned, however, the obstacle arises quickly.

Even with a phenomenon as tangible as visual experience, the issue arises
in a number of ways. Visual experiences as a whole usually have a rich and

detailed structure, for example, but how can subjects investigate and characterize that detail? Most subjects have great difficulty in introspecting and reporting this detail more than superficially. Particular difficulties arise in investigating the character of consciousness outside attention. To introspect and report this structure would seem to require attending to the relevant sort of experience, which may well change the character of the experience.

Here we can expect that at least some progress can be made by developing better methods for the gathering of first-person data. It may be reasonable to pay attention to traditions where the study of experience has been explored in detail. These traditions include those of Western phenomenology, introspectionist psychology, and even Eastern meditative traditions. Even if one is skeptical of the theories put forward by proponents of these traditions, one might still benefit from attending to their data-gathering methods. This research strategy has been pursued most notably in the "neurophenomenology" of Francisco Varela and colleagues (Varela 1997; Lutz et al. 2002), in which neurophysiological investigation is combined with phenomenological investigation in the tradition of Husserl. A number of other attempts at refining first-person methods are discussed in the papers collected in Varela and Shear (2001).

Of course, any method has limitations. Subjects' judgments about their subjective experiences are not infallible, and although training may help, it also introduces the danger that observations may be corrupted by theory. The introspectionist program of experimental psychology in the nineteenth century famously fell apart when different schools could not agree on the introspective data (Boring 1929). Still, our ambitions need not be as grand as those of the introspectionists. For now, we are not aiming for a perfect characterization of the structure of consciousness but simply for a better characterization. Furthermore, we are now in a position where we can use third-person data as a check on first-person investigation. Experimental investigation has helped us to distinguish circumstances in which first-person reports are unreliable from those in which they are more reliable (Schooler and Fiore 1997), and there is room for much more investigation of this sort in the future. So it is reasonable to hope that at least a modest refinement of our methods for the reliable investigation of first-person data will be possible.

3. Formalisms

A final obstacle is posed by the absence of general formalisms with which first-person data can be expressed. Formalisms are important for two purposes. First, they are needed for data gathering: it is not enough to simply know what one is experiencing; one also has to write it down. Second, they are needed for theory construction: to formulate principles that connect first-person data with third-person data, we need to represent the data in a way that such principles can exploit.

The main existing formalisms for representing first-person data are quite primitive. Researchers typically rely either on simple qualitative characterizations of data (as in "an experience of red in the center of the visual field") or on simple parameterization of data (as when color experiences are parameterized by hue, saturation, and brightness). These simple formalisms suffice for some purposes, but they are unlikely to suffice for the formulation of systematic theories.

It is not at all clear what form a proper formalism for the expression of first-person data about consciousness should take. The candidates include (1) parametric formalisms, in which various specific features of conscious experience are isolated and parameterized (as in the case of color experience); (2) geometric and topological formalisms, in which the overall structure of an experience (such as a visual experience) is formalized in geometric or topological terms; (3) informational formalisms, in which one characterizes the informational structure of an experience, specifying it as a sort of pixel-by-pixel state that falls into a larger space of informational states; and (4) representational formalisms, in which one characterizes an experience by using language for the states of the world that the experience represents (one might characterize an experience as an experience as of a yellow cup, for example). While each of these formalisms may have limitations, a detailed study of various alternative formalisms is likely to have significant benefits.

5. Conclusion

Overall, the prospects for a science of consciousness are reasonably bright. There are numerous clear projects for a science of consciousness that take first-person data seriously. One can recognize the distinctive problems that consciousness poses and still do science. Of course, there are many obstacles, and it is an open question how far we can progress. But the last ten years have seen many advances, and the next fifty years will see many more. For now, it is reasonable to hope that we may eventually have a theory of the fundamental principles that connect physical processes to conscious experience.

Afterword: First-Person Data and First-Person Science

The very idea of first-person data and of first-person methods in science makes some philosophers and scientists queasy. A common reaction is to say that first-person data are private, and science is public, so first-person data cannot be part of science.[3] Now, demarcation disputes over what counts as "science" are usually verbal and sterile. What matters is whether we have good reasons to accept certain conclusions, not whether those reasons count as scientific reasons. Still, it is worth noting that first-person data are private only in a very limited sense, one that is compatible with the most important elements of the publicity of science.

The sense in which first-person data are private is that a given datum that concerns the experience of a given subject is *directly* accessible only to one person—that subject. Still, that datum will be indirectly accessible to many others, for example when it is expressed through verbal report: "I experienced a small cross inside a large circle." So first-person data are certainly communicable in the way that scientific data are required to be.

One might worry that, for scientific purposes, an individual datum should be jointly observable by many parties, but this requirement is largely irrelevant to the ordinary practice of science. One does not standardly require five scientists to crowd around the same oscilloscope. Rather, what matters for publicity is that data be replicable. If someone reports a datum, from observing an oscilloscope or an animal for example, we expect that others will be able to observe other data of the same sort, using their own oscilloscopes or looking at different animals of the same species. That is publicity enough for the purposes of science.

First-person data can straightforwardly have this sort of publicity. Experiments on consciousness typically have many subjects reporting data of the same sort. In many cases, scientists can replicate the first-person data in their own case by direct observation. Indeed, this is standard practice in the field of psychophysics. To be convinced of the reality of a putative illusion, for example, scientists just need to experience it for themselves. Even when this sort of direct validation is not possible (say, because the data pertain to a group to which the scientist does not belong), it is usually straightforward to cross-validate observations with reports from many subjects. As in any science, occasional one-off observations involve unique or hard-to-replicate conditions. In these cases, as in any science, the putative observation need not be ignored, but one will be more cautious about its use. So first-person data appear to be quite compatible with scientific methods.

Of course, there are cases in which the privacy of first-person data poses a much more serious obstacle. In many cases involving infants, machines, and nonhuman animals, any first-person data cannot easily be communicated to

3. *See, for example, Piccinini (2009), who says that my view of first-person data involves an unacceptable "privatism", and who recommends instead a view on which first-person data are public records of mental states.

others. Because of this, theorists cannot be said to have access to these data. This situation is akin to the situation in the historical sciences (such as evolutionary biology), in which there were data accessible in the past to which current scientists do not have access. This means that the availability of data is limited, making the science more difficult. Still, in all of these cases, we have access to enough data (data concerning the present, in the historical case; data concerning human experience, in the case of consciousness) that one can build a reasonably robust science all the same.

Daniel Dennett responds to the ideas in an early version of this chapter (and to related claims by Alvin Goldman) in an article called "The Fantasy of First-person Science" (2001). Where Goldman and I think a science of consciousness needs to explain both third-person and first-person data, Dennett thinks that explaining the third-person data is enough: once we have explained these—including verbal reports—we have explained everything. This is Dennett's method of "heterophenomenology." A key idea is that taking verbal reports to be the explananda turns apparently irreducible first-person data into straightforwardly explicable third-person data.

The obvious objection to Dennett's method is that the science of consciousness is not primarily about verbal reports or even about introspective judgments. It is about the experiences that the reports and judgments are reports and judgments of. Explaining our reports and judgments may be useful for many purposes, but to explain our reports and judgments is not to explain experience.

Dennett's central argument for heterophenomenology proceeds by making a case that heterophenomenology is guaranteed to be at least as good a guide to first-person data as first-person phenomenology. In cases where reports about consciousness go wrong, introspection will also go wrong, so heterophenomenology misses nothing that first-person phenomenology covers. This way of proceeding mislocates the debate, however. The central problem with heterophenomenology has nothing to do with the fallibility of reports. Even if reports were infallible, the same problem would arise: to explain reports is not to explain the experiences that the reports are reports of.

Dennett says that my view requires a nonneutral attitude toward a subject's reports, taking them uncritically as a guide to their subject matter. And he says that scientists have to take a neutral attitude (taking reports themselves as data but making no claims about their truth) because reports can go wrong. But this misses the natural intermediate option that Max Velmans (2007) has called *critical phenomenology*: accept verbal reports as a prima facie guide to a subject's conscious experience except where there are specific reasons to doubt their reliability.

Critical phenomenology seems to capture most scientists' attitudes toward verbal reports and consciousness. The attitude is not "uncritical acceptance," but it is also far from the "neutrality" of heterophenomenology. On this view, we do not treat reports merely as data to be explained in their own right (though we might regard them in this way for some purposes). Rather, we are interested in them as a (fallible) guide to the first-person data about consciousness that we really want to explain. This way of thinking about the phenomena accommodates a major role for reports while preserving the distinction between explaining the reports (and third-person data in general) and explaining the experiences (first-person data) that they are reports of.

The issue is clouded just a little by Dennett's occasional blurring of the line between heterophenomenology and critical phenomenology. At one point in his reply to Goldman, he appears to allow that researchers on blindsight can give prima facie credence to subjects' claims that they have no experience in a given area as long as they do not give the subjects infallible authority. Clearly, to adopt this attitude would be to give up on the strict "neutrality" of heterophenomenology and to move beyond treating verbal reports and introspective judgments as mere third-person data. But I think Dennett's attitude is best captured by the suggestion that researchers are analogous to anthropologists listening to subjects' folk tales: they play along to obtain the subject's judgments without ever accepting them, unless those judgments are later validated by an independent investigation.

It is clear that this anthropological attitude is not the attitude of most researchers toward blindsight subjects. Even in the absence of a good theory of blindsight, the results are generally taken to be very strong (although not infallible) evidence for a conclusion concerning visual experience. The conclusion is not just that the subjects *judge* that they do not visually experience objects in a part of their visual field; it is that subjects do not visually experience objects in a part of their visual field. Likewise, in psychophysics, experiments are usually taken to be strong evidence not just that subjects judge that they visually experience a certain illusion but also that they visually experience a certain illusion. Dennett may be right that the anthropological attitude is the typical attitude of researchers toward subjects' reports about their cognitive *mechanisms*: about whether they rotated a mental image using mechanisms of symbolic representations or analog imagery, for example. But when it comes to reports about experience, by far the most common attitude is nonneutral. Reports are given prima facie credence as a guide to conscious experience.

Another relevant illustration is provided by the debate about unconscious perception among cognitive psychologists. A central part of this debate has concerned precisely which third-person measures (direct report, discrimination, etc.) are the best guide to the presence and absence of conscious perception. Here, third-person data are being used as a (fallible) guide to first-person data about consciousness, which are of primary interest. Given the heterophenomenological view, this debate is without much content: some states subserve report, some subserve discrimination, and that is about all there is to say. I think that something like this is Dennett's attitude toward those debates, but it is not the attitude of most of the scientists working in the field.

Dennett makes something of the fact that his method appeals to a subject's beliefs rather than just to reports, but the same issues arise. On Dennett's account of beliefs, to believe that such-and-such is roughly to be disposed to report that such-and-such and to behave in appropriate ways, and to explain such beliefs is in large part to explain the associated dispositions. If one takes this view of beliefs, everything I have said earlier applies to beliefs, as well as to reports: explaining the beliefs does not suffice to explain the experiences. If one does not take this view, it is no longer obvious that third-person methods can explain our specific beliefs about consciousness, as these beliefs may themselves have a phenomenal element: see chapter 9 for much more on this.

Dennett "challenges" me to name an experiment that "transcends" the heterophenomenological method, but of course both views can accommodate experiments equally. For any experiment in which I say that we are using a verbal report or an introspective judgment as a guide to first-person data, Dennett can say that we are using it as third-person data and vice versa. So the difference between the views does not lie in the range of experiments "compatible" with them. Rather, it lies in a philosophical difference concerning the way that experimental results are interpreted: should verbal reports be seen as reports of data about the subject's experience or just as data points to be explained in their own right?

In any case, the fundamental reasons for rejecting the heterophenomenological view lie prior to these questions about experiments. The fundamental question is, does explaining behavior and other third-person data suffice on its own to explain conscious experience? I think there are overwhelming grounds to say no (as argued in the previous chapter and in the response to Dennett there). The question is then, given that this is so, can there be a science of consciousness anyway? The answer provided by this chapter is yes, as long as we accept that science can deal with first-person data and as long as we allow that verbal reports and the like can be used as an indirect guide to the first-person data about consciousness.

Given this basic orientation, we can see the role of verbal reports in the science of consciousness as analogous to the role of perceptual experiences and perceptual judgments in ordinary third-person science. Roughly speaking, verbal reports stand to others' experiences as our own perceptual experiences stand to the external world. Suppose a physicist sees an object in a certain location and judges it to be in that location. One *could* take the "anthropological" view that the datum to be explained here is always just the perceptual experience or the perceptual judgment. Then one's science would be a science of explaining experiences and judgments, and the external-world hypothesis would be one hypothesis among many that are competing with various skeptical hypotheses to explain the data. Alternatively, one could take the attitude that the datum to be explained here is that the object is in the location. Then skeptical hypotheses will not really be on the table when doing the science, and instead the competition will be among different physical hypotheses for explaining the external datum.

Whatever the merits of the two views, the second corresponds to the way that science is usually practiced. On this view, perceptual states themselves do not exhaust the data. Rather, the states of affairs that they report (or represent) are taken as data. It is not unquestioned that perception is accurate. If there are conflicts among the apparent data or specific reasons to believe that perception may be unreliable, then one might retreat to taking the experiences and judgments as data in a given case and look for alternative explanations. But in the absence of positive reasons to question these data, one takes for granted that perception functions as a guide to the external world. Doing this enables science to proceed, even in the absence of decisive rejoinders to skeptical worries about the external world.

Likewise, in the science of consciousness, verbal reports do not exhaust the data. Rather, the states of affairs that they report are taken as data. It is not unquestioned that introspection is accurate. If there are conflicts among the apparent data or specific reasons to believe that introspection may be unreliable, then one might retreat to taking the reports and judgments as data in a given case and look for alternative explanations. But in the absence of positive reasons to question these data, one takes for granted that introspection and report function as a guide to consciousness. Doing this enables the science of consciousness to proceed, even in the absence of decisive rejoinders to skeptical worries about other minds.

One might say that just as a certain degree of trust in perception is a precondition for the science of physics, a certain degree of trust in introspection is a precondition for the science of consciousness. Of course, in both cases one would also like to have some reason to believe that this trust is reasonable, over and above the pragmatic justification that the science does not work as well without it. Here we enter familiar philosophical territory. For example, one might try to discredit skeptical hypotheses concerning the external world on the grounds that they are more complex than alternative explanations, or in some other way (see chapter 13 for my own take on this issue), and one might try to discredit skeptical hypotheses concerning other minds in analogous ways (I think that the best justification here may come from abduction from regularities observed in one's own case). Such philosophical justifications for ordinary practices are almost invariably partial and questionable. Still, the science seems to go on successfully all the same.

From this perspective, the most worrying obstacle for the science of consciousness comes from specific reasons to doubt the accuracy of introspection even in one's own case. It is well known that the introspective approach to psychology a century ago collapsed in part because of disagreement about the putative data: most famously, some theorists discerned an experience of imageless thought where others did not. A number of disagreements of this sort can still be found among scientists and philosophers today, and there is good reason to believe that introspection is very far from infallible. Schwitzgebel (2008), among others, has used considerations of this sort to cast doubt on the possibility of a science of consciousness.

Still, we can distinguish hard cases from easy cases. Just as we can isolate conditions under which we have specific reason not to trust perception, we can also isolate conditions under which we have specific reason not to trust introspection. There are good reasons for worrying about introspection of nonsensory experience, of consciousness outside attention, and so on, but these reasons do not obviously extend to core sensory experiences within the focus of attention. When a normal subject claims to experience a vivid red square, for example, there is usually little reason to disbelieve the subject. And it is experiences of this sort that are the bread and butter of the current science of consciousness. So for now, the science of consciousness is making considerable progress by focusing largely on these easy cases, and there is reason to believe that there will be much more progress ahead. Progress of that sort could well yield the core of a fruitful theory of consciousness. Eventually the science of consciousness will have to say something about the hard cases, too. New methods might well be required then, and it is difficult to know how far things will go. But in the meantime, one can predict that the science of consciousness will continue to thrive.

3

WHAT IS A NEURAL CORRELATE OF CONSCIOUSNESS?

1. Introduction

In this chapter and the next I discuss the role that neuroscience plays in the search for a theory of consciousness. Even if neuroscience cannot solve all of the problems of consciousness singlehandedly, it unquestionably has a major role to play. Recent years have seen striking progress in neurobiological research bearing on the problems of consciousness. The conceptual foundations of this sort of research, however, are only beginning to be laid. In these chapters I look at some of the things that are going on, from a philosopher's perspective, and try to say something helpful about these foundations.

The cornerstone of recent work in the neuroscience of consciousness has been the search for the "neural correlate of consciousness." This phrase is intended to refer to the neural system or systems primarily associated with conscious experience. The associated acronym is NCC. The hypothesis is that all of us have an NCC inside our head. The project is to find out what the NCC is. In recent years there have been quite a few proposals about the identity of the NCC. One of the most famous ones is Crick and Koch's 1990 suggestion that the neural basis of consciousness involves 40-hertz neural oscillations. That proposal has lost some favor since then, but many other suggestions have surfaced. The picture is almost reminiscent of particle physics, which now involves so many different sorts of particles that people talk about the "particle zoo." In studying consciousness, one might talk about the "neural correlate zoo."

Here are a few proposals that have been put forward:[1]

- 40-hertz oscillations in the cerebral cortex (Crick and Koch 1990)
- intralaminar nuclei in the thalamus (Bogen 1995a)
- reentrant loops in thalamocortical systems (Edelman 1989)
- 40-hertz rhythmic activity in thalamocortical systems (Llinas et al. 1994)
- extended reticular-thalamic activation system (Newman 1997)
- neural assemblies bound by NMDA (Flohr 1995)
- certain neurochemical levels of activation (Hobson 1997)
- certain neurons in the inferior temporal cortex (Sheinberg and Logothetis 1997)
- neurons in the extrastriate visual cortex projecting to prefrontal areas (Crick and Koch 1995)
- visual processing within the ventral stream (Milner and Goodale 1995)

This work raises a number of difficult conceptual and foundational issues. I can see at least five foundational questions in the vicinity:

1. What do we mean by "consciousness"?
2. What do we mean by "neural correlate of consciousness"?
3. How can we find the neural correlate(s) of consciousness?
4. What will a neural correlate of consciousness explain?
5. Is consciousness reducible to its neural correlate(s)?

The first two questions here are conceptual questions, the third is an epistemological or methodological question, the fourth is an explanatory question, and the fifth is an ontological question. The first, fourth, and fifth are versions of general questions that philosophers have discussed for a long time, and I give my own view on them elsewhere in this book. The second and third questions are more specific to the NCC investigation. I focus on the second question in this chapter and on the third question in the following chapter.

What does it mean to be a neural correlate of consciousness? At first glance, the answer might seem to be so obvious that the question is hardly worth asking. An NCC is just a neural state that directly correlates with a

---

1. *Some more recent proposals concerning the neural correlates of consciousness include those by Block (2006b), Dehaene and Changeux (2004), Lamme (2006), and Zeki (2007). Koch (2004) and Kouider (2009) provide useful reviews, as do older works by Crick and Koch (1998) and Milner (1995). Bayne, Cleeremans, and Wilken (2009), Dehaene (2001), Metzinger (2000), and Velmans and Schneider (2007) are excellent collections of relevant material.

conscious state or that directly generates consciousness or something like that. One might have a simple image: when your NCC is active, your consciousness turns on correspondingly. But a moment's reflection suggests that this idea is not completely straightforward and that the concept needs some clarification.

Here I undertake a little conceptual spadework in clarifying the concept of an NCC. This may not be the deepest problem in the area, but if we are looking for an NCC, it makes sense to get clear on what we are looking for. On the way I touch on some of the empirical work in the area and see what concept of NCC is at play in some of the central research. I also draw some consequences for the methodology of empirical work in the search. Most of this is intended as a first step rather than a last word. Much of what I say will need to be refined, but I hope at least to draw attention to some interesting issues in the vicinity.

2. States of consciousness

As a first pass, we can use the definition of a neural correlate of consciousness given in the program of the 1998 conference of the Association for the Scientific Study of Consciousness on "Neural Correlates of Consciousness" (where this chapter was first presented). This definition says that a neural correlate of consciousness is a "specific system in the brain whose activity correlates directly with states of conscious experience." This yields something like the following:

A neural system N is an NCC if the state of N correlates directly with states of consciousness.

There are at least two things to get clear on here. First, what are the relevant "states of consciousness"? Second, what does it mean for a neural state to "correlate directly" with states of consciousness? I look into both of these things in turn.

The states of consciousness we are concerned with here are all states of subjective experience, or equivalently, states of phenomenal consciousness. But what *sorts* of states of consciousness are relevant? In the NCC literature I can see a few different classes of states that are sometimes considered.

(i) Being Conscious

The first option is that the states in question are just those of being conscious and of not being conscious. The corresponding notion of an NCC will be that of a neural system whose state directly correlates with whether a subject is conscious or not. If the NCC is in a particular state, the subject will be conscious. If the NCC is not in that state, the subject will not be conscious.

This is perhaps the idea that first comes to mind when we think about an NCC. We might think about it as the "neural correlate of creature consciousness," where creature consciousness is the property a creature has when it is conscious and lacks when it is not conscious.

Although this is an interesting notion, it does not seem to capture the sort of NCC that most work in the area is aimed at. As we will see, most of the current work is aimed at something more specific. Some ideas can be taken as aiming at least in part at this notion, though. For example, Bogen's (1995a) ideas about the intralaminar nucleus seem to be directed at least in part at this sort of NCC.

Examining current work, we find that insofar as there is any consensus at all about the location of this sort of NCC, the dominant view seems to be that it should be in or around the thalamus or at least that it should involve interactions between the thalamic and cortical systems in a central role. Penfield (1937) argued that "the indispensable substratum of consciousness" lies outside the cerebral cortex and probably lies in the diencephalon (thalamus, hypothalamus, subthalamus, epithalamus). This theme has been taken up in recent years by Bogen, Newman, and Baars (1993) and others.

(ii) Background State of Consciousness

A related idea is that of the neural correlate of what we might call the *background state* of consciousness. A background state is an overall state of consciousness such as being awake, being asleep, dreaming, or being under hypnosis. Exactly what counts as a background state is not entirely clear, as one can divide things up in a number of ways and with coarser or finer grains, but presumably the class will include a range of normal and of "altered" states.

We can think of this as a slightly more fine-grained version of the previous idea. Creature consciousness is the most coarse-grained background state of consciousness: it is just the state of being conscious. Background states will usually be more fine-grained than this, but they still will not be defined in terms of specific contents or modalities.

A neural correlate of the background state of consciousness, then, will be a neural system N such that the state of N directly correlates with whether a subject is awake, dreaming, under hypnosis, and so on. If N is in state 1, the subject is awake; if N is in state 2, the subject is dreaming; if N is in state 3, the subject is under hypnosis; and so on.

It may well be that some of the thalamocortical proposals discussed earlier are intended as or might be extended into proposals concerning this sort of NCC. A more direct example is given by Hobson's (1997) ideas about neurochemical levels of activation. Hobson holds that these levels can be grouped into a three-dimensional state space and that different regions in this space correspond to different overall states of consciousness: wakefulness, REM sleep, non-REM sleep, and so on. When chemical levels are in a particular region in this space, the subject will be awake; when in another region, the subject will be in REM sleep; and so on. On this reading, one might see the neurochemical system as an NCC of the sort characterized earlier, with the different regions in state space corresponding to correlates of the various specific background states.

(iii) Contents of Consciousness

There is much more to consciousness than the mere state of being conscious or the background state of consciousness. Arguably the most interesting states of consciousness are *specific* ones: the fine-grained states of subjective experience that one is in at any given time. These might include the experience of a particular visual image, of a particular sound pattern, of a detailed stream of conscious thought, and so on. A detailed visual experience, for example, might include the experience of certain shapes and colors in one's environment, of specific arrangements of objects, of various relative distances and depths, and so on.

Specific states like these are most often individuated by their *content*. Most conscious states seem to have some sort of specific representational content that represents the world as being one way or another. Much of the specific nature of a visual experience, for example, can be characterized in terms of content. A visual experience typically represents the world as containing various shapes and colors, as containing certain objects standing in certain spatial relations, and so on. If the experience is veridical, the world will be the way the experience represents it as being. If the experience is an illusion or is otherwise misleading, the world will be other than the experience represents it as being. Either way, however, it seems that visual experiences typically have detailed representational content. The same goes for experiences in other sensory modalities and arguably for many or most nonsensory experiences as well.

Much of the most interesting work on NCCs is concerned with states like these. This is work on the neural correlates of the contents of consciousness. Much of the work on the neural correlates of visual consciousness has this character, for example. This work is not concerned merely with the neural states that determine that one *has* visual consciousness; it is concerned with the neural states that determine the specific contents of visual consciousness.

A nice example is supplied by the work of Logothetis and colleagues on the NCC of visual consciousness in monkeys (Logothetis and Schall 1989; Leopold and Logothetis 1996; Sheinberg and Logothetis 1997). In this work (discussed briefly in chapter 2), a monkey is trained to press various bars when it is confronted with various sorts of images: horizontal and vertical gratings, for example, or gratings drifting left and right, or faces and sunbursts. Let us use horizontal and vertical gratings for the purposes of illustration. After training is complete, the monkey is presented with two stimuli at once, one to each eye. In humans, this usually produces binocular rivalry, with alternating periods of experiencing a definite image and occasionally partial overlap. The monkey responds by pressing bars, in effect "telling" the experimenter what it is seeing: a horizontal grating, a vertical grating, or an interlocking grid.

At the same time, neurons in the monkey's cortex are being monitored by electrodes. It is first established that certain neurons respond to certain stimuli: to horizontal lines, for example, or to flowers. Then these neurons are monitored in the binocular rivalry situation to see how well they correlate with what the monkey seems to be seeing. It turns out that cells in the primary visual cortex (V1) do not correlate well. When the monkey is stimulated with horizontal and vertical gratings but "sees" horizontal, a large number of both "vertical" and "horizontal" cells in V1 fire. At this point, most cells seem to correlate with retinal stimulus, not with visual percept. Further into the visual system, however, the correlation increases until in the inferior temporal (IT) cortex, there is a very strong correlation. When the monkey is stimulated with horizontal and vertical grating but "sees" horizontal, almost all of the relevant horizontal cells in IT fire, and almost none of the vertical cells do. When the monkey's response switches, indicating that it is now "seeing" vertical, the cell responses switch accordingly.

These results lend themselves naturally to speculation about the location of a visual NCC. It seems that V1 is unlikely to be or to involve an NCC, for example, due to the failure of V1 cells to correlate with the contents of consciousness. Of course, there are still the possibilities that some small subset of V1 is an NCC or that V1 is a neural correlate of some aspects of visual consciousness but not of others, but I leave those aside for now. On the other hand, IT seems to be a natural candidate for the location of an NCC due to the strong correlation of its cells with the content of consciousness. At least it is natural to suppose that IT is a "lower bound" on the location of a visual NCC (due to the failure of strong correlation before then), though the NCC itself may be farther in. None of this evidence is conclusive (and Logothetis and colleagues are appropriately cautious), but it is at least suggestive.

It is clear that this work is concerned with the neural correlates of the *contents* of visual consciousness. We are interested in finding cortical areas whose neural activity correlates with and predicts specific contents of consciousness, such as experiences of horizontal or vertical lines or of flowers or sunbursts. The ideal is to find a neural system from whose activity we might determine the precise contents of a visual experience or at least its contents in certain respects (shape, color, and the like).

Interestingly, it seems that in doing this we are crucially concerned with the representational contents of the neural systems themselves. In the Logothetis work, for example, it is important to determine the receptive fields of the cells (whether they respond to horizontal or vertical gratings, for example) in order to see whether the receptive fields of active cells match up with the apparent contents of visual consciousness. In essence, the receptive field is acting at least as a heuristic way of getting at representational content in the neurons in question. Then, the crucial question is whether the representational content in the neural system matches up with the representational content in visual consciousness.

This suggests a natural definition of a neural correlate of the contents of consciousness:

> A neural correlate of the contents of consciousness is a neural representational system N such that representation of a content in N directly correlates with representation of that content in consciousness.

Or, more briefly:

> An NCC for content is a neural representational system N such that the content of N directly correlates with the content of consciousness.

For example, the Logothetis work lends itself to the speculation that IT might contain a content NCC for visual consciousness since the content of cells in IT seems to directly correlate (at least in these experiments) with the contents of visual consciousness. (Much more investigation is required to see whether this correlation holds across the board, of course.)

This definition requires that we have some way of defining the representational content of a neural system independent of the contents of consciousness. There are various ways to do this. Using a cell's receptive field to define its representational content is probably the simplest. A more refined definition might also give a role to the sort of behavior that activity in that system typically leads to. In addition, there may be more complex notions of representational content still, based on complex correlations with environment, patterns of behavior, and activity in other cells, but even a crude definition of representational content (e.g., the receptive field definition) is good enough for many purposes and can yield informative results about the visual NCC.

It is arguable that much work on the visual NCC tacitly invokes this sort of definition. Another example is Milner and Goodale's (1995) work on the two pathways of visual perception. They suggest that the ventral stream is largely for cognitive identification and decision, while the dorsal stream is largely for online motor response, and that visual consciousness correlates with activity in the ventral stream.

Much of the support for this work lies with patients who have dissociations between specific contents of conscious perception and the contents involved in motor response. For example, a subject with visual form agnosia (e.g., Milner and Goodale's patient D.F.) cannot consciously identify a vertical slot but can "post" an envelope through it without problem; while subjects with optic ataxia can identify an object but cannot act appropriately toward it. The dissociations here appear to go along with damage to the ventral and dorsal pathways, respectively.

What seems to be going on, on a natural interpretation of these results and of Milner and Goodale's hypothesis, is that for these subjects, there is a dissociation between the contents represented in the ventral pathway and those represented in the dorsal pathway. In these cases, the character of a motor response appears to be determined by the contents represented in the dorsal pathway, but the character of conscious perception appears to be determined by the contents represented in the ventral pathway.

Thus, one can see Milner and Goodale's hypothesis as involving the suggestion that the ventral stream contains the neural correlates of the contents of visual consciousness. The hypothesis is quite speculative, of course (though it is interesting to note that IT lies in the ventral stream), but it seems that the content-based analysis provides a natural interpretation of what the hypothesis is implicitly claiming regarding the visual NCC and of what may follow if the hypothesis turns out to be correct.

One could give a similar analysis of much or most work on the visual NCC. When Crick and Koch (1998) propose that the visual NCC lies outside V1, for example, much of the experimental evidence they appeal to involves cases where some content is represented in consciousness but not in V1 or vice versa. For example, Gur and Snodderly (1997) show that for some quickly alternating isoluminant color stimuli, color cells in V1 flicker back and forth even though a single fused color is consciously perceived. In addition, results by He, Cavanagh, and Intriligator (1996) suggest that the orientation of a grating can fade from consciousness even though orientation cells in V1 carry the information. The results are not entirely conclusive, but they suggest a mismatch between the representational content in V1 and the content of consciousness.

One can apply this sort of analysis equally to NCCs in other sensory modalities. An NCC of auditory consciousness, for example, might be defined as a neural representational system whose contents correlate directly with the contents of auditory consciousness: loudness, direction, pitch, tone, and the like. The analysis can arguably be applied to defining the neural correlates of bodily sensations, of conscious mental imagery, and perhaps of conscious emotion and of the stream of conscious thought. All these aspects of consciousness can be naturally analyzed (at least in part) in terms of their content. In looking for their respective NCCs, we may ultimately be looking for neural systems whose content correlates with the contents of these aspects of consciousness.

(iv) Arbitrary Phenomenal Properties

(This section is more abstract than the preceding sections and might be skipped by those not interested in philosophical details.)

One might try to give a general definition of an NCC of various states of consciousness, of which each of the foregoing would be a special case. To do this, one would need a general way of thinking about arbitrary states of consciousness. Perhaps the best way is to think in terms of arbitrary *phenomenal properties*. For any distinctive kind of conscious experience, there will be a corresponding phenomenal property: in essence the property of having a conscious experience of that kind. For example, being in a hypnotic state of consciousness is a phenomenal property; having a visual experience of a horizontal line is a phenomenal property; feeling intense happiness is a phenomenal property; feeling a throbbing pain is a phenomenal property; being conscious is a phenomenal property. Phenomenal properties can be as coarse grained or as fine grained as

you like as long as they are wholly determined by the current conscious
state of the subject.

Using this notion, one might try to define the neural correlate of an
arbitrary phenomenal property P:

> A state N_1 of system N is a neural correlate of phenomenal property P
> if N's being in N_1 directly correlates with the subject having P.

Note that we here talk of a *state* being an NCC. Given a *specific* phenomenal property—experiencing a horizontal line, for example—it is no
longer clear that it makes sense to speak of a given system being the NCC
of that property. Rather, it will be a particular state of that system. Neural
firing in certain horizontal cells in IT (say) might be a neural correlate of
seeing a horizontal line, for example. On Hobson's hypothesis, having
one's neurochemical system in a certain region of state space might be a
neural correlate of waking consciousness. These are specific states of the
neural systems in question.

Most of the time we are not concerned with neural correlates of single
phenomenal properties but of *families* of phenomenal properties. Hobson
(1997) is concerned not just with the neural correlate of waking consciousness, for example, but also with the neural correlate of the whole family of
background states of consciousness. Work on the visual NCC is not concerned with just the neural correlate of horizontal experience but also with
the neural correlates of the whole system of visual experiential contents.

We might say a *phenomenal family* is a set of mutually exclusive phenomenal properties that jointly partition the space of conscious experiences or
at least some subset of that space. That is, any subject having an experience
(of a certain relevant kind) will have a phenomenal property in the family
and will not have more than one such property. Specific contents of visual
consciousness make for a phenomenal family, for example. Any visually
conscious subject will have some specific visual content, and they will not
have two contents at once (given that we are talking about *overall* visual
content). The same goes for contents at a particular location in the visual
field. Anyone with an experience of a certain location will have some specific content associated with that location (a red horizontal line, say) and
not more than one. (Ambiguous experiences are not counterexamples here
as long as we include ambiguous contents as members of the family in question.) The same again goes for color experience at any given location. There
will be a phenomenal family (one property for each color quality) for any
such location. And the same goes for background states of consciousness.
All these sets of phenomenal properties make phenomenal families.

We can then say the following:

A neural correlate of a phenomenal family S is a neural system N such that the state of N directly correlates with the subject's phenomenal property in S.

For any phenomenal family S, a subject will have at most one property in S (one background state or one overall state of visual consciousness or one color quality at a location). A neural system N will be an NCC of S when there are a corresponding number of states of N, one for every property in P such that N's being in a given state directly correlates with the subject's having the corresponding phenomenal property. This template applies to most of the definitions given earlier.

For the neural correlate of creature consciousness, we have a simple phenomenal family with two properties: being conscious and not being conscious. An NCC here will be a system with two states that correlate with these two properties.

For the neural correlate of a background state of consciousness, we have a phenomenal family with a few more properties: dreaming, being in an ordinary waking state, being under hypnosis, and so on. An NCC here will be a neural system with a few states that correlate directly with these properties. Hobson's neurochemical system would be an example.

For the neural correlate of contents of consciousness, one will have a much more complex phenomenal family (overall states of visual consciousness, states of color consciousness at a location, particular conscious occurrent thoughts, and so on) and a neural representational system to match. The state of the NCC will directly correlate with the specific phenomenal property.

In the content case, there is an extra strong requirement on the NCC. In the other cases, we have accepted an arbitrary match of neural states to phenomenal states—any state can serve as the neural correlate of a dreaming state of background consciousness, for example. But where content is concerned, not any neural state will do. The content of the neural state in question must match the content of consciousness. This is a much stronger requirement.

It is arguable that this requirement delivers much greater explanatory and predictive power in the case of neural correlates of conscious content. The systematicity in the correlation means that it can be extended to predict the presence or absence of phenomenal features that may not have been present in the initial empirical data set, for example, and it also will dovetail more nicely with finding a mechanism and a functional role for the NCC that matches the role that we associate with a given conscious state.

It is this systematicity in the correlation that makes the current work on the neural correlate of visual consciousness particularly interesting. Without it, things would be much more untidy. Imagine that we find arbitrary neural states that correlated directly with the experience of horizontal and vertical lines such that there was no corresponding representational content in the neural state. Instead, we match seemingly arbitrary states N_1 with horizontal, N_2 with vertical, and so on. Would we count this as a neural correlate of the contents of visual consciousness? If we did, it would be in a much weaker sense, and in a way that would lead to much less explanatory and predictive power.

One might then hope to extend this sort of systematicity to other, non-content-involving phenomenal families. For example, one might find among background states of consciousness some pattern or some dimension along which they systematically vary (some sort of intensity dimension, for example, or a measure of alertness). If we could then find a neural system whose states do not just arbitrarily correlate with the phenomenal states in question but vary along a corresponding systematic dimension, then the NCC in question will have much greater potential explanatory and predictive power. So this sort of systematicity in phenomenal families is something that we should look for and something that we should look to match in potential neural correlates.

Perhaps one could define a "systematic NCC" as a neural correlate of a phenomenal family such that states correlate with each other in some such systematic way. I will not give a general abstract definition here as things are getting complex enough already, but I think one can see a glimmer of how it might go. I will, however, keep using the case of the neural correlate of the contents of consciousness (especially visual consciousness) as the paradigmatic example of an NCC precisely because its definition builds in such a notion of systematicity.

3. Direct Correlation

The other thing that we need to clarify is the notion of "direct correlation." We have said that an NCC is a system whose state directly correlates with a state of consciousness, but exactly what does direct correlation involve? Is it required that the neural system be necessary and sufficient for consciousness, for example, or merely sufficient? And over what range of cases must the correlation obtain for the system to count as an NCC? Any possible case? A relevantly constrained set of cases? And so on.

The paradigmatic case will involve a neural system N with states that correlate with states of consciousness. So we can say the following:

state of $N \leftrightarrow$ state of consciousness

and specifically

N is in state $N_1 \leftrightarrow$ subject has conscious state C_1.

In the case of the contents of consciousness, we have a system N such that representing a content R in N directly correlates with representation in consciousness. So we can say:

representing R in $N \leftrightarrow$ representing R in consciousness.

The question in all of these cases concerns the nature of the required relation (here represented as "$\leftrightarrow$"). How strong a relation is required for N to be an NCC?

(A) Necessity, Sufficiency?

The first question is whether the NCC state is required to be necessary and sufficient for the conscious state, merely sufficient, or something else in the vicinity.

(A1) *Necessity and sufficiency.* The first possibility is that the state of N is necessary and sufficient for the corresponding state of consciousness. This is an attractive requirement for an NCC, but it is arguably too strong. It might turn out that there is more than one neural correlate of a given conscious state. For example, it may be that there are two systems, M and N, such that a certain state of M suffices for being in pain and a certain state of N also suffices for being in pain, where these two states are not themselves always correlated. In this case, it seems that we would likely say that both M and N (or their corresponding states) are neural correlates of pain. But it is not the case that activity in M is necessary and sufficient for pain (as it is not necessary), and the same goes for N. If both M and N are to count as NCCs here, we cannot require an NCC to be necessary and sufficient.

(A2) *Sufficiency.* From the foregoing, it seems plausible that we require only that an NCC state be *sufficient* for the corresponding state of consciousness, not necessary. But is any sufficient state an NCC? If it is, then it seems that the whole brain will count as an NCC of any state of consciousness. The whole brain will count as an NCC of pain, for example, since being in a certain total state of the whole brain will suffice for being in pain. Perhaps there is some very weak sense in which this makes sense, but it does not seem to capture what researchers in the field are after when looking for an NCC. So something more than mere sufficiency is required.

(A3) *Minimal sufficiency.* The trouble with requiring mere sufficiency, intuitively, is that it allows irrelevant processes into an NCC. If N is an NCC, then the system obtained by conjoining N with a neighboring system M will also qualify as an NCC by the previous definition since the state of $N+M$ will suffice for the relevant states of consciousness.

The obvious remedy is to require that an NCC be a *minimal sufficient system*: that is, a *minimal* system whose state is sufficient for the corresponding conscious state. By this definition, N will be an NCC when (1) the states of N suffice for the corresponding states of consciousness and (2) no proper part M of N is such that the states of M suffice for the corresponding states of consciousness. In this way, we pare down any potential NCC to its core. Any irrelevant material will be whittled away, and an NCC will be required to contain only the core processes that suffice for the conscious state in question.

On this definition, there may be more than one NCC for a given conscious state. It may be that there is more than one minimal sufficient system for a given state (or for a given system of states), and both of these will count as a neural correlate of that state. This seems to be the right result. We cannot know a priori that there will be only one NCC for a given state or system of states. Whether there will actually be one or more than one for any given state is something that can be determined only empirically.

There is a technical problem for the minimality requirement. It may turn out that there is significant redundancy in a neural correlate of consciousness, such that, for example, a given conscious visual content is represented redundantly in many cells in a given area. If this is so, then that visual area as a whole might not qualify as a minimal sufficient system, as various smaller components of it might all themselves correlate with the conscious state. In this case the preceding definition would imply that various such small components would each be an NCC. One could deal with this sort of case by noting that the problem arises only when the states of the various smaller systems are themselves wholly correlated with each other. (If their mutual correlation can be broken, so will their correlation with consciousness, so that the overall system or some key subsystem will again emerge as the true NCC). Given this, one could stipulate that where states of minimal sufficient systems are wholly correlated with each other, it is the union of the system that should be regarded as an NCC rather than the individual systems. So an NCC would be a minimal system whose state is sufficient for a given conscious state and whose state is not wholly correlated with the state of any other system. I pass over this complication in what follows, however.

(B) What Range of Cases?

An NCC will be a minimal neural system N such that the state of N is sufficient for a corresponding conscious state. This is to say that if the system is in state N_1, the subject will have conscious state C_1. However, the question now arises: over what range of cases must the correlation in question hold?

There is sometimes a temptation to say that this question does not need to be answered: all that is required is that *in this very case*, neural state N_1 suffices for or correlates with conscious state C_1. But this does not really make sense. There is no such thing as a single-case correlation. Correlation is always defined with respect to a range of cases. The same goes for sufficiency. To say that neural state N_1 suffices for conscious state C_1 is to say that in a range of cases, neural state N_1 will always be accompanied by conscious state C_1. But what is the range of cases?

(B1) *Any possible case.* It is momentarily tempting to suggest that the correlation should range across any possible case: if N is an NCC, it should be impossible to be in a relevant state of N without being in the corresponding state of consciousness. But a moment's reflection suggests that this is incompatible with the common usage in the field. NCCs are often supposed to be relatively limited systems, such as the inferior temporal cortex or the intralaminar nucleus, but nobody (or almost nobody) holds that if one excises the entire inferior temporal cortex or intralaminar nucleus and puts it in a jar and puts the system into a relevant state, it will be accompanied by the corresponding state of consciousness.

That is to say, for a given NCC, it certainly seems *possible* that one can have the NCC state without the corresponding conscious state, for example by performing sufficiently radical lesions. So we cannot require that the correlation range over all possible cases.

Of course, one could always insist that a *true* NCC be such that it is impossible to have the NCC state without the corresponding conscious state. The consequence of this would be that an NCC would almost certainly be far larger than it is on any current hypothesis as we would have to build in a large amount of the brain to make sure that all of the background conditions are in place. Perhaps it would be some sort of wide-ranging although skeletal brain state involving aspects of processes from a number of regions of the brain. This might be a valid usage, but it is clear that this is not what researchers in the field are getting at when they are talking about an NCC.

We might call the notion just defined a *total* NCC as it builds in the totality of physical processes that are absolutely required for a given conscious state. The notion that is current in the field is more akin to that of a *core* NCC. (I adapt this terminology from Shoemaker's [1981] notion of a "total realization" and a "core realization" of a functional mental state.) A total NCC builds in everything and thus automatically suffices for the corresponding conscious states. A core NCC, on the other hand, contains only the "core" processes that correlate with consciousness. The rest of the total NCC will be relegated to some sort of background conditions that are required for the correct functioning of the core.

(Philosophical note: the sort of possibility being considered here is natural or nomological possibility or possibility compatible with the laws of nature. If we required correlation across all *logically* possible cases, there might be no total NCC at all, as it is arguably logically possible or coherently conceivable to instantiate any physical process at all without consciousness. If we require correlation across naturally possible cases, the problem goes away, as these cases are probably not naturally possible. It is almost certainly naturally necessary that a being with my brain state will have the same sort of conscious state as I do, for example.)

The question is then how to distinguish the core from the background. It seems that what is required for an NCC (in the "core" sense) is not that it correlate with consciousness across any possible conditions but rather that it correlate across some constrained range of cases in which some aspects of normal brain functioning are held constant. The question then becomes, what is to be held constant? Across just what constrained range of cases do we require than an NCC correlate with consciousness?

(B2) *Ordinary-functioning brain in ordinary environments.* One might take the moral of the foregoing to be that one cannot require an NCC to correlate with consciousness in "unnatural" cases. What matters is that the NCC correlates with consciousness in "natural" cases, that is, those that actually occur in the functioning of a normal brain. The most conservative strategy would be to require correlation only across cases involving a normally functioning brain in a normal environment, receiving "ecologically valid" inputs of the sort received in a normal life.

The trouble with this criterion is that it seems too weak to narrow down the NCC. It may turn out that this way we find NCCs at all stages of the visual system, for example. In a normal visual environment, we expect that the contents of visual systems from V1 through IT will all correlate with the contents of visual consciousness and that even the contents of the retina will do so to some extent. The reason is that in normal cases all of these will be linked in a straightforward causal chain, and the systems in question will not be dissociated. Nonetheless, it seems wrong to say that, merely because of this, all of the systems (perhaps even the retina) should count as an NCC.

The moral of this is that we need a more fine-grained criterion to dissociate these systems and to distinguish the core NCC from processes that are merely causally linked to it. To do this, we have to require correlation across a range of *unusual cases* as well as across normal cases, as it is these that yield interesting dissociations.

(B3) *Normal brain, unusual inputs.* The next most conservative suggestion is that we still require a normal brain for our range of cases but that we allow any possible inputs, including "ecologically invalid" inputs. This would cover the Logothetis experiments, for example. The inputs that evoke binocular rivalry are certainly unusual and not encountered in a normal environment. However, it is precisely these that allow the experiments to make more fine-grained distinctions than we normally can. The experiments suggest that IT is more likely than V1 to be an NCC precisely because it correlates with consciousness across the wider range of cases. If states of V1 truly do not match up with states of consciousness in this situation, then it seems that V1 cannot be an NCC. If that reasoning is correct, then it seems that we require an NCC to correlate with consciousness across all unusual inputs and not just across normal environments.

The extension of the correlation requirement from normal environments to unusual inputs is a relatively "safe" extension and seems a reasonable requirement, though those who place a high premium on ecological validity might contest it. Yet it is arguable that this is still too weak to do the fine-grained work of distinguishing an NCC from systems linked to it. Presumably unusual inputs will go only so far in yielding interesting dissociations, and some systems (particularly those well down the processing pathway) may well stay associated on any unusual inputs. So it is arguable that we will need more fine-grained tools to distinguish the NCC.

(B4) *Normal brain, vary brain stimulation.* The next possibility is to allow cases involving not just unusual inputs but also direct stimulation of the brain. Such direct stimulation might include both electrode stimulation and transcranial magnetic stimulation. On this view, we will require that an NCC correlate with consciousness across all cases of brain stimulation, as well as normal functioning. So if we have a potential NCC state that does not correlate with consciousness in the right way in a brain-stimulation condition, that state will not be a true NCC.

This requirement seems to fit some of the methods used in the field. Penfield (e.g., Penfield and Rasmussen 1950) pioneered the use of brain stimulation to draw conclusions about the neural bases of consciousness. Libet (1982) has also used brain stimulation to good effect, and more recently Newsome and colleagues (e.g., Salzman, Britten, and Newsome 1990) have used brain stimulation to draw some conclusions about neural correlates of motion perception in monkeys.

Brain stimulation can clearly be used to produce dissociations that are more fine grained than can be produced merely with unusual inputs. One might be able to dissociate activity in any system from that in a preceding system by stimulating that system directly, for example, as long as there are not too many backward connections. Given a candidate NCC—inferior temporal cortex, say—one can test the hypothesis by stimulating an area immediately following the candidate in the processing pathway. If that yields a relevant conscious state without relevant activity in IT (say), that indicates that IT is probably not a true NCC after all. Rather, the NCC may lie in a system further down the processing chain. (I leave aside the possibility that there might be two NCCs at different stages of the chain.)

This reasoning seems sound, suggesting that we may tacitly require an NCC to correlate with consciousness across brain stimulation conditions. There is no immediately obvious problem with the requirement, at least when the stimulation in question is relatively small and localized. If one allows arbitrary large stimulation, there may be problems. For example, one could presumably use brain stimulation at least in principle to disable large areas of the brain (by overstimulating those areas, for example) while leaving NCC activity intact. In this case, it is not implausible to expect that one will have the relevant NCC activity without the usual conscious state (just as in the case where one lesions the whole NCC and puts it in a jar), so the correlation will fail in this case. Intuitively, this does not seem to disprove the claim that the NCC in question is a true NCC, at least before the stimulation. If so, then we cannot allow unlimited brain stimulation in the range of cases relevant to the correlation, and more generally, some of the problems for lesions (discussed later) may apply to reasoning involving brain stimulation. Nevertheless, in the absence of strong reason to believe otherwise, one might well require that an NCC correlate with consciousness at least across cases of limited stimulation.

(B5) *Abnormal functioning due to lesions.* In almost all of the preceding cases, we have retained a normally functioning brain; we have just stimulated it in unusual ways. The next logical step is to allow cases where the brain is not functioning normally due to lesions in brain systems. Such lesions might be either natural (e.g., due to some sort of brain damage) or artificial (e.g., induced by surgery). On this view, we will require that an NCC correlate with states of consciousness not just across cases of normal functioning but across cases of abnormal functioning as well.

This certainly squares with common practice in the field. Lesion studies are often used to draw conclusions about the neural correlates of consciousness. In Milner and Goodale's (1995) work, for example, the fact that consciousness remains much the same upon lesions to the dorsal stream but not to the ventral stream is used to support the conclusion that the NCC lies within the ventral stream. More generally, it is often assumed that if some aspect of consciousness survives relatively intact when a given brain area is damaged, then that brain area is unlikely to be or to contain an NCC.

The tacit premise in this research is that an NCC should correlate with consciousness not just in cases of normal functioning but in cases of abnormal functioning as well. Given this premise, it follows that if we find an abnormal case in which neural system N is damaged but a conscious state C is preserved, then N is not a neural correlate of C. Without this premise or a version of it, it is not clear that any such conclusion can be drawn from lesion studies.

The premise may sound reasonable, but we already have reason to be suspicious of it. We know that for any candidate NCC, sufficiently radical changes can destroy the correlation. Preserving merely system N cut off from the rest of the brain, for example, is unlikely to yield a corresponding conscious state, but intuitively, this does not imply that N was not an NCC in the original case.

Less radically, one can imagine placing lesions immediately downstream from a candidate NCC so that its effects on the rest of the brain are significantly reduced. In such a case, it is probable that the system in question can be active without the usual behavioral effects associated with consciousness and quite plausibly without consciousness itself. It is not implausible that an NCC supports consciousness largely in virtue of playing the right functional role in the brain (perhaps in virtue of mediating global availability, as discussed in chapter 4). If so, then if the system is changed so that the NCC no longer plays that functional role, then NCC activity will no longer correlate with consciousness. However, the mere fact that correlation can be destroyed by this sort of lesion does not obviously imply that the system is not an NCC in a normal brain. If that inference could be made, then almost any candidate NCC could be ruled out by the right sort of lesion.

It may be that even smaller lesions can destroy a correlation in this way. For example, it is not implausible that for any candidate NCC N, there is some other local system in the brain (perhaps a downstream area) whose proper functioning is required for activity in N to yield the usual effects that go with consciousness and for N to yield consciousness itself. This second system might not itself be an NCC in any intuitive sense; it might merely play an enabling role in the way that proper functioning of the heart plays an enabling role for functioning of the brain. If so, then if one lesions this single area downstream, then activity in N will no longer correlate with consciousness. In this way, any potential NCC might be ruled out by a localized lesion elsewhere.

The trouble is that lesions change the architecture of the brain, and it is quite possible that changes to brain architecture can change the very location of an NCC, so that a physical state that was an NCC in a normal brain will not be an NCC in the altered brain. Given this possibility, it seems too strong to require that an NCC correlate with consciousness across arbitrary lesions and changes in brain functioning. We should expect an NCC to be architecture dependent, not architecture independent.

So an NCC should not be expected to correlate with consciousness across arbitrary lesion cases. There are now two alternatives. Either we can require correlation across some more restricted range of lesion cases or we can drop the requirement of correlation in abnormal cases altogether.

For the first alternative to work, we would have to find some way to distinguish a class of "good" lesions from the class of "bad" lesions. An NCC would be expected to correlate with consciousness across the good lesions but not the bad lesions. If one found a "good" lesion case where activity in system N was present without the corresponding consciousness state, this would imply that N is not an NCC. But no such conclusion could be drawn from a "bad" lesion case.

The trouble is that it is not at all obvious that such a distinction can be drawn. It might be tempting to come up with an after-the-fact distinction, defined as the range of lesions in which correlation with any given NCC N is preserved, but this will not be helpful, as we are interested in precisely the criterion that makes N qualify as an NCC in the first place. So a distinction will have to be drawn on relatively a priori grounds (it can then be used to determined whether a given correlation pattern qualifies an arbitrary system as an NCC or not). But it is not clear how to draw the distinction. One might suggest that correlation should be preserved across small lesions but not large ones; however, we have already seen that even small lesions might destroy a potential NCC. Or one might suggest that lesions in downstream areas are illegitimate, whereas upstream and parallel lesions are legitimate. Even here, however, it is not clear whether indirect interaction with an upstream or parallel area might be required to support the proper functioning of an NCC. Perhaps with some ingenuity one might be able to come up with a criterion, but it is not at all obvious how.

The second alternative is to hold that correlation across cases of normal functioning (perhaps with unusual inputs and brain stimulation) is all that is required to be an NCC. If this is so, one can never infer directly from the fact that N fails to correlate with consciousness in a lesion case to the conclusion that N is not an NCC. On this view, the location of an NCC is wholly architecture dependent, that is, entirely dependent on the normal functioning of the brain. One cannot expect an NCC to correlate with consciousness in cases with abnormal functioning or different architecture, so no direct conclusion can be drawn from failure of correlation across lesion cases. Of course, one can still appeal to cases with unusual inputs and brain stimulation to make fine-grained distinctions among NCCs.

The main objection to the second alternative is that one might *need* lesion cases to make the most fine-grained distinctions that are required. Consider a hypothetical case in which we have two linked systems N and M that correlate equally well with consciousness across all normal cases, including all unusual inputs and brain stimulation, but such that in almost all relevant lesion cases, consciousness correlates much better with N than with M. In this case, might we want to say that N rather than M is an NCC? If so, we have to build in some allowance for abnormal cases into the definition of an NCC. An advocate of the second alternative might reply by saying that such cases will be very unusual and that if N and M are dissociable by lesions, there is likely to be some unusual brain stimulation that will bring out the dissociation as well. In the extreme case where no brain stimulation leads to dissociation, one might simply bite the bullet and say that both N and M are equally good NCCs.

Taking everything into consideration, I am inclined to think the second alternative is better than the first. It seems right to say that "core" NCC location depends on brain architecture and normal functioning, and it is unclear that correlation across abnormal cases should be required, especially given all of the associated problems. A problem like the one just mentioned might provide some pressure to investigate the first alternative further, and I do not rule out the possibility that some way of distinguishing "good" from "bad" lesions might be found, but all in all it seems best to say that an NCC cannot be expected to correlate with consciousness across abnormal cases.

Of course, this has an impact on the methodology in the search for an NCC. As we have seen, lesion studies are often used to draw conclusions about NCC location (as in the Milner and Goodale research, for example, and also in much research on blindsight), and failure of correlation in lesion cases is often taken to imply that a given system is not an NCC. Still, we have seen that the tacit premise of this sort of research—that an NCC must correlate across abnormal, as well as normal, cases—is difficult to support and leads to significant problems. So it seems that lesion studies are methodologically dangerous here. One should be very cautious in using them to draw conclusions about NCC location.

This is not to say that lesion studies are irrelevant in the search for an NCC. Even if correlation across abnormal cases is not *required* for system N to be an NCC, it may be that correlation across abnormal cases can provide good *evidence* that N is an NCC and that failure of such correlation in some cases provides good evidence that N is not an NCC. Say that, as I have suggested, we define an NCC as a system that correlates with consciousness across all normal cases (including unusual input and stimulation). It may nevertheless be the case that information about correlations across all these normal cases with unusual stimulation is difficult to come by (due to problems in monitoring brain systems at a fine grain, for example) and that information about correlation across lesion cases is easier to obtain. In this case, one might sometimes take correlation across abnormal cases as *evidence* that a system will correlate across the normal cases in question and thus as evidence that the system is an NCC. Similarly, one might take failure of correlation across abnormal cases as evidence that a system will fail to correlate across certain normal cases and thus as evidence that the system is not an NCC.

The question of whether a given lesion study can serve as evidence in this way needs to be considered on a case-by-case basis. It is clear that some lesion studies will not provide this sort of evidence, as is witnessed by the cases of severe lesions and downstream lesions discussed earlier. In these cases, failure of correlation across abnormal cases provides no evidence of failure of correlation across normal cases. On the other hand, it does not seem unreasonable that the Milner and Goodale studies should be taken as evidence that, even in normal cases, the ventral stream will correlate better with visual consciousness than the dorsal stream. Of course, the real "proof" would come from a careful investigation of the relevant processes across a wide range of "normal" cases involving standard environments, unusual inputs, and brain stimulation.

But in the absence of such a demonstration, the lesion cases at least provide suggestive evidence.

In any case, the moral is that one has to be very cautious when drawing conclusions about NCC location from lesion studies. At best these studies serve as indirect evidence rather than as direct criteria, and even as such there is a chance that the evidence can be misleading. One needs to consider the possibility that the lesion in question is changing brain architecture in such a fashion that what was once an NCC is no longer an NCC, and one needs to look very closely at what is going on to rule out the possibility. It may be that this can sometimes be done, but it is a nontrivial matter.

4. Overall Definition

With all of this, we have come to a more detailed definition of an NCC. The general case is something like the following:

> An NCC is a minimal neural system N such that there is a mapping from states of N to states of consciousness, where a given state of N is sufficient, under conditions C, for the corresponding state of consciousness.

The central case of the neural correlate of the content of consciousness can be put in more specific terms:

> An NCC for content is a minimal neural representational system N such that representation of a content in N is sufficient, under conditions C, for representation of that content in consciousness.

One might also give a general definition of the NCC for an arbitrary phenomenal property or for a phenomenal family, but I leave those aside here.

The "conditions C" clause here represents the relevant range of cases. If the reasoning earlier is on the right track, then conditions C might be seen as conditions involving normal brain functioning, allowing unusual inputs and limited brain stimulation, but not lesions or other changes in architecture. Of course, the precise nature of conditions C is still debatable. Perhaps one could make a case for including a limited range of lesion cases in the definition. In the other direction, one might make a case that the requirement of correlation across brain stimulation or unusual inputs is too strong due to the abnormality of those scenarios. But I think the conditions C proposed here are at least a reasonable first pass, pending further investigation.

Of course, to some extent, defining what "really" counts as an NCC is a terminological matter. One could quite reasonably say that there are multiple different notions of NCC depending on just how one understands the relevant conditions C or the matter of necessity and sufficiency and so on, and not much really rests on which of these is the "right" definition. Still, we have seen that different definitions give very different results. Many potential definitions have the consequence that systems that intuitively seem to qualify as an NCC do not qualify after all and that NCC hypotheses put forward by researchers in the field could be ruled out on trivial a priori grounds. Those consequences seem undesirable. It makes sense to have a definition of NCC that fits the way the notion is generally used in the field and that can make sense of empirical research in the area. At the same time we want a definition of NCC to be coherent and well motivated in its own right such that an NCC is something worth looking for and such that the definition can itself be used to assess various hypotheses about the identity of an NCC. The definition I have given here is at least a first pass in this direction.

5. Methodological Consequences

The discussion so far has been somewhat abstract, and the definitions given here may look like mere words. But from these definitions and the reasoning that went into them one can straightforwardly extract some concrete methodological recommendations for the NCC search. Many of these recommendations are plausible or obvious in their own right, but it is interesting to see them emerge from the analysis.

(i) *Lesion studies are methodologically dangerous.* Lesion studies are often used to draw conclusions about neural correlates of consciousness, but we have seen that their use can be problematic. The identity of an NCC is arguably always relative to specific brain architecture and normal brain functioning, and correlation across abnormal cases should not generally be expected. In some cases, lesion studies can change brain architecture so that a system that was previously an NCC is no longer an NCC. So one can never infer directly from failure of correlation between a system and consciousness in a lesion case to the conclusion that that system is an NCC. Sometimes one can infer this indirectly by using the failure of correlation here as evidence for failure of correlation in normal cases, but one must be cautious.

(ii) *There may be many NCCs.* On the definition given earlier, an NCC is a system whose activity is *sufficient* for certain states of consciousness. This allows for the possibility of multiple NCCs in at least two ways. First, different sorts of conscious states may have different corresponding NCCs; there may be different NCCs for visual and auditory consciousness, for example, and perhaps even for different aspects of visual consciousness. Second, even for a particular sort of conscious state (such as pain), we cannot rule out the possibility that there will be two different systems whose activity is sufficient to produce that state.

Of course, it *could* turn out that there are only a few NCCs or perhaps even one. In the next chapter I discuss the possibility of some central system that represents the contents of visual consciousness, auditory consciousness, emotional experience, the stream of conscious thought, the background state of consciousness, and so on. Such a system might be seen as a sort of "consciousness module," a "Cartesian theater" (Dennett 1991), or a "global workspace" (Baars 1988) depending on whether one is a foe or a friend of the idea. However, it is by no means obvious that there will be such a system, and the empirical evidence so far is against it. In any case, the matter cannot be decided a priori, so our definition should be compatible with the existence of multiple or many NCCs.

(3) *Minimize the size of an NCC.* We have seen that an NCC should be understood as a *minimal* neural system that correlates with consciousness. Given this, we should constrain the search for the NCC by aiming to find a neural correlate that is as small as possible. Given a broad system that appears to correlate with consciousness, we need to isolate the core parts and aspects of that system that underlie the correlation. Given the rival hypotheses that consciousness correlates with a broad system or a narrower system contained within it, we might first investigate the "narrow" hypothesis. If the narrow system correlates well enough with consciousness, the broad system cannot be a true NCC.

It follows that to some extent it makes sense to "start small" in the search for an NCC. This fits the working methodology proposed by Crick and Koch (1998), who suggest that an NCC may perhaps involve a very small number of neurons (perhaps in the thousands) with certain distinctive properties. There is no guarantee that this is correct (and my own money is against it), but it makes a good working hypothesis in the NCC search. Of course, one should simultaneously investigate broad systems for correlation with consciousness so that one can then focus on those areas and try to narrow things down.

(4) *Distinguish NCC for background state and for content.* We have seen that there may be different NCCs for different sorts of states of

consciousness. An important distinction in this class is that between the neural correlate of background states of consciousness (wakefulness, dreaming, etc.) and the neural correlate of specific contents. It may be that these are quite different systems. It is not implausible on current evidence that an NCC for background states involves processes in the thalamus or thalamocortical interactions, while an NCC for specific contents of consciousness involves processes in the cortex. These different sorts of NCC will require quite different methods for their investigation.

(5) *NCC studies need to monitor neural representational content.* Arguably the most interesting part of the NCC search is the search for neural determinants of specific contents of consciousness, such as the contents of visual consciousness. We have seen that an NCC here will be a neural representational system whose contents are correlated with the contents of consciousness. To determine whether such a system is truly an NCC, then, we need methods that monitor the representational content of the system. This is just what we find in Logothetis's work, for example, where it is crucial to keep track of activity in neurons with known receptive fields.

This gets at a striking aspect of the NCC search, mentioned in the last chapter: the most informative and useful results usually come from neuron-level studies on monkeys. Large claims are sometimes made for brain imaging on humans, but it is generally difficult to draw solid conclusions from such studies, especially where an NCC is concerned. We can trace the difference to the fact that neuron-level studies can monitor representational content in neural systems, whereas imaging studies cannot (or at least usually do not). The power of single-cell studies in the work of Logothetis, Andersen, and Newsome and colleagues (e.g., the works of Logothetis and Newsome already cited, and Bradley, Chang, and Andersen 1998) comes precisely from the way that cells can be monitored to keep track of the activity profile of neurons with known representational properties, such as receptive and projective fields. This allows us to track representational content in these neural systems and to correlate it with the apparent contents of consciousness. This is much harder to do in a coarse-grained brain-imaging study, which generally tells one that there is an activity in a region while saying nothing about specific contents.

To deal with this problem, we need better methods for tracking neural representational content, especially in humans (where invasive studies are much more problematic but where evidence for conscious content are much more straightforward). There has been some recent work on the use of imaging methods to get at certain aspects of the content of visual consciousness, such as colors and shapes in the visual field (e.g., Engel, Zhang, and Wandell 1997), and different sorts of objects that activate different brain areas (e.g., Tong et al. 1998). There is also some current work on using invasive methods in neurosurgery patients to monitor the activity of single cells. One can speculate that if a noninvasive method for monitoring single-cell activity in humans is ever developed, the search for an NCC (like most of neuroscience) will be transformed almost beyond recognition.

(6) *Correlation across a few situations is limited evidence.* According to the earlier definition, an NCC is a system that correlates with consciousness across arbitrary cases of normal functioning in any environment and with any unusual input or limited brain stimulation. In practice, though, evidence is far weaker than this. Typically one has a few cases involving either a few subjects with different lesions or a study in which subjects are given different stimuli, and one notes an apparent correlation. This is only to be expected, given the current technological and ethical constraints on experimental methods, but it does mean that the evidence that current methods give is quite weak. To truly demonstrate that a given system is an NCC, one would need to demonstrate correlation across a far wider range of cases than is currently feasible. Of course, current methods may give good *negative* evidence about systems that fail to correlate and thus are not NCCs, but strong positive evidence is harder to find. Positive hypotheses based on current sorts of evidence should probably be considered suggestive but highly speculative.

(7) *We need good criteria for the ascription of consciousness.* To find an NCC, we need to find a neural system that correlates with certain conscious states. To do this, we first need a way to know when a system is in a given conscious state. This is famously problematic, given the privacy of consciousness and the philosophical problem of other minds. In general, we rely on indirect criteria for the ascription of consciousness, such as verbal reports or other behavioral signs. The need for these criteria raises a number of further methodological issues, which are the focus of chapter 4.

Methodological summary. We can use all of this to sketch a general methodology for the NCC search. First, we need methods for determining the contents of conscious experience in a subject, presumably by indirect behavioral criteria or by first-person phenomenology. Second, we need methods to monitor neural states in a subject and in particular to monitor neural representational contents. Then we need to perform experiments in a variety of situations to determine which neural systems correlate with conscious states and which do not. Experiments involving normal brain functioning with unusual inputs and limited brain stimulation are particularly crucial here. Direct conclusions cannot be drawn from systems with lesions, but such systems can sometimes serve as indirect evidence. We need to consider multiple hypotheses in order to narrow down to a set of minimal neural systems that correlate with consciousness across all relevant scenarios. We may well find many different NCCs in different modalities and different NCCs for background states and conscious contents, although it is not out of the question that there will be only a small number. If all goes well, we might expect to eventually isolate systems that correlate strongly with consciousness across any normally functioning brain.

6. Should We Expect an NCC?

One might well ask the following: given the notion of an NCC as I have defined it, is it guaranteed that there will *be* a neural correlate of consciousness?

In answering, I assume that states of consciousness depend systematically in some way on overall states of the brain. If this assumption is false, as is held by some Cartesian dualists (e.g., Eccles 1994) and some phenomenal externalists (e.g., Dretske 1995), then there may be no NCC as defined here, as any given neural state might be instantiated without consciousness. (Even on these positions, an NCC *could* be possible if it were held that brain states at least correlate with conscious states in ordinary cases). But if the assumption is true, then there will at least be some minimal correlation of neural states with consciousness.

Does it follow that there will be an NCC as defined here? This depends on whether we are talking about neural correlates of arbitrary conscious states or about the more constrained case of neural correlates of conscious contents. In the first case, it is guaranteed that the brain as a whole will be a neural system that has states that suffice for arbitrary conscious states. So the brain will be one system whose state is sufficient for a given conscious state, and given that there is at least one such system for a given state, there must be at least one such *minimal* system for that state. Such a system will be an NCC for that state. Of course, this reasoning does not guarantee that there will be only one NCC for a given state, that the NCC for one state will be the same as the NCC for another, or that an NCC will be simple. But we know that an NCC will exist.

In the case of neural correlates of the content of consciousness, things are more constrained since a neural correlate is required not just to map to a corresponding state of consciousness but also to match it in *content.* This rules out the whole brain as even a nonminimal neural correlate, for example, since representing a content in the brain does not suffice to represent that content in consciousness (much of the brain's representational content is unconscious). Of course, we may hope that there will be more constrained neural systems whose content systematically matches that of some aspect of consciousness. But it is not obvious that such a system *must* exist. It might be held, for example, that the contents of consciousness are an emergent product of the contents of various neural systems, which together suffice for conscious content in question but none of which precisely mirrors the conscious content.

One can plausibly argue that there is reason to expect that conscious contents will be mirrored by the contents of a neural representational system at *some* level of abstraction. In creatures with language, for example, conscious contents correspond well with contents that are made directly available for verbal report, and in conscious creatures more generally, one can argue (as I do in chapter 4) that the contents of consciousness correspond to contents that are made directly available for the global voluntary control of behavior. So there is a correlation between the contents of consciousness and contents revealed or exhibited in certain functional roles within the system.

Given that these contents are revealed in verbal report and are exhibited in the control of behavior, there is reason to believe that they are represented at some point within the cognitive system. Of course, this depends to some extent on just what "representation" comes to. On some highly constrained notions of representation—if it is held that the only true representation is symbolic representation, for example—then it is far from clear that the content revealed in behavior must be represented. But on less demanding notions of representation—on which, for example, systems are assigned representational content according to their functional role—then the content revealed in a functional role will straightforwardly be represented in a system that plays that functional role.

This does not guarantee that there will be any single neural system whose content always matches that of consciousness. It may be that the functional role in question is played by multiple systems and that a given system may sometimes play the role and sometimes not. If this is so, we may have to move to a higher level of abstraction. If there is no localizable neural system that qualifies as a correlate of conscious content, we may have to look at a more global system—the "global availability" system, for example, whereby contents are made available for report and global control—and argue that the contents of consciousness correspond to the contents made available in this system. If so, it could turn out that what we are left with is more like a "cognitive correlate of consciousness" (CCC?) since the system may not correspond to any neurobiological system whose nature and boundaries are independently carved out, but it can still function as a correlate in some useful sense.

In this context, it is important to note that an NCC need not be a specific anatomical area in the brain. Some of the existing proposals regarding NCCs involve less localized neurobiological properties. For example, Libet (1993) argues that the neural correlate of consciousness is temporally extended neural firing; Crick and Koch (1998) speculate that the NCC might involve a particular sort of cell throughout the cortex; Edelman (1989) suggests that the NCC might involve reentrant thalamocortical loops and so on. In these cases, NCCs are individuated by temporal properties or by physiological rather than anatomical properties or by functional properties, among other possibilities. If so, the "neural representational system" involved in defining a neural correlate of conscious content might also be individuated more abstractly. The relevant neural representational contents might be those represented by temporally extended firings or by certain sorts of cells or by reentrant loops and so on. So abstractness and failure of localization are not in themselves a bar to a system's qualifying as an NCC.

It seems, then, that a range of possibilities exists for the brain-based correlates of conscious states, ranging from specific anatomical areas through more abstract neural systems to purely "cognitive" correlates such as Baars's (1988) global workspace. Just how specific an NCC may turn out to be is an empirical question. One might reasonably expect that there will be some biological specificity. Within a given organism or species, one often finds a close match between specific functions and specific physiological systems, and it does not seem unlikely that particular neural systems and properties in the brain should be directly implicated in the mechanisms of availability for global control. If so, then we may expect specific neural correlates even of conscious contents. If not, we may have to settle for more abstract correlates, individuated at least partly at the cognitive level, though even here one would expect that some neural systems will be much more heavily involved than others. In any case it seems reasonable to expect that we will find informative brain-based correlates of consciousness at some level of abstraction in cognitive neurobiology.

Some have argued that we should not expect neural correlates of consciousness. For example, in their discussion of neural "filling in" in visual perception, Pessoa, Thompson, and Noë (1998) argue against the necessity of what Teller and Pugh (1984) call a "bridge locus" for perception, which closely resembles the notion of a neural correlate of consciousness. Much of their argument is based on the requirement that such a locus involve a spatiotemporal isomorphism between neural states and conscious states (so a conscious representation of a checkerboard would require a neural state in a checkerboard layout, for example). These arguments do not affect neural correlates of conscious contents as I have defined them since a match between neural and conscious content does not require such a spatiotemporal correspondence (a neural representation of a shape need not itself have that shape). Pessoa et al. also argue more generally against a "uniformity of content" thesis, holding that one should not expect a match between the "personal" contents of consciousness and the "subpersonal" contents of neural systems. It is true that the existence of such a match is not automatic, but as before, the fact that conscious contents are mirrored in specific functional roles gives reason to believe that they will be subpersonally represented at least at some level of abstraction.[2]

It has also been argued (e.g., by Güzeldere 1999) that there is probably no neural correlate of consciousness, as there is probably no area of the brain that is specifically dedicated to consciousness as opposed to vision, memory, learning, and so on. One may well agree that there is no such area, but it does not follow that there is no neural correlate of consciousness as defined here. An NCC (as defined here) requires only that a system be correlated with consciousness, not that it be dedicated solely or mainly to consciousness. The alternative notion of an NCC is much more demanding than the notion at issue in most empirical work on the subject, where it is often accepted that an NCC may be closely bound up with visual processing (e.g., Logothetis, Milner, and Goodale), memory (e.g., Edelman), and other processes. This becomes particularly clear once one gives up on the requirement that there be a single NCC and accepts that there may be multiple NCCs in multiple modalities.

7. Conclusion

The discussion in the previous section helps bring out what an NCC is not, or at least what it might turn out not to be. An NCC is defined as a *correlate* of consciousness. From this, it does not automatically follow that an NCC will be a system solely or mainly dedicated to consciousness or even that an NCC will be the brain system most responsible for the generation of consciousness. It certainly does not follow that an NCC will itself yield an explanation of consciousness, and it is not even guaranteed that identifying an NCC will be the key to understanding the processes underlying

2. *Noë and Thompson (2004) respond to the current article by saying that the "content matching" doctrine is false: subpersonal contents such as receptive fields will never match personal contents such as the contents of perception. However, the current framework is not committed to neural contents as simple as a receptive field, and the general considerations here about availability for report suggest that some functionally individuated system ought to bear the relevant contents.

consciousness. If we were to define an NCC in these stronger terms, it would be far from obvious that there must be an NCC, and it would also be much less clear how to search for one.

Defining an NCC solely in terms of correlation seems to capture standard usage best, and it also makes the search more clearly defined and the methodology clearer. Correlations are easy for science to study. It also means that the search for an NCC can be to a large extent theoretically neutral rather than theoretically loaded. Once we have found an NCC, one might hope that it will turn out to be a system dedicated to consciousness or that it will yield an explanation of consciousness, but these are further questions. In the meantime the search for an NCC as defined poses a tractable empirical project with relatively clear parameters, one that researchers of widely different theoretical persuasions can engage in.

One might reasonably expect the search for an NCC to yield certain rewards. For example, these systems might be used to monitor and predict the contents of consciousness in a range of novel situations. For example, we may be able to use them to help reach conclusions about conscious experience in patients under anesthesia and in subjects with "locked-in syndrome" or in an apparent vegetative state. In cases where brain architecture differs significantly from the original cases (perhaps some coma cases, infants, and animals), the evidence will be quite imperfect, but it will at least be suggestive.

These systems might also serve as a crucial step toward a full science of consciousness. Once we know which systems are NCCs, we can investigate the mechanisms by which they work and how they produce various characteristic functional effects. Just as isolating the DNA basis of the gene helped explain many of the functional phenomena of life, isolating NCC systems may help explain many functional phenomena associated with consciousness. We might also systematize the relationship between NCCs and conscious states and the abstract general principles governing that relationship. In this way we might be led to a much greater theoretical understanding.

In the meantime, the search for a neural correlate of consciousness provides a project that is relatively tractable, clearly defined, and theoretically neutral, whose goal seems to be visible somewhere in the middle distance. Because of this, the search makes an appropriate centerpiece for a developing science of consciousness and an important springboard in the quest for a general theory of the relationship between physical processes and conscious experience.

4

ON THE SEARCH FOR THE NEURAL CORRELATE OF CONSCIOUSNESS

How *can* one search for the neural correlate of consciousness? As we all know, measuring consciousness is problematic because the phenomenon is not directly and straightforwardly observable. It would be much easier if we had a way of getting at consciousness directly—if we had, for example, a consciousness meter.

If we had such an instrument, searching for the NCC would be straight-forward. We would wave the consciousness meter and measure a subject's consciousness directly. At the same time, we would monitor the underlying brain processes. After a number of trials, we would say such-and-such brain processes are correlated with conscious experiences of various kinds, so these brain processes are the neural correlates of consciousness.

Alas, we have no consciousness meter, and for principled reasons it seems we cannot have one. Consciousness is just not the sort of thing that can be measured directly. What, then, do we do without a consciousness meter? How can the search go forward? How does all the experimental research on neural correlates of consciousness proceed?

I think the answer is as follows. We get there with principles of *interpretation*, which we use to interpret physical systems to judge the presence of consciousness. We might call these *pre-experimental bridging principles.* They are the criteria that we bring to bear in looking at systems to say (1) whether or not they are conscious now and (2) which information they are conscious of and which they are not. We cannot reach in directly and grab those experiences, so we rely on external criteria instead.

That is a perfectly reasonable thing to do. But something interesting is going on. These principles of interpretation are not themselves experimentally determined or experimentally tested. In a sense they are pre-experimental assumptions. Experimental research gives us a lot of information about processing; then we bring in the bridging principles to interpret the experimental results, whatever they may be. They are the principles by which we make *inferences* from facts about processing to facts about consciousness, and so they are conceptually prior to the experiments themselves. We cannot actually refine them experimentally (except perhaps by first-person experimentation) because we have no independent access to the independent variable. Instead, these principles will be based on some combination of (1) conceptual judgments about what counts as a conscious process and (2) information gleaned from our first-person perspective on our own consciousness.

We are all stuck in this boat. The point applies whether one is a reductionist or an antireductionist about consciousness. A hard-line reductionist might put some of these points a little differently, but either way the experimental work will require pre-experimental reasoning to determine the criteria for ascribing consciousness. Of course, such principles are usually left implicit in empirical research. We do not usually see papers saying "Here is the bridging principle, here are the data, and here is what follows," but it is useful to make them explicit. The very presence of these principles has strong and interesting consequences in the search for the NCC.

In a sense, in relying on these principles we are taking a leap into the epistemological unknown. Because we do not measure consciousness directly, we have to make something of a leap of faith. It may not be a big leap, but it nevertheless suggests that everyone doing this work is engaged in philosophical reasoning. Of course, one can always choose to stay on solid ground, talking about the empirical results in a neutral way, but the price of doing so is that one gains no particular insight into consciousness. Conversely, as soon as we draw any conclusions about consciousness, we have gone beyond the information given. So we need to pay careful attention to the reasoning involved.

What are these principles of interpretation? The first and by far the most prevalent is the principle of verbal report. When someone says, "Yes, I see that table now," we infer that the subject is conscious of the table. When someone says, "Yes, I see red now," we infer that the subject is having an experience of red. Of course, one might always say, "How do you know?"— a philosopher might suggest that we may be faced with a fully functioning zombie—but in fact most of us do not believe that the people around us are zombies, and in practice we are quite prepared to rely on this principle. As pre-experimental assumptions go, this one is relatively safe—it does not require a huge leap of faith—and it is very widely used.

The principle here is that when information is verbally reported, it is conscious. One can extend this principle slightly, for no one believes an *actual* verbal report is required for consciousness; we are conscious of much more than we report on any given occasion. An extended principle might say that when information is directly *available* for verbal report, it is conscious.

Experimental researchers do not rely only on these principles of verbal report and reportability. The principles can be somewhat limiting when we want to do broader experiments. In particular, we do not want to restrict our studies of consciousness to subjects that have language. The work of Nikos Logothetis and his colleagues discussed in the last two chapters (e.g., Logothetis and Schall 1989; Leopold and Logothetis 1996; Sheinberg and Logothetis 1997) provides a beautiful example of experimental work on consciousness in nonhuman animals. This work uses experiments on monkeys to draw conclusions about the neural processes associated with consciousness. How do Logothetis et al. manage to draw conclusions about a monkey's consciousness without getting any verbal reports? They rely on the monkey's pressing bars. If the monkey can be made to press a bar in an appropriate way in response to a stimulus, we can say that that stimulus was consciously perceived.

The criterion at play seems to require that the information be available for an arbitrary response. If it turned out that the monkey could press a bar in response to a red light but could do nothing else, we would be tempted to say that it was not a case of consciousness at all but some sort of subconscious connection. If, on the other hand, we find information that is available for response in all sorts of different ways, then we will say that it is conscious.

The underlying general principle is something like this: when information is *directly available for global control* in a cognitive system, then it is conscious. If information is available for response in many motor modalities, we will say it is conscious, at least in a range of relatively familiar systems such as humans, other primates, and so on. This principle squares well with the preceding one in cases where the capacity for verbal report is present. Availability for verbal report and availability for global control seem to go together in such cases: report is one of the key aspects of control, after all, and it is rare to find information that is reportable but not available more widely. But this principle is also applicable when language is not present.

A correlation between consciousness and global availability (for short) seems to fit the first-person evidence—that gleaned from our own conscious experience—quite well. When information is present in my consciousness, it is generally reportable, and it can generally be brought to bear in controlling behavior in all sorts of ways. I can talk about it, I can point in the general direction of a stimulus, I can press bars, and so on. Conversely, when we find information that is directly available in this way for report and other aspects of control, it is generally conscious information. One can bear out this idea by considering cases.

There are some tricky puzzle cases to consider, such as blindsight, where one has *some* availability for control but arguably no conscious experience. Those cases might best be handled by invoking the directness of availability. Insofar as the information here is available for report and other control processes at all, the availability is indirect by comparison to the direct and automatic availability in standard cases. To exclude cases of involuntary unconscious response, one might also restrict the criterion to availability for *voluntary* control, although that is a complex issue.[1]

In any case, the resulting principle remains at best a first-order approximation of the functional criteria that come into play. Here, I am less interested in getting all of the fine details right than in exploring the consequences of the idea that some such functional criterion is required and is implicit in all of the empirical research on the neural correlate of consciousness. If you disagree with the criterion I have suggested—presumably because you can think of counterexamples—you may want to use those examples to refine it or to come up with a better criterion of your own. The crucial point is that in the very act of experimentally distinguishing conscious from unconscious processes, *some* such criterion is always at play.

If something like this is right, then what follows? That is, if some such bridging principles are implicit in the methodology for the search for the NCC, then what are the consequences? I use global availability as my main functional criterion in this discussion, but many of the points should generalize.

The first thing one can do is produce what philosophers might call a *rational reconstruction* of the search for the neural correlate of consciousness.

---

1. *Some further refinements: reflection on the Milner and Goodale (1995) method for ascribing consciousness suggests that availability to conceptual processing carries more weight than availability for motor processing. The process dissociation procedure of Jacoby, Lindsay, and Toth (1992) suggests a central role for availability for recollection. It is arguable that a criterion of availability for higher-order thought (cf. Carruthers 2000) can subsume most of the criteria at work in humans. Certainly, reporting an experience requires that one has formed higher-order beliefs about it, and when one forms such beliefs, one can usually report them.

With a rational reconstruction we can say: maybe things do not work exactly like this in practice, but the rational underpinnings of the procedure have something like this form. That is, if one were to try to *justify* the conclusions one has reached as well as possible, one's justification would follow the shape of the rational reconstruction. In this case, a rational reconstruction might look something like this.

1. Consciousness ↔ global availability (bridging principle)
2. Global availability ↔ neural process N (empirical work)

_____

3. Consciousness ↔ neural process N (conclusion)

According to this reconstruction, one implicitly embraces some sort of pre-experimental bridging principle that one finds plausible on independent grounds, such as conceptual or phenomenological grounds. Then one does the empirical research. Instead of measuring consciousness directly, we detect the functional property. We see that when this functional property (e.g., global availability) is present, it is correlated with a specific neural process (e.g., 40-hertz oscillations). Combining the pre-empirical premise and the empirical result, we arrive at the conclusion that this neural process is a candidate for the NCC.

Of course, it does not work nearly so simply in practice. The two stages are highly intertwined; our pre-experimental principles may themselves be refined as experimental research goes along. Nevertheless, I think one can make a separation into pre-experimental and experimental components for the sake of analysis. With this rational reconstruction in hand, what sort of conclusions follow? We can draw out at least the following six consequences.

(1) The first conclusion is a characterization of the neural correlates of consciousness. If the NCC is arrived at via this methodology, then whatever it turns out to be, it will be a *mechanism of global availability*. The presence of the NCC wherever global availability is present suggests that it is a mechanism that *subserves* global availability in the brain. The only alternative is that it might be a *symptom* rather than a *mechanism* of global availability, but in principle that possibility ought to be addressable by dissociation studies, lesioning, and so on. If a process is a mere symptom of availability, we ought to be able to empirically dissociate it from global availability while leaving the latter intact. The resulting data would suggest to us that consciousness can be present even when the neural process in question is not, thus indicating that it was not a perfect correlate of consciousness after all.

(A related line of reasoning supports the idea that a true NCC must be a mechanism of *direct* availability for global control. In principle, mechanisms of indirect availability will be dissociable from the empirical evidence for consciousness, for example by directly stimulating the mechanisms of direct availability. The indirect mechanisms will be "screened off" by the direct mechanisms in much the same way as the retina is screened off as an NCC by the visual cortex.)

In fact, if one looks at the various proposals, this template seems to fit them fairly well. For example, the 40-hertz oscillations discussed by Crick and Koch were put forward precisely because of the role they might have in binding and integrating information into working memory, and working memory is of course a major mechanism whereby information is made available for global control in a cognitive system. Similarly, it is plausible that Libet's extended neural activity is relevant precisely because the temporal extendedness of activity gives certain information the capacity to dominate later processes that lead to control. Baars's global workspace is a particularly clear example of such a mechanism: it is put forward explicitly as a mechanism whereby information can be globally disseminated. All of these mechanisms and many of the others seem to be candidates for mechanisms of global availability in the brain.

(2) This reconstruction suggests that a full story about the neural processes associated with consciousness will do two things. First, it will *explain* global availability in the brain. Once we know all about the relevant neural processes, we will know precisely how information is made directly available for global control in the brain, and this will be an explanation in the full sense. Global availability is a functional property, and as always the problem of explaining a function's performance is a problem to which mechanistic explanation is well suited. So we can be confident that within a century or two, global availability will be straightforwardly explained. Second, this explanation of availability will do something else: it will isolate the processes that *underlie* consciousness itself. If the bridging principle is granted, then mechanisms of availability will automatically be correlates of phenomenology in the full sense.

Unsurprisingly, I do not think this is a full *explanation* for consciousness. One can always ask why these processes of availability should give rise to consciousness in the first place. As yet we cannot explain why they do so, and it may well be that even full details about the processes of availability will not answer this question. Certainly, nothing in the standard methodology I have outlined answers the question; that methodology assumes a relation between availability and consciousness and therefore does nothing to explain it. The relationship between the two is instead taken as something of a primitive. So the hard problem remains. But who knows? Somewhere along the line we may be led to the relevant insights that show why the link is there, and the hard problem may then be solved. In the meantime, whether or not we have solved the hard problem, we may nevertheless have isolated the *basis* for consciousness in the brain. We just have to keep in mind the distinction between correlation and explanation.

(3) Given this paradigm, it is likely that there will be many neural correlates of consciousness. This suggestion mirrors an unsurprising suggestion in the last chapter, but this time the rational reconstruction illustrates just why such a multiplicity of correlates should exist. There will be many neural correlates of consciousness because there will be many mechanisms of global availability. There will be mechanisms in different modalities. The mechanisms of visual availability may be quite different from the mechanisms of auditory availability, for example. (Of course, they *may* be the same in that we could find a system that integrates and disseminates all of this information, but that is an open question.) There will also be mechanisms at different stages in the processing path whereby information is made globally available: early mechanisms and later ones. All of these may be candidates for the NCC. Furthermore, we will find mechanisms at many levels of description. For example, 40-hertz oscillations may well be redescribed as high-quality representations or as part of a global workspace at a different level of description. It may therefore turn out that a number of the animals in the zoo, so to speak, can coexist because they are compatible in one of these ways.

I will not speculate much further on just what the neural correlates of consciousness are. No doubt some of the ideas in the initial list will prove to be entirely off track, and some of the others will prove closer to the mark, but I hope the conceptual issues are becoming clearer.

(4) This way of thinking about things allows one to make sense of an idea that is sometimes floated: that of a *consciousness module*. Sometimes this notion is disparaged; sometimes it is embraced. The analysis given here suggests that it is at least possible that such a module exists. What would it take? It would require some sort of functionally localizable, internally integrated system through which all global availability runs. The system need not be anatomically localizable, but to qualify as a module it would need to be localizable in some broader sense. For example, the parts of the module would have to have high-bandwidth communication among themselves, compared to the relatively low-bandwidth communication that they have with other areas. Such a thing

could turn out to exist. It does not strike me as especially likely that things will turn out this way; it seems just as likely that we will find multiple independent mechanisms of global availability in the brain, scattered around without much mutual integration. If that is the result, we will probably say that there is no consciousness module after all. But that is an empirical question.

If something like this module did turn out to exist in the brain, it would resemble Baars's conception of a global workspace: a functional area responsible for integrating information in the brain and disseminating it to multiple nonconscious, specialized processes. Many of the ideas I put forward here are compatible with things that Baars has said about the role of global availability in the study of consciousness. Indeed, this way of looking at things suggests that some of his ideas are direct consequences of the methodology. The special epistemological role of global availability helps explain why the idea of a global workspace is a useful way of thinking about almost any empirical proposal about consciousness. If NCCs are identified as such precisely because of their role in global control, then at least on a first approximation, we should expect the global workspace idea to be a natural fit.

(5) We can apply this picture to the question of whether the neural correlates of *visual* consciousness are to be found in V1, in the extrastriate visual cortex, or elsewhere. If our picture of the methodology is correct, then the answer depends on which visual area is most directly implicated in global availability.

Crick and Koch (1995) have suggested that the visual NCC is not to be found within V1, because V1 does not contain neurons that project to the prefrontal cortex. This reasoning has been criticized by Ned Block for conflating access consciousness and phenomenal consciousness (see Block 1995). Interestingly, the picture I have developed suggests that it may be good reasoning. The prefrontal cortex is known to be associated with control processes, so *if* a given area in the visual cortex projects to prefrontal areas, then it may well be a mechanism of direct availability. If it does not project in this way, it is less likely to be such a mechanism; at best it might be *indirectly* associated with global availability. Of course, we still have plenty of room to raise questions about the empirical details. The broader point is that for the sort of reasons discussed in (2) earlier, it is likely that the neural processes involved in *explaining* access consciousness will simultaneously be involved in a story about the *basis* of phenomenal consciousness. If something like this idea is implicit in their reasoning, Crick and Koch might escape the charge of conflation. Of course, the reasoning depends on these somewhat shaky bridging principles, but then all work on the neural correlates of consciousness must appeal to such principles somewhere, so this limitation cannot be held against Crick and Koch in particular.[2]

(6) Sometimes the neural correlate of consciousness is conceived of as a holy grail for a theory of consciousness. It will make everything fall into place. For example, once we discover the NCC, then we will have a definitive test for consciousness, enabling us to discover consciousness wherever it arises. That is, we might use the neural correlate itself as a sort of consciousness meter. If a system has 40-hertz oscillations (say), then it is conscious; if it has none, then it is not conscious. Or if a thalamocortical system turns out to be the NCC, then a system without such a system is unlikely to be conscious. This sort of reasoning is not usually put quite so baldly, but I think one finds some version of it quite frequently.

This reasoning can be tempting, but one should not succumb to the temptation. Given the very methodology that comes into play here, we have no way of definitely establishing a given NCC as an independent test for consciousness. The primary criterion for consciousness will always remain the functional property we started with: global availability or verbal report or whatever. That is how we discovered the correlations in the first place. In other words, 40-hertz oscillations (or whatever) are relevant *because* of their role in satisfying this criterion. True, in cases where we know that this association between the NCC and the functional property is present, the NCC might itself function as a sort of "signature" of consciousness, but once we dissociate the NCC from the functional property, all bets are off. To take an extreme example, if we have 40-hertz oscillations in a test tube, that condition almost certainly will not yield consciousness, but the point applies equally in less extreme cases. Because it was the bridging principles that gave us all the traction in the search for an NCC in the

---

2. *In Chalmers (1997a), I used reasoning of this sort to argue that there is a sort of access consciousness that cannot be experimentally dissociated from phenomenal consciousness. Block (2007, 485) terms this view "epistemic correlationism" and appears to argue against it in maintaining that phenomenal and access consciousness can be dissociated. Here the idea is that data beyond verbal reports could break the correlation. However, all of the data that Block points to (in discussing the results of Sperling 1960, for example) are broadly functional data that suggest a sort of availability. As Block ultimately acknowledges (2007, 489), while the data may suggest that phenomenal consciousness can exist without a strong sort of accessibility, they are quite compatible with the thesis that phenomenal consciousness always involves the weaker sort of accessibility that is at issue here. Block's conclusion is that that the machinery of phenomenology is distinct from that of accessibility. I prefer to conclude that the neural correlates of phenomenology are distinct from those of *access*, and that there is nevertheless likely to be a tight link between the two, in that the former are likely to serve as input to the latter. Of course, this is compatible with the view that the neural correlates of visual experience are in the visual cortex (perhaps outside V1), while the neural correlates of access are largely in the prefrontal cortex.

first place, it is not clear that anything follows in cases where the functional criterion is thrown away. So there is no free lunch here. One cannot get something for nothing.

Once we recognize the central role of pre-experimental assumptions in the search for the NCC, we realize that there are limitations on just what we can expect this search to tell us. Still, whether or not the NCC is the holy grail, it is clear that the quest for it is likely to enhance our understanding considerably. I hope to have made a case that in this area, philosophy and neuroscience can come together to help clarify some of the deep problems involved in the study of consciousness.

Part III

THE METAPHYSICS OF CONSCIOUSNESS

5

CONSCIOUSNESS AND ITS PLACE IN NATURE

1. Introduction

Consciousness fits uneasily into our conception of the natural world. On the most common conception of nature, the natural world is the physical world. But on the most common conception of consciousness, it is not easy to see how it could be part of the physical world. So it seems that to find a place for consciousness within the natural order, we must either revise our conception of consciousness or revise our conception of nature.

In twentieth-century philosophy, this dilemma is posed most acutely in C. D. Broad's *The Mind and Its Place in Nature* (1925). For Broad, the phenomena of mind are the phenomena of consciousness. The central problem is that of locating mind with respect to the physical world. Broad's exhaustive discussion of the problem culminates in a taxonomy of seventeen different views of the mental-physical relation.[1] In Broad's taxonomy, a view might see the mental as nonexistent ("delusive"), as reducible, as emergent, or as a basic property of a substance (a "differentiating" attribute). The physical might be seen in one of the same four ways. So a four-by-four matrix of views results. (The seventeenth entry arises from Broad's division of the substance/substance view according to whether one or two substances are involved.) At the end, three views are left standing: those on

---

1. The taxonomy is in the final chapter, chapter 14, of Broad's book (set out on pp. 607–11, and discussed up to p. 650). The dramatization of Broad's taxonomy as a 4x4 matrix is illustrated on Andrew Chrucky's website devoted to Broad (http://consc.net/broad.html).

which mentality is an emergent characteristic of either a physical substance or a neutral substance, where in the latter case, the physical might be either emergent or delusive.

In this chapter I take my cue from Broad, approaching the problem of consciousness by a strategy of divide and conquer. I do not adopt Broad's categories: our understanding of the mind-body problem has advanced in the last seventy-five years, and it would be nice to think that we have a better understanding of the crucial issues. On my view, the most important views on the metaphysics of consciousness can be divided into six classes, which I label "type A" through "type F." Three of these (A through C) involve broadly reductive views, which see consciousness as a physical process that requires no expansion of a physical ontology. The other three (D through F) involve broadly nonreductive views, according to which consciousness involves something irreducible in nature and requires expansion or reconception of a physical ontology.

The discussion in this chapter is cast at an abstract level, giving an overview of the metaphysical landscape. Rather than engaging the empirical science of consciousness or detailed philosophical theories of consciousness, I examine some general classes into which theories of consciousness might fall. I do not pretend to be neutral in this discussion. I think that each of the reductive views is incorrect, while each of the nonreductive views holds some promise. So the first part of this chapter is an extended argument against reductive views of consciousness, while the second part is an investigation of where we go from there.

2. The Problem

A being is conscious in the sense I am concerned with when there is something it is like to be that being. A mental state is conscious when there is something it is like to be in that state. Conscious states include states of perceptual experience, bodily sensation, mental imagery, emotional experience, occurrent thought, and more. There is something it is like to see a vivid green, to feel a sharp pain, to visualize the Eiffel tower, to feel a deep regret, and to think that one is late. Each of these states has a *phenomenal character*, with *phenomenal properties* (or *qualia*) that characterize what it is like to be in the state.[2]

---

2. In my usage, qualia are simply those properties that characterize conscious states according to what it is like to have them. The definition does not build in any further substantive requirements such as the requirement that qualia are intrinsic or nonintentional. If qualia are intrinsic or nonintentional, this will be a substantive rather than a definitional point (so the claim that the properties of consciousness are nonintrinsic or that they are wholly intentional should not be taken to entail that there are no

The hard problem of consciousness (chapter 1) is that of explaining how and why physical processes give rise to phenomenal consciousness. A solution to the hard problem would involve an account of the relation between physical processes and consciousness, explaining on the basis of natural principles how and why it is that physical processes are associated with states of experience. A *reductive explanation* of consciousness will explain this wholly on the basis of physical principles that do not themselves make any appeal to consciousness.[3] A *materialist* (or physicalist) solution is a solution on which consciousness is itself seen as a physical process. A *nonmaterialist* (or nonphysicalist) solution is a solution on which consciousness is seen as nonphysical (even if closely associated with physical processes). A *nonreductive* solution is one on which consciousness (or principles involving consciousness) is admitted as a basic part of the explanation.

It is natural to hope that there will be a materialist solution to the hard problem and a reductive explanation of consciousness, just as there have been reductive explanations of many other phenomena in many other domains. But we have already seen that consciousness seems to resist materialist explanation in a way that other phenomena do not. This resistance can be encapsulated in three related arguments against materialism, summarized in what follows.

3. Arguments against Materialism

3.1 The Explanatory Argument

The first argument is grounded in the difference between the easy problems and the hard problem: the easy problems concern the explanation of behavioral and cognitive functions, but the hard problem does not. One can argue that by the character of physical explanation, physical accounts

---

qualia). Phenomenal properties can also be taken to be properties of individuals (e.g., people) rather than of mental states, characterizing aspects of what it is like to be them at a given time; the difference will not matter much for present purposes.

3. Note that I use "reductive" in a broader sense than it is sometimes used. Reductive explanation requires only that high-level phenomena can be explained wholly in terms of low-level phenomena. This is compatible with the "multiple realizability" of high-level phenomena in low-level phenomena. For example, there may be many different ways in which digestion could be realized in a physiological system, but one can nevertheless reductively explain a system's digestion in terms of underlying physiology. Another subtlety concerns the possibility of a view on which consciousness can be explained in terms of principles that do not appeal to consciousness but cannot themselves be physically explained. These definitions count such a view as neither reductive nor nonreductive. It could reasonably be classified either way, but I generally assimilate it with the nonreductive class.

explain *only* structure and function, where the relevant structures are spatiotemporal structures, and the relevant functions are causal roles in the production of a system's behavior. Furthermore, one can argue as in chapter 1 and 2 that explaining structures and functions does not suffice to explain consciousness. If so, no physical account can explain consciousness.

We can call this the explanatory argument[4] (formalized here as a mild variant on the three-premise argument in chapter 2):

1. Physical accounts explain at most structure and function.
2. Explaining structure and function does not suffice to explain consciousness.

_____

3. No physical account can explain consciousness.

If this is right, then while physical accounts can solve the easy problems (which involve only explaining functions), something more is needed to solve the hard problem. It would seem that no reductive explanation of consciousness could succeed. And if we add the premise that what cannot be physically explained is not itself physical (this can be considered an additional final step of the explanatory argument), then materialism about consciousness is false, and the natural world contains more than the physical world.

Of course, this sort of argument is controversial. But before examining various ways of responding, it is useful to examine two closely related arguments that also aim to establish that materialism about consciousness is false.

3.2 The Conceivability Argument

According to this argument, it is conceivable that there be a system that is physically identical to a conscious being but that lacks at least some of that being's conscious states.[5] Such a system might be a *zombie*: a system that is physically identical to a conscious being but that lacks consciousness entirely. It might also be an *invert*, with some of the original being's experiences

_____

4. For more on the explanatory argument, see chapter 1 and the section on type-C materialism in this chapter, as well as Levine (1983) on the "explanatory gap," Nagel (1974), and the papers in Shear (1997).

5. Versions of the conceivability argument are put forward by Bealer (1994), Campbell (1970), Chalmers (1996), Kirk (1974), and Kripke (1980), among others. Important predecessors include Descartes' conceivability argument about disembodiment and Leibniz's "mill" argument. For much more on the conceivability argument, see chapter 6.

replaced by different experiences, or a *partial zombie*, with some experiences absent, or a combination thereof. These systems will look identical to a normal conscious being from the third-person perspective. In particular, their brain processes will be molecule-for-molecule identical with the original, and their behavior will be indistinguishable. But things will be different from the first-person point of view. What it is like to be an invert or a partial zombie will differ from what it is like to be the original being. And there is nothing it is like to be a zombie.

There is little reason to believe that zombies exist in the actual world, but many hold that they are at least conceivable: we can coherently imagine zombies, and there is no contradiction in the idea that reveals itself even on reflection. As an extension of the idea, many hold that the same goes for a *zombie world*: a universe physically identical to ours but in which there is no consciousness. Something similar applies to inverts and other duplicates.

From the conceivability of zombies, proponents of the argument infer their *metaphysical possibility*. Zombies are probably not naturally possible: they probably cannot exist in our world with its laws of nature. But the argument holds that zombies *could have* existed, perhaps in a very different sort of universe. For example, it is sometimes suggested that God could have created a zombie world if he had so chosen. From here, it is inferred that consciousness must be nonphysical. If there is a metaphysically possible universe that is physically identical to ours but that lacks consciousness, then consciousness must be a further, nonphysical component of our universe. If God could have created a zombie world, then (as Kripke puts it) after creating the physical processes in our world, he had to do more work to ensure that it contained consciousness.

We can put the argument in its simplest form as follows:

1. It is conceivable that there are zombies.
2. If it is conceivable that there are zombies, it is metaphysically possible that there are zombies.
3. If it is metaphysically possible that there are zombies, then consciousness is nonphysical.

---

4. Consciousness is nonphysical.

A somewhat more general and precise version of the argument appeals to P, the conjunction of all microphysical truths about the universe, and Q, an arbitrary phenomenal truth about the universe. (Here, '&' represents 'and' and '~' represents 'not.')

1. It is conceivable that $P\&\sim Q$.
2. If it is conceivable that $P\&\sim Q$, it is metaphysically possible that $P\&\sim Q$.
3. If it is metaphysically possible that $P\&\sim Q$, then materialism is false.

———————

4. Materialism is false.

3.3 The Knowledge Argument

According to the knowledge argument, there are facts about consciousness that are not deducible from physical facts.[6] Someone could know all of the physical facts, be a perfect reasoner, and still be unable to know all of the facts about consciousness on that basis.

Frank Jackson's canonical version of the argument (Jackson 1982) provides a vivid illustration. In this version, Mary is a neuroscientist who knows everything there is to know about the physical processes relevant to color vision. But she has been brought up in a black-and-white room (in an alternative version, she is colorblind[7]) and has never experienced red. Despite all her knowledge, it seems that there is something very important about color vision that Mary does not know. She does not know what it is like to see red. Even complete physical knowledge and unrestricted powers of deduction do not enable her to know this. Later, if she comes to experience red for the first time, she will learn a new fact of which she was previously ignorant: she will learn what it is like to see red.

Jackson's version of the argument can be put as follows (here the premises concern Mary's knowledge when she has not yet experienced red):

1. Mary knows all the physical facts.
2. Mary does not know all the facts.

———————

3. The physical facts do not exhaust all the facts.

6. Sources for the knowledge argument include Jackson (1982), N. Maxwell (1968), Nagel (1974), and others. Predecessors of the argument are present in Broad's discussion of a "mathematical archangel" who cannot deduce the smell of ammonia from physical facts (Broad 1925, 70–71), and in Feigl's discussion of a "Martian superscientist" who cannot know what colors look like and what musical tones sound like (Feigl 1958/1967, 64, 68, 140). For more on the knowledge argument, see the afterword to chapter 6.

7. This version of the thought experiment had a real-life exemplar in Knut Nordby, a Norwegian sensory biologist who was a rod monochromat (lacking cones in his retina for color vision) and who worked on the physiology of color vision. See Nordby (1990) and Nordby (2007), in which he discusses the Mary scenario explicitly.

One can put the knowledge argument more generally:[8]

1. There are truths about consciousness that are not deducible from physical truths.
2. If there are truths about consciousness that are not deducible from physical truths, then materialism is false.

---

3. Materialism is false.

3.4 The Shape of the Arguments

These three sorts of argument are closely related. They all start by establishing an *epistemic gap* between the physical and the phenomenal domains. Each denies a certain sort of close epistemic relation between the domains: a relation involving what we can know or conceive or explain. In particular, each of them denies a certain sort of *epistemic entailment* from physical truths P to the phenomenal truths Q: deducibility of Q from P or explainability of Q in terms of P or conceiving of Q upon reflective conceiving of P.

Perhaps the most basic sort of epistemic entailment is a priori entailment, or *implication*. On this notion, P implies Q when the conditional 'If P then Q' is a priori—that is, when a subject can know that if P is the case, then Q is the case with justification independent of experience. All of these three arguments can be seen as making a case against the claim that P implies Q. If a perfect reasoner who knows only P cannot deduce that Q (as the knowledge argument suggests), or if one can rationally conceive of P without Q (as the conceivability argument suggests), then it seems that P does not imply Q. The explanatory argument can be seen as turning on the claim that an implication from P to Q would require a functional analysis of consciousness and that the concept of consciousness is not a functional concept.

After establishing an epistemic gap, these arguments proceed by inferring an ontological gap, where ontology concerns the nature of things in the world. The conceivability argument infers from conceivability to metaphysical possibility; the knowledge argument infers from failure of deducibility to difference in facts; and the explanatory argument infers from failure of physical explanation to nonphysicality. One might say that these

---

8. *For more on these and other formulations of the knowledge argument, see the afterword to chapter 6.

arguments infer from a failure of epistemic entailment to a failure of onto-logical entailment. The paradigmatic sort of ontological entailment is *necessitation*: P necessitates Q when the conditional 'If P then Q' is meta-physically necessary or when it is metaphysically impossible for P to hold without Q holding. It is widely agreed that materialism requires that P necessitates all truths (perhaps with minor qualifications). So if there are phenomenal truths Q that P does not necessitate, then materialism is false.

We might call these arguments *epistemic arguments* against materialism. Epistemic arguments arguably descend from Descartes' arguments against materialism (although these have a slightly different form). As a class, they are given their first thorough airing in Broad's book, which contains elements of all three earlier arguments.[9] The general form of an epistemic argument against materialism is as follows:

1. There is an epistemic gap between physical and phenomenal truths.
2. If there is an epistemic gap between physical and phenomenal truths, then there is an ontological gap, and materialism is false.

_____

3. Materialism is false.

Of course, this way of looking at things oversimplifies matters and abstracts away from the differences between the arguments.[10] The same goes for the precise analysis in terms of implication and necessitation. Nevertheless, this analysis provides a useful lens through which we can see what the arguments have in common and analyze various responses to them.

There are roughly three ways that a materialist might resist the epistemic arguments. A type-A materialist denies the existence of the relevant sort of epistemic gap. A type-B materialist accepts the existence of an unclosable epistemic gap but denies that there is an ontological gap. A type-C materialist

9. For limited versions of the conceivability argument and the explanatory argument, see Broad (1925, 614–15). For the knowledge argument, see pp. 70–72, where Broad argues that even a "mathe-matical archangel" could not deduce the smell of ammonia from microscopic knowledge of atoms. Broad is arguing against "mechanism," which is roughly equivalently to contemporary materialism. To contemporary eyes, perhaps the biggest lacuna in Broad's argument is any consideration of the possi-bility that there is an epistemic but not an ontological gap.

10. For a discussion of the relationship between various anti-materialist arguments, see the after-word to chapter 6.

accepts the existence of a deep epistemic gap but holds that it will eventually be closed. In what follows, I discuss all three of these strategies.

4. Type-A Materialism

According to type-A materialism, there is no epistemic gap between physical and phenomenal truths, or at least any apparent epistemic gap is easily closed. According to this view, it is not conceivable (at least on reflection) that there are duplicates of conscious beings that have absent or inverted conscious states. On this view, there are no phenomenal truths of which Mary is ignorant in principle from inside her black-and-white room (when she leaves the room, she gains at most an ability). And on this view, on reflection there is no hard problem of explaining consciousness that remains once one has solved the easy problems of explaining the various cognitive, behavioral, and environmental functions.[11]

Type-A materialism sometimes takes the form of eliminativism, holding that consciousness does not exist and that there are no phenomenal truths. It sometimes takes the form of analytic functionalism or logical behaviorism, which holds that consciousness exists, where the concept of "consciousness" is defined in wholly functional or behavioral terms (e.g., where to be conscious might be to have certain sorts of access to information and/or certain sorts of dispositions to make verbal reports). For our purposes, the difference between these two views is terminological. Both agree that we are conscious in the sense of having the functional capacities of access, report, control, and the like, and they agree that we are not conscious in any further (nonfunctionally defined) sense. The analytic functionalist thinks that ordinary terms such as 'conscious' should be used in the first sense (expressing a functional concept), while the eliminativist thinks that it should be used in the second. Beyond this terminological disagreement about the use of existing terms and concepts, the substance of the views is much the same.

Some philosophers and scientists who do not explicitly embrace eliminativism, analytic functionalism, and the like are nevertheless recognizably type-A materialists. The characteristic feature of the type-A materialist is the view that on reflection there is nothing in the vicinity of consciousness that needs explaining over and above explaining the various functions: to explain these things is to explain everything that needs to be explained.

---

11. Type-A materialists include Dennett (1991), Dretske (1995), Harman (1990), Lewis (1988), Rey (1995), and Ryle (1949).

The relevant functions may be quite subtle and complex, involving fine-grained capacities for access, self-monitoring, report, control, and their interaction, for example. They may also be taken to include all sorts of environmental relations. Furthermore, the explanation of these functions will probably involve much neurobiological detail, so views that are put forward as rejecting functionalism on the grounds that it neglects either biology or the role of the environment may still be type-A views.

One might think that there is room in logical space for a view that denies even this sort of broadly functionalist view of consciousness but still holds that there is no epistemic gap between physical and phenomenal truths. In practice, there appears to be little room for such a view for reasons that I discuss under type C, and there are few examples of such views in practice.[12] So I take it for granted that a type-A view is one that holds that explaining the functions explains everything, and I class other views that hold that there is no unclosable epistemic gap under type C.

The obvious problem with type-A materialism is that it appears to deny the manifest. It is an uncontested truth that we have the various functional capacities of access, control, report, and the like, and these phenomena pose uncontested explananda (phenomena in need of explanation) for a science of consciousness. In addition, it seems to be a further truth that we are conscious, and this phenomenon seems to pose a further explanandum, one that raises the interesting problems of consciousness. To flatly deny the further truth, or to deny without argument that there is a hard problem of consciousness over and above the easy problems, would be to make a highly counterintuitive claim that begs the important questions. This is not to say that highly counterintuitive claims are always false, but they need to be supported by extremely strong arguments. So the crucial question is whether there are any compelling *arguments* for the claim that, on reflection, explaining the functions explains everything.

Type-A materialists often argue by analogy. They point out that in other areas of science, we accept that explaining the various functions explains the phenomena, so we should accept the same here. And they suggest that with phenomena such as life and heat, thinkers in the past have pointed

12. Two specific views may be worth mentioning: (i) Some views (e.g., Dretske 1995) deny an epistemic gap while at the same time denying functionalism by holding that consciousness involves not just a functional role but also causal and historical relations to objects in the environment. I count these as type-A views: we can view the relevant relations as part of a functional role, broadly construed, and exactly the same considerations arise. (ii) Some views (e.g., Stoljar 2001b and Strawson 2000) deny an epistemic gap not by functionally analyzing consciousness but by expanding our view of the physical base to include underlying intrinsic properties. These views are discussed under type F.

out analogous epistemic gaps and that these phenomena turned out to be physically explained all the same. For reasons discussed in chapter 1 and the afterword there, however, these analogies carry little force. In other domains, it has long been clear (even to vitalists) that the central explananda all involve structure and function, except perhaps for those tied directly to consciousness itself.[13] So the type-A materialist needs to address the apparent further explanandum in the case of consciousness head on: either flatly denying it or giving substantial arguments to dissolve it.

Some arguments for type-A materialists proceed indirectly by pointing out the unsavory metaphysical or epistemological consequences of rejecting the view: for instance, that the rejection leads to dualism or to problems involving knowledge of consciousness.[14] An opponent will either embrace the consequences or deny that they are consequences. As long as the consequences are not completely untenable, then for the type-A materialist to make progress, this sort of argument needs to be supplemented by a substantial direct argument against the further explanandum.

Such direct arguments are surprisingly hard to find. Many arguments for type-A materialism end up presupposing the conclusion at crucial points. For example, it is sometimes argued (e.g., Rey 1995) that there is no reason to postulate qualia since they are not needed to explain behavior, but this argument presupposes that only behavior needs explaining. The opponent will hold that qualia are an explanandum in their own right. Similarly, Dennett's use of "heterophenomenology" (verbal reports) as the primary data to ground his theory of consciousness (Dennett 1991) appears to rest on the assumption that these reports are what need explaining or that the only "seemings" that need explaining are dispositions to react and report.

One way to argue for type-A materialism is to argue that there is some intermediate X such that (i) explaining functions suffices to explain X and (ii) explaining X suffices to explain consciousness. One possible X here is *representation*. It is often held both that conscious states are representational states, representing things in the world, and that we can

---

13. The disanalogy is very clear in Broad's case. Broad was a vitalist about life, holding that the functions would require a nonmechanical explanation. At the same time, though, he held that, in the case of life, unlike the case of consciousness, the only evidence we have for the phenomenon is behavioral and that "being alive" means exhibiting certain sorts of behavior.

14. For an argument from unsavory metaphysical consequences, see White (1986). For an argument from unsavory epistemological consequences, see Shoemaker (1975). The metaphysical consequences are addressed in the second half of this chapter. The epistemological consequences are addressed in Chalmers (2002b).

explain representation in functional terms. If so, it may seem to follow that we can explain consciousness in functional terms. On examination, though, this argument appeals to an ambiguity in the notion of representation. There is a notion of *functional representation*, on which *p* is represented roughly when a system responds to *p* and/or produces behavior appropriate for *p*. In this sense, explaining functioning may explain representation, but explaining representation does not explain consciousness. There is also a notion of *phenomenal representation*, on which *p* is represented roughly when a system has a conscious experience as if *p*. In this sense, explaining representation may explain consciousness, but explaining functioning does not explain representation. Either way, the epistemic gap between the functional and the phenomenal remains as wide as ever. Similar sorts of equivocation can be found with other examples of *X* that might be appealed to here, such as "perception" or "information."

Perhaps the most interesting arguments for type-A materialism are those that maintain that we can give a physical explanation of our *beliefs* about consciousness, such as the belief that we are conscious, the belief that consciousness is a further explanandum, and the belief that consciousness is nonphysical. From here it is argued that once we have explained the belief, we have done enough to explain (or to explain away) the phenomenon (e.g., Clark 2000; Dennett 2001). Here it is worth noting that this works only if the beliefs themselves are functionally analyzable; in chapter 8 I give some reasons to deny this. But even if one accepts that beliefs are ultimately functional, this claim then reduces to the claim that explaining our dispositions to talk about consciousness (and the like) explains everything. An opponent will deny this claim: explaining the dispositions to report may remove the third-person warrant (based on observation of others) for accepting a further explanandum, but it does not remove the crucial first-person warrant (from one's own case). Still, this is a strategy that deserves extended discussion.

At a certain point, the debate between type-A materialists and their opponents usually comes down to intuition: most centrally, the intuition that consciousness (in a nonfunctionally defined sense) exists or that there is something that needs to be explained (over and above explaining the functions). This claim does not gain its support from argument but from a sort of observation, along with rebuttal of counterarguments. The intuition appears to be shared by the large majority of philosophers, scientists, and others, and it is so strong that to deny it, a type-A materialist needs exceptionally powerful arguments. The result is that even among materialists, type-A materialists are a distinct minority.

5. Type-B Materialism

According to type-B materialism, there is an epistemic gap between the physical and phenomenal domains, but there is no ontological gap.[15] According to this view, zombies and the like are conceivable, but they are not metaphysically possible. On this view, Mary is ignorant of some phenomenal truths from inside her room, but nevertheless these truths concern an underlying physical reality (when she leaves the room, she learns old facts in a new way). And on this view, while there is a hard problem distinct from the easy problems, it does not correspond to a distinct ontological domain.

The most common form of type-B materialism holds that phenomenal states can be *identified* with certain physical or functional states. This identity is held to be analogous in certain respects (although perhaps not in all respects) with the identity between water and H_2O or between genes and DNA.[16] These identities are not derived through conceptual analysis but are discovered empirically. The concept *water* is different from the concept H_2O, but they are found to refer to the same thing in nature. On the type-B view, something similar applies to consciousness: the concept of consciousness is distinct from any physical or functional concepts, but we may discover empirically that these refer to the same thing in nature. In this way, we can explain why there is an epistemic gap between the physical and phenomenal domains while still denying any ontological gap. This yields the attractive possibility that we can acknowledge the deep epistemic problems of consciousness while retaining a materialist worldview.

Although such a view is attractive, it faces immediate difficulties. These stem from the fact that the character of the epistemic gap with consciousness seems to differ from that of epistemic gaps in other domains. For a start, there do not seem to be analogs of the earlier epistemic arguments in the cases of water, genes, and so on. To explain genes, we merely have to explain why systems function a certain way in transmitting hereditary characteristics; to explain water, we have to explain why a substance has a certain objective structure and behavior. Given a complete physical

---

15. Type-B materialists include Block and Stalnaker (1999), Hill (1997), Levine (1983), Loar (1990/1997), Lycan (1996), Papineau (1993), Perry (2001), and Tye (1995).

16. In certain respects, where type-A materialism can be seen as deriving from the logical behaviorism of Ryle and Carnap, type-B materialism can be seen as deriving from the identity theory of Place and Smart. The matter is complicated, however, by the fact that the early identity theorists advocated "topic-neutral" (functional) analyses of phenomenal properties, suggesting an underlying type-A materialism.

description of the world, Mary would be able to deduce all of the relevant truths about water and about genes by deducing which systems have the appropriate structure and function. Finally, it seems that we cannot coherently conceive of a world physically identical to our own, in which there is no water or in which there are no genes. So there is no epistemic gap between the *complete* physical truth about the world and the truth about water and genes that is analogous to the epistemic gap with consciousness—except perhaps for epistemic gaps that derive from the epistemic gap for consciousness. For example, perhaps Mary could not deduce or explain the perceptual *appearance* of water from the physical truth about the world, but this would just be another instance of the problem we are concerned with and so cannot help the type-B materialist.

So it seems that there is something unique about the case of consciousness. We can put this by saying that while the identity between genes and DNA is empirical, it is not *epistemically primitive*: the identity is itself deducible from the complete physical truth about the world. By contrast, the type-B materialist must hold that the identification between consciousness and physical or functional states is epistemically primitive: the identity is not deducible from the complete physical truth. (If it were deducible, type-A materialism would be true instead.) So the identity between consciousness and a physical state will be a sort of primitive principle in one's theory of the world.

Here, one might suggest that something has gone wrong. Elsewhere, the only place that one finds this sort of primitive principle is in the fundamental laws of physics. Indeed, it is often held that this sort of primitiveness—the inability to be deduced from more basic principles—is the mark of a fundamental law of nature. In effect, the type-B materialist recognizes a principle that has the epistemic status of a fundamental law but gives it the ontological status of an identity. An opponent will hold that this move is more akin to theft than to honest toil. Elsewhere, identifications are grounded in explanations, and primitive principles are acknowledged as fundamental laws.

It is natural to suggest that the same should apply here. If one acknowledges the epistemically primitive connection between physical states and consciousness as a fundamental law, it will follow that consciousness is distinct from any physical property since fundamental laws always connect distinct properties. So the usual standard will lead to one of the nonreductive views discussed in the second half of this chapter. By contrast, the type-B materialist takes an observed connection between physical and phenomenal states, unexplainable in more basic terms, and suggests that it is an identity. This suggestion is made largely in order to preserve a prior commitment to materialism. Unless there is an independent case for primitive identities, the suggestion will seem at best ad hoc and mysterious and at worst incoherent.

A type-B materialist might respond in various ways. First, some (e.g., Papineau 1993) suggest that identities do not *need* to be explained and are always primitive. However, we have seen that identities in other domains can at least be *deduced* from more basic truths and so are not primitive in the relevant sense. Second, some (e.g., Block and Stalnaker 1999) suggest that even truths involving water and genes cannot be deduced from underlying physical truths. I argue in chapter 7 that these responses are unsuccessful. For now, one can note that the epistemic arguments outlined at the beginning suggest a very strong disanalogy between consciousness and other cases.

There is another line that a type-B materialist can take. One can first note that an *identity* between consciousness and physical states is not strictly required for a materialist position. Rather, one can plausibly hold that materialism about consciousness simply requires that physical states *necessitate* phenomenal states in that it is metaphysically impossible for the physical states to be present while the phenomenal states are absent or different. That is, materialism requires that entailments $P \supset Q$ be necessary, where P is the complete physical truth about the world and Q is an arbitrary phenomenal truth.

At this point, a type-B materialist can naturally appeal to the work of Kripke (1980), which suggests that some truths are necessarily true without being a priori. For example, Kripke suggests that 'water is H_2O' is necessary—true in all possible worlds—but not knowable a priori. Here, a type-B materialist can suggest that $P \supset Q$ may be a Kripkean a posteriori necessity, like 'water is H_2O' (though Kripke himself denies this claim). If so, then we would *expect* there to be an epistemic gap since there is no a priori entailment from P to Q, but at the same time there will be no ontological gap. In this way, Kripke's work can seem to be just what the type-B materialist needs.

Here, some of the issues that arose previously arise again. One can argue that in other domains, necessities are not epistemically primitive. The necessary connection between water and H_2O may be a posteriori, but it can itself be deduced from a complete physical description of the world (one can deduce that water is identical to H_2O, from which it follows that water is necessarily H_2O). The same applies to the other necessities that Kripke discusses. By contrast, the type-B materialist must hold that the connection between physical states and consciousness is epistemically primitive in that it cannot be deduced from the complete physical truth about the world. Again, one can suggest that this sort of primitive necessary connection is mysterious and ad hoc and that the connection should instead be viewed as a fundamental law of nature.

I discuss these necessities and their problems at much greater length in chapter 6. For now, it is worth noting that there is a sense in which any type-B materialist position gives up on reductive explanation. Even if type-B materialism is true, we cannot give consciousness the same sort of explanation that we give genes and the like in purely physical terms. Rather, our explanation will always require explanatorily primitive principles to bridge the gap from the physical to the phenomenal. The *explanatory* structure of a theory of consciousness, on such a view, will be very much unlike that of a materialist theory in other domains and very much like the explanatory structure of the nonreductive theories described later. If one labels these principles identities or necessities rather than laws, the view may preserve the letter of materialism, but by requiring primitive bridging principles, one sacrifices much of materialism's spirit.

Perhaps the most interesting response from a type-B materialist is to acknowledge that the epistemic gap is unique to the case of consciousness and to try to explain this uniqueness in terms of special features of our conceptual system. I discuss this response in chapter 10, where I argue that the strategy cannot help the materialist. For the special features of our conceptual system to explain the unique epistemic gap in the case of consciousness, these features will themselves pose an explanatory gap that is as large as the original.

7. Type-C Materialism

According to type-C materialism, there is a deep epistemic gap between the physical and phenomenal domains, but it is closable in principle. On this view, zombies and the like are conceivable for us now, but they will not be conceivable in the limit. The view holds that while it currently seems that Mary lacks information about the phenomenal, in the limit there would be no information that she lacks. And while we cannot see now how to solve the hard problem in physical terms, the problem is solvable in principle.

This view is initially very attractive. It seems to acknowledge the deep explanatory gap with which we are faced while at the same time allowing that the apparent gap may be due to our own limitations. There are different versions of the view. Nagel (1974) has suggested that just as the pre-Socratics could not have understood how matter could be energy, we cannot understand how consciousness could be physical, but a conceptual revolution might allow the relevant understanding. Churchland (1997) suggests that even if we cannot now imagine how consciousness could be a physical process, that is simply a psychological limitation on our part that further progress in science will overcome. Van Gulick (1993) suggests that conceivability arguments are question-begging since once we have a good explanation of consciousness, zombies and the like will no longer be conceivable. McGinn (1989) has suggested that the problem may be unsolvable by humans due to deep limitations in our cognitive abilities but that it nevertheless has a solution in principle. Stoljar (2007) argues that zombies are conceivable for us because we are ignorant of some crucial fact but that once we learn that fact they may no longer be conceivable.

One way to put the view is as follows. Zombies and the like are prima facie conceivable (for us now, with our current cognitive processes), but they are not *ideally* conceivable (under idealized rational reflection). Alternatively, we could say that phenomenal truths are deducible in principle from physical truths, but the deducibility is akin to that of a complex truth of mathematics. It is accessible in principle (perhaps accessible a priori) but is not accessible to us now, perhaps because the reasoning required is currently beyond us or perhaps because we do not currently grasp all of the required physical truths. If this is so, then there will appear to us that a gap exists between physical processes and consciousness, but there will be no gap in nature.

Despite its appeal, the type-C view is inherently unstable. Upon examination, it turns out either to be untenable or to collapse into one of the other views on the table. In particular, I think that the view must collapse into a version of type-A materialism, type-B materialism, type-D dualism, or type-F monism and so is not ultimately a distinct option.

One way to hold that the epistemic gap might be closed in the limit is to hold that in the limit we will see that explaining the functions explains everything and that there is no further explanandum. It is at least coherent to hold that we currently suffer from some sort of conceptual confusion or unclarity that leads us to believe that there is a further explanandum and that this situation could be cleared up by better reasoning. I count this position as a version of type-A materialism, not type-C materialism. The position is obviously closely related to standard type-A materialism (the main difference is whether we have yet had the relevant insight), and the same issues arise. Like standard type-A materialism, this view ultimately stands or falls with the strength of (actual and potential) first-order arguments that dissolve any apparent further explanandum.

Once type-A materialism is set aside, the potential options for closing the epistemic gap are highly constrained. These constraints are grounded in the nature of physical concepts and in the nature of the concept of consciousness. The basic problem has already been mentioned. First, physical descriptions of the world characterize the world in terms of structure and dynamics. Second, from truths about structure and dynamics, one can deduce only further truths about structure and dynamics. Third, truths about consciousness are not truths about structure and dynamics. We can take these steps one at a time.

First: a microphysical description of the world specifies a distribution of particles, fields, and waves in space and time. These basic systems are characterized by their spatiotemporal properties and properties such as mass, charge, and quantum wave function state. These latter properties are ultimately defined in terms of spaces of states that have a certain abstract structure (e.g., the space of continuously varying real quantities or of Hilbert space states), such that the states play a certain causal role with respect to other states. We can subsume spatiotemporal descriptions and descriptions in terms of properties in these formal spaces under the rubric of *structural* descriptions. The state of these systems can change over time in accord with dynamic principles (perhaps involving laws of nature) defined over the relevant properties. The result is a description of the world in terms of its underlying spatiotemporal and formal structure and dynamic evolution over this structure.[17]

Some type-C materialists hold that we do not yet have a complete physics, so we cannot know what such a physics might explain. But here we do not need to have a complete physics. We simply need the claim that physical descriptions are in terms of structure and dynamics. This point is general across physical theories. Novel theories such as relativity and quantum mechanics may introduce new structures and new dynamics over those structures, but the general point (and the gap with consciousness) remains.

A type-C materialist might hold that there could be new physical theories that go beyond structure and dynamics, but given the character of physical explanation, it is unclear what sort of theory this could be. Novel physical properties are postulated for their potential in explaining existing physical phenomena, themselves characterized in terms of structure and dynamics, and it seems that structure and dynamics always suffice here.

---

17. *In formal terms, a structural-dynamic description is one that is equivalent to a Ramsey sentence whose O-terms include at most spatiotemporal expressions, nomic expressions, and logical and mathematical expressions.

One possibility is that instead of postulating novel properties, physics might end up appealing to consciousness itself in the way that some theorists hold that quantum mechanics does. This possibility cannot be excluded, but it leads to a view on which consciousness is itself irreducible and is therefore to be classed in a nonreductive category (type D or type F).

There is one appeal to a "complete physics" that should be taken seriously. This is the idea that current physics characterizes its underlying properties (such as mass and charge) in terms of abstract structures and relations, but it leaves open their intrinsic natures. According to this view, a complete physical description of the world must also characterize the intrinsic properties that ground these structures and relations, and once such intrinsic properties are invoked, physics will go beyond structure and dynamics in such a way that truths about consciousness may be entailed. The relevant intrinsic properties are unknown to us, but they are knowable in principle. This is an important position, but it is precisely the position discussed under type F, so I defer discussion of it until then.

Second: what can be inferred from this sort of description in terms of structure and dynamics? A low-level microphysical description can entail all sorts of surprising and interesting macroscopic properties, as with the emergence of chemistry from physics, of biology from chemistry, or more generally of complex emergent behaviors in complex systems theory. In all of these cases, however, the complex properties that are entailed are nevertheless structural and dynamic. They describe complex spatiotemporal structures and complex dynamic patterns of behavior over those structures, so these cases support the general principle that, from structure and dynamics, one can infer only structure and dynamics.[18]

A type-C materialist might suggest there are some truths that are not themselves structural-dynamic but are nevertheless implied by a structural-dynamic description. It might be argued, perhaps, that truths about *representation* or *belief* have this character. As we saw earlier, however, it seems clear that any sense in which these truths are implied by a structural-dynamic description involves a tacitly functional sense of representation or belief. This is what we would expect: if claims involving these can be seen (on conceptual grounds) to be true *in virtue* of structural-dynamic

18. *Stoljar (2007) identifies structural properties with relational properties and responds to the argument by arguing that relational properties can entail intrinsic properties. For example, being married is a relational property of an individual but arguably an intrinsic property of a couple. As I am understanding structural properties, however, they should not be identified with relational properties (though they are properties definable in terms of certain relations, especially spatiotemporal and formal relations), and claims about intrinsic properties play no role in the argument I have given.

description holding, then the notions involved must themselves be structural-dynamic at some level.

One might hold that there is some intermediate notion X, such that truths about X hold in virtue of structural-dynamic descriptions and such that truths about consciousness hold in virtue of X. As in the case of type-A materialism, however, either X is functionally analyzable (in the broad sense), in which case the second step fails, or X is not functionally analyzable, in which case the first step fails. This is brought out clearly in the case of representation. For the notion of functional representation, the first step fails, and for the notion of phenomenal representation, the second step fails. So this sort of strategy can only work by equivocation.

Third: does explaining or deducing complex structure and dynamics suffice to explain or deduce consciousness? For the usual reasons, it seems clearly not. Mary could know from her black-and-white room all about the spatiotemporal structure and dynamics of the world at all levels, but this will not tell her what it is like to see red. For any complex macroscopic structural or dynamic description of a system, one can conceive of that description's being satisfied without consciousness. And explaining the structure and dynamics of a human system is only to solve the easy problems while leaving the hard ones untouched. To resist this last step, an opponent would have to hold that explaining structure and dynamics *thereby* suffices to explain consciousness. The only remotely tenable way to do this would be to embrace type-A materialism, which we have set aside.

A type-C materialist might suggest that instead of leaning on dynamics (as a type-A materialist does), one could lean on structure. Here, spatiotemporal structure seems unpromising. To explain a system's size, shape, position, motion, and so on is clearly not to explain consciousness. A final possibility is to lean on the structure present in conscious states themselves. Conscious states have structure: there is internal structure within a single complex conscious state, and there are also patterns of similarities and differences between conscious states. But this structure is a distinctively *phenomenal* structure that is quite different in kind from the spatiotemporal and formal structure present in physics. The structure of a complex phenomenal state is not spatiotemporal structure (although it may involve the representation of spatiotemporal structure), and the similarities and differences between phenomenal states are not formal similarities and differences but differences between specific phenomenal characters.[19] This is reflected

19. *Using the Ramsey-theoretic construal of structural-dynamic descriptions given earlier: it may be that phenomenal descriptions can involve structural-dynamic descriptions (in their representational contents, for example), but given the falsity of type-A materialism, they will not themselves be structural-dynamic descriptions.

in the fact that one can conceive of any spatiotemporal structure and formal structure without any associated phenomenal structure; one can know about the first without knowing about the second; and so on. So the epistemic gap is as wide as ever.

The basic problem with any type-C materialist strategy is that epistemic implication from A to B requires some sort of *conceptual hook* by virtue of which the condition described in A can satisfy the conceptual requirements for the truth of B. When a physical account implies truths about life, for example, it does so in virtue of implying information about the macroscopic functioning of physical systems of the sort required for life. Here, broadly functional notions provide the conceptual hook. In the case of consciousness, by contrast, no such conceptual hook is available, given the structural-dynamic character of physical concepts and the quite different character of the concept of consciousness.

Ultimately, it seems that any type-C strategy is doomed for familiar reasons. Once we accept that the concept of consciousness is not itself a functional concept and that physical descriptions of the world are structural-dynamic descriptions, there is simply no conceptual room for it to be implied by a physical description. The only room left is to hold that consciousness is a broadly functional concept after all (accepting type-A materialism), or that there is more in physics than structure and dynamics (accepting type-D dualism or type-F monism), or that the truth of materialism does not require an implication from physics to consciousness (accepting type-B materialism).[20] So in the end, there is no separate space for the type-C materialist.

8. Interlude

Are there any other options for the materialist? One further option is to reject the distinctions on which this taxonomy rests. For example, some philosophers, especially followers of Quine (1951), reject any distinction between conceptual truth and empirical truth or between the a priori and the a posteriori or between the contingent and the necessary. One who is

---

20. Of those mentioned earlier as apparently sympathetic with type-C materialism, I think McGinn is ultimately a type-F monist, Nagel is either a type-B materialist or a type-F monist, Patricia Churchland is either a type-B materialist or a type-Q materialist (see later), and Stoljar is either a type-F monist (insofar as he appeals to "elemental ignorance") or a type-A or type-B materialist (insofar as he appeals to "compositional ignorance").

sufficiently Quinean might therefore reject the distinction between type-A and type-B materialism, holding that talk of epistemic implication and/or modal entailment is ungrounded but that materialism is true nevertheless. We might call such a view type-Q materialism.[21] Still, even on this view, similar issues arise. Some Quineans hold that explaining the functions explains everything (Dennett may be an example); if so, all the problems of type-A materialism arise. Others hold that we can postulate identities between physical states and conscious states in virtue of the strong isomorphic connections between them in nature (Paul Churchland may be an example); if so, the problems of type-B materialism arise. Others may appeal to novel future sorts of explanation; if so, the problems of type-C materialism arise. So the Quinean approach cannot avoid the relevant problems.

Leaving this sort of view aside, it looks as if the only remotely viable options for the materialist are type-A materialism and type-B materialism. Other views are either ultimately unstable or collapse into one of these (or the three remaining options).[22] It seems to me that the costs of these views—denying the manifest explanandum in the first case and embracing primitive identities or strong necessities in the second case—suggest very strongly that they are to be avoided unless there are no viable alternatives.

So the residual question is whether there are viable alternatives. If consciousness is not necessitated by physical truths, then it must involve something ontologically novel in the world. To use Kripke's metaphor, after fixing all the physical truths, God had to do more work to fix all the truths about consciousness. That is, there must be ontologically fundamental features of the world over and above the features characterized by physical theory. We are used to the idea that some features of the world are fundamental. In physics, features such as space-time, mass, and charge are taken as fundamental and not further explained. If the arguments against materialism are correct, these features from physics do not exhaust the fundamental

---

21. *For an explicit endorsement of type-Q materialism, see Mandik and Weisberg (2008).

22. One might ask about specific reductive views, such as representationalism (which identifies consciousness with certain representational states) and higher-order thought theory (which identifies consciousness with the objects of higher-order thoughts). How these views are classified depends on how a given theorist regards the representational or higher-order states (e.g., functionally definable or not) and their connection to consciousness (e.g., conceptual or empirical). Among representationalists, I think that Dretske (1995) and Harman (1990) are type-A materialists, while Lycan (1996) and Tye (1995) are type-B materialists. Among higher-order thought theorists, Carruthers (2000) is clearly a type-B materialist, while Rosenthal (1997) is either type-A or type-B. One could also in principle hold nonmaterialist versions of each of these views.

features of the world. We need to expand our catalog of the world's basic features.

There are two possibilities here. First, it could be that consciousness is itself a fundamental feature of the world, like space-time and mass. In this case, we can say that phenomenal properties are fundamental. Second, it could be that consciousness is not itself fundamental but is necessitated by some more primitive fundamental feature X that is not itself necessitated by physics. In this case, we might call X a *protophenomenal* property, and we can say that protophenomenal properties are fundamental. I typically put things in terms of the first possibility for ease of discussion, but the discussion that follows applies equally to the second. Either way, consciousness involves something novel and fundamental in the world.

The following question then arises. How do these novel fundamental properties relate to the already acknowledged fundamental properties of the world, namely, those invoked in microphysics? In general, where there are fundamental properties, there are fundamental laws. So we can expect that there will be some sort of fundamental principles—psychophysical laws—connecting physical and phenomenal properties. Like the fundamental laws of relativity or quantum mechanics, these psychophysical laws will not be deducible from more basic principles but instead will be taken as primitive.

But what is the character of these laws? An immediate worry is that the microphysical aspects of the world are often held to be causally closed in that every microphysical state has a microphysical sufficient cause. How are fundamental phenomenal properties to be integrated with this causally closed network?

There seem to be three main options for the nonreductionist here. First, one could deny the causal closure of the microphysical, holding that there are causal gaps in microphysical dynamics that are filled by a causal role for distinct phenomenal properties. This is type-D dualism. Second, one could accept the causal closure of the microphysical and hold that phenomenal properties play no causal role with respect to the physical network. This is type-E dualism. Third, one could accept that the microphysical network is causally closed but hold that phenomenal properties are nevertheless integrated with it and play a causal role by virtue of constituting the intrinsic nature of the physical. This is type-F monism.

In what follows, I discuss each of these views. The discussion is necessarily speculative in certain respects, and I do not claim to establish that any one of the views is true or completely unproblematic. But I do suggest that none of them has clear fatal flaws and that each deserves further investigation.

9. Type-D Dualism

Type-D dualism holds that microphysics is not causally closed and that phenomenal properties play a causal role in affecting the physical world.[23] On this view, usually known as *interactionism*, physical states cause phenomenal states, and phenomenal states cause physical states. The corresponding psychophysical laws run in both directions. On this view, the evolution of microphysical states is not determined by physical principles alone. Psychophysical principles specifying the effect of phenomenal states on physical states also play an irreducible role.

The most familiar version of this sort of view is Descartes' substance dualism (hence D for Descartes), according to which there are separate interacting mental and physical substances or entities. But this sort of view is also compatible with a property dualism on which there is just one sort of substance or entity. On a type-D property dualism, there will be both physical and phenomenal fundamental properties, and the phenomenal properties will play an irreducible role in affecting the physical properties. This view is compatible with an "emergentist" view such as Broad's, according to which phenomenal properties are ontologically novel properties of physical systems (not deducible from microphysical properties alone) and have novel effects on microphysical properties (not deducible from microphysical principles alone). Such a view would involve basic principles of "downward" causation of the mental on the microphysical (hence also D for downward causation).

It is sometimes objected that distinct physical and mental states could not interact since there is no causal nexus between them. However, one lesson from Hume and from modern science is that the same goes for any fundamental causal interactions, including those found in physics. Newtonian science reveals no causal nexus by which gravitation works, for example; rather, the relevant laws are simply fundamental. The same goes for basic laws in other physical theories, and the same presumably applies to fundamental psychophysical laws. There is no need for a causal nexus distinct from the physical and mental properties themselves.

By far the most influential objection to interactionism is that it is incompatible with physics.[24] It is widely held that science tells us that the microphysical

23. Type-D dualists include Foster (1991), Hodgson (1991), Popper and Eccles (1977), Sellars (1981), Stapp (1993), and Swinburne (1986).

24. *Papineau (2002) suggests that the evidence from physics and chemistry is quite compatible with interactionism, as existing physical and chemical theories could easily be supplemented with further forces. He argues that it is only evidence from neurobiology in recent years that has rendered interactionism implausible. I think that this suggestion reflects an overly optimistic view of the state of

realm is causally closed, so that there is no room for mental states to have any effects. An interactionist might respond in various ways. For example, it could be suggested that although no experimental studies have revealed these effects, none have ruled them out. It might further be suggested that physical theory allows any number of basic *forces* (four as things stand, but there is always room for more) and that an extra force associated with a mental field would be a reasonable extension of existing physical theory. These suggestions would invoke significant revisions to physical theory, so are not to be made lightly, but one could argue that nothing rules them out.

By far the strongest response to this objection is to suggest that, far from ruling out interactionism, contemporary physics is positively encouraging to the possibility. On the standard formulation of quantum mechanics, the state of the world is described by a wave function, according to which physical entities are often in a superposed state (e.g., in a superposition of two different positions), even though superpositions are never directly observed. According to the standard dynamics, the wave function can evolve in two ways: linear evolution by the Schrödinger equation (which tends to produce superposed states) and nonlinear collapses from superposed states into nonsuperposed states. Schrödinger evolution is deterministic, but collapse is nondeterministic. Schrödinger evolution is constantly ongoing, but on the standard formulation, collapses occur only occasionally, on measurement.

The collapse dynamics leaves a door wide open for an interactionist interpretation. Any physical nondeterminism might be held to leave room for nonphysical effects, but the principles of collapse do much more than that. Collapse is supposed to occur on measurement. There is no widely agreed definition of what a measurement is, but there is one sort of event that everyone agrees is a measurement: observation by a conscious observer. Further, it seems that no purely physical criterion for a measurement can work since purely physical systems are governed by the linear Schrödinger dynamics. As such, it is natural to suggest that a measurement is precisely a conscious observation and that this conscious observation causes a collapse.

The claim should not be too strong. Quantum mechanics does not force this interpretation of the situation on us, and there are alternative interpretations of quantum mechanics on which there are no collapses or on which

---

neurobiology, where there are still many gaps in our understanding of even the basic mechanisms of neural firing and where relatively complete causal explanations are much rarer than in physics and chemistry.

measurement has no special role in collapse.[25] Nevertheless, quantum mechanics appears to be quite *compatible* with such an interpretation. In fact, one might argue that if one were to design elegant laws of physics that allow a role for the conscious mind, one could not do much better than the bipartite dynamics of standard quantum mechanics: one principle governing deterministic evolution in normal cases and one principle governing nondeterministic evolution in special situations that have a prima facie link to the mental.

Of course, such an interpretation of quantum mechanics is controversial. Many physicists reject it precisely because it is dualistic, giving a fundamental role to consciousness. This rejection is not surprising, but it carries no force when we have independent reason to hold that consciousness may be fundamental. There is some irony in the fact that philosophers reject interactionism on largely physical grounds[26] (it is incompatible with physical theory), while physicists reject an interactionist interpretation of quantum mechanics on largely philosophical grounds (it is dualistic). Taken conjointly, these reasons carry little force, especially in light of the arguments against materialism elsewhere in this chapter.

This sort of interpretation needs to be formulated in detail in order to be assessed.[27] I think that the most promising version of such an interpretation allows conscious states to be correlated with the total quantum state

---

25. No-collapse interpretations include Bohm's "hidden-variable" interpretations and Everett's "many-worlds" (or "many-minds") interpretation. A collapse interpretation that does not invoke measurement is the Ghirardi-Rimini-Weber interpretation (with random occasional collapses). Each of these interpretations requires a significant revision to the standard dynamics of quantum mechanics, and each is controversial, although each has its benefits. (See Albert 1993 for discussion of these and other interpretations.) It is notable that, aside from the interpretation involving consciousness, there seems to be no remotely tenable interpretation that preserves the standard claim that collapses occur upon measurement.

26. I have been as guilty of this as anyone, setting aside interactionism in *The Conscious Mind* partly for reasons of compatibility with physics. I am still not especially inclined to endorse interactionism, but I now think that the argument from physics is much too glib. Three further reasons for rejecting the view are mentioned in *The Conscious Mind*. First, if consciousness is to make an interesting qualitative difference to behavior, it must act nonrandomly, in violation of the probabilistic requirements of quantum mechanics. I think there is something to this, but one could bite the bullet on nonrandomness in response, or one could hold that even a random causal role for consciousness is good enough. Second, I argued that denying causal closure yields no special advantage, as a view with causal closure can achieve much the same effect via type-F monism. Again there is something to this, but the type-D view has the significant advantage of avoiding the "combination problem" of the type-F view. Third, it is not clear that the collapse interpretation yields the *sort* of causal role for consciousness that we expect it to have. This is an important open question that requires detailed investigation.

27. Consciousness-collapse interpretations of quantum mechanics have been put forward by Wigner (1961), Hodgson (1991), and Stapp (1993). Only Stapp goes into much detail, with an interesting but somewhat idiosyncratic account that goes in a direction different from the direction I suggest here earlier.

of a system, with the extra constraint that conscious states (unlike physical states) can never be superposed. In a conscious physical system such as a brain, the physical and phenomenal states of the system will be correlated in a (nonsuperposed) quantum state. Upon observation of a superposed external system, Schrödinger evolution at the moment of observation would cause the observed system to become correlated with the brain, yielding a resulting superposition of brain states and so (by psychophysical correlation) a superposition of conscious states. At this point, however, a fundamental constraint holds that such a superposition cannot occur, so one of the potential resulting conscious states is somehow selected (presumably by a nondeterministic dynamic principle at the phenomenal level). The result is that (by psychophysical correlation) a definite brain state and a definite state of the observed object are also selected. The same might apply to the connection between consciousness and nonconscious processes in the brain: when superposed nonconscious processes threaten to affect consciousness, there will be some sort of selection. In this way, there is a causal role for consciousness in the physical world.

Interestingly, such a theory may be empirically testable. In quantum mechanics, collapse theories yield predictions slightly different from no-collapse theories, and different hypotheses about the location of collapse yield predictions that differ from each other, although the differences are extremely subtle and are currently impossible to measure. If the relevant experiments can one day be performed, some outcomes would give us strong reason to accept a collapse theory and might in turn give us grounds to accept a role for consciousness. As a bonus, this could even yield an empirical criterion for the presence of consciousness.

There are any number of further questions concerning the precise formulation of such a view, its compatibility with physical theory more generally (e.g., relativity and quantum field theory), and its philosophical tenability (e.g., does this view yield the sort of causal role that we are inclined to think consciousness must have?). But at the very least, it cannot be said that physical theory immediately rules out the possibility of an interactionist theory. Those who make this claim often raise their eyebrows when a specific theory such as quantum mechanics is invoked, but this is quite clearly an inconsistent set of attitudes. If physics is supposed to rule out interactionism, then careful attention to the detail of physical theory is required.

All of this suggests that there is at least room for a viable interactionism to be explored and that the most common objection to interactionism has little force. Of course, it does not entail that interactionism is true. There is much that is attractive about the view of the physical world as causally closed, and there is little direct evidence from cognitive science of the hypothesis that behavior cannot be wholly explained in terms of physical causes. Still, if we have independent reason to think that consciousness is irreducible, and if we wish to retain the intuitive view that consciousness plays a causal role, then this is a view to be taken very seriously.

10. Type-E Dualism

Type-E dualism holds that phenomenal properties are ontologically distinct from physical properties and that the phenomenal has no effect on the physical.[28] This is the view usually known as *epiphenomenalism* (hence type E): physical states cause phenomenal states, but the converse is not true. On this view, psychophysical laws run in one direction only—from physical to phenomenal. The view is naturally combined with the view that the physical realm is causally closed. This further claim is not essential to type-E dualism, but it provides much of the motivation for the view.

As with type-D dualism, type-E dualism is compatible with a substance dualism with distinct physical and mental substances or entities and is also compatible with a property dualism with one sort of substance or entity and two sorts of properties. Again, it is compatible with an emergentism such as Broad's, according to which mental properties are ontologically novel emergent properties of an underlying entity, but in this case, although there are emergent qualities, there is no emergent downward causation.

Type-E dualism is usually put forward as respecting both consciousness and science: it simultaneously accommodates the anti-materialist arguments about consciousness and the causal closure of the physical. At the same time, type-E dualism is frequently rejected as deeply counterintuitive. If type-E dualism is correct, then phenomenal states have no effect on our actions, physically construed. For example, a sensation of pain will play no causal role in my hand's moving away from a flame; my experience of decision will play no causal role in my moving to a new country; and a sensation of red will play no causal role in my producing the utterance "I am experiencing red now." These consequences are often held to be obviously false or at least unacceptable.

Still, the type-E dualists can reply that there is no direct *evidence* that contradicts their view. Our evidence reveals only regular connections between phenomenal states and actions, so that certain sorts of experiences

---

28. Type-E dualists include Campbell (1970), Huxley (1874), Jackson (1982), and Robinson (1988).

are typically followed by certain sorts of actions. Being exposed to this sort of constant conjunction produces a strong *belief* in a causal connection (as Hume pointed out in another context), but it is nevertheless compatible with the absence of a causal connection. Indeed, it seems that if epiphenomenalism *were* true, we would have exactly the same evidence and be led to believe that consciousness has a causal role for much the same reasons. So if epiphenomenalism is otherwise coherent and acceptable, it seems that these considerations do not provide strong reasons to reject it.[29]

Another objection holds that if consciousness is epiphenomenal, it could not have evolved by natural selection. The type-E dualist has a straightforward reply, however. On the type-E view, there are fundamental psychophysical laws associating physical and phenomenal properties. If evolution selects appropriate physical properties (perhaps involving physical or informational configurations in the brain), then the psychophysical laws will ensure that phenomenal properties are instantiated, too. If the laws have the right form, one can even expect that, as more complex physical systems are selected, more complex states of consciousness will evolve. In this way, physical evolution will carry the evolution of consciousness along with it as a sort of byproduct.

Perhaps the most interesting objections to epiphenomenalism focus on the relation between consciousness and representations of consciousness. It is certainly at least strange to suggest that consciousness plays no causal role in my utterances of "I am conscious." Some have suggested more strongly that this rules out any *knowledge* of consciousness. It is often held that, if a belief about X is to qualify as knowledge, the belief must be caused in some fashion by X. But if consciousness does not affect physical states, and if beliefs are physically constituted, then consciousness cannot cause beliefs. Even if beliefs are not physically constituted, it is not at all clear how epiphenomenalism can accommodate a causal connection between consciousness and belief.

In response, an epiphenomenalist can deny that knowledge always requires a causal connection. One can argue (as I do in chapter 9) that there is a stronger connection between consciousness and beliefs about consciousness: consciousness plays a role in *constituting* phenomenal concepts and phenomenal beliefs. A red experience plays a role in constituting

---

29. Some accuse the epiphenomenalist of a double standard: relying on intuition in making the case against materialism but going counter to intuition in denying a causal role for consciousness. But intuitions must be assessed against the background of reasons and evidence. To deny the relevant intuitions in the anti-materialist argument (in particular, the intuition of a further explanandum) appears to contradict the available first-person evidence, but denying a causal role for consciousness appears to be compatible on reflection with all of our evidence, including first-person evidence.

a belief that one is having a red experience, for example. If so, there is no causal distance between the experience and the belief. Additionally, one can argue (as I do in chapter 10) that this immediate connection to experience and belief allows for the belief to be justified. If this is right, then epiphenomenalism poses no obstacle to knowledge of consciousness.

A related objection holds that my zombie twin would produce the same reports (e.g., 'I am conscious'), caused by the same mechanisms, and that these reports are unjustified; if so, my own reports are unjustified. In response, one can hold that the true bearers of justification are beliefs and that my zombie twin and I have *different* beliefs, involving different concepts, because of the role that consciousness plays in constituting my concepts but not the zombie's. Further, the fact that we produce isomorphic reports implies that an observer might not be any more justified in believing that I am conscious than that the zombie is conscious, but it does not imply a difference in first-person justification. The first-person justification for my belief that I am conscious is not grounded in any way in my reports but rather in my experiences themselves, experiences that the zombie lacks.

For these reasons, I think that there is no knockdown objection to epiphenomenalism here. Still, it must be acknowledged that the situation is at least odd and counterintuitive. The oddness of epiphenomenalism is exacerbated by the fact that the relationship between consciousness and reports about consciousness seems to be something of a lucky coincidence, according to the epiphenomenalist view. After all, if psychophysical laws are independent of physical evolution, then there will be possible worlds where physical evolution is the same as ours but the psychophysical laws are very different, so that there is a radical mismatch between reports and experiences. It seems lucky that we are in a world whose psychophysical laws match them up so well. In response, an epiphenomenalist might try to argue that these laws are somehow the most "natural" and are to be expected, but there is at least a significant burden of proof here.

Overall, I think that epiphenomenalism is a coherent view without fatal problems. At the same time, it is an inelegant view, producing a fragmented picture of nature, in which physical and phenomenal properties are only very weakly integrated in the natural world. And, of course, it is a counterintuitive view that many people find difficult to accept. Inelegance and counterintuitiveness are better than incoherence, so if good arguments force us to epiphenomenalism as the most coherent view, then we should take it seriously. At the same time, however, we have good reason to examine other views very carefully.

11. Type-F Monism

Type-F monism is the view that consciousness is constituted by the intrinsic properties of fundamental physical entities: that is, by the categorical bases of fundamental physical dispositions.[30] On this view, phenomenal or protophenomenal properties are located at the fundamental level of physical reality and in a certain sense underlie physical reality itself.

We might call this view *Russellian monism* because it takes its cue from Bertrand Russell's discussion of physics in *The Analysis of Matter*. Russell pointed out that physics characterizes physical entities and properties by their relations to one another and to us. For example, a quark is characterized by its relations to other physical entities, and a property such as mass is characterized by an associated dispositional role, such as the tendency to resist acceleration. At the same time, physics says nothing about the intrinsic nature of these entities and properties. Where we have relations and dispositions, we expect some underlying intrinsic properties that ground the dispositions, characterizing the entities that stand in these relations.[31] As I noted in chapter 1, however, physics is silent about the intrinsic nature of a quark and about the intrinsic properties that play the role associated with mass. So this is raises a metaphysical puzzle: what are the intrinsic properties of fundamental physical systems?

At the same time, there is another metaphysical puzzle: how can phenomenal properties be integrated with the physical world? Phenomenal properties seem to be intrinsic properties that are hard to fit in with the structural-dynamic character of physical theory, and arguably, they are the only intrinsic properties that we have direct knowledge of. Russell's insight was that we might solve both these puzzles at once. Perhaps the intrinsic properties of the physical world are themselves phenomenal properties. Or perhaps the intrinsic properties of the physical world are not phenomenal properties but nevertheless constitute phenomenal properties: that is, perhaps they are protophenomenal properties. If so, then consciousness and physical reality are deeply intertwined.

This view holds the promise of integrating phenomenal and physical properties very tightly in the natural world. Here, nature consists of entities

---

30. Versions of type-F monism have been put forward by Russell (1927), Feigl (1958/1967), G. Maxwell (1979), Lockwood (1989), Chalmers (1996), Griffin (1998), Strawson (2000), and Stoljar (2001b).

31. There is philosophical debate over the thesis that all dispositions have categorical bases. If the thesis is accepted, the case for type-F monism is particularly strong since microphysical dispositions must have a categorical basis, and we have no independent characterization of that basis. Even if the thesis is rejected, however, type-F monism is still viable. We need only the thesis that microphysical dispositions *may* have a categorical basis to open room for intrinsic properties here.

with intrinsic (proto)phenomenal qualities standing in causal relations within a space-time manifold. Physics as we know it emerges from the relations between these entities, whereas consciousness as we know it emerges from their intrinsic nature. As a bonus, this view is perfectly compatible with the causal closure of the microphysical and indeed with existing physical laws. The view can retain the *structure* of physical theory as it already exists; it simply supplements this structure with an intrinsic nature. Furthermore, the view acknowledges a clear causal role for consciousness in the physical world: (proto)phenomenal properties serve as the ultimate categorical basis of all physical causation.

This view has elements in common with both materialism and dualism. From one perspective, it can be seen as a sort of materialism. If one holds that physical terms refer not to dispositional properties but to the underlying intrinsic properties, then the protophenomenal properties can be seen as physical properties, thus preserving a sort of materialism. From another perspective, it can be seen as a sort of dualism. The view acknowledges phenomenal or protophenomenal properties as ontologically fundamental, and it retains an underlying duality between structural-dispositional properties (those directly characterized in physical theory) and intrinsic protophenomenal properties (those responsible for consciousness). One might suggest that while the view arguably fits the letter of materialism, it shares the spirit of anti-materialism.

In its protophenomenal form, the view can be seen as a sort of neutral monism: there are underlying neutral properties X (the protophenomenal properties), such that the X properties are simultaneously responsible for constituting the physical domain (by their relations) and the phenomenal domain (by their collective intrinsic nature). In its phenomenal form, the view can be seen as a sort of idealism, such that mental properties constitute physical properties, although these need not be mental properties in the mind of an observer, and they may need to be supplemented by causal and spatiotemporal properties in addition. One could also characterize this form of the view as a sort of panpsychism, with phenomenal properties ubiquitous at the fundamental level. One could give the view in its most general form the name *panprotopsychism*, with either protophenomenal or phenomenal properties underlying all of physical reality.

A type-F monist may have one of a number of attitudes to the zombie argument against materialism. Some type-F monists may hold that a complete physical description must be expanded to include an intrinsic description and may consequently deny that zombies are conceivable. (We only think we are conceiving of a physically identical system because we overlook intrinsic properties.) Others could maintain that existing physical concepts refer via dispositions to those intrinsic properties that ground the disposi-tions. If so, these concepts have different primary and secondary intensions (as discussed in chapter 6 and in the appendix), and a type-F monist could correspondingly accept conceivability but deny possibility. On this inter-pretation, we misdescribe the conceived world as physically identical to ours when in fact it is just structurally identical.[32] Finally, a type-F monist might hold that physical concepts refer to dispositional properties, so that zombies are both conceivable and possible, and the intrinsic properties are not phys-ical properties. The differences among these three attitudes seem to be ulti-mately terminological rather than substantive.

As for the knowledge argument, a type-F monist might insist that for Mary to have complete physical knowledge, she would have to have a description of the world involving concepts that directly characterize the intrinsic properties; if she had this (as opposed to her impoverished descrip-tion involving dispositional concepts), she might thereby be in a position to know what it is like to see red. Regarding the explanatory argument, a type-F monist might hold that physical accounts involving intrinsic prop-erties can explain more than structure and function. Alternatively, a type-F monist who sticks to dispositional physical concepts will make responses analogous to one of the other two responses given earlier.

The type-F view is admittedly speculative, and it can sound strange at first hearing. Many find it extremely counterintuitive to suppose that funda-mental physical systems have phenomenal properties: for example, that there is something it is like to be an electron. The protophenomenal version of the view rejects this claim but retains something of its strangeness. It seems that any properties responsible for constituting consciousness must be highly unusual properties of a sort that we might not expect to find in microphysical reality. Still, it is not clear that this strangeness yields any strong objections. Like epiphenomenalism, the view appears to be compat-ible with all our evidence, and there is no direct evidence against it. One can argue that if the view were true, things would appear to us just as they in fact appear. And we have learned from modern physics that the world is a strange place. We cannot expect it to obey all of the dictates of common sense.

One might also object that we do not have any conception of what pro-tophenomenal properties might be like or of how they could constitute

32. Grover Maxwell (1979) exploits this sort of loophole in replying to Kripke's argument. Note that such a world must involve either a corpus of intrinsic properties different from those in our world or no intrinsic properties at all. A type-F monist who holds that the only coherent intrinsic properties are protophenomenal properties might end up denying the conceivability of zombies even under a struc-tural-functional description of their physical state—for reasons very different from those of the type-A materialist. The issues here are discussed at more length in chapter 6.

phenomenal properties. This is true, but one could suggest that this merely a product of our ignorance. In the case of familiar physical properties, there were principled reasons (based on the character of physical concepts) for denying a constitutive connection to phenomenal properties. Here, there are no such principled reasons. At most, there is ignorance of a connection. Of course, it would be very desirable to form a positive conception of protophenomenal properties. Perhaps we can do this indirectly by some sort of theoretical inference from the character of phenomenal properties to their underlying constituents, or perhaps knowledge of the nature of protophenomenal properties will remain beyond us. Either way, this is no reason to reject the truth of the view.[33]

There is one sort of principled problem in the vicinity, pointed out by William James (1890, chapter 6). Our phenomenology has a rich and specific structure. It is unified, bounded, and differentiated into many different aspects but with an underlying homogeneity to many of the aspects, and it appears to have a single subject of experience. It is not easy to see how a distribution of a large number of individual microphysical systems, each with its own protophenomenal properties, could somehow add up to this subject of experience with a rich and specific structure. Should one not expect something more like a disunified, jagged collection of phenomenal spikes?

This is a version of the *combination problem* for panpsychism (Seager 1995) or what Stoljar (2001b) calls the *structural mismatch* problem for the Russellian view (see also Foster 1991, 119–30). To answer it, we need a much better understanding of the *compositional* principles of phenomenology: that is, the principles by which phenomenal properties can be composed or constituted from underlying phenomenal properties, or protophenomenal properties. We have a good understanding of the principles of physical composition but no real understanding of the principles of phenomenal composition. This is an area that deserves much close attention. The combination problem is easily the most serious problem for the type-F monist view, and at this point, it is an open question whether or not it can be solved.

Some type-F monists appear to hold that they can avoid the combination problem by holding that phenomenal properties are the intrinsic properties of *high-level* physical dispositions (e.g., those involved in neural states) and need not be constituted by the intrinsic properties of microphysical states (hence, they may also deny panprotopsychism). But this seems to be

---

33. McGinn (1989) can be read as advocating a type-F view while denying that we can know the nature of the protophenomenal properties. His arguments rest on the claim that these properties cannot be known either through perception or through introspection. However, this does not rule out the possibility that they might be known through some sort of inference to the best explanation of (introspected) phenomenology, subject to the additional constraints of (perceived) physical structure.

untenable. If the low-level network is causally closed and the high-level intrinsic properties are not constituted by low-level intrinsic properties, the high-level intrinsic properties will be epiphenomenal all over again, for familiar reasons. The only way to embrace this position would seem to be in combination with a denial of microphysical causal closure, holding that there are fundamental dispositions above the microphysical level, which have phenomenal properties as their grounds, but such a view would be indistinguishable from type-D dualism.[34] So a distinctive type-F monism will have to face the combination problem directly.

Overall, type-F monism promises a deeply integrated and elegant view of nature. No one has yet developed any sort of detailed theory in this class, and it is not yet clear whether such a theory can be developed. At the same time, however, there appear to be no strong reasons to reject the view. As such, type-F monism is likely to provide fertile grounds for further investigation, and it may ultimately provide the best integration of the physical and the phenomenal within the natural world.

12. Conclusions

Are there any other options for the nonreductionist? There are two views that may not fit straightforwardly into the preceding categories.

First, some nonmaterialists hold that phenomenal properties are ontologically wholly distinct from physical properties, that microphysics is causally closed, but that phenomenal properties nevertheless play a causal role with respect to the physical. One way this might happen is by a sort of causal overdetermination: physical states causally determine behavior, but phenomenal states cause behavior at the same time. Another is by causal mediation: it might be that in at least some instances of microphysical causation from A to B, there is actually a causal connection from A to the mind to B, so that the mind enters the causal nexus without altering the structure of the network. There may be still further strategies here. We might call this class type-O dualism (taking overdetermination as a paradigm case). These views share much of the structure of the type-E view (causally closed physical

---

34. In this way, we can see that type-D views and type-F views are quite closely related. We can imagine that if a type-D view is true and there are microphysical causal gaps, we could be led through physical observation alone to postulate higher-level entities to fill these gaps—"psychons," say—where these are characterized in wholly structural-dispositional terms. The type-D view adds to this the suggestion that psychons have an intrinsic phenomenal nature. The main difference between the type-D view and the type-F view is that the type-D view involves fundamental causation above the microphysical level. This will involve a more radical view of physics, but it might have the advantage of avoiding the combination problem.

world, distinct phenomenal properties) but escape the charge of epiphenomenalism. The special causal setups of these views may be hard to swallow, and they share some of the same problems as the type-E view (e.g., the fragmented view of nature and the "lucky" psychophysical laws), but this class should nevertheless be put on the table as an option.[35]

Second, some nonmaterialists are *idealists* (in a Berkeleyan sense), holding that the physical world is itself constituted by the conscious states of an observing agent. We might call this view type-I monism. It shares with type-F monism the property that phenomenal states play a role in constituting physical reality, but on the type-I view this happens in a very different way: not by having separate "microscopic" phenomenal states underlying each physical state but rather by having physical states constituted holistically by a "macroscopic" phenomenal mind. This view seems to be nonnaturalistic in a much deeper sense than any of the earlier views and in particular seems to suffer from an absence of causal or explanatory closure in nature. Once the natural explanation in terms of the external world is removed, highly complex regularities among phenomenal states have to be taken as unexplained in terms of simpler principles. But again, this sort of view should at least be acknowledged.

As I see things, the best options for a nonreductionist are type-D dualism, type-E dualism, or type-F monism: that is, interactionism, epiphenomenalism, or panprotopsychism. If we acknowledge the epistemic gap between the physical and the phenomenal and we rule out primitive identities and strong necessities, then we are led to a disjunction of these three views. Each of the views has at least some promise, and none has clear fatal flaws. For my part, I give some credence to each of them. I think that in some ways the type-F view is the most appealing, but this sense is largely grounded in aesthetic considerations whose force is unclear.

The choice between these three views may depend in large part on the development of specific theories within these frameworks. Especially for the type-D view and type-F view, further theoretical work is crucial in assessing the theories (e.g., in explicating quantum interactionism or in understanding phenomenal composition). It may also be that the empirical science of consciousness will give some guidance. As the science progresses, we will be led to infer simple principles that underlie correlations between physical and phenomenal states. It may be that these principles turn out to point strongly toward one or the other of these views. For example, if simple principles connecting microphysical states to phenomenal or protophenomenal states can do the explanatory work, then we may have reason to favor a

---

35. Type-O positions are advocated by Bealer (2007), Lowe (1996), and Mills (1996).

type-F view, while if the principles latch onto the physical world at a higher level, then we may have reason to favor a type-D or type-E view. Moreover, if consciousness has a specific pattern of effects on the physical world, as the type-D view suggests, then empirical studies ought in principle to be able to find these effects, although perhaps only with great difficulty.

Not everyone will agree that each of these views is viable. It may be that further examination will reveal deep problems with some of them, but this further examination needs to be performed. There has been little critical examination of type-F views to date, for example. We have seen that the standard arguments against type-D views carry very little weight. And while arguments against type-E views carry some intuitive force, they are far from making a knockdown case against the views. I suspect that even if further examination reveals deep problems for some of the views in this vicinity, it is very unlikely that all of them will be eliminated.

In any case, this gives us some perspective on the mind-body problem. It is often held that even though it is hard to see how materialism could be true, materialism *must* be true since the alternatives are unacceptable. As I see it, there are at least three prima facie acceptable alternatives to materialism on the table, each of which is compatible with a broadly naturalistic (even if not materialistic) worldview and none of which has fatal problems. So given the clear arguments against materialism, it seems to me that we should at least tentatively embrace the conclusion that one of these views is correct. Of course, all of the views discussed in this chapter need to be developed in much more detail and examined in light of all relevant scientific and philosophical developments in order to be comprehensively assessed. But as things stand, I think that we have good reason to suppose that consciousness has a fundamental place in nature.[36]

36. *A further choice point for the nonreductionist is whether to adopt substance dualism or mere property dualism. In *The Conscious Mind* I argued for property dualism, but here I understood property dualism in a weak sense (there is at least a dualism of properties) compatible with substance dualism, as opposed to a strong sense (there is only a dualism of properties) which is incompatible with substance dualism. The anti-materialist arguments I consider here get us only to property dualism in the weak sense, and the choice between substance dualism and property dualism in the strong sense rests on further considerations. The issue between these latter views is somewhat obscure, but I take the key question to be whether there is a dualism of objects as well as of properties, and in particular whether there are fundamental objects over and above the objects in physics or whether there are merely further fundamental properties that attach to existing fundamental or nonfundamental objects. On the type-F view, it is natural to hold that there is a dualism of properties but not of objects. The type-D and type-E views can in principle be combined with either, but if one rules out panpsychist or panprotopsychist versions of these views and also rules out fundamental properties attaching to non-fundamental objects, it is most natural to combine these views with a dualism of objects. I remain neutral on the issue myself, but I am certainly not opposed to a substance dualism (construed as the existence of fundamental nonphysical individuals), and there are some considerations (including issues about the combination problem and the unity of consciousness) that tend to favor it.

THE TWO-DIMENSIONAL ARGUMENT
AGAINST MATERIALISM

A number of popular arguments for dualism start from a premise about an epistemic gap between physical truths and truths about consciousness and infer an ontological gap between physical processes and consciousness. Arguments of this sort include the conceivability argument, the knowledge argument, the explanatory-gap argument, and the property dualism argument. Such arguments are often resisted on the grounds that epistemic premises do not entail ontological conclusions.

My view is that one can legitimately infer ontological conclusions from epistemic premises if one is careful about how one reasons. To do so, the best way is to reason first from epistemic premises to modal conclusions (about necessity and possibility) and from there to ontological conclusions. Here, the crucial issue is the link between the epistemic and modal domains. How can one reason from theses about what is knowable or conceivable to theses about what is necessary or possible?

To bridge the epistemic and modal domains, the framework of two-dimensional semantics can play a central role. I have used this framework in earlier work (Chalmers 1996) to mount an argument against materialism. Here I revisit the argument, laying it out in a more explicit and careful form and responding to a number of objections. In what follows I concentrate mostly on the conceivability argument. Similar considerations apply to the other anti-materialist arguments, however, and in the afterword to this chapter, I show how this analysis might yield a unified treatment of many of these arguments.

1. The Conceivability Argument

The most straightforward form of the conceivability argument against materialism runs as follows:

    1. $P\&\sim Q$ is conceivable.
    2. If $P\&\sim Q$ is conceivable, $P\&\sim Q$ is metaphysically possible.
    3. If $P\&\sim Q$ is metaphysically possible, materialism is false.

    _____

    4. Materialism is false.

Here P is the conjunction of all microphysical truths about the universe, specifying the fundamental features of every fundamental microphysical entity in the language of microphysics, as well as fundamental microphysical laws. Q is an arbitrary phenomenal truth: perhaps the truth that someone is phenomenally conscious, or perhaps the truth that a certain individual (that is, an individual satisfying a certain description) instantiates a certain phenomenal property. $P\&\sim Q$ ("P and not Q") conjoins the former with the denial of the latter.

If Q is the truth that someone is phenomenally conscious, then $P\&\sim Q$ is the statement that everything is microphysically as in our world, but no one is phenomenally conscious. In this version, $P\&\sim Q$ says that the world is a _zombie world_ (see chapter 5). If Q is the truth that a certain individual instantiates a certain phenomenal property, then $P\&\sim Q$ is the statement that everything is microphysically as in our world but that it is not the case that the individual in question instantiates the relevant phenomenal property. In this case, it suffices for the truth of $P\&\sim Q$ that the world is a zombie world or simply that the individual in question is a zombie in a physically identical world. It also suffices that the individual in question is an _invert_, who has an experience that differs slightly from the corresponding experience of the corresponding individual in our (physically identical) world.

The first premise of this argument asserts an epistemic thesis, about what can be conceived. The second premise steps from the epistemic thesis to a modal thesis, about what is possible. The third premise steps from the modal thesis to a metaphysical thesis, about the nature of our world.

The third premise is relatively uncontroversial. It is widely accepted that materialism has modal commitments. Some philosophers question whether materialism is equivalent to a modal thesis, but almost all accept that materialism at least _entails_ a modal thesis. Here one can invoke Kripke's metaphor: if it is possible that there is a world physically identical to our world but phenomenally different, then after God fixed the physical facts about our world, he had to do more work to fix the phenomenal facts.

A familiar complication arises from the observation that physicalism about our world is compatible with the possibility of dualism in other worlds and in particular is compatible with the possibility of a physically identical world that contains extra, nonphysical phenomenology. This means that if Q is a negative truth about our world—say, the truth that no one instantiates a certain phenomenal property—then materialism about our world is compatible with the possibility of $P\&\sim Q$. To finesse this point, we can ensure that in this argument, Q is a positive truth (one that holds in all worlds that contain a duplicate of our world; see Chalmers 1996, 40). If Q is a positive truth, such as 'Someone is conscious,' then materialism is incompatible with the possibility of $P\&\sim Q$. Alternatively, we can conjoin P with a "that's-all" statement T, stating that the world is a *minimal* world that satisfies P (see Jackson 1998, 26). Then even when Q is a negative truth, materialism is not compatible with the possibility of $PT\&\sim Q$ (where PT is the conjunction of P and T).

The real work in the argument is done by the first and second premises. The second premise is particularly controversial: a number of examples have led many philosophers to deny that there is an entailment from conceivability to metaphysical possibility. To assess these premises, we need to understand the notion of conceivability.

2. Varieties of Conceivability

Conceivability is to be understood as an epistemic notion, defined in epistemological (and perhaps psychological) terms. To a first approximation, we can say that a sentence S is conceivable when S expresses a coherent hypothesis: one that cannot be ruled out a priori. To refine this understanding, it is useful to make some distinctions. (These distinctions are discussed at much greater length in Chalmers 2002b.)

We can say that S is prima facie conceivable (for a subject) when that subject is unable to rule out the hypothesis expressed by S by a priori reasoning on initial consideration. We can say that S is *ideally* conceivable when the hypothesis expressed by S cannot be ruled out a priori even on ideal rational reflection. The main difference here is that prima facie conceivability is tied to a subject's contingent cognitive limitations, while ideal conceivability abstracts away from those limitations.

Here are some examples: (1) '2+2=5' is neither prima facie conceivable nor ideally conceivable; (2) where S is a highly complex but provable mathematical truth, $\sim S$ will be prima facie conceivable for most subjects, but it is not ideally conceivable; (3) where S is 'There is a flying pig,' S is prima facie conceivable and is almost certainly ideally conceivable.

These notions of conceivability are versions of *negative* conceivability, which is defined in terms of what a subject can *rule out* through a priori reasoning. We can say that S is negatively conceivable when S cannot be ruled out through a priori reasoning. The notions of prima facie and ideal conceivability defined here can then be seen as prima facie negative conceivability and ideal negative conceivability, respectively.

It is also possible to define notions of *positive* conceivability, which is characterized in terms of what subjects can form a positive conception of. We can say that S is positively conceivable when one can coherently imagine a situation in which S is the case. Where negative conceivability requires merely entertaining a hypothesis and being unable to rule it out, positive conceivability involves being able to form some sort of clear and distinct conception of a situation in which the hypothesis is true. One can then say that S is *prima facie positively conceivable* when a subject can imagine a situation that the person takes to be coherent and also takes to be one in which S is the case. Furthermore, one can say that S is *ideally positively conceivable* when its prima facie positive conceivability cannot be defeated on ideal rational reflection (in particular, when arbitrary details can be filled in in the imagined situation without any contradiction revealing itself and when ideal reflection reveals the imagined situation as one in which S is the case).

Traditional notions of conceivability (Descartes' clear and distinct conceivability, for example) are arguably varieties of positive rather than negative conceivability. At the same time, the notion of positive conceivability is more complex than that of negative conceivability, and a rigorous characterization of the notion requires saying much more about just what it is to imagine a situation and so on. I characterize positive conceivability in more depth in Chalmers 2002b. In this chapter the roles of positive and negative conceivability are often interchangeable (I will be clear when the difference is relevant), so the preceding informal account suffices for present purposes. For much of the discussion one can focus on negative conceivability without much loss, but positive conceivability is available as an alternative if there turn out to be any problems with theses tied to negative conceivability.

Insofar as there is a gap between prima facie conceivability and ideal conceivability, it is ideal conceivability that is the better guide to possibility. This is especially clear in the case of prima facie negative conceivability. We have seen that the negation of a complex mathematical truth may be prima facie negatively conceivable, but it is not ideally conceivable, and it is not possible. It is less easy to find cases of prima facie positive conceivability without ideal positive conceivability (see Chalmers 2002b for some potential cases), but insofar as there are such cases, there will be little reason to think that they are possible.

Correspondingly, some familiar purported counterexamples to the claim that conceivability entails possibility are really counterexamples to the claim that prima facie conceivability entails possibility. For example, it is sometimes said that both Goldbach's conjecture and its negation are conceivable, while only one of them is possible. Here the relevant notion of conceivability is something like prima facie negative conceivability. There is no reason to believe that both Goldbach's conjecture and its negation are ideally conceivable, so there is no reason to think that this is a counterexample to the claim that ideal conceivability entails possibility. So from here onward, talk of "conceivability" simpliciter should always be understood to be talk of ideal conceivability (either positive or negative).

The other familiar class of purported counterexamples arises from Kripke's analysis of the necessary a posteriori. It is often said that sentences such as 'water is not H_2O' provide counterexamples to the claim that conceivability entails possibility: it is conceivable that water is not H_2O, but it is not metaphysically possible.

Here one has to be careful. There is a *sense* of 'conceivable' in which 'water is not H_2O' is not conceivable (given that water is H_2O in the actual world). In this sense, any conceivable situation in which it seems that water is not H_2O (a Twin Earth world, say) should better be described as a conceivable situation in which water is still H_2O but in which there is watery stuff that is not H_2O. Using the term 'conceivable' this way (as Kripke seems to do), one might say that 'water is not H_2O' seems conceivable (or that it is prima facie conceivable to one without relevant empirical knowledge) but that it is not really conceivable. We might call this sense of conceivability *secondary conceivability* (for reasons familiar from a two-dimensional analysis and discussed in Chalmers 2002b). Then the Kripkean cases are compatible with the claim that secondary conceivability entails metaphysical possibility. At the same time, however, this claim is not very useful for present purposes, as whether a sentence is secondarily conceivable will typically depend on a variety of empirical factors, and an opponent might deny that zombies are secondarily conceivable on the grounds that there is an a posteriori identity between phenomenal and physical properties. So a link between secondary conceivability and possibility does not offer an a priori route to conclusions about metaphysical possibility.

Instead, what is relevant here is *primary conceivability*: the sense in which 'water is not H_2O' can correctly be said to be conceivable. The notion of negative conceivability defined earlier is a sort of primary conceivability as it is defined in terms of what can be ruled out a priori, and 'water is H_2O' cannot be established a priori. (One might define a distinct notion of negative secondary conceivability, but I will set that aside here.) One can likewise define a notion of positive primary conceivability, so that S is positively primarily conceivable when the subject can imagine a coherent situation that verifies S, where a situation verifies S when, under the hypothesis that the situation actually obtains, the subject should conclude that S. If the subject imagines a Twin Earth situation with XYZ in the oceans and lakes and assumes that the situation obtains in the subject's own environment, then the subject should conclude that water is XYZ rather than H_2O. So 'water is not H_2O' is positively primarily conceivable, as well as negatively primarily conceivable.

Unlike secondary conceivability, matters of primary conceivability are plausibly in the a priori domain: whether S is primarily conceivable turns on matters of a priori reasoning. But primary conceivability does not entail metaphysical possibility: 'water is not H_2O' is primarily conceivable, but it is not metaphysically possible.

Still, there remains a link between primary conceivability and metaphysical possibility in these cases. When we conceive that water is not H_2O, we imagine (for example) a Twin Earth situation in which the watery liquid in the oceans and lakes is XYZ. This situation is metaphysically possible, so there is a sense in which our conceiving involves access to a possible world. Under the usual way of describing possible worlds, this world is not one in which water is not H_2O. But the world still stands in a strong relation to the sentence 'water is not H_2O.' In particular, if we came to accept that our own world had the character of this world (with XYZ in the oceans and lakes), we should then endorse the claim 'water is not H_2O.'

This can be put in two-dimensional terms by saying that while the Twin Earth does not *satisfy* 'water is not H_2O' ('water is not H_2O' is not true of that world considered as counterfactual), the Twin Earth world *verifies* 'water is not H_2O' ('water is not H_2O' is true of that world considered as actual). Equivalently, we can say that while the *secondary intension* of 'water is not H_2O' is false at w, the sentence's *primary intension* is true there. To a first approximation, a world w verifies S (or S is true at w considered as actual, or the primary intension of S is true at w) when, if we came to accept that our own world is qualitatively like w, we should then endorse S. Strictly speaking, the worlds that are relevant to primary intensions are *centered* worlds: worlds that come with a marked "center" consisting of an individual and time. When we consider a centered world w as actual, we consider the hypothesis that we are currently in the situation of the individual at the center. (For much more on these notions, see the appendix to this book.)

We can say that when the primary intension of S is true at some centered world (i.e., when some centered world verifies S), S is *primarily possible*, or *1-possible*. When the secondary intension of S is true at some world (i.e., when some world satisfies S), S is *secondarily possible*, or *2-possible*. Then 'water is not H_2O' is not 2-possible, but it is 1-possible.

The observation that sentences such as 'water is not H_2O' are conceivable but not possible in these terms comes to the claim that these sentences are primarily conceivable (1-conceivable) but are not secondarily possible (2-possible). So there is good reason to believe that 1-conceivability does not entail 2-possibility. However, these cases are entirely compatible with a link between 2-conceivability and 2-possibility, and more important for present purposes, they are entirely compatible with a link between 1-conceivability and 1-possibility.

In fact, it is not hard to argue that all of the standard Kripkean a posteriori necessities ('heat is the motion of molecules,' 'Hesperus is Phosphorus,' and so on) have this structure. For each of these necessities, one might say that its negation is conceivable but not possible, meaning that it is 1-conceivable but not 2-possible. But in each of these cases, the sentence in question is 1-possible. For example, 'heat is not the motion of molecules' is verified by a world in which something other than molecules causes sensations as of heat. 'Hesperus is not Phosphorus' is verified by a world in which the objects visible in the morning and evening skies are entirely distinct. Furthermore, it is plausible that worlds such as these are just what one is conceiving of when one conceives that heat is not the motion of molecules or that Hesperus is not Phosphorus. So in these cases, there remains a strong link between conceivability and metaphysical possibility.

To summarize, we have seen that the standard counterexamples to a conceivability-possibility link are accommodated by noting that (i) prima facie conceivability is an imperfect guide to possibility and that (ii) primary conceivability is an imperfect guide to secondary possibility. But (i) is entirely consistent with a link between ideal conceivability and possibility, and (ii) is entirely consistent with a link between primary conceivability and primary possibility. Putting the pieces together: all of these counterexamples are compatible with the thesis that ideal primary conceivability entails primary possibility.

There are two versions of this thesis, depending on whether one interprets the relevant sort of conceivability as positive or negative:

(CP+) Ideal primary positive conceivability entails primary possibility.

(CP−) Ideal primary negative conceivability entails primary possibility.

Ideal primary positive conceivability entails ideal primary negative conceivability: if S can be ruled out a priori, then no coherent imagined situation will verify S. It follows that CP− entails CP+. It is not obvious whether or not CP+ entails CP− as it is not obvious whether ideal primary negative conceivability entails ideal primary positive conceivability. That is, it is not obvious whether there is an S that cannot be ruled out a priori but such that no coherent imagined situation verifies S. (In Chalmers 2002b I argue that there is no such S so that ideal primary negative conceivability entails ideal primary positive conceivability.) So CP− is at least as strong as CP+ and is possibly somewhat stronger.

Most important for present purposes, however, both CP+ and CP− are compatible with all of the familiar purported counterexamples to the conceivability-possibility link. Furthermore, it seems that there are no clear counterexamples to either thesis (though later in the chapter I discuss some potential counterexamples that have been put forward). In particular, both theses are entirely compatible with the existence of Kripkean a posteriori necessities, so while the existence of these necessities is often used to cast doubt on conceivability-possibility theses, they cannot be used to cast doubt on CP+ or CP−.

So for now, I take these theses as reasonable conceivability-possibility theses that might be used in mounting a refined conceivability argument against materialism. Later in the chapter I return to the question of their truth.

3. A Refined Conceivability Argument

Henceforth, unqualified uses of "conceivability" and "conceivable" should be understood as invoking ideal primary conceivability. I will often be inexplicit about whether positive or negative conceivability is involved. In effect, the argument forms that follow can be understood as generating two different arguments, depending on whether one understands conceivability as ideal primary positive conceivability or as ideal primary negative conceivability. For many purposes the distinction will not matter. When it does matter, I will be explicit.

Given the preceding discussion, one might try to generate an anti-materialist argument by simply substituting primary possibility for metaphysical possibility in the original argument:

1. $P\&\sim Q$ is conceivable.
2. If $P\&\sim Q$ is conceivable, $P\&\sim Q$ is 1-possible.

3. If $P\&{\sim}Q$ is 1-possible, materialism is false.

---

4. Materialism is false.

On this reading, premises 1 and 2 are both plausible theses, but premise 3 is not obviously plausible. The reason is that materialism requires not the 1-impossibility of $P\&{\sim}Q$ but the 2-impossibility of $P\&{\sim}Q$. That is, materialism requires that it *could not have been the case* that P is true without Q also being true. This is a subjunctive claim about ordinary metaphysical possibility and so invokes 2-impossibility rather than 1-impossibility.

A materialist might reasonably question premise 3 by holding that even if there is a world w verifying $P\&{\sim}Q$, w might be a world with quite different ingredients from our own. For example, it might be that w does not instantiate true microphysical properties (those instantiated in our world) such as mass and charge but instead instantiates quite different properties, say, pseudo-mass and pseudo-charge, which stand to mass and charge roughly as XYZ stands to H_2O. Likewise, it might be that w does not lack true phenomenal properties but instead lacks quite different properties, say, pseudophenomenal properties. If so, then the possibility of w has no bearing on whether true microphysical properties necessitate true phenomenal properties, and it is the latter that is relevant for materialism.

Still, it may be that the gap between 1-possibility and 2-possibility could be closed. If P has the same primary intension and secondary intension, then a world will verify P iff it satisfies P, so P will be 1-possible iff it is 2-possible. The same goes for Q, and for $P\&{\sim}Q$. We could then run the following argument:

1. $P\&{\sim}Q$ is conceivable.
2. If $P\&{\sim}Q$ is conceivable, $P\&{\sim}Q$ is 1-possible.
3. If $P\&{\sim}Q$ is 1-possible, $P\&{\sim}Q$ is 2-possible.
4. If $P\&{\sim}Q$ is 2-possible, materialism is false.

---

5. Materialism is false.

Here, the truth of premise 3 requires that both P and Q have primary and secondary intensions that coincide. In the case of Q, this claim is quite plausible (although as I note later, this claim is not required for a refined conceivability argument to go through). As Kripke noted, there does not seem to be the same strong dissociation between appearance and reality in the case of consciousness as in the cases of water and heat. While it is not the case that anything that looks like water is water or that anything that feels like heat is heat, it is plausibly the case that anything that feels like consciousness is consciousness. So it is not clear that the notion of "pseudo-consciousness," something that satisfies the primary intension of 'consciousness' without being consciousness, is coherent. The same holds for other, more specific phenomenal properties. So there is a strong case that the primary and secondary intensions of phenomenal terms coincide. (For more on this case, see chapter 8.)

However, in the case of P, this claim is less plausible. A materialist might reasonably hold that microphysical terms (such as 'mass' and 'charge') have primary intensions that differ from their secondary intensions. In particular, it is plausible that the primary intensions of these terms are tied to a certain theoretical role. We might say that the primary intension of 'mass' picks out whatever property plays the mass role (e.g., resisting acceleration in certain ways, being subject to mutual attraction in a certain way, and so on) and that the primary intension of 'charge' picks out whatever property plays the charge role (e.g., obeying certain electromagnetic principles, being subject to attraction and repulsion in certain ways, and so on).

By contrast, one might reasonably hold that the secondary intension of microphysical terms is tied to the property that actually plays the role. For example, if property M plays the mass role in the actual world, then one might hold that in any world in which mass is instantiated, mass is M. It follows that if there are worlds in which some *other* property M' plays the mass role, then M' is not mass in that world (at best, it is pseudomass). If so, then the primary and secondary intensions of 'mass' will not coincide. The primary intension of 'mass' will pick out whatever plays the mass role in such a world, but the secondary intension will not.

There are other views of the semantics and metaphysics of microphysical terms that may reject this argument for the distinctness of the primary and secondary intensions of 'mass.' In particular, the argument will not go through on views according to which it is necessary that mass is the property that plays the mass role. (These include views on which 'mass' is a nonrigid designator whose secondary intension picks out different properties that play the role in some worlds, as well as views on which it is necessary that M is the property that plays the mass role, where M is the property rigidly designated by 'mass.') Still, the view sketched in the previous paragraph is a quite reasonable view—more plausible than the alternatives, in my opinion—and it is the view that best grounds resistance to an inference from the 1-possibility of $P\&\sim Q$ to its 2-possibility. So we can suppose that the view is correct in order to see what follows.

According to this view, a world may verify P without satisfying P. The secondary intension of P requires that certain specific properties such as mass, spin, and charge are distributed in a certain specific way across space-time, with appropriate causal and nomic relations among them. The primary intension of P requires only that whatever properties play the mass role, the spin role, and the charge role are distributed in this way. If w is a world where these roles are played by properties other than mass, spin, and charge (we might say that they are played by "schmass," "schmin," and "schmarge"), which are otherwise distributed in the right way over space-time and have appropriate causal and nomic relations among them, then w will verify P, but it will not satisfy P. Here, we might say that the physics of w has the same *structural* profile as physics in the actual world, but that it has a different *intrinsic* profile, in that it differs in the intrinsic properties that fill this structure. To verify P, a world must have the right structural profile, while to satisfy P, a world must have the right structural and intrinsic profiles.

It follows that premise 3 is not guaranteed to be true. Because a world can verify P without satisfying P, it may be that $P\&\sim Q$ is 1-possible but not 2-possible. However, this requires that P and Q be related in a certain specific way. In particular, it requires that some worlds that verify P also verify $\sim Q$, while no worlds that satisfy P also satisfy $\sim Q$. This requires in turn that some worlds that have the same structural profile as the actual world verify $\sim Q$, while no worlds that have the same structural and intrinsic profiles as the actual world satisfy $\sim Q$. We can assume for the moment that the primary and secondary intensions of Q coincide. Then we can put all of this by saying that for premise 3 to be false, it is required that the structural profile of physics in the actual world does not necessitate Q but that the combined structural and intrinsic profiles of physics in the actual world do necessitate Q.

This idea—that the structural properties of physics in the actual world do not necessitate the existence and/or nature of consciousness but that the intrinsic properties of physics combined with the structural properties do—corresponds to a familiar view in the metaphysics of consciousness. This view is the type-F monism of the last chapter, or *Russellian monism*. On this view, consciousness is closely tied to the intrinsic properties that serve as the categorical bases of microphysical dispositions. Russell and others held that the nature of these properties is not revealed to us by perception (which reveals only their effects) or by science (which reveals only their relations). But it is coherent to suppose that these properties have a special nature that is tied to consciousness. They might themselves be phenomenal properties, or they might be *protophenomenal* properties: properties that collectively constitute phenomenal properties when organized in the appropriate way.

Russellian monism is an important view on the mind-body problem. It is certainly not ruled out by the conceivability argument and related arguments. If Russellian monism is true, then when we conceive of zombies, we hold fixed the structural properties of physical systems in the actual world but not their intrinsic properties (which are protophenomenal properties). If these intrinsic protophenomenal properties qualify as physical properties, then the zombies we conceive of are not full physical duplicates, and any full physical duplicates will also be phenomenal duplicates. On this understanding, Russellian monism qualifies as a form of physicalism. However, because it relies on speculation about the special nature of the fundamental properties in microphysics, it is a highly distinctive form of physicalism that has much in common with property dualism and that many physicalists will want to reject.[1]

In any case, we can now close the loophole in the previous argument as follows:

1. $P\&\sim Q$ is conceivable.
2. If $P\&\sim Q$ is conceivable, then $P\&\sim Q$ is 1-possible.
3. If $P\&\sim Q$ is 1-possible, then $P\&\sim Q$ is 2-possible or Russellian monism is true.
4. If $P\&\sim Q$ is 2-possible, materialism is false.

———————————

5. Materialism is false or Russellian monism is true.

This argument is valid. I discussed the case for premises 1, 2, and 4 earlier, and I have just now argued for premise 3. I think that (5) is the proper conclusion of the conceivability argument. For the reasons given earlier, such arguments (and also related arguments such as the knowledge argument and the property dualism argument) cannot exclude Russellian

———————————

1. A related position arises from views on which laws of nature are necessary (e.g., Shoemaker 1998) and on which there is a lawful connection between physical properties and phenomenal properties in our world. Such a view may hold that it is essential to physical properties that they have this nomic profile, so that there is no world that satisfies $P\&\sim Q$. Some versions of this view will deny (2) in the refined argument and are discussed later in the chapter. Other versions may accept (2), holding that there is a world that verifies $P\&\sim Q$, while holding that this world involves distinct "schmysical" properties that lack the nomic profile of physical properties. The resulting view resembles Russellian monism in some respects but differs from the usual form in taking the connection between physical and phenomenal properties to be nomic in the first instance. Because it turns on this nomic connection, this view does not provide any loophole for materialism. At best, it yields a version of property dualism on which the laws of nature connecting physical and phenomenal properties are necessary. See objection 12 in section 8 for more on related issues.

monism, and Russellian monism is arguably a form of physicalism, if a distinctive and radical kind. So the possibility of Russellian monism needs to be explicitly acknowledged as an option in the conclusion.

A couple of minor notes on the argument. First, to be fully explicit, the argument might take the truth of Q as a premise. If Q were false, the ground for accepting premise 4 would collapse. In the less explicit version of the preceding argument, we can consider the truth of Q as part of the case for accepting premise 4. In fact, for reasons given earlier, the case for 4 requires that Q be a *positive* truth about consciousness. Alternatively, one can remain silent on whether Q is a positive or negative truth and handle this matter by conjoining P with a that's-all clause asserting that the world is a minimal world in which P (or equivalently, by building such a that's-all clause into P).

Second, it is worth noting that (contrary to a common supposition) the assumption that Q has the same primary and secondary intensions is not necessary for the argument for 5 to go through. To see this, we can consider the version of the argument where we adjoin a that's-all clause to P. From premises 1 and 2 we can derive the conclusion that there is a minimal world verifying P in which the primary intension of Q is false. If P has the same primary and secondary intensions, then this world will be a minimal P world in which the primary intension of Q is false. This world must differ from our world because the primary intension of Q is true in our world. (There is a small loophole here arising from the possibility that this world differs merely in the location of the center of the relevant centered world. I discuss this loophole in section 5.) It follows that there is a minimal P-world that is not a duplicate of our world, so that physicalism is false with regard to our world. It could be that, strictly speaking, physicalism will be true of *consciousness* because P necessitates Q, but physicalism will be false of properties closely associated with consciousness, namely those associated with the primary intension of Q. We might think of this sort of view as one on which phenomenal properties are physical properties that have nonphysical properties as modes of presentation.

Alternatively, if P has different primary and secondary intensions, then by the reasoning given in the earlier discussion of premise 3, one can conclude that either there is a minimal world satisfying P in which the primary intension of Q is false (which again entails the falsity of physicalism), or that the primary intension of Q is necessitated by the structural and intrinsic profiles of physics in our world but not by the structural profile alone. This view can be considered another form of Russellian monism in that the intrinsic properties of physics in our world are crucial for constituting the properties associated with the modes of presentation of consciousness. So if Q has distinct primary and secondary intensions, then one will have to formalize premises 3 and 4 somewhat differently, but the argument for 5 will still work just as well.

This completes the exposition of the two-dimensional argument against materialism. In what follows I address some objections to the final version of the argument (p. 152) that arise from the recent literature. I have already said what needs to be said about premises 3 and 4, and I do not anticipate significant objections to them (with one exception that I discuss). I discuss some objections to premise 1 and some hard-to-classify objections relatively briefly, and then I focus on objections to the crucial premise 2.

4. Objections to Premise 1

Premise 1 says that $P\&\sim Q$ is conceivable: that is, that we can conceive a world physically identical to ours containing zombies and/or inverts. It is worth noting that such a world need not be an entire zombie world. One might worry that there are complications associated with imagining *oneself* to be zombie at the center of a centered world. For the purpose of the argument, it usually suffices to conceive of a physically identical world in which some other being, corresponding to a conscious being in this world, is a zombie or an invert.

The premise can be understood as invoking ideal primary negative conceivability or ideal primary positive conceivability. The first version makes a somewhat weaker claim (positive conceivability entails negative conceivability, but the reverse is not obviously the case) and is slightly more straightforward. In this version, the premise simply says that $P\&\sim Q$ cannot be ruled out a priori: that a priori reasoning cannot rule out the hypothesis that P obtains and that someone else is a zombie, for example. The second version makes the somewhat stronger claim that we can (in principle) clearly and distinctly imagine a situation in which P holds and in which someone is a zombie or an invert (where the hypothesis that this situation obtains cannot be ruled out by a priori reasoning). Of course, any difference in strength here will be balanced by an inverse difference in strength for the corresponding versions of premise 2.

I discussed the strong prima facie case for these claims in Chalmers (1996) and will not recapitulate it here. The zombie hypothesis is at least prima facie coherent and imaginable. To reject the premise, one needs to find something that undermines the prima facie coherence and imaginability, such as some sort of a priori incoherence, contradiction, or unimaginability in the hypothesis that emerges on reflection. A detailed defense of the premise involves arguing that no candidate for this sort of undermining can succeed. Here I consider various candidates.

(1) *Analytic functionalism.* One way to reject the conceivability premise would be to accept an analytic functionalist view of consciousness on which to say that someone is conscious is that to say they have a state that functions in an appropriate way in their cognitive system and their behavior. If consciousness were defined in this way, then any functionally identical being would be conscious by definition, so zombies would be ruled out. Analytic functionalism about consciousness is widely rejected, however, and I have argued against it in the last chapter (under the discussion of type-A materialism), so I will not argue against it further here.

(2) *Prima facie but not ideal conceivability.* It is natural to suggest that zombies may be prima facie but not ideally conceivable (see van Gulick 1999 and Worley 2003 for suggestions along these lines). This corresponds to the type-C materialism of the last chapter, according to which there is a prima facie epistemic gap between physical and phenomenal truths that may be closed on ideal reflection, perhaps because of new discoveries about physical processes or perhaps because of novel reasoning. As I argued there, to render zombies incoherent even on ideal reflection requires some sort of conceptual link between physical and phenomenal concepts. Given that physics and physical concepts are all structural-dynamic in character (and new scientific developments are unlikely to change this, although see option 3), phenomenal concepts must have a character that is linked to structural-dynamic concepts in an appropriate way. Upon examination, the only candidate that is remotely tenable is the hypothesis that phenomenal concepts are functional concepts, but we have already seen that there is good reason to reject that view.

A related objection (e.g., Bailey forthcoming) holds that arguments from ideal conceivability are toothless since nonideal creatures such as ourselves cannot know whether or not a given statement is ideally conceivable. I think that there is little reason to accept this claim. Although we are nonideal, we can know that it is not ideally conceivable that 0=1 and that it is ideally conceivable that someone exists. We know that certain things about the world (say, that all philosophers are philosophers) are knowable a priori and that certain things about the world (say, that there is a table in this room) are not so knowable even by an ideal reasoner. Likewise, reasoning of this sort gives us very good reason to think that there is no a priori entailment from physical to phenomenal truths and that zombie hypotheses are conceivable even for an ideal reasoner.

(3) *Expanding the conception of the physical.* Stoljar (2001a) argues that whether zombies are conceivable depend on how we understand physical

properties. When we conceive of zombies, we hold fixed *t-physical* properties, or properties as characterized in physical theory. But we do not hold
fixed *o-physical* properties, or the underlying properties of physical objects,
including the intrinsic properties that play the roles characterized in physical theory. So the position is left open that o-physical zombie duplicates
are both inconceivable and impossible: if we adequately conceived of
the o-physical properties, we would see that any o-physical duplicate of a
conscious being is conscious. Furthermore, if we expanded P to include
hypothetical o-physical concepts of these intrinsic properties (characterizing their intrinsic nature), then $P\&\sim Q$ would be inconceivable. I think
that this is an important position, but it is clearly a version of Russellian
monism, so I take it to be compatible with the overall argument given
earlier.

(4) *Zombies presuppose epiphenomenalism.* John Perry (2001) has suggested
that the assertion that zombies are conceivable presupposes epiphenomenalism, the thesis that consciousness plays no causal role. If we thought that
consciousness plays a causal role, we would not find zombies conceivable.
In Chalmers (2004b) I argue that this claim is simply false. Its falsity is
demonstrated by the fact that many nonepiphenomenalist views are compatible with the conceivability of zombies. For example, many type-B
materialists (such as Hill, Loar, and Papineau) accept that zombies are conceivable and that consciousness plays a causal role. These philosophers deny
that zombies are possible, but that denial comes at a different stage of the
argument. Furthermore, the Russellian monist view is a nonepiphenomenalist view that we have seen is compatible with the conceivability of zombies in the relevant sense. Finally, even Cartesian interactionist dualism, in
which consciousness certainly plays a causal role, is compatible with the
conceivability (and possibility) of zombies. On such a view, physically identical beings without consciousness will presumably have large causal gaps in
their functioning (or else will have some new element to fill those gaps), but
there is nothing obviously inconceivable about such causal gaps. (For more
on this see Chalmers 2004b.)

(5) *The judgments of zombies.* It is an admittedly strange feature of zombies that they appear to make *claims* about consciousness that are indistinguishable from the claims of conscious beings and that they even make
parallel *judgments*, if judgments are functionally understood. In *The
Conscious Mind* I called this "the paradox of phenomenal judgment" and
argued that, while it is strange (many strange things happen in other possible worlds), it does nothing to undermine the coherence of zombies.
Thomas (1998) argues that we have to choose between saying that zombies'
claims are true, meaningless, insincere, or mistaken and that each of these

options is untenable. Others (Kirk 1999; Lynch 2006) have argued that the coherence of zombies undermines our *knowledge* of consciousness since we will then be unable to distinguish ourselves from zombies. In chapter 9 I argue that an appropriate account of the content and epistemology of our phenomenal judgments shows that there is no problem here.

(6) *Zombies are not positively conceivable.* Some (e.g., Ashwell 2003; Marcus 2004) have argued that while zombies may be negatively conceivable, they are not positively conceivable. To positively conceive another creature, one must conceive of some combination of physical processes and conscious states. But conceiving of physical processes clearly does not suffice to conceive of a zombie (since conscious beings may have the same processes), and in conceiving of a zombie it is out of the question to conceive of conscious states. So we can form no positive conception of a zombie.

In response, I think it is clear that when we conceive of zombies we conceive of the *absence* of consciousness. There is no more problem with clearly and distinctly imagining a situation in which there is no consciousness than in imagining a world in which there are no angels or in imagining a world with one particle and nothing else. The argument here appears to require that absences are never positively conceivable or at least that to positively conceive an absence always requires conceiving something else in its place. But these cases suggest that such a claim is clearly false. The claim may turn on misinterpreting the notion of positive conceivability. Presumably there is a sense in which conceiving of an absence is negative conceiving, but this is not the sense that is relevant here.

A general point about the preceding arguments: many of these arguments, especially 4–6, turn on considerations that are specific to the conceivability of zombies and do not apply to the conceivability of inverts and the like. One should keep in mind that for the anti-materialist argument, one does not need to consider beings as remote from us as zombies or even as remote as full-scale inverts. It suffices if we can conceive of a being whose conscious experience is for just a moment slightly different from that of an actual physical duplicate: perhaps they experience a slightly different shade at a point in the background of their visual field. Any problems that are specific to zombies then will not apply.

5. Hard-to-Classify Objections

Here I consider three objections to the argument that are not straightforwardly classifiable as objections to premise 1 or premise 2.

(1) *The conditional-concepts objection.* David Braddon-Mitchell (2003), John Hawthorne (2002a), and Robert Stalnaker (2002) have independently presented versions of the following intriguing objection. The conceivability of zombies is compatible with materialism if the concept of consciousness has a certain conditional structure. Suppose that 'consciousness' functions as follows. If dualism is true in the actual world (that is, if a relevant sort of nonphysical property is instantiated), then 'consciousness' picks out a nonphysical property, and if physicalism is true in the actual world (that is, if no relevant nonphysical property is instantiated but a relevant sort of physical property is instantiated), then 'consciousness' picks out a physical property. Then if dualism is actually true, we should accept that zombies are possible, and it is at least conceivable that dualism is actually true in that we cannot rule out the truth of dualism a priori. It follows that it is conceivable that zombies are possible. But this conceivability is entirely compatible with the claim that dualism is actually false, so that in fact zombies are impossible.

In response, let us say that S is *metaconceivable* when it is conceivable that S is possible. Then this objection shows that the *metaconceivability* of zombies may be compatible with materialism. But the relevant premise of the conceivability argument was not that zombies are metaconceivable but that zombies are conceivable. That is, the premise (at least in the negative conceivability version) asserts that we cannot rule out a priori that $P\&\sim Q$ obtains in the actual world, not that we cannot rule out a priori that $P\&\sim Q$ obtains in some possible world. There are good reasons to accept this premise, and the preceding considerations do nothing to undermine them. So these considerations do not threaten the argument.

Hawthorne and Stalnaker do not discuss the claim that zombies are conceivable (as I am understanding that claim here), and they say nothing to undermine either that claim or the claim that conceivability in this sense entails possibility, so their discussion leaves all the premises in the argument I have discussed intact. Braddon-Mitchell, by contrast, makes it clear that he accepts premise 2 but denies premise 1. He says that the apparent conceivability of zombies is just a "shadow" of their metaconceivability. That is, we are apt to conflate the claim that zombies are conceivable with the claim that they are metaconceivable, and we mistakenly take the good reasons for the latter to be reasons for the former. He does not say anything to argue directly that zombies are inconceivable, however. On the face of it, even once we distinguish the two notions, the grounds for saying that zombies are conceivable (e.g., that there is no a priori contradiction in the idea) are as strong as ever.

These proponents could suggest that the conditional account predicts that zombies are inconceivable and that it has independent support. At least on Braddon-Mitchell's version of the account (Hawthorne and Stalnaker are not explicit about this), it is an a priori conceptual truth that if PT is the case, then Q is the case, as he takes the conditional account to be an a priori conceptual analysis of phenomenal concepts. Braddon-Mitchell supports this claim by arguing that if an oracle told us that the world is purely physical, we would respond by accepting physicalism about phenomenal consciousness rather than denying that it exists. (Hawthorne makes a similar observation.)

In response, I think that although the observation about our reaction to oracles is correct, it gives no support to the conditional concepts analysis. As Alter (2006) has noted, the observation is grounded in the fact that we are more certain that we are conscious than we are of any philosophical thesis about consciousness. Furthermore, our certainty that we are conscious is plausibly a posteriori knowledge, justified by experience. If so, then (as Alter argues), our inference from PT to Q in the oracle situation is partly grounded in this a posteriori knowledge rather than being a priori. So the oracle observation does not support the thesis that it is a priori that if PT is the case, Q is the case. Furthermore, that thesis is undermined by both the zombie intuition itself and the knowledge-argument intuition that someone who knows PT would not thereby be in a position to know (through a priori reflection) what it is like to see red. So we have good reason to reject the conditional analysis of phenomenal concepts.

(2) *The zombie parity objection.* Balog (1999) has suggested that there must be something wrong with the conceivability argument on the grounds that if zombies are possible, zombies could make a parallel argument to the conclusion that materialism is false in their world. This conclusion would be incorrect, as materialism is true in their world. So something must be wrong with the zombies' argument. As the argument is valid, it must have a false premise. Balog argues that if the premises of the original argument are true, then the premises of the zombies' argument are true. It follows that one of the premises of the original argument is false. Balog locates the problem in the equivalent of premise 2, the inference from conceivability to possibility, but this specific claim is not needed to undermine the original argument.

In response, I think it is not correct that if the premises of the original argument are true, the premises of the zombies' arguments are true. A tacit premise of the original argument is Q itself, stating, for example, that someone is phenomenally conscious. (As discussed earlier, either this could be built in as an explicit premise, or it can function as part of the support for premise 4.) The corresponding premise of the zombies' argument will be the claim 'Someone is phenomenally conscious.' I think that this claim is false. For example, in a debate between zombie realists and zombie eliminativists, the zombie eliminativists (who say 'No one is phenomenally conscious') are correct. (For support for this claim, based in an analysis of phenomenal concepts, see chapter 9.) If this is right, then the zombies' argument has a false premise where the original argument has a true premise, and the failure of the zombies' argument does nothing to undermine the original argument.

(3) *The indexical objection.* A fairly common move in response to the conceivability argument (see, e.g., Ismael 1999; Perry 2001) is to suggest that it is undermined by an analogy with indexicals. Even if I have complete objective knowledge of the world, I may lack indexical knowledge, such as the knowledge that it is now 8 PM. So it is conceivable that all of those objective truths obtain and that it is not now 8 PM. However, it does not follow that the fact that it is now 8 PM is some ontologically further fact about the world and that materialism is false. Likewise, it does not follow from the conceivability of zombies that materialism is false.

One might take this to be an objection to premise 2, the inference from conceivability to possibility. But in fact the point is compatible with premise 2. Premise 2 says that if $P\&{\sim}Q$ is conceivable, it is 1-possible. The analog version for time says that if $P\&{\sim}N$ is conceivable (where N is 'It is now 8 PM'), then $P\&{\sim}N$ is 1-possible. However, $P\&{\sim}N$ *is* 1-possible in that there is a centered world verifying $P\&{\sim}N$: a world physically identical to our world, with the center placed somewhere else. In terms of the current argument, the objection is rather that from the fact that there is a *centered* world verifying $P\&{\sim}N$, it does not follow that there is an *uncentered* world satisfying $P\&{\sim}N$ (or satisfying anything in the vicinity), and such an uncentered world is what is needed for materialism to be false. By analogy, something similar goes for $P\&{\sim}Q$. So if we accept the analogy, we should deny premise 3.

In my main argument for premise 3, I assume the thesis that Q has the same primary and secondary intension. If that thesis is correct, the indexical objection does not apply as centering is irrelevant to the intensions of such sentences. If there is a centered world verifying $P\&{\sim}Q$, then the corresponding uncentered world will also satisfy ${\sim}Q$ (and any difference between the primary and secondary intensions of P will lead at worst to Russellian monism). However, a proponent of the indexical objection may hold that phenomenal concepts are themselves indexical concepts, which have distinct primary and secondary intensions (for example, the primary intension of 'I' picks out the individual at the center of a centered world, while the secondary intension of 'I' picks out the same individual in all worlds). If so, then Q will have distinct primary secondary intensions. When I considered this possibility earlier, I noted that the argument still goes through but that there is a small loophole in the argument due to centering. In effect, the proponent of the indexical objection is exploiting this loophole in order to resist the argument.

To make considerations about indexical concepts maximally explicit, one can modify the formal argument. The modified argument invokes the sentence PTI, a conjunction of P, T, and I. Here P and T are understood as before (the "that's-all" truth T is built in explicitly here for completeness), while I is a conjunction of relevant indexical truths, such 'I am x,' 'Now is y,' and so on. Here, x and y are descriptions picking out unique individuals and times (see chapter 7 for more on this). The modified argument runs as follows:

1. $PTI\&{\sim}Q$ is conceivable.
2. If $PTI\&{\sim}Q$ is conceivable, then $PTI\&{\sim}Q$ is 1-possible.
3. If $PTI\&{\sim}Q$ is 1-possible, then $PT\&{\sim}Q$ is 2-possible or Russellian monism is true.
4. If $PT\&{\sim}Q$ is 2-possible, materialism is false.

_____

5. Materialism is false or Russellian monism is true.

Here premise 2 is an instance of the general principle discussed earlier, and premise 4 is as before. The case for the modified premise 3 is more or less the same as that for the earlier premise 3. The main difference is that this version removes the residual loophole in the case for premise 3 at the end of section 3, after we relaxed the assumption that Q has the same primary and secondary intensions. That loophole involved the suggestion that a centered world w^* verifying $PT\&{\sim}Q$ need not differ in any objective respect from the actual centered world w since it might differ only in the location of the center. That loophole is now removed. If both w and w^* verify PTI, then they cannot differ only in the location of the center because I specifies that location.[2] So w and w^* will differ in objective

_____

2. Strictly speaking, there is an exception for cases of wholly symmetrical worlds where individuals cannot be picked out by any unique objective descriptions. But there is no reason to think that the actual world is such a world, and any such symmetries play no role in the judgment that $PTI\&{\sim}Q$ is conceivable.

respects despite both verifying PT, and the rest of the argument will go through as before.

As for the modified premise 1, this premise follows from the observation that adding indexical information does not close the epistemic gap between PT and Q. For example, I can coherently conceive that PT is the case, that I am x, that now is y, and that someone else is a zombie. (Note that this is a disanalogy with indexical cases: $PTI\&\sim N$ is not conceivable where N is a claim about what time it is now.) Likewise, if we give Mary in her black-and-white room the same sort of indexical information, she will still not be in a position to know what it is like to see red. The epistemic gaps are just as wide as they were before. So the modified premise 1 is as plausible as the earlier version.

At this point, an opponent may suggest that phenomenal concepts are primitive indexical concepts that are quite independent of other indexical concepts such as I and *now*. For example, phenomenal concepts might involve a primitive phenomenal indexical E, which picks out a phenomenal state of the experiencer in a way analogous to that in which 'I' and 'now' pick out the speaker and the time. If so, then the full indexical truth I must include claims of the sort 'E is such-and-such,' where the right-hand side is an independent specification of the referent. The opponent might further suggest that this right-hand side could specify a physical or functional property. That is, the indexical truth I might include a claim of the form 'E is PP,' where PP picks out a physical or functional property instantiated by the subject. (Hawthorne 2002a makes a suggestion along these lines.) But if so, $PTI\&\sim Q$ may well be contradictory. Say that Q is 'Someone instantiates E.' P will entail that 'Someone instantiates PP' and in conjunction with I will entail 'Someone instantiates E.' If so, then $PTI\&\sim Q$ is not conceivable after all.

I think that this interesting suggestion founders at the first stage. There is good reason to believe that our core phenomenal concepts are not index-icals. It is plausible that there are indexical phenomenal concepts such as E that we might gloss as *this phenomenal property*, picking out a phenomenal property that the subject is currently having. But as I argue in chapter 8, these concepts are distinct from our core phenomenal concepts, such as the pure phenomenal concept of phenomenal redness. Crucially, any identity claim involving pairs of such concepts is cognitively significant. For example, the thought *this phenomenal property is R*, involving an indexical concept and a phenomenal concept of phenomenal redness, is as cognitively significant as a thought such as *this shape is circle*, involving an indexical and a geometric concept of circularity. If so, the phenomenal concept is distinct from the indexical concept.

One can also make a direct case against any analysis of phenomenal knowledge as indexical or demonstrative knowledge as follows. The epistemic gaps associated with indexicals always disappear from an objective perspective. Say that I am physically omniscient but do not know whether I am in the United States or Australia (we can imagine that there are appropriate qualitative twins in both places). Then I am ignorant of the truth of 'I am in Australia,' and discovering that I am in Australia will constitute new knowledge. However, if other people are watching from the third-person point of view and are also physically omniscient, they will have no corresponding ignorance concerning whether I am in Australia. They will know that A is in Australia and that B is in the United States, and that is that. There is no potential knowledge that they lack. From their perspective, they know everything there is to know about my situation. So my ignorance is essentially indexical and evaporates from the objective viewpoint. The same goes for indexical ignorance concerning what time it is. When I am ignorant of the truth of 'It is now 3 AM,' a physically omniscient historian in later years will have no corresponding ignorance about whether it was then 3 AM. Demonstrative ignorance concerning the referent of "this" works in a similar way. In all of these cases, the ignorance disappears from the objective viewpoint. Objectively omniscient observers can know everything there is for them to know about my situation, and there will be no doubts left for them to settle.

The epistemic gaps associated with phenomenal knowledge behave quite differently. Consider Mary in her black-and-white room, ignorant of what it will be like for her to see red for the first time. In this case, a physically omniscient observer may have precisely analogous ignorance: even given the observer's complete physical knowledge, that person may have no idea what it will be like for Mary to see red for the first time, so this ignorance does not evaporate from the objective viewpoint. The same goes even more strongly for knowledge of what it is like for others to see red. For any observers, regardless of their viewpoint, there will be an epistemic gap between complete physical knowledge and this sort of phenomenal knowledge.

This suggests strongly that phenomenal knowledge is not a variety of indexical or demonstrative knowledge at all. Rather, it is a sort of objective knowledge of the world, not essentially tied to any viewpoint. If so, then any analysis of phenomenal concepts as indexical concepts will fail.

(4) *The objection from blockers.* Leuenberger (2008) argues that on a certain conception of physicalism, along with certain views about what is possible, the conceivability argument will not go through. Suppose that P

is such that it suffices for consciousness in any metaphysically possible world unless that world contains "blockers" (cf. Hawthorne 2002a) that prevent consciousness from arising. In this circumstance, we can say that the truth of P is *ceteris absentibus* ("other things being absent") sufficient for the truth of Q for all relevant Q. Leuenberger suggests that this condition suffices for an interesting sort of physicalism, which he calls *ceteris absentibus* physicalism. On this view, one can allow the conceivability and even the metaphysical possibility of zombies while denying the inference to the falsity of physicalism. Any world with zombies is also a world with blockers, so it is not a world that falsifies *ceteris absentibus* physicalism.

As it stands, the argument denies a version of premise 3: the claim that if $P\&\sim Q$ is possible, then physicalism is false. Now, strictly speaking, the argument I have given requires only the weaker premise that if $PT\&\sim Q$ is possible, physicalism is false, where T is a that's-all clause saying that our world is a minimal world in which P is true. But Leuenberger will also deny this premise. On his view, our world and the zombie world are both minimal worlds in which P is true (one contains consciousness; the other contains blockers; neither contains both), so that $PT\&\sim Q$ is true in the zombie world, so once again he will deny the relevant version of premise 3.

I could respond by denying that *ceteris absentibus* is strong enough to count as physicalism or in any case by saying that the argument here still establishes the falsity of physicalism in the sense that I am concerned with. But one can also respond to the argument for *ceteris absentibus* physicalism in its own right. I think it is clear that when we conceive of the zombie world, we do not conceive of a world with blockers. We conceive of a world with physics and *nothing else*: no blockers, no consciousness. That is, it is conceivable that $P\&\sim Q\&\sim B$, where B is 'There are blockers.' Leuenberger must deny that such a world is metaphysically possible. So it appears that Leuenberger must deny instances of the relevant conceivability-possibility principle, sending us back to the key issues concerning premise 2.

Leuenberger responds to an objection like this by denying that $P\&\sim Q\&\sim B$ is positively conceivable on the grounds that blockers are too unfamiliar for their absence to be positively conceivable. One can respond to this denial by extending my response to objection (6) in the previous section. Absences are positively conceivable, and absences of unfamiliar entities (aliens, ghosts, blockers) are not different in principle (Leuenberger does not give a reason to believe that if we were familiar with blockers, the situation would be any different). Furthermore, even if Leuenberger were right about this, it seems obvious that $P\&\sim Q\&\sim B$ is negatively conceivable.

Leuenberger does not deny this claim but says only that he thinks the argument from negative conceivability is less threatening to physicalism. So one can respond to this objection by defending the entailment from negative conceivability to possibility, as I do in the next section.

(5) *Objections to two-dimensional semantics.* One general sort of resistance to the two-dimensional argument comes from resistance to the two-dimensional framework as I have set it out. If one does not think that the notion of a primary intension is coherent, then most of the premises of the argument will not even be meaningful, let alone true. This sort of objection is too broad in scope to be covered in this chapter; see the appendix for some replies to objections. Here I just note that much prominent resistance to two-dimensional semantics is really resistance to the claims that the intensions it postulates are the semantic content of utterances or that they are what is said or that they are what is ascribed in propositional attitude ascriptions or some such similar thesis. It is worth noting that the arguments in this chapter need no such thesis. All they need is that sentences or utterances can be associated with primary intensions in the way I describe. Nothing turns on whether this association yields a sort of "semantic content," can be used for attitude ascriptions, and so on. All that matters is that the relation of verification between worlds and utterances is well defined and that it makes the premises true.

For example, a critical work by Bealer (2002) focuses all of its arguments on the semantic theses and gives no argument against the claim that statements can be associated with primary intensions or against the claim that they satisfy the CP theses. Something similar applies to a book on two-dimensionalism by Soames (2004), which is mostly devoted to arguing against certain two-dimensional analyses of attitude ascriptions and spends very little time arguing against the underlying association of statements with primary intensions. Setting arguments of this sort aside, the majority of other arguments against two-dimensionalism are really arguments against specific theses such as the associated conceivability-possibility premise and are addressed in the following sections. So henceforth, I assume the coherence of the framework and defend the specific theses.

6. Objections to Premise 2

Finally, we come to the crucial premise 2. It is this premise that bridges the epistemic and modal domains, and it is this premise and associated principles that have attracted the most in-depth philosophical discussion.

Premise 2 says that if $P\&\sim Q$ is conceivable, $P\&\sim Q$ is 1-possible. This premise can be seen as an instance of the general conceivability-possibility thesis CP:

CP: If S is conceivable, S is 1-possible.

Here, "conceivability" should be understood as ideal primary conceivability of either the negative or positive variety (I always take "ideal primary" as understood from here on). The two versions of the thesis that result are equivalent to theses CP– and CP+, discussed earlier. Thesis CP– is equivalent to the claim that if $\sim S$ is not a priori, S is 1-possible. The positive version, CP+, holding that if S is positively conceivable, S is 1-possible, is somewhat weaker than the negative version because positive conceivability entails negative conceivability but the reverse is not obviously the case. Much of my discussion applies equally to both CP+ or CP–, so I often just speak of CP except where the distinction is relevant.

The case for premise 2 largely derives from the case for CP, and from here on I mostly focus on the general principle rather than the specific premise. Of course, if it turns out that the general principle needs to be restricted to a certain class of sentences to be plausible, then the question will arise as to whether $P\&\sim Q$ falls into that class.

Why believe CP? In the first instance, the thesis is plausible because there are no clear counterexamples to it. Principles linking conceivability and possibility have been widely accepted in the history of philosophy but have more recently been questioned because of various counterexamples, such as the Goldbach case (both Goldbach's conjecture and its negation are conceivable, but only one is possible) and especially the Kripke cases ('Hesperus is not Phosphorus' is conceivable but not possible). CP accommodates these examples straightforwardly, with the idealization accommodating Goldbach cases, and the primary/secondary distinction accommodating Kripke cases. If it handles these cases, then the central sources of resistance to conceivability-possibility principles is undermined. But of course, there may be other possible sources of resistance.

7. Strong Necessities

Before proceeding, it is useful to clarify CP by making clear what a counterexample to it would involve.

According to the two-dimensional analysis, ordinary Kripkean a posteriori necessities such as 'water is H_2O' and 'Hesperus is Phosphorus' have
a necessary secondary intension but a contingent primary intension. That
is, such statements are 2-necessary but 1-contingent: there are centered
possible worlds (a Twin Earth world or a world with distinct morning and
evening stars) that verify their negations. When S is an a posteriori necessity of this sort, with a contingent primary intension, we might say that S
is a *weak a posteriori necessity.*

By contrast, we can say that an a posteriori necessity is a *strong a posteriori necessity* or just a *strong necessity* iff S has a necessary primary intension. Strong necessities are a posteriori necessities that are verified by all
centered metaphysically possible worlds. It is not easy to give examples of
strong necessities, because all of Kripke's a posteriori necessities appear to
be weak necessities. But I discuss some putative candidates in what follows.

It is easy to see that CP– is equivalent to the thesis that there are no
strong necessities. If S is negatively conceivable but not 1-possible, then $\sim S$
will be a strong necessity. If S is a strong necessity, then $\sim S$ will be negatively conceivable but not 1-possible.

Insofar as CP+ is potentially weaker than CP–, the relationship between
CP+ and the thesis that there are no strong necessities is not as clear.
Certainly any counterexample to CP+ will yield a strong necessity, but the
reverse is not obviously the case. To handle this, we might define two
classes of strong necessities, according to whether they provide counterexamples to CP+ or merely to CP–. Let us say that a *negative strong necessity*
is a statement S such that S is 1-necessary and 2-necessary but $\sim S$ is negatively conceivable. The latter condition is equivalent to the requirement
that S is not a priori, so negative strong necessities are equivalent to strong
necessities as defined earlier. A *positive strong necessity* is a statement S such
that S is 1-necessary and 2-necessary while $\sim S$ is positively conceivable.
Then all positive strong necessities are negative strong necessities, but the
reverse is not trivially the case. Then CP– and CP+ are equivalent to the
theses that there are no negative strong necessities and that there are no
positive strong necessities, respectively.

What would a strong necessity involve? To get an idea, consider a philosophical view on which it is metaphysically necessary that an omniscient
being (e.g., God) exists but on which it is not a priori that such a being
exists. Then, according to this view, 'An omniscient being exists' (or O) is
an a posteriori necessity. Like all a posteriori necessities, O is 2-necessary,
and $\sim O$ is negatively conceivable (and also positively conceivable if we
add the plausible claim that it is positively conceivable that there is no

omniscient being). If O were an ordinary a posteriori necessity, then O would be 1-contingent: there would be a metaphysically possible world verifying $\sim O$. However, on the philosophical view in question, there is no such world. 'There is an omniscient being' does not seem to have any difference in its primary and secondary intensions, so if a world satisfies O, it verifies O. So, given that O is 2-necessary, O is 1-necessary. It follows that if this philosophical view is correct, then O is a strong necessity. It is at least a negative strong necessity, and given the positive conceivability claim, it is a positive strong necessity.

One could put the matter by saying that there is an epistemically possible *scenario* verifying $\sim O$ but no metaphysically possible *world* verifying $\sim O$. Here a scenario can be understood as corresponding to a maximal a priori coherent hypothesis in the way that worlds correspond to maximal, metaphysically possible hypotheses. I give a formal treatment of scenarios in Chalmers (2004a, 2011), but here I leave the notion intuitive. (One might call this sort of scenario a *negative scenario* since it corresponds to a maximal, negatively conceivable hypothesis. One could also define a *positive scenario* so that it corresponds to a maximal, positively conceivable hypothesis.) The notion of scenarios is not defined in terms of metaphysical possibility, and in particular it is not assumed that scenarios correspond to metaphysically possible worlds. Nevertheless, it is plausible that there is an intimate relationship.

For any a posteriori necessity S, there will be a scenario verifying $\sim S$. For example, as 'water is H_2O' is not a priori, there will be a scenario verifying 'water is not H_2O.' That is, there will be some maximal a priori coherent hypothesis H (perhaps involving the assumption that the watery stuff is made of XYZ and so on) such that if we accept H, we should accept 'water is not H_2O.' For ordinary a posteriori necessities, these scenarios will correspond closely to centered, metaphysically possible worlds, so that there will be a centered world verifying $\sim S$. For example, 'water is not H_2O' is verified by a centered XYZ world, where the individual at the center is and has always been surrounded by clear, drinkable XYZ in the oceans and lakes. There is little reason to doubt that such a world is metaphysically possible, and there is an intuitive sense in which it qualitatively matches the scenario that we imagine when we entertain the hypothesis that water is not XYZ.

(I leave the notion of correspondence [or of qualitative matching] between scenarios and worlds at an intuitive level here because it is not needed to play a formal role in the arguments. One might formalize it by requiring that scenarios be described in a limited vocabulary consisting of semantically neutral terms and indexicals in the form $D\&I$, where D is a semantically neutral statement, and I is a conjunction of indexical statements. Then a scenario characterized by $D\&I$ will correspond to a centered world w iff D is true of w and iff I is true (in the obvious sense) of the individuals at the center of w.)

When S is a strong necessity, by contrast, there will be a scenario verifying $\sim S$, but this scenario will correspond to no metaphysically possible world. (When S is a positive strong necessity, there will be a positive scenario verifying $\sim S$; when S is a negative strong necessity, there will be a negative scenario verifying $\sim S$.) For example, given the theist view outlined earlier, there will be a (negative and positive) scenario verifying 'There is no omniscient being' involving some maximally detailed hypothesis under which there is no such being. But on this view, there is no centered world that corresponds to this scenario, and there is no centered world that itself verifies 'There is no omniscient being.' We might put this intuitively by saying that on this view, the space of (centered) metaphysically possible worlds is *smaller* than the space of epistemically possible scenarios, at least in the relevant respect. Given this view, there are scenarios that correspond to no world.

To bring this back to the mind-body case, take the paradigmatic type-B materialist who holds that premise 1 is true, premise 2 is false, and materialism is true. On this view, the material conditional $P \supset Q$ (which is itself the negation of $P\&\sim Q$) is a strong necessity. The truth of materialism implies that it is 2-necessary, the truth of premise 1 implies that it is a posteriori and its negation is 1-conceivable, but the falsity of premise 2 implies that its negation is 1-necessary. According to the type-B materialist, there are *scenarios* verifying $P\&\sim Q$, including various specific zombie scenarios, but these scenarios correspond to no metaphysically possible world.

Note that the analog of CP with scenarios instead of worlds is close to trivial. If S is conceivable in the relevant sense, there will automatically be a scenario verifying S (at least if the notions of a scenario and of verification are unproblematic). Even a type-B materialist and a believer in strong necessities can accept that principle. They must simply deny that all scenarios correspond to worlds. So CP might be seen as equivalent to the thesis that, for every scenario, there is a corresponding world.

(In Chalmers 2004a, the "core thesis" of epistemic two-dimensional semantics says that S is a priori iff S has a necessary 1-intension. If 1-intensions are defined over scenarios, then the resulting weak core thesis is independent of CP, makes no claim about metaphysical possibility, and need not be disputed by believers in strong necessities. If 1-intensions are defined over centered worlds, then the resulting strong core thesis is equivalent to CP and must be disputed by believers in strong necessities. The strong core thesis can also be understood as the thesis of metaphysical plenitude: that every negatively conceivable statement is verified by some centered world. So the nexus of the debate over premise 2 might be phrased in terms of either CP, the strong core thesis, or the thesis of metaphysical plenitude.)

My view is that for every scenario there is a corresponding world and that there are no strong necessities. In *The Conscious Mind* I gave the following reasons for this: (i) strong necessities cannot be supported by analogy with other a posteriori necessities; (ii) they involve a far more radical sort of a posteriori necessity than Kripke's, requiring a distinction between conceptual and metaphysical possibility at the level of worlds; (iii) they lead to an ad hoc proliferation of modalities; (iv) they raise deep questions of coherence; (v) strong necessities will be brute and inexplicable; and (vi) the only motivation to posit a strong necessity in the mind-body case is the desire to save materialism. I still accept most of these reasons, but there is more to say.

In the last decade or so, numerous objections to CP have been proposed. These objections fall into a number of classes. The first, and largest, involves attempts at exhibiting clear cases of strong necessities. The second involves attempts at explaining how there might be strong necessities in the phenomenal case (if not elsewhere) by analyzing the nature of phenomenal concepts. The third involves general philosophical objections. I will consider these three classes in turn.

8. Are There Strong Necessities? I: Examples

We can start with fourteen putative counterexamples to CP. The first five involve a posteriori identities. The next four are tied to issues about the a priori and a priori entailment and involve potential challenges to CP–. The last five, suggested especially by Yablo (1999, 2002), involve challenges to CP– and CP+.

(1) *Kripke cases.* It is occasionally proposed that some Kripkean a posteriori necessities are in fact strong necessities. In particular, it is sometimes proposed that coextensive names such as 'Cicero' and 'Tully' may have the same primary intension, as well as the same secondary intension. If so, 'Cicero is Tully' is a strong necessity (as it is clearly a posteriori).

In response: when we entertain the hypothesis that Cicero is not Tully, this hypothesis corresponds to specific scenarios that we can elaborate. In particular, the relevant scenarios may involve the hypothesis that the causal chains associated with the names 'Cicero' and 'Tully' pick out different historical individuals. A scenario like this certainly corresponds to a centered, metaphysically possible world: there are certainly worlds where the causal chains associated with these words function as described. And it seems clear that if we discovered that our world were such a world, we would reject the hypothesis that Cicero is Tully. So such a world seems to verify 'Cicero is not Tully' (although it may not satisfy 'Cicero is not Tully'). Worlds like this can be found for any Kripkean a posteriori necessity S (as Kripke himself pointed out, in effect), and such worlds will always verify $\sim S$.

One might resist the claim that the world in question verifies S by rejecting the claim that there is an a priori entailment (for the speaker in question) from a description of the world in question to S. In response, I think that the sort of considerations in chapter 7 strongly suggest that these entailments are a priori at least in principle. Even if one rejects this claim, however, there clearly remains *some* distinctive epistemic relation between the world in question and 'Cicero is not Tully'. In particular, it remains the case that if one accepts (hypothetically) that the actual world is qualitatively just like the world in question and reflects on this hypothesis, then one will accept the claim that Cicero is not Tully. (Note that this is quite unlike the situation that the theist thinks obtains in the God case, where there is no world that stands in this inferential relation to 'There is no God.') So if one rejects a priori entailments, one can use this sort of inferential relation to define primary intensions, and ordinary Kripkean necessities will always have a primary intension that is false at some world.

(2) *Essential modes of presentation.* Block (2006a) and Tye (1997) have suggested that one might get counterexamples to CP via identities in which each expression picks out an identity via an essential property. For example, let Q be a quantum-mechanical description that happens to pick out H_2O. Then '$Q=H_2O$' is a posteriori (since the quantum-mechanical and chemical descriptions are not conceptually connected), but each picks out the referent via an essential property (which corresponds to the primary intension), so '$Q=H_2O$' will be 2-necessary. Kallestrup (2006) also argues that a posteriori microphysical identities such as '$Q=H_2O$' will be strong necessities on the grounds that microphysical terms have identical primary and secondary intensions.

In response: it is arguable that microphysical and chemical expressions pick out their referents by *contingent* properties for reasons described earlier.

Further, an entity can have more than one essential property, so that if a substance is picked out by *distinct* essential properties, the corresponding primary intensions will differ, and the sentence will not be 1-necessary. Finally, it is pretty clear that the scenario one has in mind when one conceives of the falsity of '$Q=H_2O$' (say, a world where something with the structure of Q yields quite different chemical-level properties due to different quantum-mechanical laws) will itself correspond to a possible world w that verifies 'Q is not H_2O.' So, unless one gives independent reason to think that there is no such world w (perhaps because one holds the strong view of the necessity of laws of nature, discussed later under objection (12)), there is little reason to deny the natural view that 'Q' and 'H_2O' have distinct primary intensions. If so, there is no counterexample here.

(3) *Distinct homophonous expressions.* Block (2006a) has suggested a case analogous to the 'Cicero=Tully' case, except that the same orthographic expression is used on each side. For example, perhaps one has acquired the term 'chat' on two separate occasions for what one takes to be two separate species. As it happens, the two expressions 'chat' pick out the same referent, so that 'chat=chat' is necessary. Over time, one loses any associated information while still recognizing that these are distinct expressions. Then 'chat=chat' is not a priori. But according to Block, both sides will have the same primary intension. At least, the preceding explanation, suggesting a primary intension along the lines of "the thing causally connected to my use of 'chat,'" suggests that the two intensions are the same and the sentence is 1-necessary.

In response: even here, there will be a centered world corresponding to the scenario one has in mind when one entertains the falsity of the hypothesis one expresses with 'chat=chat'. Such a centered world involves distinct causal chains from each of the two uses of 'chat' to distinct entities. Here the two uses can at least be distinguished *indexically*, with a primary intension along the lines of "the thing causally connected to *this* use of 'chat.'" (If necessary, these indexicals can be grounded in direct indexical reference to token mental states, as with the case of demonstratives discussed below.)

(4) *Demonstratives.* Schiffer (2003) suggests a objection that turns on identities involving perceptual demonstratives, such as 'that=that'. In most such cases, there is no problem: the conceivable falsity of such a claim corresponds to a scenario in which the item causing a certain sort of experience in one differs from the item causing a different sort of experience, and this scenario will correspond to a centered world such that if one discovered this world to be actual, then one would reject 'that=that'. But there are cases in which the relevant experiences are indistinguishable, such as Austin's "two tubes" case (1990), in which one simply sees two red dots in

a symmetrical visual field, or a case where one sees many dots and has no way to pick out any one of them by description. Then the preceding model involving different sorts of experience will not apply.

In response: again one will have to invoke indexicals here so that the primary intension of each 'that' will be roughly equivalent to that of "the cause of *this* experience" for different phenomenal indexicals 'this.' In this case, the phenomenal indexical must be considered a primitive indexical akin to 'I' and 'now.' Formally, evaluating the primary intension of such an indexical requires a centered world where the center includes not just a subject and a time but also certain marked experience tokens to which the distinct phenomenal indexicals are linked. Then 'that=that' will be false at centered worlds where the two relevant experience tokens marked at the center are caused by different objects. For more on this, see chapter 8.

(5) *Dancing qualia.* Hawthorne (2006) suggests a case involving phenomenal concepts based on the dancing qualia case in *The Conscious Mind*. Say that Fred starts with identical red experiences in the left and right half of his visual field, forms concepts R_1 and R_2 (pure phenomenal concepts in the language of chapter 8) of the relevant phenomenal property (phenomenal redness), and judges $R_1 = R_2$. After this the experiences in the right half of his visual field "dance" between red and blue every minute, while they continue to play the same functional role (in *The Conscious Mind* I argue that this is naturally impossible but allow that it is logically possible). Fred has been told that this may happen, but when a change happens he is unable to notice it. After four minutes his right-field experience is back to red, and he once again entertains the thought $R_1 = R_2$. According to Hawthorne, he is unable to know $R_1 = R_2$ by any amount of a priori reasoning, so R_1 *is not* R_2 is at least negatively conceivable. But both R_1 and R_2 have the same primary intension, so $R_1 = R_2$ is 1-necessary. If so, this is a counterexample to CP–.

In response: this case should be treated analogously to a case in which Fred's cognitive processes are tampered with so that he first judges $7+5=12$ (with normal processes), then $7+5=14$ with abnormal cognition, then back again. If Fred knows this is happening, then when he entertains $7+5=12$, he will be unable to know that truth through any amount of a priori reasoning. Nevertheless, his thought is still a priori. This is simply a situation in which tampering with cognitive processes renders him less than ideal, so that he is unable to know all a priori knowable truths. (Or, in a closely related version, it is a situation where misleading empirical evidence undercuts his ability to know these truths.) The dancing qualia case should be treated the same way.

(6) *Ordinary macroscopic truths.* Another class of examples comes from the suggestion that consciousness is not alone in its failure to be a priori entailed by microphysical truths. Block and Stalnaker (1999) have suggested that many ordinary macroscopic truths such as 'Water boils at 100 degrees' (or W) are not a priori entailed in this way. If so, then $P\&\sim W$ is at least negatively conceivable. But $P\&\sim W$ is not 2-possible (at least if water and its properties supervene on the microphysical), and it is not clearly 1-possible, either. If it is not, then $P\&\sim W$ is a counterexample to CP–.

In response: chapter 7 makes the case that these macroscopic truths are a priori entailed by P or at least by $PQTI$, the conjunction of P with Q (all phenomenal truths), T (a that's-all truth) and I (indexical truths). Now, $P\&\sim Q$, $P\&\sim T$, and $P\&\sim I$ may be negatively conceivable, but the latter two are clearly also 1-possible, so they do not yield strong necessities; and the 1-possibility of $P\&\sim Q$ is precisely the current topic of dispute. So any failures of a priori entailment by P associated with the failure of entailment of Q, T, or I give no independent support to the existence of strong necessities. Such support would require at least a truth M such that $PQTI$ does not a priori entail M and such that $PQTI \supset M$ is 2-necessary and 1-necessary. The arguments in the next chapter suggest that no ordinary macroscopic truths M are like this.

In any case, even if one rejects the a priori entailment thesis here, these cases will yield at best exceptions to CP– (i.e., negative strong necessities), not exceptions to CP+ (i.e., positive strong necessities). Even if W is like Q in that $P\&\sim W$ and even $PQTI\&\sim W$ is negatively conceivable, $PQTI\&\sim W$ is not positively conceivable: "water-zombies" are not positively conceivable in the way that zombies are positively conceivable. So this sort of case leaves CP+ unthreatened.

(7) *Unknowable mathematical truths.* Perhaps the most challenging cases for CP– are mathematical truths M such that M is true (and therefore necessarily true and 1-necessarily true) but not knowable, and so not knowable a priori. If there are such cases, M is a negative strong necessity (though not a positive strong necessity, as $\sim M$ is not positively conceivable). Here one might appeal to unprovable true mathematical sentences, such as those whose existence is entailed by Gödel's theorem.

In response: unprovability in a given system does not entail nonapriority. For example, the consistency of Peano arithmetic is not provable in Peano arithmetic but is still plausibly knowable a priori. One can make the case (see Chalmers 2002b) that all true statements of arithmetic are knowable a priori at least under an idealization (i.e., our failure to know them a priori is due to certain limitations of our cognitive systems). One might worry about sentences of higher set theory, such as the continuum hypothesis, but here it is far from clear that such sentences are determinately true or false, and it is also far from clear that they are not knowable a priori under an idealization. So although these cases provide an interesting challenge to CP–, they do not provide clear counterexamples to CP–. And as in the previous case, there is no challenge to CP+ here.

(8) *Inscrutable truths.* A related class of potential counterexamples to CP– includes special sorts of true sentences M such that, according to certain philosophical views, M is not a priori entailed by any underlying qualitative truths but such that it is necessitated by such truths. In Chalmers (2002b) I call these *inscrutable truths.* Such sentences might include vague sentences such as 'John is bald' under some versions of the epistemic theory of vagueness, according to which such sentences can be true but unknowable even in principle on the basis of underlying qualitative information. Others might include certain moral or metaphysical truths, on views according to which there are true such sentences with no a priori link to underlying qualitative truths.

In response: in Chalmers (2002b) I argue that there are no compelling counterexamples here, as the philosophical views in question should all be rejected. In any case, these cases do not typically go along with the positive conceivability of $PQTI \supset {\sim}M$, so they at best challenge CP–, not CP+.

(9) *The deeply contingent a priori.* Hawthorne (2002a) suggests that some truths may be a priori even though they are false in some possible worlds considered as actual. For example, let $E \supset H$ be a conditional from one's total evidence to a hypothesis it supports. Then there are some grounds for holding $E \supset H$ to be a priori, since the inference from E to H transmits justification and arguably cannot itself be a posteriori. If this is right, then it seems to follow that $E\&{\sim}H$ is ruled out a priori, so it counts as inconceivable by the earlier definition. But $E\&{\sim}H$ is certainly 1-possible: it is verified by many worlds where the evidence E is misleading. So $E \supset H$ is not 1-necessary. Strictly speaking, this sort of case does not challenge CP– but rather challenges the associated "right-to-left" principle that 1-possibility entails 1-conceivability. This is still a worry for the framework, however, and addressing it helps to clarify an important issue.

In response: there may be a sense in which $E \supset H$ is a priori here, in that it has some justification independently of experience. But there is also a sense in which it is not, or at least in which its justification is much weaker than that of many other a priori truths. Intuitively, one cannot *conclusively* rule out the possibility that $E\&{\sim}H$, whereas one can conclusively rule out the hypothesis that $2+2=5$, for example. One can get conclusive justification from proof and analysis (among other methods), but not from abduction and induction. In the uses of the a priori in the current context, it is always the conclusive a priori that is relevant. By this standard, $E\&\sim H$ is not ruled out a priori. This allows one to accommodate the clear intuition that $E\&\sim H$ is not just 1-possible but also 1-conceivable. It is always conclusive apriority that is relevant to matters of conceivability.

(10) *Disquotational truths.* Yablo (2002) suggests that certain disquotational truths, such as "'sister' means sister," are a priori but are not 1-necessary. It could turn out that 'sister' does not mean sister in worlds where the term is used differently, and such worlds verify "'sister' does not mean sister."

In response: the treatment of this case differs depending on whether one sees "'sister'" picking out its referent orthographically (so that just a certain orthographic form is required) or semantically (so that a certain meaning is required). If "'sister'" is understood orthographically, then "'sister' means sister" is not a priori: it is substantive a posteriori knowledge that the orthographic item means anything at all. If "'sister'" is understood semantically, then "'sister' means sister" may be a priori, but it is also 1-necessary: cases where the orthographic item is used with a different meaning will be irrelevant to the primary intension of "'sister.'"

(11) *Response-enabled concepts.* Yablo (2002) argues that certain geometric terms such as 'oval' may pick out certain shapes according to the way they trigger certain responses rather than through a substantive independent grasp. In the actual world the extension of 'oval' includes cassinis (where 'cassini' is defined mathematically), but 'cassinis are ovals' is not knowable a priori. However, 'cassinis are ovals' is nevertheless necessary and 1-necessary (a world where cassinis do not cause oval experiences is not a world where it would have turned out that cassinis are not ovals, according to Yablo), so it is a strong necessity.

In response: I think that the actual term 'oval' may embody a geometric understanding so that 'cassinis are ovals' (or something like it) is a priori. But there might be other terms that could work in Yablo's response-enabled way, though, so I will go along with his treatment of 'oval' as one of them. Under this assumption, we should say that 'cassinis are ovals' is not 1-necessary. If w is a world where Hs cause oval experiences, then (under this model of 'oval') it is a priori that if w is actual, so that Hs cause oval experiences, then Hs are ovals. (What matters for evaluating a primary intension is the a priori connection, not the "turns out" claim above.)

(12) *Laws of nature.* According to some philosophical views, laws of nature are not just naturally necessary but metaphysically necessary. Shoemaker (1999) holds such a view and suggests that it may provide a counterexample to CP.

In response: on some versions of this view, laws of nature follow a version of the Kripkean model. That is, if mass in the actual world obeys certain laws, then nothing in any counterfactual world counts as mass unless it obeys exactly those laws, so any law involving mass will be necessary. On one model, this pattern obtains because of the semantics of 'mass', and in particular because a counterfactual property must have the same nomic role as actual mass in order to qualify as the referent of 'mass'. On another model, the pattern obtains because of the metaphysics of mass, and in particular because properties such as mass have their nomic profile essentially (as on Shoemaker's view). On these models, we need not deny that there are worlds that correspond to the scenario we conceive when we conceive that mass obeys different laws. It is just that such worlds will contain "schmass" rather than mass. I think that it is implausible that the modal profile of 'mass' and/or the essential properties of mass are this precise (see Fine 2002 and Sidelle 2002 for arguments to this effect), but in any case, this model does not provide a counterexample to CP. On these models, a schmass world may verify the hypothesis that the relevant law of nature is false, so laws of nature are not strong necessities.

To yield strong necessities, this sort of view must hold not only that there are no worlds where mass obeys different laws but also that there are no related worlds where something else (schmass) obeys those different laws. Here, the relevant sort of view is one according to which the fundamental properties and laws of all worlds are the fundamental properties and laws of our world (where these laws are not knowable a priori). In effect, this restricts the space of metaphysically possible worlds to the space of naturally possible worlds. If this view is correct, then a fundamental law will be a strong necessity: there will be no world corresponding to the scenario that we conceive when we conceive that it is false.

I think there are no good reasons to accept this extremely strong view of laws of nature and there are good reasons to reject it. The best reasons to take seriously the hypothesis that laws of nature are necessary come from the Kripke and Shoemaker models just mentioned. But nothing in these models supports the strong view or yields a strong necessity. Rather, the CP thesis can itself be taken as reason to reject the view.

(13) *A necessary god.* I have already noted that the existence of strong necessities is entailed by theist views on which an omniscient being (or an omnipotent being or a perfect being) exists necessarily but on which the existence of such a being is not knowable a priori. If we say that a god is by definition an omniscient being (or a perfect being or whatever), then 'A god exists' will be a strong necessity.

In response: I think that theist views of this sort are to be rejected. If the existence of such a god were knowable a priori, then such a god might exist necessarily, but if it is not, then one should conclude that such a being exists at best contingently. I cannot respond to every argument for believing in a necessary god here, but they all rest on highly contentious premises, and once again, CP itself provides an argument against these views. The best way to defend the existence of a necessary god is to argue that a world without such a being is not even conceivable.

Even if one believes that the existence of a god provides a strong necessity, it is not clear that this sort of strong necessity undermines the case against materialism. The debate over materialism uses necessity as a criterion of ontological distinctness: the question of whether physical truths necessitate phenomenal truths is relevant precisely insofar as it bears on the question of whether the phenomenal involves nothing ontologically over and above the physical. A variety of necessity in which the existence of a god is necessary will not be well suited to this ontological role. On such a view, the existence of a god will be necessitated by physical truths, but such a god will presumably nevertheless be ontologically nonphysical. So if the only strong necessities are strong necessities of this sort, connecting ontologically distinct existences, their existence is no help to physicalism. Given that $P\&\sim Q$ is conceivable, Q will be something over and above the physical, either because it is necessitated by the physical or because it is tied to the physical only by this sort of strong necessity.

Something similar applies to views on which laws of nature are strong necessities. Even on such views, laws presumably connect ontologically distinct properties: if there is a fundamental law connecting properties A and B, this will not ground any sort of ontological reduction of one property to the other. Indeed, if this view is correct, then a dualist view with fundamental phenomenal properties and fundamental laws connecting them to the physical will itself be a view on which the phenomenal is necessitated by the physical. So again, strong necessities of this sort are no help to the physicalist.

(14) *Metamodal claims.* Yablo (1999) adapts the god case to provide an intriguing argument against CP. According to Yablo, it is at least *conceivable* that there is a necessarily existing god. It is also conceivable that there is no necessarily existing god. So, if G is 'It is necessary that there is an omniscient being,' then both G and $\sim G$ are conceivable. If so, then by CP, both G and $\sim G$ are 1-possible. There appears to be no relevant distinction between the primary and secondary intensions of the expressions involved, so it follows that G and $\sim G$ are 2-possible, or (metaphysically) possible simpliciter. So it is possible that it is necessary that there is an omniscient

being, and it is possible that it is not necessary that there is an omniscient being. But this is a contradiction, at least given S5 as the logic of the metaphysical modality. If it is possible that S is necessary, then S is necessary, so it is not possible that S is not necessary.

In response: one might reply by denying S5 or by finding relevant two-dimensional structure, but I think these moves are unpromising. One could also respond, more promisingly, by making the observation about the ontological relevance of this sort of necessity. But I think it is best to deny that it is conceivable that there is a necessarily existing god, at least in the relevant sense of conceivability. Perhaps it is prima facie negatively conceivable that there is such a being, in that we cannot obviously rule it out a priori, but I do not think it is conceivable in any stronger sense. I can certainly form no clear and distinct conception of such a god (like many, I was suspicious of the idea the moment I heard about it as a student), and continued rational reflection reveals all sorts of problems with the idea. Once one accepts that it is conceivable that there is no god (and this seems like a much stronger intuition, at least to me), this has a strong tendency to undermine the coherence of the hypothesis that a god exists necessarily.

The problematic issues here arise because of the double modality. We are conceiving not just of nonmodal qualitative features of worlds but also of what is possible or necessary within those worlds. Conceiving of a god (an omnipotent, omniscient, and omnibenevolent being, say) is arguably not too hard. But to conceive in addition that the being exists necessarily, we have to conceive that the space of possible worlds is such that this god exists in each of them, despite the conceivability of a godless world. That is, we have to conceive that CP is itself false. This is what does all the work in the example: if it is conceivable that CP is false, then (by CP!) it is possible that CP is false. CP is surely necessarily true if it is true at all, so it follows from the possible falsity of CP that CP is false. (Howell 2008 argues against the current framework directly in this way.)

One way to respond to this sort of argument is to restrict the conceivability/possibility thesis to claims about the distribution of nonmodal properties within worlds, leaving double modals outside its scope. I think this response would not be entirely ad hoc (CP would then apply to worlds considered nonmodally but not to "cosmoses" of possible worlds), but I prefer to hold on to the stronger thesis by denying that it is conceivable that CP is false. I hold that CP is a priori, although highly nontrivial, like many theses in philosophy. In fact, I sketch an a priori argument for CP later in this chapter. If this is correct, then CP is not conceivably false on ideal rational reflection, and it is not ideally conceivable that a necessarily existing god exists.

(15) *The conceivability of materialism.* A closely related metamodal argument (Marton 1998; Sturgeon 2000; Frankish 2007; Brown 2010; Balog forthcoming) that is specific to the mind-body domain proceeds as follows: (i) it is at least conceivable that materialism is true about consciousness. Therefore (ii) it is conceivable that $P \supset Q$ is necessary. By CP (and setting aside two-dimensional structure), it follows that (iii) it is possible that $P \supset Q$ is necessary. From this it follows using S5 that (iv) $P \supset Q$ is necessary. Using CP and S5, one can equally infer from the fact that (v) it is conceivable that $P \supset Q$ is not necessary to the conclusion that (vi) $P \supset Q$ is not necessary. But (iv) and (vi) are contradictory. So one should reject CP.

My response here parallels the response to the previous objection. It may be prima facie negatively conceivable that materialism is true about consciousness, but this is not obviously conceivable in any stronger sense. Many people have noted that it is very hard to imagine that consciousness is a physical process. I do not think this unimaginability is so obvious that it should be used as a *premise* in an argument against materialism, but likewise, the imaginability claim cannot be used as a premise, either. Furthermore, if I am right that CP is a priori, then there is an a priori argument that $P \supset Q$ is not necessary, so that it is not even ideally negatively conceivable that $P \supset Q$ is necessary.

Overall. We have seen that while there are many putative counterexamples to CP, none of these provides a clear counterexample. In most cases, there are reasonably straightforward independent grounds for rejecting the claim that the cases in question provide strong necessities. Perhaps the most serious challenges come from mathematical cases such as the continuum hypothesis and from metamodal cases. These are the cases where, in advance of commitment to CP, independent reasoning does not clearly settle the question of whether strong necessities are involved. Still, these are cases where the initial situation is unclear rather than cases where there is a clear counterexample. If one can make the case for CP independently, then these cases are not too much of a threat.

It is also worth noting that cases such as these seem to work best as challenges to CP– rather than to CP+, so that CP+, which is all that is required for the argument against materialism, is relatively unthreatened. We have also seen at various points along the way that even if one takes certain cases to involve strong necessities, the existence of such strong necessities will still be compatible with modified versions of CP (say, a version involving ontological necessities in the law/god cases or a version involving non-modal sentences in the metamodal cases) that will be strong enough for the anti-materialist argument to go through. So where the consideration of counterexamples is concerned, the anti-materialist argument seems to be on reasonably strong ground.

9. Are There Strong Necessities? II: Explanations

In the previous section, I considered attempts on behalf of type-B materialism to establish that there are strong necessities outside the mind-body domain and I argued that these attempts fail. Other type-B materialists adopt an alternative strategy: they accept that there are no strong necessities outside the mind-body domain but argue that there are nevertheless strong necessities inside the mind-body domain. To avoid postulating an ad hoc exception, such a view must provide an *explanation* of why the mind-body domain is exceptional.

By far the most common way to explain such exceptions is to appeal to the special nature of phenomenal concepts, the concepts that we use to think about consciousness. Proponents argue that because of this nature, we should expect that there are strong necessities involving consciousness, ones that reflect not an ontological gap in nature but rather a merely epistemic gap in our cognitive processes.

I think that this strategy is the most interesting and attractive strategy for the defense of type-B materialism. However, I do not think that the strategy can work. In chapter 10, I argue that no such strategy can succeed in supporting type-B materialism against the arguments considered here. Here, I briefly consider two versions of the strategy and offer some different arguments (drawn from Chalmers 1999) against them.

(1) *Independent cognitive processes.* Hill (1997) and Hill and McLaughlin (1999) offer a psychological explanation of why we can conceive of zombies, appealing to the cognitive processes by which we conceive of physical processes and by which we conceive of experiences. On their view, these processes involve independent faculties, and the mental representations involved have independent cognitive roles, so it is to be expected that there is no conceptual connection between them. The psychological explanation is consistent with physicalism. So the conceivability of zombies does not entail the falsity of physicalism.

In response: the crucial question is whether a psychological explanation of the independence of physical and phenomenal concepts suffices to explain the existence of strong necessities. On the face of it, it seems not. After all, one can also give a psychological explanation of why we can conceive of red squares, in terms of the distinct cognitive processes involved in conceiving of color and shape. One can give a psychological explanation of why we can conceive of five-horned animals, or of silicon-based life, but no one would infer that there are strong necessities denying the metaphysical possibility of red squares or five-horned animals or silicon-based life.

An explanation of a strong necessity has to do two things: it has to show us why a state of affairs should be conceivable while at the same time being impossible. To put matters differently, it should explain why conceivability is an *unreliable* guide to the possibility of such states of affairs. This is what Kripke (1980) does in "explaining away" the intuition that heat might not have been molecular motion: he explains why and how the conceivability of this state of affairs is compatible with its impossibility. Hill (1997) likens his strategy to Kripke's, but it discharges only half of the burden. It explains why zombies might be conceivable, but it does nothing to explain why and how this conceivability coexists with the impossibility of zombies. If we do not demand such an explanation, a strategy like Hill and McLaughlin's could be used to "explain away" any conceivability intuition at all. Presumably, there will always be a psychological explanation of the processes involved in a modal intuition, but one should not infer that these intuitions are always unreliable. If one did, then one might likewise find a psychological explanation of our mathematical beliefs and infer that these beliefs are no guide to mathematical truth.

Hill and McLaughlin (1999) come close to addressing this issue by saying: "Given these differences between sensory concepts and physical concepts, a sensory state and its nomologically correlated brain state would seem contingently connected even if they were necessarily one." However, this may well be a deeply "per impossibile" counterfactual. ("Given mathematical concepts, 1+1 would seem to be 2 even if it were 3".) What we need is an explanation of how the two states could be necessarily one. Or ascending to the level of concepts, we need an explanation of how two such distinct concepts could pick out the same property. As it stands, Hill and McLaughlin's strategy does not provide such an explanation.

(2) *Recognitional concepts.* Loar (1990/1997, 1999) attempts to fill this gap by explaining how physical and phenomenal concepts can be conceptually distinct but nevertheless pick out the same property, without distinct properties serving as modes of presentation. If one could do this, one would thereby explain why identities involving such concepts are strong necessities.

Loar appeals to two theses about phenomenal concepts. First, he appeals to the thesis that they are recognitional concepts, picking out their referent through a direct process of recognition. Second, he appeals to the thesis that they have the same primary and secondary intensions. (Loar puts this in his own terminology by saying that phenomenal concepts have the same property as both referent and reference-fixer, but for ease of discussion I translate into my terminology.) The significance of the first thesis is that a recognitional concept ("*that* sort of cactus") may refer to the same property as a physical-theoretical concept even though the two concepts are cognitively distinct. On its own, this is not enough to yield a strong necessity. Recognitional concepts and physical-theoretical concepts typically have quite different primary intensions, partly because the recognitional concept picks out its referent under a contingent mode of presentation (e.g., a cactus might be picked out by relying on the sort of experience it produces). So Loar adds the second thesis, holding that phenomenal concepts are unique among recognitional concepts in having the same primary and secondary intensions. Loar also holds that theoretical physical concepts have coinciding primary and secondary intensions, an assumption that I will go along with here for the purpose of simplifying discussion. (As usual, relaxing the assumption only opens up the possibility of Russellian monism.)

From the first thesis, Loar infers that phenomenal concepts may corefer with physical concepts even though they are cognitively distinct (in such a way that zombies are conceivable). Both concepts are rigid, so they will have coinciding secondary intensions. From the second thesis (combined with the same claim about physical concepts), he infers, in effect, that the two concepts have coinciding primary intensions. So an identity involving the concepts will be 1-necessary despite being a posteriori and counterconceivable. Such an identity will be a strong necessity.

The problem with this is straightforward. The truth of the second thesis undercuts Loar's inference from the first thesis. It may be true that recognitional concepts are cognitively distinct from theoretical concepts, and it may be true that they *often* corefer with those concepts. However, the cases in which they do are all cases where the recognitional concepts have non-trivial two-dimensional structure, typically picking out their referent as the cause of a certain sort of experience (or by some similar contingent mode of presentation), so that they have distinct primary and secondary intensions. Furthermore, this two-dimensional structure provides a clear *explanation* of how and why the recognitional concept corefers with a theoretical concept. If we remove this feature of recognitional concepts (as we do in accepting the second thesis), we no longer have any reason to believe that recognitional concepts and distinct theoretical concepts should corefer.

Loar's two theses, if accepted, should lead one to accept that phenomenal concepts and physical concepts are (i) cognitively distinct and (ii) have the same primary and secondary intensions. But nothing here begins to justify the coreference of phenomenal and physical concepts. In fact, the situation is the opposite: in every other case of concepts satisfying (i) and (ii), they have distinct referents. One might suppose that recognitionality is doing some extra work here (thus distinguishing this case from other cases involving nonrecognitional concepts), but it merely supports (i), and supports the possibility of coreference when (i) is true but (ii) is false. So nothing here supports the possibility of coreference when (i) and (ii) are both true. Rather, given the truth of (i) and (ii), one should more naturally infer that the referents of the concepts differ.

Loar suggests that his two theses are themselves neutral between physicalism and dualism and therefore can equally be conjoined with the claim that phenomenal concepts pick out physical properties as with the claim that they pick out nonphysical properties. But this is far from obvious: the reasoning above suggests that Loar's two theses support the claim that phenomenal concepts pick out nonphysical properties. Perhaps Loar could build in the further claim that phenomenal concepts pick out physical properties as part of his explanation, but then this claim will be doing all the work. Loar's opponent will deny the possibility of this claim, so Loar still needs an explanation of how phenomenal concepts *could* pick out physical properties, given the earlier situation. As things stand, the model will then require that physical properties have their phenomenal mode of presentation noncontingently. But this means that the explanation is building in a necessary connection between physical and phenomenal properties from the start and so is assuming strong necessities in order to explain strong necessities.

It appears that neither Hill and McLaughlin's nor Loar's account can explain the existence of strong psychophysical necessities. Instead, both accounts need to assume such necessities at a key point as a kind of primitive. One might think that some more refined account will avoid this problem, but I think that the problem is inevitable. For an in-depth discussion of problems that afflict all appeals to phenomenal concepts to support physicalism, see chapter 10.

10. Modal Rationalism

So far I have argued that there are no clear counterexamples to the conceivability-possibility thesis and no good explanations of how it could be false. Most type-B materialists support their view either by potential counterexamples to the conceivability-possibility thesis or by potential explanations of its falsity, so I think that this removes the central plank of support from the view. Still, one might wonder why CP *has* to be true. Why *couldn't* there be strong necessities, so that some scenarios correspond to no metaphysically possible world?

The first thing one can say at this point is that in the absence of an explanation, these strong necessities will be brute and inexplicable.

Epistemically, they must be taken as primitive in the same way that we take the fundamental laws of nature as primitive. We might consider them to be either "fundamental laws of metaphysics" or laws grounded in related fundamental laws involving properties, essences, and the like. I think that there is good reason to doubt that there are a posteriori fundamental laws of this sort. Rather, where there are a posteriori fundamental laws, these should always be taken as laws of nature and therefore as metaphysically contingent.

The most fundamental reason for rejecting strong necessities comes from conceptual analysis of modal notions and an analysis of the reasons that lead us to believe in modality in the first place. This analysis is itself an extended project, but here I give the sketch of an argument.

The argument involves locating the roots of our modal concepts in the rational domain. When one looks at the purposes to which modality is put (e.g., in the first chapter of Lewis 1986), it is striking that many of these purposes are tied closely to the rational and the psychological: analyzing the contents of thoughts and the semantics of language, giving an account of counterfactual thought, and analyzing rational inference. It can be argued that for a concept of possibility and necessity to be truly useful in analyzing these domains, it must be a rational modal concept that is tied constitutively to consistency, rational inference, or conceivability.

It is not difficult to argue that even if not all conceivable worlds are metaphysically possible worlds, we *need* a modal concept tied to rational consistency, apriority, or conceivability to best analyze the phenomena in question. We might call this modality the *logical* modality. We can say that S is logically necessary when S is a priori, and we can define corresponding notions of possibility and entailment. (Note that, as defined here, the logical modality has no special connection to formal logic; the terminology is imperfect, but alternatives such as "epistemic" and "conceptual" modality also have obvious imperfections.) We can then argue that a space of logically possible *worlds* will be vital for many of the explanatory needs for which possible worlds are needed in the first place.

To see this, let us pretend for a moment that all worlds with laws of nature that differ from ours are metaphysically impossible. Even so, it will still be tremendously useful to appeal to a wider space of logically possible worlds (or worldlike entities) with different laws to help analyze and explain the hypotheses and inferences of a scientist investigating the laws of nature. Such a scientist will be considering all sorts of rationally coherent possibilities involving different laws; she will make conditional claims and engage in counterfactual thinking about these possibilities; and she may have terms and concepts that are coextensive at all worlds with our laws but that intuitively differ in meaning because they come apart at worlds with different laws. To analyze these phenomena, the wider space of worlds is needed to play the role that possible worlds usually play.

Something similar applies to zombie worlds. Even on a type-B materialist view, we can think counterfactually (and rationally) about the possibility of a different distribution of phenomenal properties with the same physical properties. We need worlds that correspond to these possibilities to make sense of counterfactual thought, of the semantics of counterfactual utterances, of rational inferences involving consciousness, of the contents of rational beliefs about consciousness, and so on. We can write coherent science fiction about zombies and speak coherently about the truth in such fictions. Talk of logically possible zombie worlds is justified in the usual way by their role in these uses.

Further, there is no bar to a space of such worlds. If one does not want simply to postulate them, one can easily construct them in an "ersatz" way, perhaps by using equivalence classes of sets of semantically neutral sentences. (If one has qualms about using the term *world* for these entities, nothing turns on the word: one can call them "scenarios" or something similar instead.) One can then introduce means of semantically evaluating expressions at these worlds, by considering these worlds as actual (considering what to infer from the hypothesis that the world actually obtains) or as counterfactual (considering what would have been the case had the world obtained). There are a few complications: one may want to add centers to the worlds for consideration as actual, and one may want to allow haecceitistic differences between worlds for consideration as counterfactual, depending on one's philosophical views. But this sort of construction is reasonably straightforward (a related construction is given in Chalmers 2011).

The two sorts of evaluation with respect to these worlds correspond to two sorts of necessity of sentences. We might say that S is *epistemically necessary* if it is true at all logically possible worlds considered as actual and that S is *subjunctively necessary* if it is true at all logically possible worlds considered as counterfactual. Truths involving the epistemic modality are in general a priori, while truths involving the subjunctive modality may be partly grounded in nonmodal truths about the actual world. When a sentence S is subjunctively but not epistemically necessary, it will be an a posteriori necessity. If property terms A and B are such that 'Something has A iff it has B' is subjunctively but not epistemically necessary, then A and B will express distinct concepts while referring to the same property. (At least this is so given a coarse-grained individuation of properties; for familiar reasons, fine-grained individuation requires going beyond possible worlds.)

On this analysis, we have two modal concepts, epistemic and subjunctive necessity. But importantly, the two concepts are constitutively linked to each other and to the rational domain. We might see both as varieties of (ideal) conceivability. Epistemic possibility involves what conceivably *might be* the case, and subjunctive possibility involves what conceivably *might have been* the case. Both are ultimately grounded in what it is rationally coherent to suppose.

These logically possible worlds and semantic evaluation over them yield a modal space that is useful for all sorts of purposes. In fact, these worlds will be useful for precisely the purposes for which possible worlds are needed in the first place. This modal space is perfectly suited to analyze such rational and psychological matters as counterfactual thought, rational inference, and the contents of thought and language. And through two-dimensional semantic evaluation, we have seen that it can yield "metaphysical" modal phenomena such as the concept/property distinction and a posteriori necessities.

At this point, opponents of the CP thesis might allow that the space of logically possible worlds is coherent and useful in its own right, but they may well suggest that we also have good reason for believing in a separate space of metaphysically possible worlds. Presumably this space will be narrower than the first space. While the space of logically possible worlds includes worlds with zombies, worlds with different laws, worlds without gods, and so on, the space of metaphysically possible worlds may exclude some or all of these.

In response, one can first argue that the space of logically possible worlds, along with the two sorts of evaluation, suffices to account for all of the modal phenomena that we have reason to believe in and that we might invoke possible worlds to explain. Certainly it accounts for the data about counterfactuals, inference, and content at least as well as the ordinary space of possible worlds does. It also accounts for the Kripkean data, concerning intuitions about a posteriori necessities and the like. While it does not account for "data" about the necessity of laws or of gods, these cannot be considered clear and untendentious data. Rather, they are theoretical claims whose status is up in the air, to be settled by the best account of modality.

One can then argue that there is no good reason to postulate a separate space of metaphysically possible worlds. There is no clear explanatory work left for such a space to do. The space of logically possible worlds, which we have independent reason to postulate, explains all of the untendentious modal data. It is not that there is no such thing as metaphysical necessity. Rather, metaphysical necessity is simply subjunctive necessity over the space of logically possible worlds. To introduce a further primitive, restricting the space of worlds, is to introduce an unnecessary wheel.

To resist, opponents might do one of four things. First, they might argue that logically possible worlds are problematic in their own right: something about their construction or the associated sorts of semantic evaluation is ill defined or incoherent. Second, they might argue that logically possible worlds cannot explain the phenomena: there are untendentious modal data that logically possible worlds cannot explain but that a separate space of metaphysically possible worlds can explain. Third, they might argue that, although logically possible worlds can explain the untendentious phenomena, there is good theoretical reason to believe in a distinct space of metaphysically possible worlds all the same. Fourth, they might argue that we have an independent pretheoretical grasp of the notion of metaphysical possibility, one to which an independent space of metaphysically possible worlds may answer.

The first strategy is unpromising, as the logical modality is well-enough behaved. Of course, a Quinean might disagree, but I think that such a Quinean then has good reason to be skeptical about the metaphysical modality in addition. The second strategy is also unpromising, as the main data that led philosophers to postulate a distinctive metaphysical modality are the Kripkean data, and these data are accommodated on the picture I have drawn.[3] As for the third strategy, the main further reasons here might be theoretical: for example, the independent reasons to believe in materialism

---

3. *One version of the second strategy (Vaidya 2008; Roca-Royes forthcoming) notes that while the two-dimensional strategy may explain intuitive Kripkean data about *de dicto* modal claims (it is necessary that water is H_2O), it does not explain Kripkean data about *de re* modal claims (this lectern is necessarily made of wood). There are at least two natural two-dimensional ways to accommodate these data, roughly depending on whether or not one allows that there can be coincident objects (like a statue and a lump of clay) with distinct modal properties. If one does not allow coincident objects, then one can hold that any apparent *de re* modal properties of an object in fact depend on the way the object is picked out (as 'Goliath' or as 'Lump,' for example) and that the different ways of picking out the object will be associated with different secondary intensions, which determine the different modal profiles. If one allows coincident objects, then one can endorse a plenitudinous ontology with arbitrarily many different coincident objects corresponding to different modal profiles. Then terms such as 'Goliath' and 'Lump' will have different primary intensions that pick out different coincident objects, with *de re* modal properties then fixed by the corresponding modal profile. Either way, the *de re* modal truths will be fixed by the two-dimensional intensions of our expressions (over logically possible worlds) along with nonmodal truths. My own view is that the choice between these two pictures is a matter of convention rather than discovery; see my "Ontological Anti-Realism" (Chalmers 2009) for more on this theme.

Vaidya (2008) argues that because the logical modality is plausibly governed by the principles of logical system S4 or S5, the modal rationalist picture cannot accommodate the violations of these principles in the *de re* cases discussed by Salmon (1989). For example, Salmon argues that while it is not possible that a given table T originated from material M (where M lies just beyond the bound of T's possible origins), it is possible that it is possible that T originated from M. Salmon's claim is far from an obvious datum, but in any case it can be accommodated on either picture. On the second picture, for example, it comes to the claim that an individual's modal profile is not essential to that individual. This claim can be accommodated by ensuring that T's modal profile picks out entities with different modal profiles in different worlds. All of this can be regarded as part of the two-dimensional structure of our concepts of table, ordinary object, and so on. A modal rationalist sympathetic with Salmon's claim might even say that it is a conceptual truth (in a broad sense tied to a priori two-dimensional structure) that if there are tables, then their modal profiles work this way.

might give one reason to take a distinct metaphysical modality seriously. These reasons count for something, but in order to have force against the analysis I have suggested, they ultimately have to be cashed out by an independent grounding for this modality.

The fourth strategy is perhaps the most interesting. Here, the idea might be that we have a pretheoretical (and perhaps primitive) grip on the notion of *a way things could have been* or of other closely related notions in the vicinity. In particular, the idea will be that we have a grip on the notion of the way things *really* could have been, such that it is at least a substantive open question whether all ways that things conceivably could have been are ways that things really could have been.

In response, I think there is good reason to doubt that we have a grip on any such notion at least insofar as the notion is distinct from rational and nomological notions. We certainly have a grip on various notions of ways things *conceivably* could have been. We also have a grip on the notion of ways things *naturally* could have been, where this notion is tied to how things could have been in our universe with its laws of nature. But there is little reason to think that we have an independent pretheoretical grip on an intermediate notion. Certainly, while there are many uses of modal phenomena in ordinary discourse that invoke broadly epistemic modalities and broadly natural modalities, it is extremely difficult to exhibit uses of modal phenomena in ordinary nonphilosophical discourse that invoke an independent metaphysical modality.

Many philosophers have been persuaded that we possess an independent concept of the metaphysical modality by Kripke's analysis. But Kripke himself simply stipulates that *p* is (metaphysically) possible if it might have been the case that *p* and goes on to make the case that this notion of possibility

---

Roca-Reyes (forthcoming, section 9) objects to the second picture on the grounds that it just relocates the problem: in order to know whether anything falls into the extension of the terms in question (whether Goliath and Lump exist, for example), we need modal knowledge which is not explained on the current account. But on this account, the existence of Goliath and Lump will be entailed a priori by underlying nonmodal truths about the world. And at least given a "lightweight" construal of existence (in the terms of Chalmers 2009), this will be a sort of conceptual entailment, so the relevant modal knowledge will be a species of broadly conceptual knowledge.

The residual issue here, perhaps, is whether the two-dimensional analysis *explains* the data concerning *de re* modality or merely *accommodates* those data. Some "heavyweight realist" opponents will hold that the phenomena here are robustly metaphysical in a way that broadly semantic and epistemological accounts such as the current one cannot explain. For example, some will hold that the existence of coincident objects or of objects with certain modal profiles requires an explanation in terms of more robustly metaphysical modal notions. These questions turn on subtle metaontological issues that I cannot settle here, but my general approach to such issues is set out in Chalmers (2009).

comes apart from apriority. That much is plausibly correct, but it does little to support a notion of metaphysical possibility that is independent of conceivability. The Kripkean reasons for believing in a distinctive metaphysical modality are all grounded in the use of subjunctive evaluation of various conceivable situations: about what could and would have been the case had various conceivable situations obtained. The corresponding notion of metaphysical possibility can be seen as the concept of subjunctive necessity over the space of logically possible worlds. So while Kripke's results make the case that the notion *it might have been that* (subjunctive) behaves differently from the notion *it might be that* (epistemic), they do little to suggest that the former is independent of conceivability and rational notions. Instead, Kripke's data can all be seen as grounded in the epistemic and subjunctive evaluation of logically possible worlds.

Overall, I think there is good reason to deny that we have an independent concept of metaphysical modality to which a separate space of worlds could answer. The believer in strong necessities must embrace a modal dualism, with distinct and independent metaphysical modalities and distinct and independent spaces of worlds that answer to them.

The picture I have sketched, in contrast, is a sort of modal monism, with a single primitive space of worlds, along with two sorts of evaluation of sentences over this space. This avoids a modal dualism with distinct primitive spaces of logically and metaphysical possible worlds. I think that this second primitive is an invention; nothing in our conceptual system requires it. It is a primitive that answers to no one and does no work.

This sort of view is occasionally described (e.g., by Sturgeon 2010) as antirealist about modality. I would not describe it that way: I think it is a view on which the metaphysical modality is perfectly real and is constitutively tied to the logical (or epistemic) modality. One is not antirealist about logic or about rational inference simply because one thinks that they are constitutively tied to the epistemic domain. The same goes for the metaphysical modality. At best, this picture is antirealist about a certain conception of the metaphysical modality, but I do not think that this conception should be taken as defining the notion. Likewise, the belief that one has a priori access to modality does not make one an antirealist about modality any more than the belief that one has a priori access to mathematical truths makes one an antirealist about mathematics.

It is also worth noting that if we postulate a metaphysical modality that is independent of conceivability, the epistemology of modality becomes quite problematic. Certainly, the most widely used route to modal conclusions goes via conceivability. The picture I have given explains why this should be so. But if metaphysical modality involves an independent primitive, then it becomes quite unclear why conceivability should be any guide to it at all. Why should there not be just one metaphysically possible world, or thirty-seven? A proponent of a distinct modality might postulate principles that entail the existence of a relatively broad space, but now the issue recurs under the guise of the question: why should we accept those principles, given that metaphysical modality is primitive? By contrast, the picture in which the metaphysical modality is grounded in the logical modality yields a simple explanation and a simple epistemology.[4]

One natural worry is this: if this modality is grounded in the rational domain, then how can it drive ontological conclusions? Why does the mere logical possibility of a zombie world entail the falsity of materialism, for example? In response, it is obvious that modal notions from the rational domain have a bearing on ontology. For example, an a priori entailment from unmarried men to bachelors gives us reason to accept that bachelors are not an ontological extra. Furthermore, materialism is itself a modal thesis, or at least a modally constrained thesis, so the analysis of modality quite reasonably drives conclusions about materialism. At this point, a type-B materialist might respond by giving up on both the modal analysis of materialism and modal constraints on materialism, instead casting the thesis in terms of (for example) metaphysical grounding or property identity. However, analogs of most of what I have said here will still be applicable. For example, there is no reason to believe in metaphysical grounding that does not have a certain relationship to conceptual or epistemic grounding. And properties themselves are constrained by their modal profiles: if two properties could possibly have come apart from one another, they are different properties. So the preceding considerations will recur as reasons to deny that the individuation of properties can come apart from the logical modality in the way that the type-B materialist requires.

According to the picture I have sketched, both the rational modal concepts (rational entailment, apriority, conceivability) and the metaphysical modal concepts (possibility, necessity, property) can be seen as part of a single family. The connection between them is subtle, but both are grounded in the rational domain. The result is modal rationalism in

---

4. *Chappell (2006) addresses this challenge by sketching a picture that grounds an entailment between conceivability and possibility while simultaneously being available to those who accept a primitive notion of metaphysical modality. This picture is grounded in two principles: "presumption of possibility," which holds that a world-candidate is metaphysically possible unless there is an explanation of why it is not, and a "consistency principle," which holds that any such explanation must be grounded in a priori coherence. These principles are intended to be a priori but substantive, so that they are compatible with the primitivist picture. Of course, one can still raise the question of how we can know these principles to be true. But in any case, Chappell's picture offers a useful alternative grounding for modal rationalism and CP, one that is available to those who accept a distinct and primitive metaphysical modality.

more senses than one: a priori access to modality and constitutive ties between the modal and rational domains.

Of course, there is much more to say about all of this. But one can discern the outlines of an account on which the link between conceivability and possibility is grounded in the rational roots of our modal concepts.

Afterword: Other Anti-Materialist Arguments

Here I discuss five other arguments against materialism through the lens of a two-dimensional analysis: the knowledge argument, the property dualism argument, Kripke's modal argument, the argument from disembodiment, and the semantic stability argument.

(1) The Knowledge Argument

The knowledge argument (Jackson 1982), concerning Mary in her black-and-white room who does not know what it is like to see red, is sometimes put as a simple deductive argument:

1. Mary knows all the physical facts.
2. Mary does not know all the phenomenal facts.

   _____

3. Some phenomenal facts are not physical facts.

Now, I think it is obvious that this simple argument on its own cannot defeat physicalism. One can put the point as follows. The expression "physical facts" is ambiguous between *narrowly physical* facts—facts about some delimited domain such as microphysics (or microphysics, chemistry, and biology) and *broadly physical* facts—including high-level physical facts that are not themselves narrowly physical facts but that supervene metaphysically on those facts. In the Mary scenario as described, it is stipulated that Mary knows all the *narrowly physical* facts, but materialism requires only that phenomenal facts are *broadly physical* facts. So if "physical facts" in the argument refers to narrowly physical facts, then the conclusion does not entail the falsity of materialism. And if "physical facts" refers to broadly physical facts, then premise 1 is unsupported by the thought experiment, since it cannot be taken for granted that Mary knows all the broadly physical facts: the premise will then beg the question against the materialist who holds that phenomenal facts are broadly physical facts.

To avoid this problem, the knowledge argument must be formulated in terms of deducibility and necessitation. One connection between narrowly and broadly physical facts is that the latter are the facts necessitated by the former. This observation on its own does not bridge the gap. But at this point we can observe that the Mary scenario supports something slightly stronger than the claim that Mary knows all the narrowly physical facts. Crucially (as emphasized in Jackson's own exposition), Mary is in a position to know all facts *deducible* from the narrowly physical facts (by a priori reasoning), as she can be taken to be an ideal a priori reasoner. Even then she will not know what it is like to see red. The premises then entitle us to the conclusion that phenomenal facts are not *deducible* from narrowly physical facts. This is now at least in the vicinity of the required conclusion that phenomenal facts are not necessitated by narrowly physical facts (and so are not broadly physical facts). To cross the gap explicitly, we can build in one more premise, yielding the following:

1. Mary is in a position to know all facts deducible from the narrowly physical facts.
2. Mary is not in a position to know all the phenomenal facts.
3. If a phenomenal fact is not deducible from the narrowly physical facts, it is not necessitated by the narrowly physical facts.

---

4. Not all phenomenal facts are necessitated by the narrowly physical facts.

I think that this is the best way to use the knowledge argument scenario to mount an argument against materialism while staying close to Jackson's original intentions. One can bring out its relationship to the arguments discussed earlier by making some cosmetic changes to simplify the argument. First, we can talk of truths rather than facts and represent the narrowly physical truths by P and the relevant phenomenal truth by Q. Second, we can identify deducibility with a priori entailment. Third, we can combine premises 1 and 2 into a single premise. Fourth, we can build in the connection between (4) and materialism explicitly. This yields the following argument:

1. $P \supset Q$ is not a priori.
2. If $P \supset Q$ is not a priori, $P \supset Q$ is not necessary.
3. If $P \supset Q$ is not necessary, materialism is false.

---

4. Materialism is false.

Reformulated this way, the argument has a familiar structure. Its structure is more or less the same as that of the conceivability argument at the beginning of the chapter. In fact, the first premise is equivalent to the claim that $P\&\sim Q$ is ideally negatively conceivable, and the second premise is equivalent to the claim that this conceivability entails that $P\&\sim Q$ is possible. So we can see the knowledge argument, formulated this way, as equivalent to a version of the conceivability argument formulated using negative conceivability. Understood this way, the role of the Mary scenario is to give support to the negative conceivability claim in the first premise.

There is one small but important difference between the knowledge argument cast in terms of deducibility and necessitation (one might call this the deducibility argument) and the negative conceivability argument. The premise that $P \supset Q$ is not a priori is slightly stronger than the premise that Mary is not in a position to know Q by a priori reasoning from P. The reason is that the latter premise could be made true by Mary's being unable to acquire the *concepts* involved in Q (such as the concept of phenomenal redness) from inside her black-and-white room. This leaves the way open for the underdiscussed *missing-concept* reply to the knowledge argument, which allows that $P \supset Q$ is a priori but holds that Mary is unable to perform the inference inside the room because she lacks the concept. To defeat this reply, one needs an argument for the stronger claim that $P \supset Q$ is not a priori, for example by arguing that even when Mary has the relevant phenomenal concepts, she cannot always deduce the relevant phenomenal truths (about other people, for example) from P. But now we are back to a version that is equivalent to the negative conceivability argument.

Comparing the arguments, we can say that the knowledge argument has the weakest first premise, the negative conceivability argument has a somewhat stronger first premise, and the positive conceivability argument has a stronger first premise again. This means that the premise behind the knowledge argument is correspondingly slightly easier to accept than the other two. This difference is reflected in the fact that some philosophers accept the claim about Mary's new knowledge while being uncertain about the conceivability claims. This advantage is balanced, however, by an inverse relationship in the strength of the premises required to get from the first premise to the failure of materialism. Here, the second premise of the positive conceivability argument is the weakest, that of the negative conceivability argument is somewhat stronger, and the corresponding premise of the knowledge argument (i.e., premise 3 linking deducibility and necessitation) is stronger again.

The missing-concept reply yields an objection to this premise of the knowledge argument but not to the corresponding premise of the conceivability argument. Also, we have seen that the second premise of the positive conceivability argument (an instance of CP+) is weaker than that of the negative conceivability argument (an instance of CP−) in that various potential counterexamples to CP− may yield objections to the latter but not to the former.

All three arguments have their place. In my view, the first premises of each are extremely plausible, so it makes sense to focus especially on the argument with the weakest second premise, namely, the positive conceivability argument. For someone who has doubts about the positive conceivability of zombies or inverts, however, the negative conceivability argument provides a somewhat weaker first premise that may be easier to accept, along with a second premise that is still plausible. As for the deducibility argument, I think its highly compelling first premise serves most effectively as part of an argument for the first premise of the negative conceivability argument, although it then requires some additional work to respond to the missing-concept reply.

In any case, once the knowledge argument is formulated in the version that is equivalent to the negative conceivability argument, the usual dialectic ensues. Most existing replies to the knowledge argument can equally be seen as replies to this argument. For example, the ability reply (holding that knowledge of what it is like to see red involves knowledge-how, not knowledge-that) can be seen as denying the claim that there are any phenomenal truths Q such that $P \supset Q$ is not a priori. The old-fact reply, which holds that Mary learns a physical fact that she already knew under a new phenomenal mode of presentation, can be seen as denying premise 2. This reply is usually inspired by analogies with cases like the water/H_2O case and the Hesperus/Phosphorus case, just as responses to the original premise 2 were.

To respond to the old-fact reply and to these analogies, one needs a link between apriority and necessity that is plausible even in light of these cases. Once again, this link can be built through the two-dimensional analysis. In effect, one can replace premise 2 by the claim that if $P \supset Q$ is not a priori, $P \supset Q$ is not 1-necessary. Then one can add further premises connecting this to the claim that $P \supset Q$ is not 1-necessary (with the loophole for Russellian monism, a loophole that is just as wide open in the original knowledge argument, as Stoljar 2001b notes) and from that claim to the conclusion that materialism is false. In my view, the resulting two-dimensional analysis of the knowledge argument is probably the most powerful way to support it.

A related way to develop the knowledge argument in response to the old-fact reply invokes what we might call the new fact thesis (Lockwood 1989, 136–37; Chalmers 1996, 141–42; Thau 2002, 127):

New fact thesis: Whenever one gains new knowledge of an old fact, one simultaneously gains knowledge of a new fact.

So when Lois, who knows that Superman can fly, learns that Clark can fly (old fact, new way), she also learns that someone working for the *Daily Planet* can fly (new fact). Strictly speaking, to make this thesis connect with the deducibility argument and to accommodate exceptions in the case of indexicals, one should invoke a modified new fact thesis (Chalmers 2005, p. 290):

Modified new fact thesis: Whenever one gains new nonindexical knowledge not deducible from previous knowledge, one simultaneously gains new knowledge (or becomes in a position to gain knowledge) of some fact that is not necessitated by the previously known facts.

This thesis then combines with the other premises of the deducibility argument to yield an argument against materialism.

I think that the resulting argument is the most powerful nontechnical version of the knowledge argument. The modified new fact thesis is roughly equivalent in strength to the CP– thesis, and any counterexamples to one are likely to be counterexamples to the other. My own view is that the best explanation of the truth of the new fact thesis is given by the two-dimensional analysis of belief and knowledge. Nevertheless, this version of the argument does not require any special technical apparatus, so it has the advantage of avoiding any objections to the apparatus itself, as well as being somewhat more accessible. So again, these two versions of the argument can work well together.

(2) The Property Dualism Argument

The property dualism argument stems from J. J. C. Smart's (1959) article advocating the mind-brain identity theory, and has more recently been developed by Stephen White (1986, 2007). Smart attributes to Max Black the objection that if mental states and physical states are contingently identical, they must still be picked out via different properties. If so, then mental terms and physical terms will be associated with distinct properties. In more contemporary terms, the underlying thesis might be put as follows:

Distinct-property thesis: When an identity claim $a=b$ is not a priori, a and b pick out their referents via distinct properties.

One might then formalize the argument as follows, where q is an arbitrary mental term:

1. For all physical terms p, $p=q$ is not a priori.
2. If $p=q$ is not a priori, p and q pick out their referent via distinct properties.

_____

3. For all physical terms p, q picks out its referent by a property distinct from the property that picks out the referent of p.

Here the conclusion is not yet the denial of materialism. One could get closer by augmenting the argument with the premise that physical terms have the same property as referent and as reference-fixer. The argument then warrants the conclusion that the reference-fixer for q is distinct from any physical property. Of course, an opponent may question the extra premise for reasons familiar from the discussion of physical terms in section 3, but as before, a proponent might respond by arguing that this loophole leads only to a Russellian version of the identity theory. Likewise, an opponent may suggest that the argument warrants only the claim that the reference-fixer for q is distinct from any narrowly physical property, not from any broadly physical property. A proponent might reply by invoking the thesis that any broadly physical property can be expressed by a physical term.

The argument can be developed in various ways; see White (1986, 2007) and Block (2006a) for versions somewhat different from the above. But it is clear that what is crucial to each is the distinct-property thesis embodied in premise 2. So here I concentrate on that thesis and on its relationship to the two-dimensional analysis.

The distinct-property thesis is closely related to the two-dimensional principle CP–. The thesis entails that when $a=b$ is not a priori, so that $a \neq b$ is negatively conceivable, $a \neq b$ will be 1-possible, which entails that a and b have distinct primary intensions. Primary intensions are not properties, but there is a close relationship. Any property corresponds to an intension (over uncentered possible worlds), picking out those individuals that have the property in a given world. Some theorists identify the property with the associated intension, and most agree that a property at least determines an intension. If so, then where there are distinct intensions, there are distinct properties.

The two-dimensional analysis also provides a natural way to determine the property or at least the intension associated with a given expression. The intension can be understood as a function that picks out what an expression picks out at a world under the hypothesis that the world in question is actual. This understanding fits naturally with the understanding in White (2007), where the distinct-property thesis is motivated by the claims that (i) when an identity is a posteriori, it can rationally be disbelieved, and (ii) for a rational belief, there will always be a possible world that rationalizes the belief: roughly, a world such that if that world were actual, the belief would be true. If we associate expressions with intensions, then these two claims (along with plausible auxiliary premises) entail that when $a=b$ is not a priori, a and b will be associated with distinct intensions.

One important difference is that where properties correspond to intensions over uncentered worlds, primary intensions are intensions over centered worlds. This difference reflects a defect in the distinct-property thesis as it stands. Indexical identity claims such as 'I am David Chalmers' are not a priori, but it is hard to find a reference-fixing property associated with indexicals such as 'I' and 'here,' and there is no obvious uncentered world that rationalizes the denial of such a claim. To fix this problem, one needs to either exclude indexicals from the scope of the distinct-property thesis or modify the thesis so that it invokes primary intensions (or perhaps reference-fixing relations) rather than properties, with centered worlds playing the role of possible worlds.

Modified in this way, the distinct-property thesis is equivalent to thesis CP–. The ensuing dialectic is also quite similar. For example, a type-B materialist might respond to White's argument by saying that rational beliefs require an *epistemically* possible situation in which the belief is true but do not require a *metaphysically* possible situation. In the terms used earlier, this comes to the claim that the identity claim in question may be false relative to some *scenario* (considered as actual) but that this scenario does not correspond to a metaphysically possible world. In effect, this response requires the existence of strong necessities, with the ensuing dialectic as before.

Likewise, Block (2006a) responds to the property dualism argument by suggesting that a posteriori identity claims always involve distinct *cognitive* modes of presentation (CMoPs) but need not involve distinct *metaphysical* modes of presentation (MMoPs, or properties). In terms of the two-dimensional framework, CMoPs might be seen as corresponding to primary intensions defined over scenarios, while MMoPs might be seen as primary intensions over centered worlds. The residual question is then, once again, the question of whether there is a centered world for every scenario. If there is, then distinct CMoPs will always entail distinct MMoPs. In any case, primary intensions are well suited to play the role of MMoPs, and the residual issue once more comes down to the question of whether there are strong necessities.

(3) The Argument from Disembodiment

One version of Descartes' conceivability argument runs as follows. Here B can stand for my body or for any physical thing:

1. It is conceivable that I am not B.
2. If it is conceivable that I am not B, it is possible that I am not B.
3. If it is possible that I am not B, then I am not B.

---

4. I am not B.

Here, the first premise is based on an intuition about disembodiment: it seems conceivable that I could exist without my body existing. The second premise is an instance of a general thesis connecting conceivability and possibility, and the third premise reflects the claim that any physical thing is essentially that physical thing. The conclusion, generalized, is that I am not any physical thing but instead am a nonphysical thing.

The soundness of this argument is often doubted, and the reasons for this doubt can be expressed straightforwardly in the current framework. The sense of conceivability in which premise 1 is plausible is primary (positive or negative) conceivability. To connect with this interpretation of premise 1, premise 2 must be interpreted as involving 1-possibility. For premise 3 to be plausible, on the other hand, it must be interpreted as involving 2-possibility. When identity statements involving rigid designators are true (or false), they are 2-necessary (or 2-impossible), but if premise 2 involves 1-possibility and premise 3 involves 2-possibility, then the argument is not valid.

One might try to find a univocal reading of the argument, but such a reading will not succeed. If premise 1 invokes secondary conceivability, then it may fail. Secondary conceivability depends on how things turn out empirically, and if it turns out that I am physical, my disembodiment will not be secondarily conceivable. If premise 1 invokes primary conceivability but premise 2 invokes 2-possibility, then it will fail, as primary conceivability does not entail 2-possibility. If premise 3 invokes

1-possibility, then it will fail, as true identity statements need not be 1-necessary. So we arrive at a familiar diagnosis of Descartes' arguments: the sort of conceivability that he is entitled to does not ground the sort of possibility that he needs.

In this case, it appears that there is no straightforward way to fix up the argument in the way that we fixed up the conceivability argument earlier. It may be that there is some way to repair the argument, but if so, it will require more than the two-dimensional tools here.

(4) Kripke's Modal Argument

The anti-materialist argument that is most closely related to the two-dimensional argument is Kripke's modal argument against the identity theory. Kripke's argument can be put as follows. Let p stand for pain and c be a term for C-fiber firing:

1. It is apparently contingent that $p=c$.
2. If it is apparently contingent that $p=c$, then there is a world with a being in an epistemic situation that is qualitatively identical to mine in which a corresponding statement is false.
3. If there is a world with a being in an epistemic situation that is qualitatively identical to mine in which a corresponding statement is false, then there is a world at which $p \neq c$.
4. If there is a world at which $p \neq c$, then $p \neq c$.

_____

5. $p \neq c$.

Here, premise 2 expresses the model that Kripke thinks works in all the usual cases of "apparently contingent" identity statements. For example, it is apparently contingent that heat is molecular motion (although this is true and necessary), and its apparent contingency is explained by a world with a being in my epistemic situation for whom a corresponding statement would be false. In particular, in a world where heat sensations are not produced by molecular motion, a corresponding utterance of 'heat is molecular motion' would be false. This model turns on there being a difference between being felt as heat and being heat. But as premise 3 suggests, Kripke holds that this model does not apply in the case of pain. Anything that is felt as pain is pain, and any epistemic situation in which something is felt as pain is an epistemic situation in which there is pain.

So if a counterpart statement is false at a world because C-fiber firing is not felt as pain in that world, then the original statement will also be false at that world because C-fiber firing cannot be pain in that world. So C-fiber firing cannot be pain anywhere.

The first premise can be seen as saying that it is conceivable in one sense that pain is not C-fiber firing. Kripke does not say a great deal about the apparent contingency of a statement, but he does say that it goes along with the sense that the statement could have turned out to be false. It seems reasonable to identify this with something like primary positive conceivability of that statement's negation. Furthermore, the second premise is closely related to the claim that '$p \neq c$' is 1-possible. Let us say that the *Kripkean primary intension* of an utterance is defined at all centered worlds where the being at the center is in the same epistemic situation and making a corresponding utterance: the intension is true at such a world if that utterance is true. Let us say that a statement is *K-possible* if its Kripkean primary intension is true at some centered world. Then premise 2 says that if a true identity statement is apparently contingent, it is K-possible. Putting all this together (and putting things using operators rather than sentence predicates to match the earlier structure), the argument can be seen as follows:

1. It is 1-conceivable that $p \neq c$.
2. If it is 1-conceivable that $p \neq c$, it is K-possible that $p \neq c$.
3. If it is K-possible that $p \neq c$, it is possible that $p \neq c$.
4. If it is possible that $p \neq c$, $p \neq c$.

———————————

5. $p \neq c$.

Interpreted this way, Kripke's argument is quite close in structure to the two-dimensional argument I have given. One obvious difference is that Kripke's argument applies only to the type identity theory, not to materialism in general. But it is clear that one might extend it, for example by replacing the identity claim $p = c$ with a conditional such as $P \supset Q$ and making some adjustments. Another difference is that Kripke's argument does not take into account the loophole for Russellian monism, which (as Maxwell 1979 observes) can itself be seen as a sort of identity theory on which $p = c$ is true because both pain and C-fiber firing are identical to a hidden intrinsic property that underlies the dispositions associated with C-fiber firing. This is because (as Maxwell also observes) Kripke's argument for premise 3 takes into account the possibility of an appearance-reality distinction for 'pain' but overlooks the possibility of a corresponding distinction for 'C-fiber firing.' When one takes this possibility into account, room for a Russellian identity theory is left open. But as before, one can always accommodate this loophole by building in Russellian monism as a disjunct in the consequent of premise 3 and in the conclusion.

The biggest problem with Kripke's argument lies with the second premise. It is not true in general that if the negation of an identity statement is 1-conceivable, it is K-possible. For example, I might introduce 'Bill' as a descriptive name that rigidly designates whatever phenomenal quality I am currently experiencing at the center of my visual field. As it happens, Bill is phenomenal blueness, but this statement seems apparently contingent in the way that any ordinary identity statement does. Like other such statements, 'Bill is not phenomenal blueness' is 1-conceivable. 'Bill is the quality at the center of my visual field' may be a priori, but 'Bill is phenomenal blueness' is not. But 'Bill is not phenomenal blueness' is not K-possible. Any being in a qualitatively identical epistemic situation to mine will be experiencing phenomenal blueness in the center of their visual field. For any such being, a statement corresponding to 'Bill is not phenomenal blueness' will be false. So 'Bill is phenomenal blueness' is K-necessary, and the generalization of premise 2 is not true in general. That is, 1-conceivability does not entail K-possibility.

This is a serious problem for Kripke's formulation of the argument. It is especially problematic because Kripke's reasoning in the case of pain and C-fibers seems to rely on just the same features that are present in the case of phenomenal blueness and Bill. It is reasonable for an opponent to say that where this argument is concerned, the identity between pain and C-fiber firing is on a par with the identity between phenomenal blueness and Bill.

One can get around this problem, but it requires dropping Kripke's framework of corresponding epistemic situations and corresponding statements. To eliminate the problem, we need to move from Kripkean primary intensions to primary intensions as I have characterized them. The two sorts of intensions resemble each other in some respects, but they are defined quite differently: Kripkean primary intensions are defined in terms of the truth of certain counterfactual statements at counterfactual worlds, whereas I have defined primary intensions in terms of the epistemic status of certain conditionals in our world. (In the terminology of Chalmers 2004a, Kripkean primary intensions are defined *contextually*, while my primary intensions are defined *epistemically*.) Correspondingly, Kripkean intensions behave like primary intensions in many but not all situations. The case of 'Bill=phenomenal blueness' is a situation where the two come apart. The Kripkean intension of my utterance of this statement is true at all centered worlds where it is defined, but the primary intension is not. In particular, the primary intension of this statement will be false at a centered world in which the individual at the center is experiencing phenomenal redness. Given the way 'Bill' functions, if I accept that my centered world is such a world, then I should accept that Bill is phenomenal redness. So while 'Bill is not phenomenal blueness' is not K-possible, it is I-possible. The case falsifies an entailment from the relevant sort of conceivability to K-possibility, but it is quite compatible with an entailment from conceivability to I-possibility.

I conclude that Kripke's argument can be modified to yield a general argument against materialism from plausible premises and that the best way to do so is to invoke the two-dimensional framework in the way that I have discussed. This is not too surprising, as the argument can itself be considered a sort of refinement of Kripke's original argument. Doing things two-dimensionally also has the advantage that many objections to Kripke's original argument can be seen straightforwardly to fail, though of course there are new objections in their place. In any case, the two-dimensional connection between the epistemic and the ontological domain seems once again to be the central locus on which many of these issues turn.

(5) The Semantic Stability Argument

Bealer (1994, 2002) gives a closely related modal argument. The key premise of Bealer's argument is something along the lines of the following:

(SS) If S is semantically stable, then if one has an a priori stable intuition that S is possible, then S is possible.

Here a term is semantically stable iff, necessarily, in any language group in an epistemic situation qualitatively identical to ours, the expression would mean the same thing. So, for example, 'two' is semantically stable, but 'water' is not. The restriction to semantic stability is intended to rule out Kripke-style a posteriori necessities such as 'water is H_2O.' As for the rest of SS, Bealer's "intuition that S is possible" seems to come to roughly the same thing as positive conceivability, and his "a priori stable" intuition of possibility comes to something like ideal positive conceivability.

An immediate problem is that Bealer's key premise SS is vulnerable to the same counterexamples as the key premise of the Kripkean argument.

For example, the term 'Bill' discussed earlier is semantically stable according to Bealer's criterion, but 'Bill is phenomenal blueness' is an a posteriori necessity. Correspondingly, there is a modal intuition that 'Bill is not phenomenal blueness' is possible, but it is not possible. Something similar applies to 'L,' a rigid designator for the number of languages actually spoken. By the definition here, 'L' is semantically stable, but '$L > 0$' is an a posteriori necessity.

To get around this problem, one can replace Bealer's notion of semantic stability by the related notion of semantic neutrality. A term T is semantically neutral iff its modal profiles are determined a priori. In two-dimensional terms, the secondary intension of T must be determined a priori: that is, for all scenarios v_1 and v_2 and all worlds w, the extensions of T at (v_1, w) and at (v_2, w) coincide. Then in our language, the reformulated thesis can be put as follows:

(SN) If S is semantically neutral, then if S is conceivable, S is possible.

Here 'conceivable' stands for ideal positive conceivability, and 'possible' can stand for ordinary metaphysical possibility, as primary/secondary distinctions do not come into play when S is semantically neutral. The counterexamples to SS involving 'Bill' and 'L' are not counterexamples to SN, as 'Bill' and 'L' are not semantically neutral: their modal profile is determined a posteriori.

The thesis SN is an immediate consequence of CP. Thesis CP tells us that when S is conceivable, it is 1-possible. When S is semantically neutral, S is 1-possible iff it is 2-possible, so thesis SN follows. On the face of it, SN is somewhat weaker than CP as it makes no commitment about the modal status of nonneutral sentences. Correspondingly, SN is perhaps slightly easier to accept, both because it is weaker and because its formulation requires less technical apparatus. At the same time, CP is more powerful in allowing an analysis of issues involving nonneutral expressions. In any case, the theses are clearly closely related, and the most important potential counterexamples to CP discussed earlier are also potential counterexamples to SN.

Because most physical expressions are arguably not semantically neutral, one cannot apply SN directly to them, and in particular one cannot use it directly to draw the conclusion that $P\&{\sim}Q$ is possible. Nevertheless, one can argue against many identity claims indirectly. For example, Bealer argues against 'pain is C-fiber firing' by applying SS to the conceivability of 'A being is in pain and has no part with more than n parts' for large n

such that a C-fiber necessarily has more than n parts. Bealer himself uses the strategy only to argue against identity physicalism, appealing to different considerations to argue against other forms, but one could go a step further to obtain a more general argument. One might apply SN to the conceivability of $S\&\sim Q$, where S is a semantically neutral characterization of the structure of microphysics, yielding (when combined with the premise that Q is semantically neutral) the conclusion that $S\&\sim Q$ is possible. One can then argue that if $S\&\sim Q$ is possible, then either $P\&\sim Q$ is possible or Russellian monism is true. What results will be a dialectic quite similar to the dialectic discussed earlier.

A recent anti-materialist argument by Nida-Rümelin (2007) raises related issues. Nida-Rümelin's key premise is a principle of cognitive transparency CT, holding that anyone who grasps a property P via two distinct concepts can in principle find out without further empirical investigation that those concepts are necessarily coextensive. Here one grasps a concept when one is in a position to know its modal profile, given one's background knowledge (so one grasps the concept *water* iff one knows that water is essentially H_2O). Nida-Rümelin uses the two-dimensional apparatus to define and analyze the notion of grasping, but at the same time she suggests that CT is weaker and less controversial than CP.

Nida-Rümelin's thesis CT is closely related to SN, however. The connection derives from the fact that, according to Nida-Rümelin's formal definitions, anyone who possesses a semantically neutral concept grasps the concept. Applying CT to this special case and making natural assumptions, one is led to CT*: any true property identity $p=q$ involving semantically neutral expressions is knowable a priori. Moreover, CT* immediately yields the following special case of SN: when (semantically) neutral $\sim(p=q)$ is ideally negatively conceivable, it is true and therefore possible. Correspondingly, potential counterexamples to SN will typically yield counterexamples to CT, as will the major potential counterexamples to CP. For example, someone such as Loar (1990/1997), who holds that there are true a posteriori property identities involving semantically neutral physical and phenomenal concepts, will deny CT* and CT. (CT* is nearly equivalent to the "semantic premise" that Loar rejects, which is in turn closely connected to the distinct-property thesis discussed earlier; see Chalmers 2005 for more discussion here.) Still, the plausibility of CT might be seen as providing one more reason to reject these views.[5]

5. For more on this matter, see http://consc.net/mnr.html.

CONCEPTUAL ANALYSIS AND REDUCTIVE EXPLANATION

[with Frank Jackson]

I. Introduction

Is conceptual analysis required for reductive explanation? If there is no a priori entailment from microphysical truths to phenomenal truths, does reductive explanation of the phenomenal fail? We say yes. Ned Block and Robert Stalnaker, in "Conceptual Analysis, Dualism, and the Explanatory Gap" (1999), say no.

Some type-B materialists respond to epistemic arguments against materialism by accepting that there is a unique epistemic gap between the domain of physical processes and the domain of consciousness, while arguing that this gap does not yield an ontological gap. Block and Stalnaker, however, argue that the gap is not unique: related epistemic gaps arise between microscopic and macroscopic processes in other domains. In particular, they argue that although there is no a priori entailment from microphysical truths to truths about consciousness, there is also no a priori entailment from microphysical truths to ordinary macroscopic truths, such as truths about water. As it is uncontroversial that water is physical, this argument is intended to undercut any inference from the failure of a priori entailment to the failure of reductive explanation or to the falsity of physicalism. Not all epistemic arguments are undercut by this strategy: arguments from positive conceivability are left standing, for example. Nevertheless, if Block and Stalnaker's arguments were successful, they would remove at least some of the sting of the epistemic gap.

A number of issues can be distinguished:

1. Is there an a priori entailment from microphysical truths to ordinary macroscopic truths?
2. If there is no a priori entailment from microphysical truths to phenomenal truths, does reductive explanation of the phenomenal fail?
3. If there is no a priori entailment from microphysical truths to phenomenal truths, is physicalism about the phenomenal false?
4. Is there an a priori entailment from microphysical truths to phenomenal truths?

We hold that the first three questions should be answered positively (with some qualifications to be outlined). Block and Stalnaker hold that the first three questions should be answered negatively. Their central strategy is to argue for a negative answer to the first question. They use this conclusion to argue for a negative answer to the second and third questions. They argue that truths about water and life, for example, are not entailed a priori by microphysical truths, and that this is no bar to the reductive explanation and physical constitution of water and of life.

In what follows, we address Block and Stalnaker's arguments for a negative answer to the first three questions, while remaining neutral on the fourth. We proceed by giving an independent defense of a positive answer to a version of the first question. This makes the ensuing reply to Block and Stalnaker more straightforward and also makes the discussion more accessible.

Because of this approach, in the bulk of this chapter we do not focus on questions about explanation or about ontology, and questions about consciousness play only a minor role. The focus is squarely on questions about conceptual analysis and a priori entailment in their own right.[1] In addition

---

1. *This bracketing of ontological issues has sometimes been overlooked by commentators on the article on which this chapter is based. For example, Levine (forthcoming) reads the article as arguing directly for ontological conclusions and responds to it as such. It is worth clarifying the dialectical situation. We think that certain epistemic gaps entail ontological gaps. Block and Stalnaker respond by arguing that epistemic gaps are ubiquitous in many domains in which there are no corresponding ontological gaps. Their argument proceeds mainly by arguing against thesis 1 about a priori entailment. We respond to them by arguing for a closely related thesis about a priori entailment. For most of the article, only these epistemological theses are at issue. Ontological and modal issues are discussed only in a brief final section of the original article, which has been deleted from this version as it recapitulates material that is discussed in much more depth in chapters 5 and 6. Levine does not engage that material, and instead reads the main sections of the article as arguing for modal rationalism and for an epistemic-ontological entailment. Arguments for these theses cannot really be found here.

to being the main locus of our disagreement with Block and Stalnaker, these questions are independently important in helping to understand the way that language and concepts relate to the rest of the world.[2]

2. Clarifying the Thesis

The initial thesis at issue is whether there is an a priori entailment from microphysical truths to ordinary macrophysical truths.[3] Before we proceed, we need to clarify and qualify this thesis to meet some obvious objections.

On our usage, P entails Q when the material conditional $P \supset Q$ is true: that is, when it is not the case that P is true and Q is false. An a priori entailment is just an a priori material conditional. For ease of usage, we will speak of a priori entailment as *implication*. On this usage, P implies Q when the material conditional $P \supset Q$ is a priori: that is, when it is possible to know that P entails Q with justification independent of experience. As defined here, entailment is a nonmodal notion, while implication involves an epistemic modality. We will assume that there are some a priori truths; general skepticism about the a priori is beyond the scope of this chapter.

As in chapter 6, let P be the conjunction of microphysical truths about the world. Microphysical truths are truths about the fundamental entities and properties of physics in the language of a completed physics. We can also stipulate that P includes the conjunction of the fundamental laws of physics. We will not engage the issue of what counts as "physics" but we stipulate that if there are any fundamental mental entities or properties, they are not part of physics. (This begs no important questions: if the mental is fundamental, it cannot be reductively explained.) We also will not engage issues arising specifically from the foundations of quantum mechanics, and we will take it for granted that microphysical truths include or imply truths about the spatiotemporal position, velocity, and mass of microscopic entities.[4] So P will likely include or imply truths about the

2. *For example, the theses about a priori entailment defended here can help serve as a foundation for the two-dimensional view of meaning and content discussed elsewhere in this book (see section 5 of the appendix for more on this theme). In part for this reason, and also for reasons discussed in section 5 of this chapter, we do not appeal to the two-dimensional apparatus in the main arguments given here.

3. Horgan (1984) puts forward a version of this thesis under the name "cosmic hermeneutics," although he qualifies the thesis to allow a role for a posteriori identities involving rigid designators in inferring macroscopic truths from microscopic truths. Chalmers (1996), Jackson (1994a, 1998), and Lewis (1994) argue for versions of the thesis.

4. To simplify, we can assume something like a Bohmian interpretation of quantum mechanics. The central claim can also be defended under other interpretations, but further complexities are involved.

distribution of fundamental entities (perhaps particles, waves, and/or fields) in space-time, truths about their fundamental properties, and truths about the fundamental laws that govern them.

Let M be a typical macroscopic truth concerning natural phenomena, such as water or life, outside the psychological, social, and evaluative domains. Some such truths are these: 'Water boils at 100 degrees centigrade,' 'Water is H_2O,' 'Water covers much of this planet,' 'Life propagates through the replication of DNA,' and 'There are many living beings'. The initial thesis at issue is that for this sort of M, P implies M. This thesis needs to be immediately qualified to handle some obvious loopholes.

(1) *Negative truths.* As described, P is compatible with the claim that there are further nonphysical entities or properties in the world: angels, perhaps, or epiphenomenal ectoplasm. So P does not imply negative truths (if they are truths) such as the truth that there are no angels or that there is no epiphenomenal ectoplasm. For similar reasons, P does not imply universally quantified truths such as the truth (if it is a truth) that all living beings contain DNA molecules.

This loophole can be closed by conjoining to P a "that's-all" statement T, asserting that our world is a *minimal* world satisfying P. Intuitively, this statement says that our world contains what is implied by P and *only* what is implied by P. More formally, we can say that world w_1 *outstrips* world w_2 if w_1 contains a qualitative duplicate of w_2 as a proper part and the reverse is not the case. Then a minimal P-world is a P-world that outstrips no other P-world.[5] It is plausible that no world containing angels is a minimal P-world: for any P-world containing angels, there is an angel-free P-world that it outstrips. So $P\&T$ implies that there are no angels. For similar reasons, $P\&T$ implies the other negative and universally quantified statements mentioned above. So the thesis at issue should be that for the relevant

5. It is well known that (just as in the case of defining intrinsic properties), some notion in this circle has to be taken as primitive: perhaps the notion of minimality or of outstripping or of containing a qualitative duplicate. One also might invoke the notion of intrinsic property itself, for example, to say that world w_1 outstrips w_2 if all the intrinsic properties and relations in w_2 are correspondingly instantiated in w_1 and if the reverse is not the case.

A complication arises in characterizing the that's-all claim in terms of minimality where a priori entailment rather than necessitation is concerned. The relevant claim must hold that the actual world is minimal among the class of *epistemic* possibilities satisfying P, where an epistemic possibility corresponds intuitively to a maximally specific hypothesis that is not ruled out a priori. On some philosophical views, this might come apart from a definition in terms of minimality among the class of metaphysical possibilities. For example, given a view on which it is necessary but not a priori that God exists, 'God exists' might be entailed by P conjoined with an assertion of metaphysical minimality, but not conjoined with an assertion of epistemic minimality. This can be handled straightforwardly by formalizing the notion of epistemic possibility (e.g., Chalmers 2011). Alternatively, where this sort of case is concerned, one can retain the intuitive characterization of the that's-all statement.

macroscopic truths M, $P\&T$ implies M. (From now on we abbreviate '$P\&T$' as 'PT' and similarly for other conjunctions among the four statements discussed in this section.)

(2) *Indexical truths.* As described, the information contained in PT specifies a world objectively. For this reason, it does not imply any indexical truths: truths such as 'I am Australian', 'life evolved in the past', or 'there is water on this planet.' It also may not imply truths such as 'water is made of H_2O.' If the universe contains an inhabited planet where there is a superficially identical liquid made of XYZ, then the information in PT alone will not allow us to decide whether we live on the H_2O planet or on the XYZ planet, so PT is at least epistemically compatible with the claim that water is made of XYZ.

This loophole can be closed by conjoining to PT some *locating* information (or *indexical* information) I, which can be thought of as a "you are here" marker added to the objective map given by PT. I can consist of the conjunction of any two truths 'I am A' and 'now is B,' where A is an identifying description of myself (or the subject in question) and B is an identifying description of the current time. (An identifying description is a description such that PT implies that there is a unique individual or time satisfying the description.) As long as PT implies all relevant objective information, then I will enable the subject to "locate" himself or herself, and PTI will imply all indexical truths.[6] So the thesis at issue should be that for the relevant macroscopic truths M, PTI implies M.

(3) *Phenomenal truths.* One of the questions at issue is whether phenomenal truths—truths concerning states of phenomenal consciousness—are implied by microphysical truths. Many hold that they are not, and also hold that adding indexical and that's-all information does not close the gap. We will not adjudicate that issue here, but we note that if phenomenal truths are not implied by PTI, then it is likely that many other macroscopic truths are not so implied either. For example, knowing whether an object is red arguably requires knowing whether it is the sort of object that causes a certain sort of color experience, and knowing whether an object is hot arguably requires knowing whether it is the sort of object that causes experiences of heat. If so, then if truths about color experience and heat experience are not implied by PTI, truths about color and heat are not implied, either.

6. Strictly speaking, to handle some cases (e.g., the "two tubes" case discussed in Austin 1990), I needs to contain further indexical information, such as information about the referent of certain special demonstratives (see Chalmers 2002b). This subtlety can be passed over for present purposes.

This loophole can be closed while remaining neutral on the important issues by conjoining Q, the conjunction of all phenomenal truths, with PTI. Q will specify the phenomenal states and properties instantiated by every subject bearing such states and properties, at every time.[7] That is, for every subject who is phenomenally conscious at a given time, Q will specify precisely what it is like to be that subject at that time. We can also stipulate that Q includes any fundamental principles that lawfully govern phenomenal states or that connect phenomenal states with physical states. The thesis at issue is then whether $PQTI$ implies the relevant macroscopic truths M, which we can now understand to include truths about color and heat, as well as phenomenal truths.

To see that this is a neutral way of posing the issue, note that if $PQTI$ implies all such M (as we shall argue), then either (i) PTI alone implies all such M or (ii) $PQTI$ implies all such M but PTI does not. In the first case, the original thesis involving PTI will be upheld. (In this case, phenomenal truths will themselves be implied by PTI.) In the second case, all failures of PTI to imply a relevant M will be associated with the failure of PTI to imply Q in the sense that adding Q will close any epistemic gaps. Putting these cases together, the thesis concerning $PQTI$ entails the crucial claim that *if* phenomenal truths are not implied by PTI, then there is a special epistemic gap in the phenomenal case.[8]

(If we combine these alternatives with the thesis that reductive explanation goes along with a priori entailment, then the first alternative leads to the view that all of the relevant macroscopic truths, including phenomenal truths, are reductively explainable. The second alternative leads to the view that phenomenal truths are not reductively explainable and that other macroscopic truths are reductively explainable "modulo phenomenology"— that is, that we can reductively explain those aspects of them for which the phenomenal plays no conceptually constitutive role. This would fit nicely with the view (articulated by Nagel 1974 and Searle 1991, among others) that the actual reductive explanation of phenomena such as color and heat has proceeded by explaining their objective aspects while leaving their subjective aspects untouched.)

7. The specification of phenomenal states in Q should use terms that express pure phenomenal concepts (chapter 8), picking out phenomenal states directly in terms of phenomenal character, as opposed to relational phenomenal concepts, which pick out phenomenal states in terms of their typical external causes or effects. We are neutral here about just what is involved in phenomenal character.

8. *Levine (forthcoming) reads "special" as building in a special metaphysical status. No such metaphysical claim is intended here: the claim is just that the epistemic gap is special in that closing it closes all other epistemic gaps.

Note that the addition of Q to the conjunction changes the way that we define T and I. (In fact, if P does not imply Q and Q is true, then the original version of PTI is false.) Given the addition of Q, T must hold that the actual world is a minimal world satisfying PQ, and I must involve identifying descriptions of a subject and a time relative to the information in PQ. So the crucial thesis is that $PQTI$, understood as the conjunction of P and Q with T and I so understood, implies M for the relevant M. Note also that the information in I depends on the specification of a subject and a time, so that strictly speaking, $PQTI$ will vary between subjects and times, and the thesis will be that $PQTI$ implies M for any given subject and time in our community. In what follows, we can assume that an arbitrary subject and time have been selected.

3. A Priori Entailment and Conceptual Analysis

It is sometimes claimed that for $A \supset B$ to be a priori, the terms in B must be definable using the terms of A. According to this view, a priori entailment requires definitions or explicit conceptual analyses: that is, finite expressions, using only terms in A, that are a priori equivalent to the original terms in B, yielding counterexample-free analyses of those terms. This is not our view. The falsity of the claim can be seen from the following.

Let G be the conjunction of the statements in the following passage: 'Smith believes with justification that Jones owns a Ford. Smith initially has no beliefs about Brown's whereabouts. Smith forms a belief that Jones owns a Ford or Brown is in Barcelona, based solely on a valid inference from his belief that Jones owns a Ford. Jones does not own a Ford, but as it happens, Brown is in Barcelona.' Let K be the statement 'John does not know that Jones owns a Ford or Brown is in Barcelona.'

It is plausible that $G \supset K$ is a priori. It is also plausible that there is no explicit analysis of the concept of knowledge using the terms involved in G. If these plausible claims are correct, a priori entailment does not require explicit analyses of the terms in the consequent using the terms in the antecedent. It is also somewhat plausible that there is no explicit analysis of the concept of knowledge at all. If this plausible claim is correct, a priori entailment does not require explicit analyses of the terms in the consequent.

The two important features of the case are the apriority of the conditional $G \supset K$ and the absence of explicit analyses of the concept of knowledge. On the first point: once general skepticism about the a priori is set aside, this conditional seems to be a typical example of an a priori truth.

Someone who knows that G is true and who possesses the concepts involved in K (in particular the concept of knowledge) is thereby in a position to know that K is true, even if they lack any further relevant empirical information. That is, a grasp of the concept of knowledge (along with a grasp of the other concepts involved) and rational reflection suffice to eliminate the possibility that G is true and K is false.

This conditional plays an essential role in Gettier's argument for the conclusion that knowledge is not justified true belief. Gettier's argument was an a priori argument in which empirical information played no essential role, and its conclusion is a paradigmatic example of a non-obvious a priori truth. The argument proceeds by presenting the possibility that G holds and appealing to the reader's concept of knowledge to make the case that if G holds, K holds (and J holds, where J is a corresponding positive claim about John's justified true belief). Empirical information plays no essential role in justifying belief in this conditional, so the conditional is a priori. The a priori conditional itself plays an essential role in deriving the a priori conclusion.

On the absence of explicit analyses of knowledge: we take it that this is a reasonable conclusion to draw from four decades of failed attempts to produce explicit analyses. Certainly no explicit analysis has met with widespread approval, and proposed analyses are always confronted quickly by plausible counterexamples. Of course, it could be that there is a correct explicit analysis that has not yet been produced or that has been produced but overlooked. But even if so, it seems clear that the a priori entailment from G to K is not *hostage* to an explicit analysis of knowledge that would support the entailment. Whether or not there is such an analysis, the entailment is a priori all the same.

So a priori entailment does not require explicit analysis. If anything, the moral of the Gettier discussion is that the reverse is often true. Explicit analyses are themselves dependent on a priori intuitions concerning specific cases, or equivalently, on a priori intuitions about certain conditionals. The Gettier literature shows repeatedly that explicit analyses are hostage to specific counterexamples, where these counterexamples involve a priori intuitions about hypothetical cases. So a priori conditionals seem to be prior to explicit analyses at least in matters of explicit justification, and in general there is no reason to hold that a priori conditionals need explicit analyses to underwrite them.

It could be argued that while these a priori entailments are not underwritten by explicit analyses, they are underwritten by explicit *sufficient* conditions for knowledge or its absence—for example, the condition that a belief based solely on inference from a false belief is not knowledge. Of course, it is trivial that there is a sufficient condition in the vicinity of such an entailment (the antecedent provides one such), so the claim will be interesting only if the complete set of sufficient conditions for knowledge is not indefinite and open-ended. But the Gettier literature suggests precisely that the set of sufficient conditions for knowledge is open-ended in this way; if it were not, we would have a satisfactory explicit analysis. And as before, the a priori entailments are not hostage to the proposed sufficient conditions; if anything, proposed sufficient conditions are hostage to a priori intuitions about specific cases.

Once an essential role for explicit definitions is eschewed, the model of conceptual analysis that emerges is something like the following. When given sufficient information about a hypothetical scenario, subjects are frequently in a position to identify the extension of a given concept, on reflection, under the hypothesis that the scenario in question obtains. Analysis of a concept proceeds at least in part through consideration of a concept's extension within hypothetical scenarios and observation of regularities that emerge. This sort of analysis can reveal that certain features of the world are highly relevant to determining the extension of a concept and that other features are irrelevant.

What emerges as a result of this process may or may not be an explicit definition, but it will at least give useful information about the features in virtue of which a concept applies to the world. It will usually be the case that one can find complex expressions whose conditions of application approximate those of the original concept to some degree, where one finds increasingly good approximations through increasingly complex expressions. In this way we can elucidate at least many important aspects of how a concept's extension depends on the world. But in general, there is no reason to suppose that a finite expression yielding a counterexample-free analysis of a concept must result from this process.[9] This pattern, whereby a conditional ability to evaluate a concept's extension yields elucidation of a concept without a finite counterexample-free analysis, is illustrated very clearly in the case of 'knowledge.'

The possibility of this sort of analysis is grounded in the following general feature of our concepts. If a subject possesses a concept and has unimpaired rational processes, then sufficient empirical information about the actual world puts a subject in a position to identify the concept's extension.

---

9. Jackson is somewhat more optimistic than Chalmers about the possibility of satisfactory finite analyses, especially if one recognizes that conceptual analysis can accommodate an element of conceptual revision to clear up confusions in a folk concept. See Jackson, Pettit, and Smith (2000) for some reasons for optimism.

For example, if a subject possesses the concept *water*,[10] then sufficient information about the distribution, behavior, and appearance of clusters of H_2O molecules enables the subject to know that water is H_2O, to know where water is and is not, and so on. This conditional knowledge requires only possession of the concept and rational reflection, and so requires no further a posteriori knowledge.[11]

Of course, this claim is trivial if the empirical information in question is allowed to include information directly involving the concept at issue (for example, *water*). But as this case and the case of knowledge suggests, the claim is often true even when that sort of information is excluded. A 'water'-free description of the world can enable one to identify the referent of *water*, and a 'knowledge'-free description of the world can enable one to decide whether a given belief is an instance of knowledge. In these cases, we can say that *nontrivially* sufficient information enables identification of a concept's extension. We will not give a precise account of what counts as nontrivially sufficient information (presumably one should also exclude near-synonymous expressions such as 'aqueous' or 'epistemic') and instead will leave the notion intuitive. There is no requirement at this point that the information in question be microphysical, or that it be about perceptual evidence, or that it be the information in *PQTI*.

This ability to identify a concept's extension is not restricted to true empirical information about the actual world. If the world had turned out differently, we could still have identified the concept's extension. Correspondingly, we can evaluate the concept's extension given *hypothetical* information about ways the actual world might be. Let us say that a hypothesis is *epistemically possible* (in the broad sense) when it is not ruled out a priori. Let us say that an epistemically possible hypothesis characterizing the total state of the world corresponds to an *epistemic possibility*: intuitively, a specific way the actual world might turn out to be, for all one can know a priori.[12] Then sufficient information about an epistemic possibility enables a subject to know what a concept's extension will be under the hypothesis that the epistemic possibility in question is actual. For

---

10. We slide between the levels of thought and language in this chapter for ease of discussion; nothing turns on this.

11. *Tye (2009, 62) reads this passage as resting on the claim that we can know a priori that something is water iff it has certain features (e.g. being a clear colorless liquid that comes out of taps), and criticizes the model for "passing the buck" from expressions such as 'water' to expressions such as 'colorless' and 'tap'. But for reasons already given, the a priori entailments in question require no such buck-passing analyses.

12. See Chalmers (2002a) for a formalization of this notion. The informal characterization suffices for present purposes.

example, in the Gettier case, it is irrelevant whether Smith's case is actual. A subject can know that *if* Smith's case as described is actual, then Smith does not know that Jones owns a Ford or Brown is in Barcelona. Or in the case of water, given appropriate information about the distribution, behavior, and appearance of clusters of XYZ molecules (information analogous to the information we have about H_2O in the actual world), a subject is in a position to conclude that *if* the information is correct, then water is XYZ.

If something like this is right, then possession of a concept such as *knowledge* or *water* bestows a *conditional ability* to identify the concept's extension under a hypothetical epistemic possibility, given sufficient information about that epistemic possibility and sufficient reasoning. That is, possession of these concepts in a sufficiently rational subject bestows an ability to evaluate certain conditionals of the form $E \supset C$, where E contains sufficient information about an arbitrary epistemic possibility and where C is a statement using the concept and characterizing its extension.[13] Conceptual analysis often proceeds precisely by evaluating conditionals like these.

In the most important cases, these conditionals will be a priori. Certainly there will be related cases in which $E \supset C$ is a posteriori. For example, it is a posteriori that if a glass contains H_2O, it contains water. However, these will be cases in which the antecedent E does not contain sufficient empirical information to identify the concept's extension given possession of the concept alone. The aposteriority of these conditionals reflects the fact that further empirical information is required for their justification. But then all we need to do is conjoin E with the relevant further empirical information F, and we will obtain a conditional $E' \supset C$ that is knowable a priori, where E' is the conjunction of E and F. For example, in the case of 'water,' identification of the concept's extension requires a great deal of further information about the distribution, behavior, and appearance of clusters of H_2O molecules in the world. Once this information F is conjoined with the original information E, we obtain a more complex conditional of the form $E' \supset C$ that is plausibly a priori.

Given sufficient empirical information in the antecedent, there is good reason to believe that the resulting conditionals will be a priori. These a priori conditionals will reflect the way in which we can identify a concept's referent. If we possess a concept, then sufficient empirical information E enables us to conclusively identify the concept's extension and to know

---

13. Determinate application of these conditionals may be restricted to epistemic possibilities that are not too far from home. When epistemic possibilities deviate greatly from our presuppositions about the actual world, some of our concepts will lose determinate application.

associated truths C, and we are in a position to do this whether the information in E is actual or hypothetical. Because all of the relevant empirical information is present in the antecedent of the con-ditional, empirical information plays no essential role in justifying belief in the conditional. So $E \supset C$ is a priori. We can call this sort of conditional an *application conditional*.

We do not claim that application conditionals with nontrivially sufficient information in the antecedent exist for all concepts. For example, it may be that there is no way to know truths about time without having empirical information that more or less explicitly invokes the concept of time. If so, there will be no antecedents with nontrivially sufficient information to imply consequents about time. Some other primitive concepts (space? cause? consciousness?) may also be like this. But for many or most concepts, there will exist application conditionals (corresponding to arbitrary epistemic possibilities) whose antecedents contain nontrivially sufficient information.

Nothing here conflicts with the conclusions of Kripke's (1980) modal arguments about names and natural kind terms. According to Kripke, it is an a posteriori necessity that water is H_2O. This modal claim is entirely compatible with there being an a priori conditional from certain (false) statements about the distribution, behavior, and role of XYZ to 'water is XYZ.' Kripke allows that a conditional can be a priori even when it is not necessary. For example, his view allows that claims such as 'heat (if it exists) is the dominant cause of heat sensations' may be a priori, although not necessary. The same goes for many claims with similar form, such as claims about the length of the meter stick in Paris. If so, then many conditionals of the same form as 'if X is such-and-such, then X is heat' may be a priori, even where it is an a posteriori necessity that heat is not X.[14]

One can put this by making the familiar observation that even if it is not metaphysically possible that water is XYZ, it is epistemically possible that

---

14. Some contemporary philosophers (e.g., Salmon 1986) go beyond Kripke's view, holding that statements such as 'heat (if it exists) is the dominant cause of heat sensations' (and the like) are *not* a priori and that many apparently empirical identities of the form 'X is Y' *are* a priori. This counterintuitive view is usually held for theory-dependent reasons. For example, if a philosophical theory holds that statements like these express singular propositions (so that 'X is Y' expresses the same singular proposition as 'Y is Y') and that the apriority of a statement is a function of the proposition it expresses, then given certain assumptions about the apriority of singular propositions the theory will be committed to these counterintuitive claims. We think that this is itself a good reason to reject the theories in question, and that there are also strong independent reasons to reject such theories, but we cannot go into that matter here. For present purposes, we simply assume that the intuitive claims about apriority are correct.

water is XYZ in the broad sense that it is not ruled out a priori that water is XYZ. It is also epistemically possible that XYZ has a certain specific distribution, behavior, and appearance (of a sort that is characteristic of water). A subject possessing the concept of 'water' can reason straightforwardly that *if* the second hypothesis obtains (in the actual world), then the first hypothesis obtains. This sort of a priori relationship among epistemic possibilities is entirely compatible with different necessary relationships among metaphysical possibilities.

There is also nothing here that contravenes Kripke's epistemological arguments against certain descriptive views of reference-fixing. Indeed, these arguments can be seen as invoking just this sort of reasoning about epistemic possibilities. In considering whether the term 'Gödel' is a priori equivalent to 'the prover of the incompleteness of arithmetic,' Kripke considers a certain epistemically possible hypothesis on which the incompleteness of arithmetic was proved by a man named 'Schmidt' and was then stolen and promulgated by a friend named 'Gödel.' Kripke suggests that if this hypothesis is actual, then our term 'Gödel' refers not to Schmidt, who proved incompleteness, but to his friend. If so, it is not a priori that Gödel (if he existed) proved the incompleteness of arithmetic. This is a straightforward example of armchair reasoning about how the extension of a concept depends on how the actual world turns out.

One observation must be made in the case of names. It is possible that two people who use a given name might use it with *different* a priori application conditionals. For example, if Leverrier uses 'Neptune' as a name for whatever planet perturbs the orbit of Uranus, then conditionals of the form 'If X is the planet that perturbs the orbit of Uranus, X is Neptune' will be knowable a priori by him. But if Leverrier's wife uses 'Neptune' knowing only that it is an astronomical object for which her husband is searching, then the conditional just mentioned will not be knowable a priori by her. She will still have an ability to know the term's extension given sufficient information about the actual world, but for her, the antecedent information will crucially require information about her husband's intentions. So possession of 'Neptune' gives the wife and the husband conditional abilities to apply the term that are somewhat different from each other. They yield different application conditionals, and they yield a different pattern of application across epistemic possibilities.

This sort of epistemic variability suggests that at least in the case of names, we should take the apriority of a sentence to be subject-relative. For example, we can say that a sentence S is a priori for a speaker when the belief that S would express for the speaker can be justified independently of experience, yielding a priori knowledge.[15] So in the case just discussed, 'Neptune (if it exists) perturbs the orbit of Uranus' is a priori for Leverrier but not for his wife. The relevant class of a priori conditionals will then be subject-relative in a similar way. But it remains the case that when a subject possesses a name, the subject will have a conditional ability to identify its extension given sufficient empirical information about the actual world, and the relevant conditionals will be a priori for the subject.

The case of names is incidental to our central purposes, but it is arguable that something similar can occur for a natural kind term such as 'water.' The most obvious cases of this will occur when a subject uses the term with deference to others in a linguistic community. Such cases will be not unlike the case of Leverrier's wife. For present purposes, it is probably best to take it that we are stipulating that the terms in question are used nondeferentially. Deference raises issues that are orthogonal to the central issues here about reductive explanation. Nothing important to those issues would change if we were dealing with a community of one speaker or with only "expert" subjects.[16]

It may be that a natural-kind term can be epistemically variable for reasons independent of deference. For example, perhaps a city dweller might use 'water' nondeferentially for the liquid that comes out of faucets (knowing nothing of oceans), and a beach dweller might use 'water' nondeferentially for the liquid in the oceans (knowing nothing of faucets). This sort of case can be treated as we suggested that cases involving names be treated: the subjects have different conditional abilities, and different associated conditionals will be knowable a priori for each of them. As before, this epistemic variability gives no reason to deny that the a priori conditionals exist. In what follows, we will usually abstract away from this sort

---

15. Alternatively, we might say that a sentence S is a priori for a subject when an assertion of S by that subject would express an a priori justifiable thought, where thoughts are the sort of propositional attitude tokens apt to be directly expressed by an assertion, including beliefs and belief-like attitudes such as entertainings. The move from beliefs to thoughts accommodates the possibility that the subject does not believe what he or she asserts. An a priori justifiable thought is a thought that can be justified independently of experience, on idealized rational reflection, yielding a priori knowledge.

16. *Díaz Leon (forthcoming b) worries that nondeferential use of an expression such as 'water' or 'H$_2$O' requires empirical knowledge of the subject matter, so that if nondeferential use is required for knowledge of the relevant conditionals, this knowledge will not be a priori. In response: it is not obvious that nondeferential use requires empirical knowledge of this sort. Perhaps mere belief in or entertaining of empirical or conditional hypotheses is enough to possess the relevant concepts. But even if empirical knowledge is required here, this should be classed with familiar cases in which empirical knowledge plays an enabling role in allowing a subject to entertain a hypothesis, rather than an epistemic role in justifying the hypothesis. Díaz Leon also suggests that we are invoking a technical notion of apriority defined in terms of expertise, but here we are using the ordinary notion involving justification independent of experience throughout.

of cross-subject variability, as the central issues about reductive explanation are largely orthogonal to these questions about variable use within a community. When necessary, all of the claims about apriority in the following can be put in subject-relative terms.

4. On the Entailment of Macroscopic Truths

We can now address the crucial question. For the relevant macroscopic truths M, does $PQTI$ imply M?

We have already made the case that for many such truths M, there is *some* nontrivially sufficient empirical information E such that E implies M. The question now is whether the specific empirical truth $PQTI$ is such an E, that is, whether $PQTI$ contains sufficient information to imply M.

A conclusive argument for this thesis would require very detailed discussion, but here we present some reasons for finding the thesis plausible. The basic argument has a two-step structure. First, $PQTI$ implies complete information (in the language of physics) about the structure, dynamics, composition, and distribution of macroscopic systems, as well as information about the actual and potential perceptual appearances that they present. Second, this information about macroscopic structure, dynamics, composition, distribution, and appearance (along with residual information from $PQTI$) implies ordinary macroscopic truths such as M. But we can take things a little more slowly. To address the question, it is useful to start by imagining that one starts with *only* the empirical information specified by $PQTI$ and by asking: could one thereby come to know the truth of M?

To start with, one can get some distance using Q alone. On a phenomenalist view, Q alone (construed as the complete truth about actual and counterfactual experiences) implies all truths. Even if phenomenalism is rejected, Q still gives a significant epistemic foothold on the world. Combining the complete phenomenal information in Q with the indexical information in I puts me in a position to determine the phenomenal character of my current experiences and of my experiences throughout my lifetime. This includes in particular the phenomenal character of a lifetime of *perceptual* experiences. This information serves as at least an epistemic guide to many macroscopic truths, just as it does in ordinary life. If V is a specific phenomenal character of a visual experience as of a large object in front of me, then if I know that I am now having an experience with phenomenal character V, then I might reasonably infer that there is a large object in front of me.[17] The same goes for many other perceptual experiences.

Of course, this information does not remotely suffice to imply all of the relevant macroscopic truths M. First, there is a vast class of truths about which my perceptual experience gives no guidance: truths concerning unperceived objects, for example. Second, for those truths M about which my perceptual experience gives guidance, it remains epistemically possible (in the broad sense) that I have these perceptual states but that M is false. Such epistemic possibilities range from traditional skeptical scenarios concerning the nonexistence of the external world to a wide range of scenarios involving perceptual illusions, false testimony, false abductive or inductive inferences, and so on.

Nevertheless, truths about which my perceptual experience gives no guidance can often be settled by further information, and skeptical scenarios can often be ruled out by further information. Starting with the further information in Q, information about others' experiences and about counterfactual experiences will give guidance about many unperceived objects. Numerous skeptical scenarios will still be left open, at least if phenomenalism and related views are rejected. But once the information in P (and T and I) is admitted, many such scenarios are immediately ruled out: those in which the physical world does not exist, for example. The residual question is whether the information in $PQTI$ suffices to derive knowledge of the unknown truths and to rule out all of the skeptical scenarios.

The information in P will play a crucial role. This includes complete information about the structure and dynamics of the world at the microphysical level: in particular, it includes or implies the complete truth about the spatiotemporal position, velocity, and mass of microphysical entities. This information suffices in turn to imply information about the structure and dynamics of the world at the macroscopic level, at least insofar as this structure and dynamics can be captured in terms of spatiotemporal structure (position, velocity, shape, etc.) and mass distribution. For example, for any given region of space at a time, the information in P implies information about the mass density in the region, the mass density in various

---

17. As before, Q characterizes the experience according to its phenomenal character alone, leaving causal relationships to the environment unspecified. So Q does not characterize V as the phenomenal character of visual experiences caused by large objects, and knowledge of Q does not build in this sort of causal knowledge. Rather, knowledge of Q builds in knowledge of phenomenal character—that is, knowledge of what it is like to have the relevant experiences. The relevant point here is that knowledge of phenomenal character alone plausibly gives some epistemic guidance about the nature of the environment even if it leaves open many skeptical hypotheses.

subregions, the causal connections among various complex configurations of matter in the region, and the extent to which the matter in the region behaves or is disposed to behave as a coherent system. This information suffices to determine which regions are occupied wholly by causally integrated systems that are disposed to behave coherently. So the information plausibly suffices for at least a geometric characterization—in terms of shape, position, mass, composition, and dynamics—of systems in the macroscopic world.

The central point here is that a macroscopic description of the world in the language of physics is implied by a microscopic description of the world in the language of physics. Such a thesis is extremely plausible. It is not subject to any worries about translation between vocabularies and it involves only a change of scale. The only worry might concern the status of bridging principles within physical vocabulary. For example, is it a priori that the mass of a complex system is the sum of the masses of its parts? If there are any concerns here, however, they can be bypassed by stipulating that the relevant physical principles are built into P.[18] In addition, P implies information about systems' microstructural composition and about the distribution of systems across space and time, including the relations between systems (characterized in macrophysical terms) and about any given system's history (characterized in macrophysical terms).

Further, the information in P and Q together will imply truths about regularities connecting the physical and phenomenal domains, and $PQTI$ will include or imply all truths about lawful covariation between the world's physical and phenomenal states. If my own phenomenal states depend directly on associated physical states, then P and Q in conjunction with I will imply information about the dependence. If there are certain regularities by which other physical systems in the world indirectly affect my perceptual phenomenal states, then P, Q, and I will imply information about those regularities. So although information about the external causes of perceptual phenomenal states is not built in to Q, $PQTI$ will imply information about these causes. It will also imply information about the perceptual phenomenal states that various external systems are disposed to cause when appropriately situated: that is, about the perceptual appearance of these systems.

---

18. In fact, for present purposes one could even stipulate that P contains a complete description of the world, both microscopic and macroscopic, in the language of physics. The central issues about consciousness and the central issues that divide us from Block and Stalnaker arise equally whether one starts with microphysics or macrophysics and so are unaffected by such a stipulation. Still, on our view such a stipulation is unnecessary.

Overall, *PQTI* implies complete information about the (geometrically characterized) structure and dynamics of macroscopic systems and objects in the world, their spatiotemporal distribution and microstructural composition, and their actual and potential perceptual appearances. This information puts a subject in a position to conclusively know (on rational reflection) the truth or otherwise of any ordinary macroscopic claim *M*. Complete knowledge of perceptual appearances yields the information that members of our community rely on in coming to know macroscopic truths, and complete structural, dynamic, distributional, and compositional information contains all the information that we need to settle the truth of claims that perceptual information does not settle.

For example, knowledge of the appearance, behavior, and composition of a certain body of matter in one's environment, along with complete knowledge of the appearance, behavior, and composition of other bodies of matter in the environment and knowledge of their relationships to oneself, puts one in a position to know (on rational reflection) whether the original system is a body of water. The same goes for knowledge of whether the system is gold, whether it is alive, whether it boils at a certain temperature, or whether it is found in the oceans. The same also applies to ordinary macroscopic truths *M* in general. Complete knowledge of structure, dynamics, composition, distribution, and appearance puts one in a position to know whether *M* is true.

Further, the information in *PQTI* serves to conclusively eliminate arbitrary skeptical hypotheses under which *M* might be false. Hypotheses involving perceptual illusions or hallucinations are eliminated by full structural and dynamic information. Hypotheses concerning differences in the past and the future are eliminated by full distributional information. Hypotheses concerning differences in underlying causal or compositional structure are eliminated by full compositional information. Even skeptical hypotheses concerning differences in others' minds are plausibly eliminated by full phenomenal information. Further skeptical hypotheses about the subject's own relation to these systems or about their exhaustiveness are removed by the indexical and that's-all information in *PQTI*. A relevant skeptical hypothesis would have to be one in which the structure, dynamics, distribution, composition, and appearance of objects and systems across space and time is preserved (along with indexical and that's-all information) but in which *M* is false. There do not seem to be any such: the knowledge outlined here suffices for conclusive knowledge of *M*.

Importantly, no other empirical information is required to justify the inference from *PQTI* to *M*. *PQTI* contains all of the information that is needed to know M. We can imagine a subject engaged in a Cartesian suspension of all empirical belief who is then given the information that $PQTI$. Given this information alone, the subject would be in a position to reconstruct knowledge of the structure, dynamics, distribution, composition, and appearance of external systems by the earlier reasoning. From there, the subject would be in a position to ascertain the truth of macroscopic claims such as M and to eliminate any relevant skeptical hypotheses. All that is required here is possession of the concepts in M, the information in $PQTI$, and rational reflection.

If so, then knowledge of $PQTI$ suffices in principle for conclusive knowledge of M, with no other empirical information required. The same reasoning applies hypothetically: even without knowing $PQTI$, a subject is in a position to know that *if $PQTI$* is true, then M is true, and is in a position to rule out any hypothesis on which $PQTI$ is true but M is not. So the subject is in a position to know the truth of the material conditional $PQTI \supset M$.[19] As before, empirical information plays no essential role in justifying knowledge of this conditional (all of the information required is present in the antecedent), so the subject is in a position to know the conditional a priori.[20] It follows that $PQTI$ implies M.

As before, a priori knowledge of $PQTI \supset M$ does not rely on any explicit analysis of the expressions involved in M or on any explicit bridging principles connecting the vocabulary of $PQTI$ with the vocabulary of M. Just as a 'knowledge'-free description of a Gettier situation implies relevant claims about knowledge without requiring an explicit bridge between the vocabularies, $PQTI$ implies the truth of M without requiring an explicit bridge between the vocabularies. Rather, $PQTI$ serves as sufficient information for determining the truth of M in the sense described earlier. In effect, this breaks down into two stages: $PQTI$ serves as sufficient information for determining complete information about structure, dynamics, distribution, composition, and appearance, and this information serves in turn as sufficient information for determining the truth of M. So $PQTI \supset M$ is an a priori application conditional.

19. One might worry that if M involves a natural kind term, belief in truths involving the term (even conditional truths) may require acquaintance with the relevant kind. In response: even if acquaintance is required for possession of the concept and so for the relevant belief, it does not enter essentially into the belief's justification for the reasons discussed here. Whatever one says about acquaintance, it is plausible that a subject competent with the terms can in principle use $PQTI \supset M$ to express a belief such that the belief is true, justified, and constitutes knowledge and such that empirical information does not enter essentially into the justification of this knowledge. So $PQTI \supset M$ will be a priori for the subject.

20. A more detailed argument against empirical justification is given in section 5, part (6).

It might be objected that we do not yet have a completed physics, so we do not yet know what P says, so we cannot know whether $PQTI$ implies M.[21] But for present purposes, we do not need to know what P says. All we have needed here is that P implies truths about the structure and dynamics of macroscopic objects in spatiotemporal terms along with truths about mass and microphysical composition. That implication is likely to be robust over physical theories: if a physical theory does not yield this implication, we are unlikely to count it as a complete physical theory. In any case, we stipulated earlier that we are assuming a physical theory that implies truths about the position, velocity, and mass of all microscopic entities. Given this assumption, the step to an analogous characterization of macroscopic systems proceeds as outlined here.

It might also be objected that no human could grasp all of the information in $PQTI$, so that no human could grasp the truth of the relevant conditional. This is surely true, but it is no bar to the apriority of the conditional. Apriority concerns what is knowable in principle, not in practice, and in assessing apriority, we idealize away from contingent cognitive limitations concerning memory, attention, reasoning, and the like. Once we idealize away from human memory and processing limitations, the problem here is removed.

We can summarize the argument in a way that makes clear the role of the idealization by appeal to a fanciful thought experiment. Imagine a human augmented by a "virtual world" machine. This is a machine containing (i) a supercomputer to store the physical information in P and to make the a priori calculations required to move from microscopic structure to macroscopic structure, (ii) a virtual reality device to produce direct knowledge of the phenomenal states described in Q, and (iii) tools that use these devices to focus on arbitrary regions of the world and to deliver information about the macroscopic structure, dynamics, composition, and perceptual appearance of systems in those regions. Using such a machine, a human with no other empirical information could straightforwardly ascertain the truth of the relevant claims M. The virtual world does no more than give access to the information contained in $PQTI$ and process this information on a priori grounds. So if a human using such a device can ascertain the truth of M, it is plausible that $PQTI \supset M$ is a priori.

---

21. Byrne (1999) makes this sort of objection against an argument for a priori entailment in Chalmers (1996). Byrne's objections pass over the two-step character of the entailment from microphysical structure and dynamics to macrophysical structure and dynamics and from there (in combination with perceptual appearances) to the relevant macroscopic truths. (This two-step structure is present in Chalmers 1996, albeit briefly.) His discussion also passes over the role of epistemological considerations regarding the elimination of skeptical scenarios.

One might ask the following. Given that $PQTI$ implies ordinary macroscopic truths, does similar reasoning suggest that PTI alone implies many such truths? Such reasoning may work for truths concerning the objective spatiotemporal structure of macroscopic systems. But for many or most macroscopic expressions (most obviously expressions such as 'green' and 'hot' but plausibly also expressions such as 'water' and 'tiger'), our application of the expressions relies essentially on associated perceptual appearances. For a typical truth M involving such an expression, PTI will imply M only if PTI implies truths about the associated perceptual appearances. This will plausibly require that PTI implies the relevant phenomenal truths in Q.

One can then ask: could reasoning such as that given earlier establish that PTI implies the truths in Q? It seems not. There are familiar reasons (e.g., Jackson 1982) to hold that information about the structure, dynamics, and composition of physical systems does not suffice for information about the character of conscious experiences. There are also familiar reasons (see chapters 5 and 6) to hold that there are conceptually coherent alternative possibilities in which things are physically just as in PTI but in which different sorts of experiences are present or in which there are no experiences at all.[22] Whether or not these reasons are sound, their existence makes it clear that there is no direct argument that PTI implies Q analogous to the present argument concerning $PQTI$. Any argument that PTI implies Q must rest on quite different considerations.[23]

Note that we have not argued here that $PQTI$ implies every truth in every domain (although we are inclined to accept this claim). Given what we have said here, it could be that certain truths in special domains—perhaps concerning mathematics, metaphysics, morality, or mentality—are not implied by $PQTI$.[24] Presumably this will be because these truths are

22. A reviewer asks whether this can be squared with knowledge of other minds. Yes: just as the information in Q can be an epistemic guide to truths about the external world without implying those truths, the information in P (and information about one's own mind) might be an epistemic guide to truths about other minds without implying those truths.

23. Jackson articulates considerations of this sort in forthcoming work.

24. One might worry in particular about mental truths concerning subjects' propositional attitudes. If these truths are not implied by $PQTI$, then it is likely that many other truths will not be: perhaps truths involving social concepts (e.g., 'money') or involving terms used deferentially (e.g., 'arthritis,' used by an nonexpert). For a more general thesis that applies to such truths, one would need to argue that $PQTI$ implies these mental truths (as we hold) or to expand $PQTI$ to include mental truths of a more general sort. This question does not affect the present discussion, as truths involving ordinary macroscopic concepts of the natural world (such as 'water' or 'gold,' used nondeferentially) do not seem to be tied to propositional attitudes in this way.

not conclusively knowable even given full information about structure, dynamics, appearance, distribution, composition and so on. Perhaps these truths are knowable only through different means, or perhaps they are not conclusively knowable at all. But we hope we have said enough to make it plausible that ordinary macroscopic truths concerning everyday macroscopic natural phenomena are implied by *PQTI*.

5. Block and Stalnaker on A Priori Entailment

Block and Stalnaker (1999) give a number of arguments against a priori entailments from microphysical truths to macroscopic truths. They do not always cast things in these terms: their discussion often suggests that the issue is whether there is an analysis of macroscopic concepts "in microphysical terms" and whether principles that cross the bridge from microphysical to macroscopic are themselves "microphysical claims." This way of putting things is unfortunate, as on a natural reading these theses are implausible and much stronger than what is needed. But it is clear from the context of Block and Stalnaker's discussion that a priori entailment is the real issue, and many of their arguments are naturally seen as arguments against a priori entailments.

(1) *Explicit analyses.* One aspect of the global structure of Block and Stalnaker's article can be seen as follows. In the first part (especially sections 4–9), they argue that there are no explicit analyses of typical macroscopic expressions (such as 'water' and 'life') of a sort that could support an a priori entailment from microphysical to macroscopic truths. In the second part (the long section 10), they discuss the use of the two-dimensional semantic framework as an alternative to explicit analyses and argue that the existence of the framework does not support the a priori entailments in question. The intended upshot is that the existence of these a priori entailments is doubtful and that reductive explanation does not require a priori entailment.

An argument with this structure cannot successfully make a case against a priori entailments. To see this, it suffices to note that if this sort of argument succeeds, it succeeds equally in making a case against the a priori Gettier entailments discussed earlier. It is at least as plausible for 'knowledge' as for 'water' and for 'life' that there is no explicit analysis to support the entailments. Moreover, the general criticisms of this use of the two-dimensional framework presumably apply equally to its use in the case of 'knowledge.' Nevertheless, the a priori Gettier entailments discussed earlier exist, or at least it is clear that this sort of argument does little to make a case against them. So by parity, this sort of argument does little to make a case against the a priori entailments we are concerned with.

We can agree with Block and Stalnaker that there are plausibly no precise, explicit conceptual analyses of concepts such as 'water' and 'life' (or at least no precise analyses of a manageable length). But as we made clear earlier (and as is also made clear in Chalmers 1996 and Jackson 1998), such explicit analyses are not required for a priori entailment.[25]

We can also agree with Block and Stalnaker that the mere existence of the two-dimensional semantic framework does not imply that the a priori entailments in question exist. As Block and Stalnaker say, the two-dimensional framework provides a good way to capture a priori connections when they exist, but the framework alone does not demonstrate specific a priori connections. Correspondingly, the two-dimensional framework plays no essential role in our arguments for a priori entailments given here. In the arguments for a priori entailment given in *The Conscious Mind* and *From Metaphysics to Ethics*, it plays only a clarifying role, in removing certain confusions that may arise from the presence of a posteriori necessary connections and in providing a convenient shorthand for discussing the patterns by which a concept applies to the world. The core of the argument for a priori entailments proceeds independently of these semantic details, just as it does in the Gettier case.[26]

Insofar as it is captured by this global structure, then, Block and Stalnaker's discussion does not engage the first-order issue of whether the a priori entailments in question exist. Still, their article also contains numerous arguments that go beyond what is suggested by this structure. We discuss these in what follows.

---

25. As part of their argument, Block and Stalnaker suggest that the most plausible conceptual analyses are restricted to connections within the same "family" of terms (as with the analysis of 'bachelor' as 'unmarried man'), so that analyses of macroscopic concepts in microphysical terms are implausible. Ned Block has suggested in correspondence that this point extends to a priori entailments, so that the only plausible a priori entailments involve connections within a family. The reasons for accepting this thesis are unclear, however. The main evidence for it seems to lie in the fact that the most familiar and uncontroversial a priori entailments involve intrafamily connections. On the view we are advocating, however, this evidence is easily explained by the fact that there are few *short* cross-family a priori entailments, since cross-family entailments usually have detailed and unwieldy antecedents.

26. For this reason, we do not address Block and Stalnaker's discussion of the two-dimensional framework in this chapter. On our use of the two-dimensional framework, the primary intension (or A-intension) of a concept reflects the a priori conditionals that capture the way a concept applies within various epistemic possibilities in the manner suggested in section 3 of this chapter. For reasons discussed in the appendix, this understanding of the framework in epistemic terms differs subtly from Block and Stalnaker's understanding in terms of context-dependence.

(2) *Conceivability.* In a discussion about conceivability, Block and Stalnaker discuss the issue (raised by Levine 1993) of whether it is conceivable that P holds without W holding, where P is the complete microphysical truth and W is 'water is boiling.' They discuss two senses of conceivability. In the first sense, conceivability is tied closely to a posteriori possibility and necessity, so that $P \& {\sim} W$ is inconceivable. This sense of conceivability is clearly irrelevant to the issue of a priori entailment. In the second sense, P without Q is conceivable if Q cannot be deduced from P using logic and conceptual truths. This sense is more clearly relevant to the issue. We would prefer that the notion be cast in the more general terms of a priori reasoning rather than explicit deduction, but this does not matter to Block and Stalnaker's discussion.[27] They say

> Let C be a complete description, in microphysical terms, of a situation in which water (H_2O) is boiling, and let T be a complete theory of physics. Can one deduce from T, supplemented with analytic definitions, that H_2O would boil in circumstances C? To see that one cannot, suppose that the deduction is taking place on Twin Earth. The stuff they call 'water' is XYZ, and the process they call 'boiling' is a process that superficially resembles boiling, but that involves a different physical process. Just as they would say (truly) "Water is XYZ, and not H_2O (and if there were H_2O, it wouldn't be water)," so they would say (truly) "If there were H_2O, and it were behaving like that, it wouldn't be boiling." They could hardly deduce "H_2O would boil in circumstances C" if on their meaning of 'boil,' H_2O can't boil at all. (We assume that boiling is a natural kind concept. If you don't agree, substitute some other process term that does express a natural kind concept.) (8)

We can agree with Block and Stalnaker that if there are residents of Twin Earth, they might truly say "If there were H_2O, and it were behaving like that, it wouldn't be boiling." However, this is irrelevant to the issue of whether there is an a priori entailment from 'H_2O is behaving like that' to 'H_2O is boiling.' The first is a subjunctive conditional about an explicitly counterfactual scenario and as such is relevant to issues concerning necessity, not apriority.

---

27. Block and Stalnaker's first sense of conceivability is a version of secondary conceivability (chapter 6). Their second sense is a version of primary conceivability and in particular is close to ideal primary negative conceivability. Block and Stalnaker note that this notion is a purely negative notion, so that the name "conceivability" is misleading. However, there is also a closely related positive notion in the vicinity, namely ideal primary positive conceivability.

Compare the following. There is plausibly an a priori entailment from something like 'molecular motion is the dominant cause of our heat sensations' (M_1) to 'molecular motion is heat' (M_2). On a Twin Earth, however, where heat sensations are caused by something very different, residents might truly say, "If molecular motion were the dominant cause of our heat sensations, it wouldn't be heat." The latter is a subjunctive claim about an explicitly counterfactual scenario, so at best its truth reflects negatively on the *necessity* of an entailment from M_1 to M_2. Its truth clearly has no bearing on the apriority of the entailment (which remains plausible for everything said here). The same goes for microphysics and the boiling of water.

(In fact, the thought experiment does not even bear directly on the necessity of the entailment since presumably the necessity of an utterance in English does not entail the necessity of the homophonic utterance in Twin English (witness 'water is H_2O'). If anything, the thought experiment bears on whether it is a priori that the entailment is necessary.)

Block and Stalnaker also say the following:

> We don't really need a Twin Earth story to make our point. Consider a person on actual Earth, who does not know the story about how water boils—perhaps she doesn't even know that water is made up of molecules. One presents her with the theory T, and a description (in microphysical terms) of a water boiling situation. Can she then deduce that if T is true and a situation met conditions C, then the H_2O would be boiling? No, since for all she knows the actual situation is like the one on Twin Earth. Perhaps, if she were told, or could figure out, that the theory was actually true of the relevant stuff in her environment, she could then conclude (using her knowledge of the observable behavior of the things in her environment) that H_2O is water, and that the relevant microphysical description is a description of boiling, but the additional information is of course not a priori, and the inference from her experience would be inductive. (8)

This example is simply an illustration of the general phenomenon whereby physical information must be supplemented by locating information ('you are here') to imply relevant conclusions. The subject needs locating information to know that the theory describes the subject's own environment and not a very different environment. So while this example may show that there is no implication from P (the complete physical truth) to W, it does nothing to show that there is no implication from PI (physical truth supplemented by locating information) to W. Of course (as is made clear in Chalmers 1996 and Jackson 1998), the latter is the more relevant claim.

(3) *Uniqueness.* In discussing the possibility of conceptual analyses of terms like 'water,' Block and Stalnaker spend a considerable amount of time discussing the possibility of analyzing this term as something like 'the waterish stuff around here,' where 'waterish' abbreviates a cluster of descriptions of familiar macroscopic properties of water (such as clarity, liquidity, and drinkability). They argue that no such analysis can succeed. The argument proceeds by considering various possible cases where there is more than one sort of stuff in the environment that satisfies the relevant descriptions. Given that we hold that explicit analysis is not required for a priori entailment, we could simply set this discussion aside as irrelevant, but there are some points that are worth discussing.

Block and Stalnaker suggest at one point that for an a priori entailment to go through, water must be analyzed as something like 'the *unique* waterish stuff in our environment.' This seems clearly false. First, it seems obviously epistemically possible (in the broad sense) that there could turn out to be two sorts of stuff with the relevant properties filling the oceans and lakes in our environment in roughly equal distributions. In such a case, it seems clear that we would say that there are two sorts of water (that is, this epistemically possible hypothesis is an instance of the epistemically possible hypothesis that there are two sorts of water). So any a priori analysis requiring uniqueness would clearly be incorrect.

Second, the falsity of an analysis involving uniqueness does nothing to rule out a priori entailment. The thought experiment just given involves largely a priori consideration of an epistemically possible hypothesis. A priori consideration of that hypothesis suggests that it counts as an instance of the epistemically possible hypothesis that there are two sorts of water. So the thought experiment is entirely compatible with an a priori entailment from specific details concerning the hypothesis (in water-free terms) to a conclusion involving water and indeed may even positively suggest the existence of such an entailment.

If one wanted to come up with an explicit analysis that handles these cases directly, one might start simply with 'the watery stuff in our environment,' which handles them well (where the phrase is naturally interpreted to cover all instances of watery stuff in our environment). There will be cases where this analysis does not work. Perhaps if there is a single dominant watery stuff and small pockets of different stuff, we will count only the dominant stuff as 'water.' We could then move to something like 'the dominant watery stuff in our environment, if there is one, or any watery stuff in our environment, if there is not.' But no doubt this analysis would itself need to be refined to handle more complex cases, just as in the case of knowledge. It is probably easier, then, to give up the aim of producing a perfect, explicit analysis and to content ourselves with the observation that we have an a priori grasp of how our concepts apply to specific epistemic possibilities when these are described in sufficient detail. Nothing about these cases contravenes this observation.

(4) *Ghost heat.* In the course of their discussion of uniqueness, Block and Stalnaker discuss a hypothetical epistemic possibility in which it turns out that there is "ghost heat." In this situation, things are microphysically just as normal (P is true), so the causal role associated with heat is filled by molecular motion. But the causal role is also filled by a nonphysical substance, which we can call "ghost heat" in a case of causal overdetermination. Block and Stalnaker say that under this epistemic possibility, it turns out that there are two sorts of heat (molecular motion and ghost heat), so that 'heat = molecular motion' turns out to be false, so P does not imply that heat is molecular motion.

We are not certain that this sort of causal overdetermination is coherent, and we are not certain that if it is coherent, then the epistemic possibility in question should be interpreted as one in which there are two kinds of heat. But even if so, the conclusion is simply an instance of the failure of the microphysical facts P to rule out epistemic possibilities in which there are further nonphysical facts. As before, ruling out these epistemic possibilities requires conjoining a that's-all statement T, holding that the actual world is a minimal P-world to P. Once T is conjoined to P (yielding PT), the hypothesis involving ghost heat is ruled out: a world with ghost heat is clearly not a minimal P-world. So the example shows at best that P does not imply H (where H is 'heat is molecular notion'); it does not show that PT does not imply H. And as is made clear in Chalmers (1996) and Jackson (1998), the latter is the more relevant claim.

Block and Stalnaker anticipate this sort of response and reply as follows:

> Recall that Jackson's definition of physicalism recognized the possibility of a world that is a microphysical duplicate of the actual world, while also containing some additional nonphysical substances and properties. In response, a "nothing but" condition is built into the definition of physicalism by requiring for the truth of physicalism only that *minimal* physical duplicates of the actual world be duplicates simpliciter. But the need for this qualification presupposes that the "nothing but" condition is not something that is entailed by microphysics *itself;* that is, *it is not a claim of microphysics that our*

world is a minimal physical duplicate of itself. To take the "nothing but" condition to be an implicit claim of microphysics would be to build the thesis of physicalism into microphysics, which philosophers such as Jackson and Chalmers, who reject physicalism, should be reluctant to do. They reject physicalism, not microphysics. The truth of what physicists write in textbooks does not depend on the mind-body problem. Even if it is a microphysical fact that H_2O is *a* waterish stuff around here, it is not a microphysical fact that it is *the* waterish stuff around here. (19)

The objection here seems to be that the that's-all statement T is not itself implied by P. This is correct but irrelevant. The thesis is not that T is part of microphysics. The theses are rather that (i) PT (perhaps in conjunction with QI) implies the relevant macroscopic truths; (ii) this sort of implication is required for reductive explanation; and (iii) an analogous claim (that PT necessitates all truths) is required for physicalism. Nothing that Block and Stalnaker say here gives any reason to reject these claims.

(5) *Methodology and simplicity.* In the background of Block and Stalnaker's specific arguments about uniqueness lie some more general worries about the role of a posteriori methodological considerations, such as simplicity, in determining the extension of our terms. These worries are not elaborated at length in Block and Stalnaker's discussion, but they come up in a number of places and in a number of different ways.

For example, in the discussion of ghost heat, Block and Stalnaker suggest that it is by using considerations of simplicity that we rule out the possibility of ghost heat. That seems roughly correct. Our observations are compatible with two hypotheses, $P\&T$ and $P\&G$, where P contains the relevant physical truths, T is a that's-all statement, and G is a claim about ghost heat. We do not decide between these hypotheses purely through observation or deduction but through the use of simplicity considerations such as Ockham's razor. Something similar goes on in inductive and abductive inference. These considerations play a common role in moving from partial information about the world to more complete information about the world.

All this is quite compatible with our position. It is no part of our position that a posteriori methods are never used in determining our concepts' extensions. They are used all the time: in particular, it is by using a posteriori methods that we form empirical hypotheses about how the world is. The information in $PQTI$ itself is knowable only a posteriori, and simplicity considerations play a central role in our coming to know aspects of this information. But nothing here bears on the claim that *given* the information about *PQTI* (which rules out the *P&G* hypothesis), the application of our concepts is determined a priori.

There is one passage that may bear directly on this claim. After considering our intuitions about how the term 'water' might apply to various epistemic possibilities, including possibilities in which there are multiple substances that play the relevant role, Block and Stalnaker write:

> It is a part of the semantics of natural kind terms that they are natural kinds, but it may also be part of the semantics of these terms that this is a defeasible condition. What is not plausibly part of the semantics, something we all know in virtue of knowing our language alone, is what to say in all the myriad cases in which the defeasible condition is defeated. In these cases, what we should say will no doubt be dictated by principles of "simplicity," conservativeness, etc. (21)

Block and Stalnaker do not say anything to back up these claims directly or to argue against an opponent who holds that these conditions of application to various epistemic possibilities are as much a (tacit) part of the concept of 'water' as the conditions of application brought out in the Gettier literature are a (tacit) part of the concept of 'knowledge.' Furthermore, even if these conditions of application are not part of the semantics of 'water' in English, this does not entail that a subject's application of the term to epistemic possibilities is not justified a priori. As we saw earlier in the case of 'Neptune,' it may be the case that the relevant conditionals involving a term may vary among the users of a term (so that the corresponding conditions of application are not built in to the term's semantics in English) but that each user's knowledge of the conditionals is justified a priori all the same. So Block and Stalnaker need to give substantive arguments against the a priori knowability of the conditionals in question.

Block and Stalnaker go on to discuss the case of 'rheumatism,' in which as scientists acquired more empirical information about various diseases underlying a central syndrome, the term began to be used for the syndrome rather than the diseases. They also discuss the case of 'jade,' in which we discovered two underlying substances and decided that there are two sorts of jade. Nothing here contravenes the claim that these decisions manifested a tacit grasp of a priori conditions of application of the terms in question and that the relevant conditionals (from a full specification of the empirical details to conclusions about jade and rheumatism) are a priori.

Of course, the claim should not be made too strong. There is almost certainly a high degree of indeterminacy in our concepts, including indeterminacy in their application to the actual world and to hypothetical epistemic possibilities. It can sometimes happen that when an epistemic possibility is found to be actual, no clear decision about the concept's application is dictated. In such a case there often ensues (explicit or implicit) terminological stipulation or refinement that is influenced by various sociological and pragmatic factors. It may be that in the 'rheumatism' case, for example, the initial extension of the concept was indeterminate between applying to the syndrome in general and applying to the most common underlying disease. If so, there is an equally rational possible history in which the term comes to be applied to the disease, but in our world, it came to be applied to the syndrome.

Such cases can naturally be seen as cases of mild conceptual change or of conceptual refinement. In these cases, a term that formerly expressed one concept comes to express a slightly different concept, so that (i) the term's extension becomes more determinate, (ii) certain sentences whose truth values were previously indeterminate come to express truths, and (iii) certain conditionals that were not a priori come to be a priori. But these changes happen in parallel, and there is no time at which a concept's extension is not determined a priori by truths about the underlying state of the world.

Conceptual change is the exception rather than the rule. Most of the time, decisions concerning a concept's extension in response to empirical developments are dictated rationally rather than arbitrarily. Cases of this sort pose no threat to the a priori entailment thesis. To see this, note that in these cases the relevant empirical developments could be presented in advance as an epistemically possible hypothesis, and decisions concerning the concept's extension under that hypothesis will themselves be rationally accessible in principle. So the empirical knowledge in question plays no essential role in justifying the conditional from the empirical developments to a conclusion about the concept's extension. So in these cases we have no argument against a priori entailment.

(6) *A priori knowledge versus armchair knowledge.* A more general worry may be lurking in the background. It may be that Block and Stalnaker are prepared to concede that in many cases a conditional from a sufficiently complete description of an epistemic possibility to a conclusion about a concept's extension is knowable "from the armchair," but they may deny that it is a priori. This view is suggested by the following passage:

> This seems to be armchair reasoning, reflection that does not include any obvious reference to real experiments, so it is tempting to conclude that this reflection just unfolds our concepts in a totally a priori way. But what this conclusion misses is that our reasoning about the

proper epistemic response in various counterfactual situations is informed not only by our concepts but by implicit and explicit theories and general methodological principles that we have absorbed through our scientific culture—by everything that the "we" who are performing these thought experiments believe. What people should rationally say in response to various hypothesized discoveries will vary depending on their experience, commitments and epistemic priorities. (43)

On this view, armchair knowledge of application conditionals depends in part on general empirical background knowledge. For example, the empirical background knowledge that the world is simple may play a role in our requiring that the extension of a concept be as simple as possible. Or perhaps the knowledge that the world contains numerous natural kinds may make us more inclined to apply terms in the manner typical of natural kinds. The view can be put as follows. For relevant truths M, (i) a subject can know an application conditional $PQTI \supset M$ from the armchair; (ii) there is some general empirical information E, acquired at some time in the past, that plays a role in justifying the subject's knowledge of the conditional; and (iii) empirical knowledge such as E plays an *essential* role in justifying knowledge of the conditional. If (i) and (ii) are correct, the conditional is not known a priori; if (iii) is also correct, the conditional is not knowable a priori.

We argued in section 4 that empirical knowledge E does not play this sort of justificatory role. It is useful, however, to examine further the roles that empirical information might play in knowledge of application conditionals. There is no question that empirical information can play a *causal* role in acquiring this knowledge. Empirical knowledge often plays a causal role in the acquisition of concepts with certain a priori connections, and it sometimes plays a role in triggering changes in the a priori connections associated with a term, as in the cases just discussed. There is also no question that E could play a *mediating* role in our knowledge of an application conditional. That is, E might itself be implied by $PQTI$, and one could then straightforwardly use E in combination with $PQTI$ to deduce M. But neither of these possibilities entails that E plays an essential role in *justifying* knowledge of the relevant conditionals. We suspect that the cases in which Block and Stalnaker think that empirical information has a justificatory role are in fact cases where the information has a causal or mediating role.

To examine this matter in the context of the current objection, we will take it for granted that considerations presented earlier in this chapter establish that for empirical truths M, the conditional $PQTI \supset M$ is at least knowable from the armchair. The same considerations suggest that the truth or falsity of conditionals of the form $X \supset M$ will be knowable from the armchair for (false) antecedents X representing specific epistemic possibilities that are analogous to but distinct from $PQTI$. (Such possibilities might include different configurations of physical and phenomenal properties, as well as possibilities involving different laws of nature.) Further, the earlier considerations suggest that the relevant armchair knowledge is sufficient to justify hypothetical reasoning from the hypothetical acceptance of X to the conclusion that M. (Note that this entails that our knowledge of these conditionals is not essentially grounded, uninterestingly, in armchair knowledge that X is false.) We can call the relevant conditionals *armchair conditionals*. Now the question is this: insofar as an empirical claim E plays a role in knowledge of armchair conditionals such as $PQTI \supset M$, does it play a justificatory role or merely a causal or mediating role?

To adjudicate this issue, we can focus on the status of E itself. By the usual reasoning, knowledge of $PQTI$ will enable a subject to know from the armchair whether E is true. For example, the information in $PQTI$ puts us in a position to know that the world is reasonably simple.[28] So there will be corresponding armchair conditionals of the form $PQTI \supset E$. Further, since E is a posteriori, there will also be epistemic possibilities (in the broad sense) under which E is *false*: for example, epistemic possibilities under which the world is not simple. So there will be antecedents X (e.g., describing a nonsimple world) such that $X \supset \sim E$ is an armchair conditional. Although the epistemic possibility specified by X falsifies E, we can nevertheless evaluate it using various ordinary concepts, yielding corresponding armchair conditionals $X \supset C$.

We can then ask: does the role played by E in knowledge of armchair conditionals $PQTI \supset M$ extend to a role in knowledge of armchair conditionals $X \supset C$ where X falsifies E? (For example, does our knowledge that the world is simple play a role in our application of concepts to a nonsimple, epistemic possibility?) If E plays a causal role in knowledge of application conditionals, we would expect the answer to be yes. If E plays a mediating role, we would expect the answer to be no. If E plays a justifying

---

28. An opponent might try to avoid this line of argument by holding that the truth or falsity of E cannot be settled even by armchair reasoning from antecedents such as $PQTI$ and X. This position would require a very different sort of argument, however, arguing directly against the considerations in favor of armchair knowledge in section 4. The position is also implausible in Block and Stalnaker's favored case of simplicity.

role, it is not clear what we would expect the answer to be. In fact, one can argue that whether the answer is yes or no, E plays no essential role in justifying the application conditionals.

If the answer is yes: then for such an X and C, $X \supset C$ and $X \supset \sim E$ are armchair conditionals, so the subject can reason hypothetically from the information that X to the conclusion that C and $\sim E$. It follows that if the subject were to discover that X were actual (assuming rationality), the subject would come to know that C and $\sim E$. Then E would play no essential role in justifying the subject's knowledge that C, because the justification for items of knowledge cannot be essentially grounded in a falsehood. A subject who rationally evaluates X as a hypothetical can come to conclude C (under that hypothesis) by the same rational process, so E plays no essential role in justifying acceptance of the conditional from X to C. So in this application of the concepts involved in C, E plays no essential justificatory role. At most, E plays a causal role in the subject's acquiring a concept with this pattern of application.

If the answer is no: then the justificatory role of E extends at most to armchair conditionals $Y \supset C$ such that there is armchair justification for $Y \supset E$. Further, if there is armchair justification for $Y \supset E$, then if E justifies $Y \supset C$, $Y \supset E$ will also justify $Y \supset C$ without antecedently assuming E (by hypothetical reasoning from Y to E to C). So justification of $Y \supset E$ is required for E-involving knowledge of $Y \supset C$, and given this justification, E plays no further essential role in justifying $Y \supset C$. In particular, justification of $PQTI \supset E$ is required for E-involving knowledge of $PQTI \supset C$, and given this justification, E plays no further essential role in justifying $PQTI \supset C$. This suggests strongly that in these cases E plays only a mediating role in knowledge of $PQTI \supset C$.

The only residual question about this second class of cases is what justifies the armchair conditional $PQTI \supset E$. Knowledge of this conditional is not essentially justified by E itself. To see this, note that a subject who is given the information in $PQTI$ and who antecedently suspends judgment about E will nevertheless be in a position to conclude that E holds. Further, the same sorts of factors are plausibly relevant in justifying $PQTI \supset E$ and in justifying $X \supset \sim E$ for those X that falsify E, but E cannot justify the latter for the reasons given earlier. Alternatively, $PQTI \supset E$ might be justified by some other empirical factor F, but then knowledge of E does not play an essential role in justifying $PQTI \supset C$, contrary to the original hypothesis. Knowledge that F is all that is required, and we can run the same argument for F. The same goes for the disjunction of E and F and indeed for any empirical claim. So no empirical claim plays an essential role in justifying knowledge of armchair conditionals of the form $PQTI \supset C$. At most, such claims play a mediating role.

To illustrate the situation, we can take the case of simplicity and the example of $PQTI \supset M$. On both alternatives described here, a posteriori simplicity considerations might play some role in adjudicating the status of M. On the first alternative, this is because these considerations have played a causal role in the subject's possessing a concept whose a priori conditions of application across all epistemic possibilities involve simplicity. On the second alternative, it is because the information that the world is simple is itself derivable from $PQTI$ and thereby plays a role in the a priori process of reasoning from antecedent to consequent. Either way, the a posteriori considerations play no role in justifying the conditional itself and are therefore no bar to its apriority.

It might be objected that if empirical considerations can play a role in affecting what is a priori involving a concept (as in the first alternative given above regarding simplicity and also in the version of the 'rheumatism' case involving terminological stipulation), then the notion of apriority is being watered down. But this seems wrong: apriority is a matter of nonempirical *justification*. Concept acquisition is usually empirically driven, and conceptual drift can occur in response to empirical factors, but neither of these is any bar to the apriority of resulting claims involving the concepts.

A related objection notes that if the apriority of various sentences can be affected by empirical developments, then there is no guarantee that claims we now regard as a priori will turn out to be a priori; as a result, any metaphysical and explanatory conclusions that rest on claims about apriority are suspect. But this is wrong. Even where the sort of conceptual drift described here occurs, the relevant claims at the first stage are still a priori; it is just that later, the same sentence is used to express something different that is not a priori. The change here is merely terminological. Whether people use 'rheumatism' for the syndrome or the disease, the substantive issues concerning the phenomenon itself are the same. More generally, whether or not people choose to use terms in a way that requires simplicity, the substantive issues concerning the phenomena are the same. The change in language simply means that we express things differently.

It may even be that in the future people may come to use a term such as 'consciousness' or 'life' with a priori application conditions that differ from ours, due to sociological or pragmatic factors or terminological stipulation or terminological drift. But this sort of future terminological change has no bearing on the truth or the apriority of claims that we currently make using the term, and has no bearing on any metaphysical or explanatory conclusions that might follow.[29] For example, it could turn out that due to this sort of drift, what someone later calls 'consciousness' can be reductively explained, but that does not imply that consciousness can be reductively explained.

We conclude that none of Block and Stalnaker's arguments against a priori entailment are compelling.[30]

6. Does Reductive Explanation Require A Priori Entailment?

Block and Stalnaker hold that reductive explanation does not require a priori entailment.[31] In arguing for this thesis, their main strategy involves arguing that in paradigm cases of reductive explanation, no a priori entailment exists. We have already rebutted these arguments. They also offer a positive model of reductive explanation with some arguments in support, so it is worth saying something here about what reductive explanation involves. We start by examining a clear way in which reductive explanation can succeed and a clear way in which it can fail.

When a concept of some natural phenomenon supports a priori entailments from the microphysical, there is a clear sense in which the phenomenon can be reductively explained. These a priori entailments might not support a *reduction* of the phenomenon in question to a microphysical phenomenon (at least in some senses of this term), perhaps because such entailments are compatible with multiple realizability. Still, in showing how any instance of the phenomenon is itself implied by microphysical phenomena, we show that there is a sort of transparent epistemic connection between the microphysical and macroscopic phenomena. Both the microphysical and the macroscopic phenomena are epistemically contingent

---

29. This objection reflects a point that occasionally arises in discussion of the two-dimensional framework. Cannot the primary intension (or A-intension) of a term change, and if so, does this not call any conclusions drawn from a priori reasoning into question? In response: yes, the primary intension of a term can change (though this sort of change is not especially common and is usually minor), and no, this terminological change has no bearing on conclusions drawn from a priori reasoning with our current concept. A related but better objection holds that we can be wrong about the primary intension of a concept because we have not reasoned sufficiently deeply about what to say about a given epistemic possibility. This can certainly happen, but it does not cast doubt on the a priori method. Rather, it suggests that the a priori method has to be practiced well.

30. Yablo (2002) gives some further arguments against the case for a priori entailment based partly on the role of "sensibility" in deriving macroscopic knowledge from microscopic knowledge. Chalmers (2002b) replies to these arguments.

31. A close tie between reductive explanation and a priori entailment is suggested by Chalmers (1996), Levine (1993), and Loar (1990/1997).

in that they involve the actualization of just one of a host of coherent epistemic possibilities. When transparent entailment is present, however, the epistemic contingency in the macroscopic phenomena is reduced to the epistemic contingency in the microphysical phenomena: there is no further epistemic contingency in the connection.

When a phenomenon is entailed a priori by $PQTI$ rather than just by P, something similar applies. To be sure, there may be some further epistemic contingency in T, I, and possibly Q so that these truths themselves may not be reductively explained. But we generally count reductive explanation "modulo totality, indexicality, and consciousness"—that is, reduction of the epistemic contingency of a phenomenon to the epistemic contingency in $PQTI$—to be reductive explanation enough. T and I are sufficiently minor additions to the reduction base that they do not change much, and while Q is a larger addition, scientists are prepared to put the explanation of the subjective aspects of a phenomenon (such as color and heat) on hold and settle for an explanation of the objective aspects. This "carving off" strategy arguably does not yield a complete reductive explanation of these phenomena, but at least we know just what we are not explaining.

So in a reductive explanation of a phenomenon such as water or life, we find that a low-level account of the physical processes involved will in principle imply and explain truths about the macroscopic structure, dynamics, behavior, and (in conjunction with Q) appearance of relevant systems. Furthermore, our concepts of water and life dictate that systems with appropriate sorts of structure, dynamics, behavior, and appearance automatically qualify as water or as alive (at least if they are appropriately situated in our environment or are relevantly related to systems in our environment). So the relevant microphysical truths (perhaps in conjunction with Q, T, and I) imply the existence of water or of life, and their existence is reductively explained. The same applies to various specific features of water and of life, which can be implied and explained in similar ways.

The corresponding view on the problem of consciousness is type-A materialism (chapter 5): the view that there is an a priori entailment from PTI to the phenomenal truths Q (perhaps because phenomenal concepts are functional concepts). It is clear that *if* type-A materialism is true, then the phenomenal can be reductively explained in terms of the physical. In this case, there will be a transparent epistemic connection from the physical to the phenomenal, and any epistemic contingency in the phenomenal truths will be reduced to epistemic contingency in physical truths. (Consequently, all other macroscopic truths that are reductively explainable "modulo consciousness" will be reductively explainable *simpliciter*.) Once again, a priori entailment supports reductive explanation.

Next consider a clear case of a failure of reductive explanation. Let us say that the property dualist is right about consciousness and that consciousness is connected to the physical only by contingent laws, perhaps ultimately by fundamental psychophysical laws. These laws might be inferred, in principle, from psychophysical regularities in the actual world. Given the presence of these laws, we can still arguably have some sort of explanation of consciousness and its properties in terms of physical processes and the psychophysical laws. From *PTI* plus psychophysical laws, the various specific phenomena of consciousness will be implied. This will not be a case of *reductive* explanation, however, precisely because of the need for principles in our explanatory base over and above what is present in *P*. The laws themselves are not explained: they are epistemically primitive, in that they are not implied by more basic truths.[32] Moreover, these substantive, epistemically primitive principles play a central role in the explanation of the phenomena. So there is no transparent explanation of the phenomena in physical terms alone, and reductive explanation fails.

Now let us consider a third sort of case, one that corresponds to the way Block and Stalnaker envisage the situation with respect to consciousness and reductive explanation in general. Here, as before, we observe numerous psychophysical regularities between brain states and states of consciousness. But on Block and Stalnaker's approach, we are led to infer an underlying *identity* between various brain states and phenomenal states. These identities are not entailed a priori by *PTI*, and correspondingly, the truths about consciousness are not entailed a priori by *PTI*, but the truths about consciousness are entailed a priori by *PTI* plus the identities (at least if truths about brain states are entailed a priori by *PTI*). So we still have a sort of explanation of consciousness and its properties, in terms of physical processes and psychophysical identities.

This third case is a version of type-B materialism, on which physical truths necessitate phenomenal truths without entailing them a priori. We think that this sort of case cannot occur, but let us set that worry aside for the moment and pretend that it can. Assuming that it can occur, is the third case more akin to the first or the second case? There are different respects in which it resembles each. Ontologically, it is more akin to the first case, involving type-A materialism, since it is compatible with a materialist ontology on which the explained phenomenon is ultimately

32. That is, they are not implied by truths that do not themselves involve phenomenal states. On a Humean view of laws, fundamental psychophysical laws will be implied by truths about the distribution of physical and phenomenal states. But this sort of implication is irrelevant to reductive explanation as phenomenal states are what we are aiming to explain. On a non-Humean view of laws, fundamental psychophysical laws will straightforwardly be epistemically primitive.

physical. Epistemically, however, it is more akin to the second case, which involves property dualism.

Like the second case, the third case yields no transparent explanation of consciousness in terms of physical processes. At best, there is an explanation in terms of physical processes *plus* psychophysical identities, and epistemically, the psychophysical identities play exactly the same role as psychophysical laws. They are inferred from regularities between brain processes and consciousness in order to systematize and explain those regularities. Most important, the identities are not themselves explained but are epistemically primitive. As with the second case, it is precisely because we need these epistemically primitive psychophysical principles to explain the phenomenon that transparent reductive explanation fails.

Ontologically, these identities may differ from laws. But epistemically, they are just like laws. They are epistemically primitive psychophysical "bridging" principles that are not themselves explained but that combine with physical truths to explain phenomenal truths. An explanation of the phenomenal will have two epistemically irreducible components: a physical component and a psychophysical component. By calling the bridging principles identities rather than laws, this view may preserve the ontological structure of materialism, but the explanatory structure of this materialist view is just like the explanatory structure of property dualism.

Identities play a role in reductive explanation in other domains, of course. Identities involving heat or temperature or genes all have some explanatory work to do, but in these cases, the identities are not epistemically primitive. The identities between heat and the motion of molecules and the identity between genes and DNA, for example, are themselves implied by *PQTI* (at least insofar as they are true) for the reasons discussed earlier in this chapter. So in these cases, both macroscopic truths about the phenomena and the identities themselves are transparently explained.

It is sometimes held that "identities do not need to be explained" (e.g., Papineau 1993). Block and Stalnaker (1999) say something similar ("Identities don't have explanations"). But this seems to conflate ontological and epistemological matters. Identities are ontologically primitive, but they are not epistemically primitive. Identities are typically implied by underlying truths that do not involve identities. The identities between genes and DNA and between water and H_2O are implied by the underlying truths in *PQTI*, for example. Once a subject knows all the truths about DNA and its role in reproduction and development, for example, the subject will be in a position to deduce that genes are DNA. So this identity is not epistemically primitive.

Of course, just as with other truths involving macroscopic phenomena, subjects do not typically come to know these identities by deducing them from microscopic truths. But the identities are deducible all the same, and their deducibility is what makes the phenomena in question reductively explainable. If the identities in question were epistemically primitive, then explanations of the macroscopic phenomena in terms of microscopic phenomena would have a primitive "vertical" element, and science would have established a far weaker explanatory connection between the microscopic and the macroscopic than it actually has.[33]

Something similar applies even to the case of 'Mark Twain is Samuel Clemens,' which Block and Stalnaker discuss. A subject who knows all of the qualitative truths in question—physical, mental, social—and who possesses the concepts 'Mark Twain' and 'Samuel Clemens' will be in a position to deduce that the identity is true, even if the subject is initially ignorant of it. The subject will be in a position to know that there was an individual who was known to his parents as 'Samuel Clemens,' who wrote books such as *Huckleberry Finn* under the name 'Mark Twain,' whose deeds were causally responsible for the current discussion involving 'Mark Twain' and involving 'Samuel Clemens,' and so on. From all of this information, the subject will easily be able to deduce that Mark Twain was Samuel Clemens, and the deduction will be a priori in the sense that it will not rely on any empirical information outside the information specified in the base. So this identity is not epistemically primitive.

We might imagine that there are eliminativists who deny the existence of Mark Twain. They accept the existence of Samuel Clemens and the descriptions of his exploits: that he went by the name 'Mark Twain,' that he published many of the works that we know of under that name, and so on. But they deny that Clemens was Twain: they say that Clemens used the name 'Twain' but Twain never really existed. The response to such an eliminativist seems clear. Once the eliminativist concedes the full description of Clemens's exploits and of his connection to our current use of the name 'Mark Twain,' we should say: if you grant all that, you grant that Clemens was Twain. Once the qualitative description is given, there is no further fact about Twain's existence of which we are ignorant. There is at most a

---

33. One could plausibly go further and argue that a scientist's warrant to accept a micro-macro identity in the first place depends on a warrant to accept in-principle deducibility of the macroscopic phenomena from underlying processes. In the absence of a warrant to accept such deducibility, scientists will be justified in accepting only correlation, not identity.

terminological decision to make, and the terminological decision seems clear. So the identity of Twain with Clemens is itself deducible from underlying truths.

It may be that there is a way in which it sounds odd to ask for an explanation of why Mark Twain is Samuel Clemens or of why water is H_2O. This is partly because we naturally interpret these phrases as asking for a causal or historical explanation. When asked why Mark Twain lived in Missouri, we will give a causal explanation of the factors that led him to be there and to stay there. It is not so easy to explain causally why H_2O is water or why Samuel Clemens is Mark Twain (although even here, historical explanation might do at least some work).

Setting aside causal/historical explanation, it seems no harder and no easier to explain *reductively* the identities that Mark Twain is Samuel Clemens or that water is H_2O than it is to explain reductively the nonidentities that Mark Twain lived in Missouri or that there is water in the Pacific Ocean.[34] The slight sense of linguistic oddness is equally present in all these cases, so there is nothing special about identities here. What matters is that in all these cases, the relevant truths are not epistemically primitive. They are implied by various underlying truths, and none of them are needed to deduce truths that cannot be deduced without them. So there is nothing here that gives support to the sort of epistemically primitive micro-macro identities that Block and Stalnaker need.

We have argued that (1) there is no reason to believe that there are epistemically primitive micro-macro identities, and that (2) even if there were any epistemically primitive micro-macro identities, they would not support transparent reductive explanation of the macroscopic phenomena of the sort found in most cases of reductive explanation.

Of course, an opponent could hold that such identities (if they existed) would support "reductive explanation" in *some* sense (e.g., a sense wherein a reductive explanation is simply an explanation that involves an ontological reduction). Nothing rests on the verbal issue,

---

34. *It is sometimes supposed that it is trivial to explain identities because identity sentences express trivial singular propositions. But explanatory contexts are epistemic contexts. Just as it is trivial to believe that Twain is Twain but not trivial to believe that Twain is Clemens, it is trivial to explain why Twain is Twain but not trivial to explain why Twain is Clemens. In these cases, the nontrivial belief and explanation in question are most naturally understood as targeted not merely at a singular proposition but rather at the associated modes of presentation. The required belief involves something like a belief that one individual falls under both Twain-associated and Clemens-associated modes of presentations. Likewise, the required explanation involves an explanation of why one individual falls under both Twain-associated and Clemens-associated modes of presentations. Something similar goes for water and H_2O. If type-B materialism were correct, something similar would go for physical processes and consciousness.

however. The significant points are (1) that this sort of explanation would be very much unlike most paradigmatic cases of reductive explanation and (2) that by invoking an epistemically primitive bridging structure, the explanatory structure of this theory would be more akin to that of property dualism than to that of standard materialism. We might say that this sort of theory would be ontologically reductive but epistemically nonreductive. With this sort of theory, as with a property dualist theory, the explanatory gap between physical and phenomenal might be bridged, but it would not be closed.

8. Conclusions

We have argued that ordinary truths about macroscopic natural phenomena are entailed a priori by the combination of physical truths, phenomenal truths, indexical truths, and a that's-all statement. We have argued that reductive explanation requires a priori entailment. If that is right, then if the phenomenal is reductively explainable in terms of the physical, then there is an a priori entailment from physical truths, indexical truths, and a that's-all statement to phenomenal truths. Contrapositively, if there is no such entailment, then the phenomenal is not reductively explainable in terms of the physical.

Part IV

CONCEPTS OF CONSCIOUSNESS

8

THE CONTENT OF PHENOMENAL CONCEPTS

1. Introduction

Experiences and beliefs are different sorts of mental states and are often taken to belong to very different domains. Experiences are paradigmatically phenomenal, characterized by what it is like to have them. Beliefs are paradigmatically intentional, characterized by their propositional content. But there are a number of crucial points where these domains intersect. One central locus of intersection arises from the existence of phenomenal beliefs: beliefs that are about experiences.

The most important phenomenal beliefs are *first-person* phenomenal beliefs: subjects' beliefs about their own experiences and especially about the phenomenal character of the experiences that they are currently having. Examples include the belief that one is now having a red experience, or that one is experiencing pain.

Phenomenal beliefs always involve *phenomenal concepts*: concepts of the phenomenal character of an experience. When one believes that one is having a red experience, one deploys a phenomenal concept of a red experience. The most important phenomenal concepts are those that we acquire directly from having experiences with that sort of phenomenal character. For example, when one first learns what it is like to experience an orgasm, one acquires a phenomenal concept of the experience of orgasm.

Phenomenal concepts and phenomenal beliefs raise important issues in the theory of content, in epistemology, and in the metaphysics of consciousness. In the theory of content, analyzing the content of phenomenal concepts and phenomenal beliefs raises special issues for a general theory of content, and content of this sort has sometimes been taken to be at the foundations of a theory of content more generally. In epistemology, phenomenal beliefs are often taken to have a special epistemic status, and are sometimes taken to be the central epistemic nexus between cognition and the external world. In the metaphysics of consciousness, it is often held that a correct account of phenomenal concepts will help us to understand the epistemic gap between physical processes and consciousness, and perhaps that it will allow us to explain away this gap in purely psychological terms, with no ontological consequences.

My project in the next three chapters is to analyze phenomenal concepts and phenomenal beliefs in a way that sheds some light on these issues.[1] In this chapter, I start by focusing on the content of phenomenal concepts and phenomenal beliefs. I then use this analysis to discuss the distinctive underlying constitution of these concepts and beliefs. In the next chapter, I apply this analysis to some central epistemological issues about consciousness: infallibility, justification, and the dialectic over the "myth of the given." In chapter 10, I focus on the role of phenomenal concepts in understanding the explanatory gap and the metaphysics of consciousness.

2. Preliminaries

The discussion that follows is premised upon what I call "phenomenal realism": the view that there are phenomenal properties (or phenomenal qualities, or qualia)—properties that type mental states by what it is like to have them—and that phenomenal properties are not conceptually reducible to physical or functional properties. On the phenomenal realist view, when Frank Jackson's Mary is inside her black-and-white room, she lacks factual knowledge concerning what it is like to see red. Views that deny this deny phenomenal realism. Likewise, on the phenomenal realist view it is coherent to suppose that a hypothetical being has the same physical, functional, and environmental properties as an existing conscious being but does not have the same phenomenal properties.[2] Phenomenal realism

---

1. The analysis presented here is a development of a brief discussion in chapter 5 (203–208) of *The Conscious Mind*.

2. What if someone holds that functional duplicates without consciousness are coherently conceivable but that physical duplicates without consciousness are not? Such a view would be in the spirit of phenomenal realism. This suggests that we could define phenomenal realism more weakly as the thesis that the phenomenal is not conceptually reducible to the functional, omitting mention of the physical.

is incompatible with type-A materialism about consciousness (see chapter 5), but it is compatible with type-B materialism and Russellian monism, as well as with nonmaterialist views.

Those who are not phenomenal realists might want to stop reading now, but there are two reasons why they might continue. First, although the arguments I give for my view of phenomenal beliefs presuppose phenomenal realism, some aspects of the view may be tenable even on some views that deny phenomenal realism. Second, some of the most important arguments *against* phenomenal realism are epistemological arguments that center on the connection between experience and belief. I use my analysis to help rebut those arguments and thus indirectly to support phenomenal realism against its opponents.

A note on modality: because I am assuming phenomenal realism but not property dualism, all references to necessity and possibility should be taken as invoking conceptual necessity and possibility. Similarly, talk of possible worlds can be taken as invoking conceivable worlds (corresponding to the epistemically constructed scenarios discussed in the appendix), and talk of constitutive relations should be taken as invoking conceptually necessary connections. If one accepts a certain sort of link between conceptual and metaphysical possibility (e.g., the thesis that ideal primary conceivability entails primary possibility), then these references can equally be taken as invoking metaphysical possibility and necessity.

A note on phenomenal properties: it is natural to speak as if phenomenal properties are instantiated by mental states and as if there are entities, namely experiences, that bear their phenomenal properties essentially. But one can also speak as if phenomenal properties are directly instantiated by conscious subjects, typing subjects by aspects of what it is like to be them at the time of instantiation. These ways of speaking do not commit one to corresponding ontologies, but they at least suggest such ontologies. In a *quality-based* ontology, the subject-property relation is fundamental. From this one can derive a subject-experience-property structure by identifying experiences with phenomenal states (instantiations of phenomenal properties) and attributing phenomenal properties to these states in a derivative sense. In a more complex *experience-based* ontology, a subject-experience-property

---

I do not define it this way for two reasons. First, if functional duplicates without consciousness are conceivable, physical duplicates without consciousness must be conceivable too, as there is no reasonable possibility of a conceptual entailment from microphysical to phenomenal that does not proceed via the functional. Second, it is not easy to give a precise account of what functional duplication consists in, and stipulating physical identity finesses that question. But if someone disagrees, everything that I say will apply, with appropriate changes, on the weaker view.

structure is fundamental (where experiences are phenomenal individuals or at least something more than property instantiations), and the subject-property relation is derivative. In what follows, I sometimes use both sorts of language and am neutral between the ontological frameworks.

3. Varieties of Phenomenal Concepts

Phenomenal beliefs involve the attribution of phenomenal properties. These properties are attributed under phenomenal concepts. To understand the content of phenomenal beliefs, we need to understand the nature and content of phenomenal concepts.

I take concepts to be mental entities rather than abstract objects. (Most of what I say can be translated into a framework in which concepts are regarded as abstract objects, however.[3]) On this understanding, concepts can be regarded as constituents of beliefs (and other propositional attitudes) in a manner loosely analogous to the way in which words are constituents of sentences. Like beliefs, concepts are tokens rather than types in the first instance. But they also fall under types, some of which I explore in what follows. In such cases it is natural to use singular expressions such as 'the concept' for a concept type, just as one sometimes uses expressions such as 'the belief' for a belief type, or 'the word' for a word type. I use italics for concepts and beliefs throughout.

I look at a red apple and visually experience its color. This experience instantiates a phenomenal quality R, which we might call phenomenal redness. It is natural to say that I am having a red experience, even though experiences are not red in the same sense in which apples are red. Phenomenal redness (a property of experiences or of subjects of experience) is a different property from external redness (a property of external objects), but both are respectable properties in their own right.[4]

I attend to my visual experience and think *I am having an experience of such-and-such quality*, referring to the quality of phenomenal redness. There are various concepts of the quality in question that might yield a true belief.

---

3. *I now think that speaking of concepts as mental entities has led to some unnecessary confusion in readers, so I provide footnotes throughout with translation into the abstract-entity framework. Speaking within the abstract-entity framework, the entities that the mental-entity framework calls "concepts" are *graspings* of concepts, or perhaps representations with concepts as their content.

4. *I am neutral throughout this and the following chapter on whether phenomenal redness is itself a representational property, but everything I say here is consistent with a view on which phenomenal redness is representational, perhaps in the fashion discussed in chapters 11 and 12.

We can first consider the concept expressed by 'red' in the public-language expression 'red experience' or the concept expressed by the public-language expression 'phenomenal redness.' The reference of these expressions is fixed via a relation to red things in the external world and ultimately via a relation to certain paradigmatic red objects that are ostended in learning the public-language term 'red.' A language learner learns to call the experiences typically brought about by these objects 'red' (in the phenomenal sense) and to call the objects that typically bring about those experiences 'red' (in the external sense). So the phenomenal concept involved here is *relational* in that it has its reference fixed by a relation to external objects. The property that is referred to need not be relational, however.[5] The phenomenal concept plausibly designates an intrinsic property rigidly, so that there are counterfactual worlds in which red experiences are never caused by red things.

One can distinguish at least two relational phenomenal concepts, depending on whether reference is fixed by relations across a whole community of subjects or by relations restricted to the subject in question. The first is what we can call the *community relational concept*, or red_C. This can be glossed roughly as *the phenomenal quality typically caused in normal subjects within my community by paradigmatic red things*. The second is what we can call the *individual relational concept*, or red_I. This can be glossed roughly as *the phenomenal quality typically caused in me by paradigmatic red things*. The two concepts red_C and red_I corefer for normal subjects, but for abnormal subjects they may yield different results. For example, a red/green-inverted subject's concept red_C will refer to (what others call) phenomenal redness, but that subject's concept red_I will refer to (what others call) phenomenal greenness.

The public-language term 'red' as a predicate of experiences can arguably be read as expressing either red_C or red_I. The community reading of 'red' guarantees a sort of shared meaning within the community in that all uses of the term are guaranteed to corefer and in that tokens of sentences such as 'X has a red experience at time t' will have the same truth-value whether uttered by normal or abnormal subjects. On the other hand, the individual reading allows a subject better access to the term's referent. On this reading, an unknowingly inverted subject's term 'red' will refer to what she thinks it refers to (unless the inversion was recent), while on the community reading, her term 'red' may refer to something quite different, and

---

5. *This does not rule out the possibility that phenomenal redness is relational in some other way. On a sense-datum view, phenomenal redness may involve a relation to sense data, and on a representational view, it may involve an intentional relation to external properties.

her utterance 'I have had red experiences' may even be unknowingly quite false.[6] In any case, we need not settle here just what is expressed by phenomenal predicates in public language. All that matters is that both concepts are available.

Phenomenal properties can also be picked out indexically. When seeing a tomato, I can refer indexically to a visual quality associated with it, using a concept I might express by saying 'this quality' or 'this sort of experience.' These expressions communicate a demonstrative concept that we might call $this_E$.[7] This concept functions in an indexical manner, roughly by picking out whatever quality the subject is currently ostending. Like other demonstratives, it has a "character" that fixes reference in a context roughly by picking out whatever quality is ostended in that context, and it has a distinct "content" that corresponds to the quality that is actually ostended—in this case, phenomenal redness. The demonstrative concept $this_E$ rigidly designates its referent, so that it picks out the quality in question even in counterfactual worlds in which no one is ostending the quality.

The three concepts red_C, red_I, and $this_E$ may all refer to the same quality, phenomenal redness. In each case, reference is fixed relationally, with the quality characterized in terms of its relations to external objects or acts of ostension. There is another crucial phenomenal concept in the vicinity, one that does not pick out phenomenal redness relationally but rather picks it out directly in terms of its intrinsic phenomenal nature. This is what we might call a *pure phenomenal concept*.

To see the need for the pure phenomenal concept, consider the knowledge that Mary gains when she learns for the first time what it is like to see red. She learns that seeing red has such-and-such a quality. Mary learns (or reasonably comes to believe) that red things will typically cause experiences of such-and-such a quality in her and in other members of her community. She learns (or gains the cognitively significant belief) that the experience she is now having has such-and-such a quality and that the quality she is now ostending is such-and-such. Call Mary's "such-and-such" concept here R. Note that the phenomenal concept R should be distinguished from the phenomenal quality R (unitalicized) that it refers to.

Mary's concept R picks out phenomenal redness, but it is distinct from the concepts red_C, red_I, and $this_E$. We can see this by using cognitive significance as a test for difference between concepts. Mary gains the belief

---

6. These cases may not be entirely hypothetical. Nida-Rümelin (1996) gives reasons, based on the neurobiological and genetic bases of color blindness, to believe that a small fraction of the population may actually be spectrum inverted with respect to the rest of us. If so, it is natural to wonder just what their phenomenal expressions refer to.

7. *I have changed notation from the less mnemonic 'E' in the original to '$this_E$' here.

$red_C = R$—that the quality typically caused in her community by red things is such-and-such—and this belief is cognitively significant knowledge. She gains the cognitively significant belief $red_I = R$ in a similar way. And she gains the belief $this_E = R$—roughly, that the quality she is now ostending is such-and-such.[8]

Mary's belief $this_E = R$ is as cognitively significant as any other belief in which the object of a demonstrative is independently characterized: for example, my belief *I am David Chalmers* or my belief *that object is tall*. For Mary, $this_E = R$ is not a priori. No a priori reasoning can rule out the hypothesis that she is now ostending some other quality entirely, just as no a priori reasoning can rule out the hypothesis that I am David Hume or that the object I am pointing to is short. Indeed, nothing known a priori entails that the phenomenal quality R is ever instantiated in the actual world.

It is useful to consider analogies with other demonstrative knowledge of types. Let $this_S$ be a demonstrative concept of a shape ("this shape"). Jill might tell Jack that she is about to show him her favorite shape. When she shows him a circle, he might form the thought *Jill's favorite shape is $this_S$*. This is a demonstrative thought, where this instance of $this_S$ picks out the shape of a circle. He might also form the thought *Jill's favorite shape is circle*. This is a nondemonstrative thought: instead of a demonstrative concept, the right-hand side uses what we might call a *qualitative* concept of the shape of a circle. Finally, he might form the thought *$this_S$ is circle*. This is a substantive, nontrivial thought, taking the form of an identity involving a demonstrative concept and a qualitative concept. Here, as in the examples in the last paragraph, one conceives the object of a demonstration *as* the object of a demonstration ("this shape, whatever it happens to be") and at the same time attributes to it substantive qualitative properties, conceived nondemonstratively.

Of course, Jack's concept *circle* (unlike Mary's concept R), is an old concept, previously acquired, but this is inessential to Jack's case. We can imagine that Jack has never seen a circle before and that he acquires the qualitative concept of circularity on seeing a circle for the first time. He will then be in a position to think the qualitative thought *Jill's favorite shape is circle* and to think the substantive demonstrative-qualitative thought *$this_S$ is circle*.

---

8. *In the abstract object framework, the same reasoning suggests that there are distinct community and individual relational phenomenal concepts, indexical phenomenal concepts, and pure phenomenal concepts. It could at least be argued that there are deferential and nondeferential grasps of pure phenomenal concepts, however. If so, instances of the former may be hard to distinguish from instances of grasping the community relational concept.

Mary's situation is analogous. Where Jack thinks the substantive thought *this*$_S$ *is circle*, Mary might think the substantive thought *this*$_E$ = R ("this quality is R"). Like Jack's thought, Mary's thought involves attributing a certain substantive, qualitative nature to a type that is identified demonstratively. This qualitative nature is attributed using a qualitative concept of phenomenal redness, acquired upon having a red experience for the first time. Her thoughts *red*$_C$ = R and *red*$_1$ = R are substantive thoughts analogous to Jack's thought *Jill's favorite shape is circle*. Her crucial thought *this*$_E$ = R is a substantive thought involving both a demonstrative and a qualitative concept and is as cognitively significant as Jack's thought *this*$_S$ *is circle*.

So the concept R is quite distinct from *red*$_C$, *red*$_1$, and *this*$_E$. We might say that unlike the other concepts, the pure phenomenal concept characterizes the phenomenal quality *as* the phenomenal quality that it is.

The concept R is difficult to express directly in language, since the most natural terms, such as 'phenomenal redness' and 'this experience,' arguably express other concepts such as *red*$_C$ and *this*$_E$. Still, one can arguably discern uses of these terms that express pure phenomenal concepts, or, if not, one can stipulate such uses. For example, Chisholm (1957) suggests that there is a "noncomparative" sense of expressions such as 'looks red'; this sense seems to express a pure phenomenal concept, whereas his "comparative sense" seems to express a relational phenomenal concept.[9] And at least informally, demonstratives are sometimes used to express pure phenomenal concepts. For example, the belief *this*$_E$ = R might be informally expressed by saying something like "this quality is *this* quality."

It may be that there is a sense in which R can be regarded as a "demonstrative" concept. I will not treat it this way. I take it that demonstrative concepts work roughly as analyzed by Kaplan (1989), so that they have a reference-fixing "character" that leaves their referent open. This is how *this*$_E$ behaves: its content might be glossed roughly as "this quality, whatever it happens to be." On the other hand, R is a substantive concept that is tied a priori to a specific sort of quality, so it does not behave the way that Kaplan suggests that a demonstrative should. Still, there is an intimate relationship between pure and demonstrative phenomenal concepts that I discuss later, and if someone wants to count pure phenomenal concepts as "demonstrative" in a broad sense (perhaps regarding *this*$_E$ as "indexical"),

---

9. The distinction also roughly tracks Nida-Rümelin's (1995, 1997) distinction between "phenomenal" and "nonphenomenal" readings of belief attributions concerning phenomenal states. "Phenomenal" belief attributions seem to require that the subject satisfies the attribution by virtue of a belief involving a pure phenomenal concept, while "nonphenomenal" attributions allow that the subject can satisfy the attribution by virtue of a belief involving a relational phenomenal concept.

there is no great harm in doing so as long as the relevant distinctions are kept clear. What matters for my purposes is not the terminological point but the more basic point that the distinct concepts $this_E$ and R exist.

The relations among these concepts can be analyzed using the two-dimensional framework (discussed in the appendix) for representing the content of concepts. The central points in what follows should be comprehensible if matters involving the two-dimensional framework are skipped, but the framework makes the analysis of some of the crucial points much clearer.

According to the two-dimensional framework, when an identity $A = B$ is a posteriori, the concepts A and B have different primary intensions. If A and B are rigid concepts and the identity is true, A and B have the same secondary intensions. So we should expect that the concepts red_C, red_I, $this_E$, and R have different primary intensions but the same secondary intension. And this is what we find. The secondary intension of each picks out phenomenal redness in all worlds. The primary intension of red_C picks out, in a given centered world, roughly the quality typically caused by certain paradigmatic objects in the community of the subject at the center of the world. The primary intension of red_I picks out roughly the quality typically caused by those objects in the subject at the center.

As for the demonstrative concept $this_E$, to a first approximation, one might hold that its primary intension picks out the quality that is ostended by the subject at the center. This characterization is good enough for most of our purposes, but it is not quite correct. It is possible to ostend two experiences simultaneously and invoke two distinct demonstrative concepts, as when one thinks *that quality differs from that quality*, ostending two different parts of a symmetrical visual field (see Austin 1990). Here no descriptive characterization such as this one will capture the difference between the two concepts. It is better to see $this_E$ as a sort of indexical, like *I* or *now*. To characterize the epistemic possibilities relevant to demonstrative phenomenal concepts, we need centered worlds whose centers contain not only a "marked" subject and time but also one or more marked experiences—in the general case, a sequence of such experiences.[10] Then a concept such as $this_E$ will map a centered world to the quality of the "marked" experience (if any) in that world. Where two demonstrative concepts $this_{E1}$ and $this_{E2}$ are involved, as in the case under discussion, the relevant epistemic possibilities will contain at least two marked experiences, and we can see $this_{E1}$ as picking out the quality of the first marked experience in a

---

10. In the experience-based framework, if experiences do not map one-to-one to instances of phenomenal properties, then instances of phenomenal properties should be marked instead.

centered world and $this_{E2}$ as picking out the quality of the second. Then the belief under discussion will endorse all worlds at which the quality of the first marked experience differs from the quality of the second. This subtlety will not be central in what follows.

The primary intension of R is quite distinct from all of these. It picks out phenomenal redness in all worlds. I analyze this matter in more depth shortly, but one can see intuitively why this is plausible. When Mary believes *roses cause R experiences* or *I am currently having an R experience*, she thereby excludes all epistemic possibilities in which roses cause some other quality (such as G, phenomenal greenness) or in which she is experiencing some other quality. Only epistemic possibilities involving phenomenal redness remain.

The cognitive significance of identities such as $red_C = R$, $red_I = R$, and $this_E = R$ is reflected in the differences between the concept's primary intensions. The first two identities endorse all epistemic possibilities in which paradigmatic objects stand in the right relation to experiences of R; these are only a subset of the epistemic possibilities available a priori. The third identity endorses all epistemic possibilities in which the marked experience at the center (or the ostended experience, on the rough characterization) is R. Again, there are many epistemic possibilities (a priori) that are not like this: centered worlds in which the marked experience is G, for example. Once again, this epistemic contingency reflects the cognitive significance of the identity.

Phenomenal realists (e.g., Loar 1997; Hawthorne 2002a) analyzing what Mary learns have occasionally suggested that her phenomenal concept is a demonstrative concept. This is particularly popular as a way of resisting anti-materialist arguments, as it is tempting to invoke the distinctive epistemic and referential behavior of demonstrative concepts in explaining why an epistemic gap does not reflect an ontological gap. But on a closer look it is clear that Mary's central phenomenal concept R (the one that captures what she learns) is *distinct* from her central demonstrative concept $this_E$, as witnessed by the nontrivial identity $this_E = R$, and is not a demonstrative concept in the usual sense. This is not just a terminological point. Those who use these analyses to rebut anti-materialist arguments typically rely on analogies with the epistemic and referential behavior of ordinary (Kaplan-style) demonstratives. Insofar as these analyses rely on such analogies, they mischaracterize Mary's new knowledge. Something similar applies to analyses that liken phenomenal concepts to indexical concepts (e.g., Ismael 1999; Perry 2001). If my analysis is correct, then pure phenomenal concepts (unlike demonstrative phenomenal concepts) are not indexical concepts at all.

4. Inverted Mary

We can now complicate the situation by introducing another thought experiment on top of the first one. Consider the case of *Inverted Mary*, who is physically, functionally, and environmentally just like Mary, except that her phenomenal color vision is red/green inverted. (I assume for simplicity that Inverted Mary lives in a community of inverted observers.) Like Mary, Inverted Mary learns something new when she sees red things for the first time, but Inverted Mary learns something different from what Mary learns. Where Mary learns that tomatoes cause experiences of (what we call) phenomenal redness, Inverted Mary learns that they cause experiences of (what we call) phenomenal greenness. In the terms given earlier, Mary acquires beliefs $red_C = R$, $red_1 = R$, and $this_E = R$, while Inverted Mary acquires beliefs $red_C = G$, $red_1 = G$, and $this_E = G$ (where G is the obvious analogue of R). So Mary and Inverted Mary acquire beliefs with quite different contents.

This is already enough to draw a strong conclusion about the irreducibility of content. Recall that Mary and Inverted Mary are physical/functional and environmental twins even after they see red things for the first time. Nevertheless, they have beliefs with different contents. It follows that belief content does not supervene conceptually on physical/functional properties. It follows from this that intentional properties are not conceptually supervenient on physical/functional properties in the general case.

This is a nontrivial conclusion. Phenomenal realists often hold that, while the phenomenal is conceptually irreducible to the physical and functional, the intentional can be analyzed in functional terms. If what I have said here is correct, then this irreducibility cannot be quarantined in this way. If the phenomenal is conceptually irreducible to the physical and functional, so too is at least one aspect of the intentional: the content of phenomenal beliefs.

At this point, there is a natural temptation to downplay this phenomenon by reducing it to a sort of dependence of belief content on reference that is found in many other cases: in particular in the cases that are central to externalism about the content of belief. Take Putnam's case of Twin Earth. Oscar and Twin Oscar are functional duplicates, but they inhabit different environments: Oscar's contains H_2O as the clear liquid in the oceans and lakes, while Twin Oscar's contains XYZ (which we count not as water but as twin water). As a consequence, Oscar's *water* concept refers to water (H_2O), while Twin Oscar's analogous concept refers to twin water (XYZ). Because of this difference in reference, Oscar and Twin Oscar seem to have different beliefs: Oscar believes that water is wet, while Twin Oscar believes that twin water is wet. Perhaps the case of Mary and Inverted Mary is just like this.[11]

The analogy does not go through, however, or rather, it goes through only to a limited extent. Oscar and Twin Oscar's *water* concepts here are analogous to Mary and Inverted Mary's relational phenomenal concepts (red_C or red_1) or perhaps to their demonstrative concepts. For example, the relational concepts that they express with their public-language expressions 'red experience' will refer to two different properties, phenomenal redness and phenomenal greenness. Mary and Inverted Mary can deploy these concepts in certain beliefs, such as the beliefs that they express by saying 'Tomatoes cause red experiences' even before they leave their monochromatic rooms for the first time. Because of the distinct referents of their concepts, there is a natural sense (Nida-Rümelin's "nonphenomenal" sense) in which we can say that Mary believed that tomatoes caused red experiences, while Inverted Mary did not; she believed that tomatoes caused green experiences. Here the analogy goes through straightforwardly.

The pure phenomenal concepts R and G, however, are less analogous to the two *water* concepts than to the chemical concepts H_2O and *XYZ*. When Oscar learns the true nature of water, he acquires the new belief *water* = H_2O, while Twin Oscar acquires an analogous belief involving *XYZ*. When Mary learns the true nature of red experiences, she acquires a new belief red_C = R, while Inverted Mary acquires an analogous belief involving G. That is, Mary and Inverted Mary's later knowledge involving R and G is fully lucid knowledge of the referents of the concepts in question, analogous to Oscar and Twin Oscar's knowledge involving the chemical concepts H_2O and *XYZ*.

But here we see the strong disanalogy. Once Oscar acquires the chemical concept H_2O and Twin Oscar acquires *XYZ*, they will no longer be twins. Their functional properties will differ significantly. By contrast, at the corresponding point Mary and Inverted Mary are still twins. Even though Mary has the pure phenomenal concept R and Inverted Mary has G, their functional properties are just the same. So the difference between the concepts R and G across functional twins is something that has no counterpart in the standard Twin Earth story.

All this reflects the fact that in standard externalist cases, the pairs of corresponding concepts may differ in reference, but they have the same or similar *epistemic* or *notional* contents. Oscar and Twin Oscar's *water* concepts have different referents (H_2O vs. XYZ), but they have the same

---

11. This sort of treatment of phenomenal belief is suggested by Francescotti (1994).

epistemic contents: both aim to refer to roughly the liquid around them with certain superficial properties. Something like this applies to Mary's and Inverted Mary's relational phenomenal concepts, which have different referents but the same epistemic content (which picks out whatever quality stands in a certain relation), and to their demonstrative concepts (which pick out roughly whatever quality happens to be ostended).

In terms of the two-dimensional framework, where epistemic contents correspond to primary intensions, Oscar's and Twin Oscar's *water* concepts have the same primary intension but different secondary intensions. A similar pattern holds in all the cases characteristic of standard externalism. The pattern also holds for Mary's and Inverted Mary's relational phenomenal concepts and their demonstrative phenomenal concepts.

But Mary's concept R and Twin Mary's concept G have *different* epistemic contents. In this way they are analogous to Oscar's concept H_2O and Twin Oscar's concept XYZ. But again, the disanalogy is that R and G are possessed by twins and H_2O and XYZ are not. So the case of Inverted Mary yields an entirely different phenomenon: a case in which *epistemic* content differs between twins.

This can be illustrated by seeing how the concepts in question are used to constrain epistemic possibilities. When Oscar confidently believes that there is water in the glass, he is not thereby in a position to rule out the epistemic possibility that there is XYZ in the glass (unless he has some further knowledge, such as the knowledge that water is H_2O). The same goes for Twin Oscar's corresponding belief. For both of them, it is equally epistemically possible that the glass contains H_2O and that it contains XYZ. Any epistemic possibility compatible with Oscar's belief is also compatible with Twin Oscar's belief. In both cases, these will be roughly those epistemic possibilities in which a sample of the dominant watery stuff in the environment is in the glass.

Epistemic content reflects the way that a belief constrains the space of epistemic possibilities, so Oscar's and Twin Oscar's epistemic contents are the same. Something similar applies to Mary and Inverted Mary, at least where their pairwise relational and demonstrative phenomenal concepts are concerned. When Mary confidently believes (under her relational concept) that her mother is having a red experience, for example, she is not thereby in a position to rule out the epistemic possibility that her mother is having an experience with the quality G. Both Mary's and Inverted Mary's beliefs are compatible with any epistemic possibility in which the subject's mother is having the sort of experience typically caused in the community by paradigmatic red objects. So their beliefs involving relational concepts have the same epistemic contents.

Mary's and Inverted Mary's pure phenomenal concepts do not work like this, however. Mary's concept R and Inverted Mary's concept G differ not just in their referents but also in their epistemic contents. When Mary leaves the monochromatic room and acquires the confident belief (under her pure phenomenal concept) that tomatoes cause red experiences, she is thereby in a position to rule out the epistemic possibility that tomatoes cause experiences with quality G. The only epistemic possibilities compatible with her belief are those in which tomatoes cause R experiences. For Inverted Mary, things are reversed. The only epistemic possibilities compatible with her belief are those in which tomatoes cause G experiences. So their epistemic contents are quite different.

Again, the epistemic situation with R and G is analogous to the epistemic situation with the concepts H_2O and XYZ. When Oscar believes (under a fully lucid chemical concept) that the glass contains H_2O, he is thereby in a position to rule out all epistemic possibilities in which the glass contains XYZ. For Twin Oscar, things are reversed. This is to say that H_2O and XYZ have different epistemic contents. The same goes for R and G.

In the case of the pure phenomenal concepts, unlike standard externalist cases, we have a situation in which two concepts in physically identical subjects differ in their epistemic content. So phenomenal concepts seem to give a case in which even epistemic content is not conceptually supervenient on the physical.

Using the two-dimensional framework, the primary intension of a concept reflects the way it applies to epistemic possibilities. We have seen that the primary intensions of Oscar's and Twin Oscar's *water* concepts are the same, as are the primary intensions of Mary's and Inverted Mary's relational and demonstrative phenomenal concepts. Still, R and G differ in the way they apply to epistemic possibilities, and their primary intensions differ accordingly. The primary intension of R picks out phenomenal redness in all worlds, and the primary intension of G picks out phenomenal greenness in all worlds. When Mary thinks *I am having an R experience now*, the primary intension of her thought is true at all and only those worlds in which the being at the center is having an R experience.

Something very unusual is going on here. In standard externalism and in standard cases of so-called "direct reference," a referent plays a role in constituting the subjunctive content (secondary intension) of concepts and beliefs, while leaving the epistemic content (primary intension) unaffected. In the pure phenomenal case, by contrast, the quality of the experiences plays a role in constituting the *epistemic* content of the concept and of the corresponding belief. One might say very loosely that in this case, the referent of the concept is somehow present inside the concept's sense in a way much stronger than in the usual cases of "direct reference."

We might say that the pure phenomenal concept is *epistemically rigid*: its epistemic content picks out the same referent in every possible world (considered as actual). By contrast, ordinary rigid concepts are merely *subjunctively rigid*, with a subjunctive content that picks out the same referent in every possible world (considered as counterfactual). Epistemically rigid concepts will typically be subjunctively rigid, but most subjunctively rigid concepts are not epistemically rigid. Pure phenomenal concepts are both epistemically and subjunctively rigid.[12]

One might see here some justification for Russell's claim that we have a special capacity for direct reference to our experiences.[13] Contemporary direct reference theorists hold that Russell's view is too restrictive and that we can make direct reference to a much broader class of entities. But the cases they invoke are "direct" only in the weak sense outlined earlier: the subjunctive content depends on the referent, but the epistemic content of the concept does not. In the phenomenal case, the epistemic content itself seems to be partly constituted by the referent. It is not hard to imagine that some such epistemic requirement on direct reference is what Russell had in mind.

5. Direct Phenomenal Concepts

We have seen that the contents of phenomenal concepts and phenomenal beliefs do not supervene conceptually on physical properties. Do these contents supervene conceptually on some broader class of properties, and if so, on which? Here I offer an analysis of how the content of pure

12. Further, epistemically rigid concepts will usually be subjunctively rigid *de jure*, which entails that they are what Martine Nida-Rümelin (2007) calls "super-rigid": they pick out the same referent relative to all pairs of scenarios considered as actual and worlds considered as counterfactual. When represented by a two-dimensional matrix, superrigid concepts have the same entry at each point of the matrix.

13. Russell also held that there can be direct reference to universals and perhaps to the self. It is arguable that for at least some universals (in the domains of mathematics or of causation, perhaps), one can form an epistemically rigid concept whose epistemic content picks out instances of that universal in all worlds. So there is at least a limited analogy here, though it seems unlikely that in these cases the content of such a (token) concept is directly constituted by an underlying instance of the universal in the manner suggested later.

There is no analogous phenomenon with the self. There may, however, be a different sense in which we can make direct reference to the self, to the current time, and to particular experiences. This is the sort of direct indexical reference that corresponds to the need to build these entities into the center of a centered world. We can refer to these "directly" (in a certain sense) under indexical concepts, but we cannot form concepts whose epistemic contents reflect the referents in question. This suggests that direct reference to particulars and direct reference to properties are quite different phenomena.

phenomenal concepts is constituted. I do not give a knockdown argument for this analysis by decisively refuting all alternatives, but I offer it as perhaps the most natural and elegant account of the phenomena and as an account that can in turn do further explanatory work.

To start with, it is natural to hold that the contents of phenomenal concepts and beliefs supervene conceptually on the combination of physical and phenomenal properties. Mary and Inverted Mary are physical twins, but they are phenomenally distinct, and this phenomenal distinctness (Mary experiences phenomenal redness, Inverted Mary experiences phenomenal greenness) precisely mirrors their intentional distinctness (Mary believes that tomatoes cause R experiences, Inverted Mary believes that tomatoes cause G experiences). It is very plausible to suppose that their intentional distinctness holds in virtue of their phenomenal distinctness.

The alternative is that the intentional content of the phenomenal concept is conceptually independent of both physical and phenomenal properties. If that is so, it should be conceivable that two subjects have the same physical and phenomenal properties, while having phenomenal beliefs that differ in content. Such a case might involve Mary and Mary* as physical and phenomenal twins who are both experiencing phenomenal redness for the first time (while being phenomenally identical in all other respects), with Mary acquiring the belief that tomatoes cause R experiences while Mary* acquires the belief that tomatoes cause G experiences. It is not at all clear that such a case is conceivable.

Another possibility is that the intentional content of Mary's phenomenal concept in question might be determined by phenomenal states *other* than the phenomenal redness that Mary is visually experiencing. For example, maybe Mary's belief content is determined by a faint phenomenal "idea" that goes along with her phenomenal "impression," where the former is not conceptually determined by the latter, and neither one is conceptually determined by the physical. In that case, it should once again be conceivable that twins Mary and Mary* both visually experience phenomenal redness upon leaving the room, with Mary acquiring the belief that tomatoes cause R experiences while Mary* acquires the belief that tomatoes cause G experiences—this time because of a difference in their associated phenomenal ideas. But again, it is far from clear that this is conceivable.

There is a very strong intuition that the content of Mary's phenomenal concept and phenomenal belief is *determined* by the phenomenal character of her visual experience in that it will vary directly as a function of that character in cases where that character varies while physical and other phenomenal properties are held fixed and also in that it will not vary independently of that character in such cases. I adopt this claim as a plausible working hypothesis.

In particular, I take it that in cases such as Mary's, the content of a phenomenal concept and a corresponding phenomenal belief is partly *constituted* by an underlying phenomenal quality, in that the content will mirror the quality (picking out instances of the quality in all epistemic possibilities), and in that across a wide range of nearby conceptually possible cases in which the underlying quality is varied while background properties are held constant, the content will co-vary to mirror the quality. Let us call this sort of phenomenal concept a *direct phenomenal concept.*[14]

Not all experiences are accompanied by corresponding direct phenomenal concepts. Many of our experiences appear to pass without our forming any beliefs about them and without the sort of concept formation that occurs in the Mary case. The clearest cases of direct phenomenal concepts arise when a subject attends to the quality of an experience and forms a concept wholly based on the attention to the quality, "taking up" the quality into the concept. This sort of concept formation can occur with visual experiences, as in the Mary case, but it can equally occur with all sorts of other experiences: auditory and other perceptual experiences, bodily sensations, emotional experiences, and so on. In each case we can imagine the analogue of Mary having such an experience for the first time, attending to it, and coming to have a concept of what it is like to have it. There is no reason to suppose that this sort of concept formation is restricted to entirely novel experiences. I can experience a particular shade of phenomenal redness for the hundredth time, attend to it, and form a direct phenomenal concept of what it is like to have that experience, a concept whose content is based entirely on the character of the experience.

6. Direct Phenomenal Beliefs

Direct phenomenal concepts can be deployed in a wide variety of beliefs and other propositional attitudes. When Mary attends to her phenomenally red experience and forms her direct phenomenal concept R, she is thereby in a position to believe that tomatoes cause R experiences, to believe that others have R experiences, to believe that she previously had no R experiences, to desire more R experiences, and so on.

---

14. *In the abstract object framework, a direct phenomenal concept corresponds to a direct *grasping* of a pure phenomenal concept. The distinction between direct phenomenal concepts and other pure phenomenal concepts is only a distinction at the level of mental entities and not at the level of the corresponding abstract objects.

Perhaps the most crucial sort of deployment of a direct phenomenal concept occurs when a subject predicates the concept of the very experience responsible for constituting its content. Mary has a phenomenally red experience, attends to it, forms the direct phenomenal concept R, and forms the belief *this experience is R*, demonstrating the phenomenally red experience in question. We can call this special sort of belief a *direct phenomenal belief*.

We can also cast this idea within an experience-free ontology of qualities. In this framework, we can say that a direct phenomenal concept is formed by attending to a quality and taking up that quality into a concept whose content mirrors the quality, picking out instances of the quality in all epistemic possibilities. A direct phenomenal belief is formed when the referent of this direct phenomenal concept is identified with the referent of a corresponding demonstrative phenomenal concept. This happens, for example, when Mary forms the belief *this quality is R*. The general form of a direct phenomenal belief in this framework is $this_E = R$, where $this_E$ is a demonstrative phenomenal concept and R is the corresponding direct phenomenal concept.

A number of subtleties arise when considering the constitution and content of direct phenomenal beliefs.

1. For a direct phenomenal belief, it is required that the demonstrative and direct concepts involved be appropriately "aligned." Say that Mary experiences phenomenal redness in both the left and right halves of her visual field, forms a direct phenomenal concept R based on her attention to the left half, forms a demonstrative concept of phenomenal redness based on her attention to the right half, and identifies the two by a belief of the form $this_E = R$. Then, even though the same quality (phenomenal redness) is referred to on both sides, this is not a direct phenomenal belief since the concepts are grounded in different instances of that quality. The belief has the right sort of content, but it does not have the right sort of constitution.

To characterize the required alignment more carefully we can note that all direct phenomenal concepts, like all demonstrative phenomenal concepts, are based in acts of attention to instances of phenomenal qualities. A direct phenomenal concept such as R does not characterize a quality *as* an object of attention, but it nevertheless requires attention to a quality for its formation. The same act of attention can also be used to form a demonstrative phenomenal concept $this_E$. A direct phenomenal belief (in the quality-based framework) will be a belief of the form $this_E = R$, where the demonstrative phenomenal concept $this_E$ and the direct phenomenal concept R are *aligned*: that is, where they are based in the same act of attention.

One can simplify the language by regarding the act of attention as a demonstration. We can then say that both demonstrative and direct phenomenal concepts are based in demonstrations and that a direct phenomenal belief is a belief of the form $this_E = R$, where the two concepts are based in the same demonstration.[15]

2. As with all acts of demonstration and attention, phenomenal demonstration and attention involve a cognitive element. Reference to a phenomenal quality is determined in part by cognitive elements of a demonstration. These cognitive elements will also enter into determining the content of a corresponding direct phenomenal concept.

Consider two individuals with identical visual experiences. These individuals might engage in different acts of demonstration (e.g., one might demonstrate a red quality experienced in the right half of the visual field, and the other a green quality experienced in the left half of the visual field) and thereby form distinct direct phenomenal concepts. Or they might attend to the same location in the visual field but demonstrate distinct qualities associated with that location (e.g., one might demonstrate a highly specific shade of phenomenal redness, and the other a less specific shade, again resulting in distinct direct phenomenal concepts). These differences will be due to differences in the cognitive backgrounds of the demonstrations in the two individuals. I am neutral here about whether such cognitive differences are themselves constituted by underlying functioning, aspects of cognitive phenomenology, or both.

One can imagine varying the visual experiences and the cognitive background here independently. Varying visual experiences might yield a range of cases in which direct phenomenal concepts of phenomenal redness, greenness, and other hues are formed. Varying the cognitive background might yield a range of cases in which direct phenomenal concepts of different degrees of specificity (for example) are formed.

Along with this cognitive element comes the possibility of failed demonstration if the cognitive element and the targeted experiential elements mismatch sufficiently. Take Nancy, who attends to a patch of phenomenal color, acting cognitively as if to demonstrate a highly specific phenomenal shade. Nancy has not attended sufficiently closely to notice that the patch has a nonuniform phenomenal color. Let us say that she has an experience of a square colored with different shades of red on its left and

---

15. Gertler (2001) has independently developed a related account of phenomenal introspection, according to which a phenomenal state is introspected when it is "embedded" in another state and when the second state constitutes demonstrative attention to the relevant content by virtue of this embedding. On my account, things are the other way around. Any "embedding" holds in virtue of demonstrative attention rather than the reverse.

right side.[16] In such a case, the demonstrative phenomenal concept will presumably refer to no quality at all. Given its cognitive structure, it could refer only to a specific quality, but symmetry prevents it from referring to either instantiated quality, and presumably uninstantiated qualities cannot be demonstrated.

What of any associated direct phenomenal concept? It is not out of the question that the subject forms *some* substantive concept where a direct phenomenal concept would normally be formed—perhaps a concept of an intermediate uninstantiated shade of phenomenal red, at least if the instantiated shades are not too different. Like a direct phenomenal concept, this concept will have a content that depends constitutively on associated qualities of experience (Inverted Nancy might form a concept of an intermediate phenomenal green), but it will not truly be a direct phenomenal concept since its content will not directly mirror an underlying quality.

This possibility of cognitive mismatch affects the path from demonstration to a demonstrated phenomenal quality, but given that a phenomenal quality is truly demonstrated, it does not seem to affect the path from demonstrated phenomenal quality to a direct phenomenal concept. That is, as long as a phenomenal quality is demonstrated, and the cognitive act typical of forming a direct phenomenal concept based on such a demonstration is present, a direct phenomenal concept will be formed.

We might call a concept that shares the cognitive structure of a direct phenomenal concept a *quasi-direct* phenomenal concept, and we can call a belief with the same cognitive structure as a direct phenomenal belief a *quasi-direct* phenomenal belief. Like a direct phenomenal concept, a quasi-direct phenomenal concept arises from an act of (intended) demonstration, along with a characteristic sort of cognitive act. Unlike a direct phenomenal concept, a quasi-direct phenomenal concept is not required to have a content that is constituted by an underlying quality. Nancy's key concept is a quasi-direct phenomenal concept but not a direct phenomenal concept.

We can call a quasi-direct phenomenal concept that is not a direct phenomenal concept a *pseudo-direct* phenomenal concept, and we can define a pseudo-direct graspings phenomenal belief similarly. If the suggestion above is correct, then the only pseudo-direct phenomenal concepts are like Nancy's in involving an unsuccessful demonstration. As long as a quasi-direct phenomenal concept is grounded in a successful demonstration, it will be a direct phenomenal concept. I return to this claim later.[17]

---

16. This sort of case was suggested to me by Delia Graff and Mark Johnston.

17. *In the abstract object framework, we can speak of quasi-direct and pseudo-direct graspings of pure phenomenal concepts.

3. All direct phenomenal concepts are pure phenomenal concepts, but not all pure phenomenal concepts are direct phenomenal concepts. To see this, note that Mary may well retain some knowledge of what it is like to see tomatoes even after she goes back into her black-and-white room, or while she shuts her eyes, or while she looks at green grass. She still has a concept of phenomenal redness than can be deployed in various beliefs, with the sort of epistemic relations to relational and demonstrative phenomenal concepts that is characteristic of pure phenomenal concepts. Inverted Mary (still Mary's physical twin) has a corresponding concept deployed in corresponding beliefs that *differ* in content from Mary's. As before, their corresponding beliefs *differ* in epistemic content, including and excluding different classes of epistemic possibilities. Mary's concept is still a concept of phenomenal redness as the quality it is, based on a lucid understanding of that quality rather than on a mere relational or demonstrative identification. So as before, it is a pure phenomenal concept. But it is not a direct phenomenal concept, since there is no corresponding experience (or instantiated quality) that is being attended to or taken up into the concept. We can call this sort of concept a *standing* phenomenal concept, since it may persist in a way that direct phenomenal concepts do not.[18]

There are some differences in character between direct and standing phenomenal concepts. Direct phenomenal concepts may be very finegrained, picking out very specific phenomenal qualities (a highly specific shade of phenomenal redness, for example). Standing phenomenal concepts are usually more coarse-grained, picking out less specific qualities. One can note this phenomenologically from the difficulty of "holding" in mind specific qualities as opposed to coarser categories when relevant visual experiences are not present, and this is also brought out by empirical results showing the difficulty of reidentifying specific qualities over time.[19] At the cost of some degree of coarse-graining, it usually seems possible for a direct phenomenal concept to yield a corresponding standing phenomenal concept as a "successor" concept once the experience in question disappears.[20]

As with direct phenomenal concepts, the content of standing phenomenal concepts does not conceptually supervene on the physical. Mary and Inverted Mary, back in their rooms, are physically identical but have

18. *In the abstract object framework, these are standing grasps of pure phenomenal concepts.

19. See Raffman (1995) for a discussion of these results in an argument for an antirepresentationalist "presentational" analysis of phenomenal concepts that is compatible with the analysis here.

20. *That is, a direct grasp of a pure phenomenal concept often leads to a standing grasp of a somewhat more coarse-grained pure phenomenal concept.

different standing phenomenal concepts. A question arises as to what determines their content. I do not analyze that matter here, but I think it is plausible that their content is determined by some combination of (1) nonsensory phenomenal states of a cognitive sort, which bear a relevant relation to the original phenomenal quality in question (e.g., a faint Humean phenomenal "idea" that is relevantly related to the original "impression"); (2) dispositions to have such states; and (3) dispositions to recognize instances of the phenomenal quality in question. It is not implausible that Mary and Inverted Mary (back in their rooms) still differ in some or all of these respects and that these respects are constitutively responsible for the difference in the content of their concepts.

One might be tempted to use the existence of standing phenomenal concepts to argue against the earlier analysis of direct phenomenal concepts (that is, of concepts akin to those Mary acquires on first experiencing phenomenal redness) as constituted by the quality of the relevant instantiated experience. Why not assimilate them to standing phenomenal concepts instead, giving a unified account of the two? In response, note first that it remains difficult to conceive of the content of direct phenomenal concepts varying independently of the phenomenal quality in question, whereas it does not seem so difficult to conceive of the content of standing phenomenal concepts varying independently. Second, note that the difference in specificity between direct and standing phenomenal concepts gives some reason to believe that they are constituted in different ways.

The lifetime of a direct phenomenal concept is limited to the lifetime of the experience (or the instantiated quality) that constitutes it. (In some cases a specific phenomenal concept might persist for a few moments due to the persistence of a vivid iconic memory, but even this will soon disappear.) Some might worry that this lack of persistence suggests that it is not a concept at all since concepthood requires persistence. This seems misguided, however. It is surely possible for a concept to be formed moments before a subject dies. The concepts in question are still predicable of any number of entities during their limited lifetimes, and these predications can be true or false (e.g., Mary may falsely believe that her sister is currently experiencing R). This sort of predicability, with assessibility for truth or falsehood, seems sufficient for concepthood; at least it is sufficient for the uses of concepthood that are required here.

4. As with pure phenomenal concepts generally, we do not have public language expressions that distinctively express the content of direct phenomenal concepts. Public reference to phenomenal qualities is always fixed relationally, it seems, by virtue of a relation to certain external

stimuli, certain sorts of behavior, or certain demonstrations. (Recall Ryle's remark that there are no "neat" sensation words.) Of course, Mary can express a pure phenomenal concept by introducing her own term, such as 'R,' or by using an old term, such as 'red,' with this stipulated meaning. But this use will not be public, at least in the limited sense that there is no method by which we can ensure that other members of the community will use the term with the same epistemic content. One can at best ensure that they pick out the same quality by picking it out under a different epistemic content (e.g., as the quality Mary is having at a certain time) or by referring through semantic deference (as the quality that Mary picks out with 'R'). In this sense it seems that any resulting language will be "private": it can be used with full competence by just one subject, and others can use it only deferentially. (An exception may arguably be made for terms that express *structural* pure phenomenal concepts, e.g., phenomenal similarity and difference and perhaps phenomenal spatial relations, which arguably do not rely on relational reference fixing.)

Of course, the view I have set out here is just the sort of view that Wittgenstein directed his "private language" argument against. The nature of the private language argument is contested, so in response I can say only that I have seen no reconstruction of it that provides a strong case against the view I have laid out. Some versions of the argument seem to fall prey to the mistake just outlined, that of requiring a strong sort of "repeatability" for concept possession (and an exceptionally strong sort at that, requiring the recognizability of correct repeated application). A certain sort of repeatability is required for concept possession, but it is merely the "hypothetical repeatability" involved in *present* predicability of the concept to actual and hypothetical cases, with associated truth conditions. Another reconstruction of the argument, that of Kripke (1981), provides no distinctive traction against my analysis of direct phenomenal concepts: any force that it has applies to concepts quite generally.

One might even argue that Kripke's argument provides *less* traction in the case of direct phenomenal concepts, as this is precisely a case in which we can see how a determinate application condition can be constituted by an underlying phenomenal quality. Kripke's remarks about associated phenomenal qualities (41–51)—for example, a certain sort of "headache"—being irrelevant to the content of concepts such as addition apply much less strongly where *phenomenal* concepts are concerned. Of course, there is more to say here, but in any case it is a curiosity of Kripke's reconstruction of the argument that it applies least obviously to the phenomena at which Wittgenstein's argument is often taken to be aimed.

7. Further Questions

I have argued that pure phenomenal concepts and phenomenal beliefs are conceptually irreducible to the physical and functional because these concepts themselves depend on the constitutive role of experience. Does this sort of irreducibility extend to other concepts or beliefs? Are concepts and beliefs irreducible to the physical and functional quite generally?

There is one class of concepts for which such a conclusion clearly follows. This is the class of concepts that have phenomenal concepts as constituents. Such concepts might include concepts of *the tallest conscious being in this room*, *the physical basis of consciousness*, and *the external cause of R*, where *R* is a pure concept of phenomenal redness. More generally, let us say that a concept is *partly phenomenal* if it has conceptual ties with phenomenal concepts, so that thoughts involving that concept conceptually entail nontrivial thoughts involving pure phenomenal concepts. Then partly phenomenal concepts will inherit the irreducibility of phenomenal concepts.

It is arguable that many or most of our perceptual concepts are partly phenomenal. At least some concepts of external colors can be analyzed roughly as *the property causally responsible for C in me*, where *C* is a pure concept of a phenomenal color. Things are more complex for community-level concepts. Here it is more plausible that an external color concept might be analyzed in terms of community-wide relations to a nonspecific phenomenal concept: perhaps *the property causally responsible for the dominant sort of visual experience caused by certain paradigmatic objects in this community* or something like that. But this still has the concept of visual experience as a constituent and so will still be partly phenomenal. The alternative is that external color concepts might be analyzed in terms of their relations to certain *judgments* or other nonexperiential responses, in which case the reducibility or irreducibility will not be so clear. I will not adjudicate this matter here, but my own view is that many or most of the perceptual concepts that we actually possess are partly phenomenal.

One might try to extend this further. In the case of theoretical concepts from science, for example, one can argue that these have conceptual ties to various perceptual concepts (as the Ramsey–Lewis analysis of theoretical concepts suggests). If so, and if the perceptual concepts in question are partly phenomenal, then it is plausible that these concepts are partly phenomenal. One might also argue for conceptual ties between intentional concepts and phenomenal concepts, as well as between social concepts and intentional concepts, so that a wide range of social concepts will turn out to be partly phenomenal. If this is right, then a being without consciousness could have at best impoverished versions of these concepts and perhaps could not have such concepts at all.

This sort of argument will not work for all concepts. Many mathematical or philosophical concepts have no obvious tie to phenomenal concepts, for example. In fact, there is good reason to think that some concepts are not partly phenomenal. If all concepts were partly phenomenal, it would be hard to avoid the conclusion that the content of all concepts is wholly analyzable in phenomenal terms, which would lead naturally to phenomenalism or idealism. My own view is that certain central concepts, such as causal and mathematical concepts, are not conceptually tied to phenomenal concepts. Once this is recognized, it becomes clear that even if a wide range of concepts have contents with a phenomenal component, only a small number of these concepts are entirely phenomenal.

Even if some concepts are conceptually independent of phenomenal concepts, it is not out of the question that their content might still be irreducible. One intriguing possibility is that phenomenology could play a crucial role in a subject's *possessing* a causal or a mathematical concept even though these concepts are conceptually independent of phenomenal concepts. (Compare a reductive view on which neural states might play a crucial role in a subject's possessing concepts that are conceptually independent of neural concepts.) There is at least some intuition that a capacity for consciousness may be required to have concepts in the first place, and it is not obviously false that phenomenology plays a role in the possession of even nonphenomenal concepts.

Such a thesis would require much further argument, of course, and I am not certain whether it is true. But even if it is false, the more limited thesis that phenomenology plays an ineliminable role in the possession of phenomenal and partly phenomenal concepts has significant consequences. If even the more limited thesis is true, then the project of giving a functional analysis of intentionality cannot succeed across the board, and a central role must be given to phenomenology in the analysis of intentional content.

9

THE EPISTEMOLOGY OF
PHENOMENAL BELIEF

1. Infallibility

A traditional thesis in the epistemology of mind holds that first-person beliefs about phenomenal states are *infallible* or *incorrigible* (I use these terms equivalently), in that they cannot be false. In recent years such a thesis has been widely rejected. This rejection stems from both general philosophical reasoning (e.g., the suggestion that if beliefs and experiences are distinct existences, there can be no necessary connection between them) and from apparent counterexamples (e.g., a case in which someone, expecting to be burned, momentarily misclassifies a cold sensation as hot).

In this light, the analysis of phenomenal concepts and phenomenal belief in the previous chapter has interesting consequences. The analysis turns out to support an infallibility thesis, albeit a very limited one. In the last chapter (which I presuppose here), I distinguished a special class of direct phenomenal beliefs. These beliefs have the form $this_E = R$, where R is a direct phenomenal concept of a currently experienced phenomenal quality (phenomenal redness, say) and $this_E$ is an appropriately aligned demonstrative phenomenal concept ("this phenomenal quality") of the same quality. It is easy to see that direct phenomenal beliefs support an infallibility thesis.

Infallibility Thesis: A direct phenomenal belief cannot be false.

The truth of this thesis is an immediate consequence of the definition of direct phenomenal belief. A direct phenomenal concept by its nature picks out instances of an underlying demonstrated phenomenal quality, and a direct phenomenal belief identifies the referent of that concept with the original demonstrated quality (or predicates the concept of the very experience that instantiated the quality), so its truth is guaranteed.

If we combine this thesis (which is true by definition) with the substantive thesis that there are direct phenomenal beliefs (which is argued in the previous chapter), then we have a substantive infallibility thesis, one that applies to a significant range of actual beliefs.[1]

The thesis nevertheless has a number of significant limitations. The first is that most phenomenal beliefs are not direct phenomenal beliefs, so most phenomenal beliefs are still corrigible. The most common sort of phenomenal belief arguably involves the application of a *pre-existing* phenomenal concept (either a relational phenomenal concept or a standing pure phenomenal concept) to a new situation, as with the beliefs typically expressed by claims such as 'I am having a red experience' or 'I am in pain.' These are not direct phenomenal beliefs and are almost certainly corrigible.

There are also cases in which a direct phenomenal concept is applied to a quality (or an experience) other than the one that constituted it, as when one forms a direct phenomenal concept R based on a quality instantiated in the left half of one's visual field and applies it to a quality instantiated in the right half. These are also not direct phenomenal beliefs and are again almost certainly corrigible.

(The second sort of case brings out a further limitation in the infallibility thesis: it does not yield infallibility in virtue of content. If the left and right qualities in the preceding case are in fact the same, then the resulting non-direct phenomenal belief will arguably have the same content as the corresponding direct phenomenal belief, but the infallibility thesis will not apply to it. The domain of the infallibility thesis is constrained not just by content but also by underlying constitution.)

It is plausible that all of the standard counterexamples to infallibility theses fall into classes such as these, particularly the first. All of the standard counterexamples appear to involve the application of pre-existing

---

1. Pollock (1986, 32–33) entertains a version of this sort of view as a way of supporting infallibility, discussing a "containment thesis," according to which experiences are constituents of beliefs about experiences. He rejects the view on the grounds that (1) it does not support the infallibility of negative beliefs about experiences (e.g., the belief that one is not having a given experience), which he holds to be required for infallibility in general, and that (2) having an experience does not suffice to have the relevant belief, so having the belief also requires thinking about the experience, which renders the infallibility thesis trivial. I discuss both of these points in what follows.

phenomenal concepts (*pain, hot, red experience*), so none of the standard counterexamples apply to the infallibility thesis articulated here.

There is a natural temptation to find further counterexamples to the infallibility thesis. For example, one might consider a case in which a subject's experience changes very rapidly, and argue that the corresponding direct phenomenal concept must lag behind. In response to these attempted counterexamples, the most obvious reply is that these cannot truly be counterexamples, since the truth of the infallibility thesis is guaranteed by the definition of direct phenomenal belief. If the cases work as described, they do not involve direct phenomenal beliefs: either they involve a concept that is not a direct phenomenal concept, or they involve a direct phenomenal concept predicated of a quality other than the one that constitutes it. At best, they involve what I earlier called pseudodirect phenomenal beliefs: beliefs that share the cognitive structure of direct phenomenal beliefs (and thus are quasi-direct phenomenal beliefs) but that are not direct phenomenal beliefs.

One need not let matters rest there, however. I think that these counterexamples can usually be analyzed away on their own terms so that the purported pseudodirect phenomenal beliefs in question can be seen as direct phenomenal beliefs and as correct. In the case of a rapidly changing experience, one can plausibly hold that the content of a direct phenomenal concept co-varies immediately with the underlying quality so that there is no moment at which the belief is false. This is just what we would expect, given the constitutive relation suggested earlier. We might picture this schematically by suggesting that the basis for a direct phenomenal concept contains within it a "slot" for an instantiated quality such that the quality that fills the slot constitutes the content. In a case where experience changes rapidly, the filler of the slot changes rapidly, and so does the content.

Something similar goes for many other examples involving quasi-direct phenomenal beliefs. Take a case in which a subject attends to two different visual qualities (demonstrating them as $this_{E1}$ and $this_{E2}$) and mistakenly accepts $this_{E1} = this_{E2}$. In this case, someone might suggest that if the subject forms specific quasi-direct phenomenal concepts R_1 and R_2 based on the two acts of attention, these must have the same content, leading to false quasi-direct phenomenal beliefs (and thus to pseudodirect phenomenal beliefs). On my account, this case is better classified as one in which R_1 and R_2 are direct phenomenal concepts with different contents, yielding two correct direct phenomenal beliefs $this_{E1} = R_1$ and $this_{E2} = R_2$. The false beliefs here are of the form $this_{E1} = R_2$, $this_{E2} = R_1$, and $R_1 = R_2$. The last of these illustrates the important point that identities involving two direct phenomenal concepts, like identities involving two pure phenomenal concepts more generally, are not infallible.

Other cases of misclassification can be treated similarly. In the case in which a subject expecting to be burned misclassifies a cold sensation as hot, someone might suggest that any quasi-direct phenomenal concept will be a concept of phenomenal hotness, not coldness. Still, one can plausibly hold that if a quasi-direct phenomenal concept is formed, it will be a concept of phenomenal coldness and will yield a correct, direct phenomenal belief. The subject's mistake involves misclassifying the experience under standing phenomenal concepts and perhaps a mistaken identity involving a direct and a standing phenomenal concept.

It is arguable that most cases involving quasi-direct phenomenal beliefs can be treated this way. The only clear exceptions are cases such as Nancy's, from the last chapter, in which no phenomenal quality is demonstrated, and so no substantive direct phenomenal concept is formed. It remains plausible that as long as a quality is demonstrated, the cognitive act in question will yield a direct phenomenal concept with the right content and a true direct phenomenal belief. If that is correct, one can then accept a broader infallibility thesis applying to any quasi-direct phenomenal belief that is based on a successful demonstration of a phenomenal quality. I do not try to establish this thesis conclusively since I do not need it and since the infallibility thesis for direct phenomenal beliefs is unthreatened either way. But it is interesting to see that it can be defended.

One might suggest that the infallibility thesis articulated here (in either the narrower or the broader version) captures the plausible core of traditional infallibility theses. A number of philosophers have had the sense that there is something correct about the infallibility theses that is not touched by the counterexamples. This is reflected, for example, in Chisholm's distinction between "comparative" and "noncomparative" uses of "appears" talk, where only the noncomparative uses are held to be infallible. I think that this is not quite the right distinction. Even noncomparative uses can be corrigible when they correspond to uses of pure phenomenal concepts outside direct phenomenal beliefs. But perhaps a thesis restricted to direct phenomenal beliefs might play this role.

Certainly the analysis of direct phenomenal beliefs shows why the most common general philosophical argument against infallibility does not apply across the board. In the case of direct phenomenal beliefs, beliefs and experiences are *not* entirely distinct existences. It is precisely because of the constitutive connection between experiential quality and belief that the two can be necessarily connected.

Another limitation involves infallibility theses that are articulated in a "reverse" or bidirectional form, holding that all phenomenal states are infallibly known or at least infallibly knowable. Such a thesis is not supported by the current discussion. Most phenomenal states are not attended to and are not taken up into direct phenomenal concepts, so they are not the subjects of direct phenomenal beliefs. Moreover, for all I have said, it may be that some phenomenal states, such as fleeting or background phenomenal states, *cannot* be taken up into a direct phenomenal concept perhaps because they cannot be subject to the right sort of attention. If so, they are not even infallibly knowable, let alone infallibly known.

Infallibility theses are also sometimes articulated in a "negative" form, requiring that subjects cannot be mistaken in their belief that they are *not* having a given sort of experience. No direct phenomenal belief is a negative phenomenal belief, so the current framework does not support this thesis, and I think that the thesis is false in general.

A final limitation is that, although direct phenomenal beliefs are infallible, subjects are not infallible about whether they are having a direct phenomenal belief. For example, if I am not thinking clearly, I might misclassify a belief involving a standing phenomenal concept as a direct phenomenal belief. In the Nancy case from the previous chapter, if Nancy is philosophically sophisticated, she might well think that she is having a direct phenomenal belief even when she is not.

One could argue that this lack of higher-order infallibility prevents the first-order infallibility thesis from doing significant epistemological work. The matter is delicate: higher-order infallibility is probably too strong a requirement for an epistemologically useful infallibility thesis. On the other hand, *some* sort of further condition is required for a useful thesis. For example, any member of the class of true mathematical beliefs is infallible (since it is necessarily true), but this is of little epistemic use to a subject who cannot antecedently distinguish true and false mathematical beliefs. A natural suggestion is that some sort of higher-order accessibility is required.

Intermediate accessibility requirements might include these: for the infallibility of a direct phenomenal belief to be epistemologically significant, a subject must know that it is a direct phenomenal belief, or at least be justified in so believing, or a subject must be capable of knowing on reflection that it is a direct phenomenal belief, or direct phenomenal beliefs must be cognitively or phenomenologically distinctive as a class relative to nondirect phenomenal beliefs.

I am sympathetic with the sufficiency of a requirement appealing to cognitive or phenomenological distinctiveness if properly articulated.

Whether such a requirement holds of direct phenomenal beliefs turns on questions about quasi-direct and pseudodirect phenomenal beliefs. If there are many pseudodirect phenomenal beliefs, and if there is nothing cognitively or phenomenologically distinctive about direct phenomenal beliefs by comparison, then direct phenomenal beliefs will simply be distinguished as quasi-direct phenomenal beliefs with the right sort of content, and the infallibility claim will be relatively trivial. On the other hand, if pseudodirect phenomenal beliefs are rare, or if direct phenomenal beliefs are a cognitively or phenomenologically distinctive subclass, then it is more likely that infallibility will be nontrivial and carry epistemological significance.

If pseudodirect phenomenal beliefs are restricted to cases in which no phenomenal quality is demonstrated, such as the case of Nancy (as I have suggested), then the infallibility thesis will hold of a class of beliefs that can be distinctively and independently characterized in cognitive and phenomenological terms: the class of quasi-direct phenomenal beliefs that are based in a successful demonstration. This would render the infallibility claim entirely nontrivial, and it would make it more likely that it could do epistemological work. I will not try to settle this matter decisively here, however, and I will not put the infallibility thesis to any epistemological work in what follows.

It might be thought that the infallibility thesis suffers from another problem: that direct phenomenal beliefs are infallible because they are *trivial*. After all, beliefs such as *I am here* or *this is this* are (almost) infallible but only because they are (almost) trivial. ('Almost' is present because of the arguable nontriviality of my existence and spatial locatedness in one case and because of the possibility of reference failure for the demonstrative in the other.)

The analogy fails, however. The trivial beliefs in question are (almost) cognitively insignificant: they are (almost) a priori, containing (almost) no cognitively significant knowledge about the world. This is reflected in the fact that they hardly constrain the class of a priori epistemic possibilities: they are true of (almost) all such possibilities, considered as hypotheses about the actual world. (Two-dimensionally, these beliefs have a primary intension that is [almost] conceptually necessary.) A direct phenomenal belief, by contrast, is cognitively significant: it heavily constrains the class of a priori epistemic possibilities and is false in most of them (considered as actual). For example, Mary's direct phenomenal belief, on leaving her room, is false of all worlds (considered as actual) in which the subject is not experiencing phenomenal redness. (Two-dimensionally: the primary intension of a direct phenomenal belief is conceptually contingent.) So direct phenomenal beliefs, unlike the beliefs in the previous paragraph, are entirely nontrivial.

So the infallibility thesis articulated here has a number of limitations, but it nevertheless applies to a significant class of nontrivial phenomenal beliefs.[2]

2. Acquaintance and Justification

At this point is natural to ask: if we can form this special class of infallible, distinctively constituted beliefs where phenomenal states and properties are concerned, why can we not do so where other states and properties are concerned? Why can we not form direct height concepts, for example, whose epistemic content is directly constituted by our height properties and which can be deployed in infallible direct height beliefs? Or similarly for direct chemical beliefs, direct age beliefs, direct color beliefs, and so on?

At one level, the answer is that we simply cannot. If one tries to form a direct height concept—one whose content depends constitutively on an instantiation of a height property—the best one can do is form a relational height concept (*my height, the height of my house*) or a demonstrative height concept. But these are not pure height concepts at all. They are analogous only to red_C or $this_E$ in that their subjunctive content may depend on the property in question, but their epistemic content does not.

It is arguable whether pure height concepts exist at all: that is, whether there is any concept whose epistemic content picks out a certain height (say, two meters) in every epistemically possible scenario. But even if there are pure height concepts, they are not direct height concepts. Perhaps one can independently form a pure height concept of a given height (two meters),

---

2. *One might worry that direct phenomenal beliefs cannot constitute knowledge, for reasons articulated by Williamson (2000) in arguing against the "luminosity" of phenomenal and other beliefs. The worry is that a direct phenomenal belief in p (e.g., that one has R) is not safe because it could easily have been false: for any such belief, there are nearby possible worlds in which one has a slightly different experience R', so that p is false in those worlds. But as Weatherson (2004) has observed, it is far from clear why this sort of safety should be required for knowledge. If safety is relevant to knowledge in these cases, the relevant sort of safety plausibly concerns not whether p is true in nearby worlds but whether what one believes in those nearby worlds is true there. According to the current framework, in worlds where one experiences a slightly different quality R', one will believe a slightly different proposition p' (that one has R') and one's belief will be true. So direct phenomenal beliefs will be safe in the relevant sense. Correspondingly, while I have not argued that propositions about phenomenal qualities are "luminous" (that when one experiences a given quality, one is in a position to know that one does), Williamson's argument does not provide a strong reason to reject that claim.

which might coincide with an instantiated height, but it will not depend constitutively on that. The best one can do is attend to an object, have an experience or judgment concerning its height, and use this experience or judgment as the epistemic content of a "pure" height concept. Here the instantiation of a height property is not constitutively relevant to the concept's content, but only causally relevant: it is the height experience or judgment that is constitutively relevant, and the experience or judgment is only causally dependent on the instantiation of the height. In no case does the epistemic content of a height concept depend constitutively on an instance of a demonstrated height property or of any height property at all.

Proponents of certain direct realist views may hold that it is possible to form a direct concept of a height property (or other perceivable external properties) by demonstrating it and taking it up into a concept in a manner analogous to the manner suggested for phenomenal properties. I think that this is implausible. In a case where an object is two meters tall but appears to be one meter tall, any "pure" height concept formed as a result will be a concept of one meter, not of two meters. There may be a demonstrative concept of two meters, but that is not enough. More generally, considering a range of cases in which height and experience are varied independently, we can see that any contribution of the height to a pure concept is "screened off" by the contribution of the experience. This suggests that if anything is playing a constitutive role in the concept's content, it is the experience and not the external property.[3]

The same goes for chemical concepts, age concepts, and external color concepts. Although we can form many such concepts, in no case is it possible to form a direct concept: that is, a concept whose epistemic content depends constitutively on a demonstrated property instance. It seems that only phenomenal properties can support direct concepts.

---

3. There may be further moves available to the direct realist. For example, a direct realist might hold that the constitutive role of external properties is restricted to cases of veridical perception and that nonveridical perception must be treated differently. This sort of restriction threatens to trivialize the constitution thesis, as any causal connection might be seen as a "constitutive" connection by a relevantly similar restriction. (If A causes B, which necessitates C, then A is usually contingently connected to C, but if we restrict our attention to cases where A causes B, then A necessitates C relative to this restriction.) And the case remains formally disanalogous to the case of direct phenomenal concepts, in which there is no factor distinct from the quality that even looks like it screens off the contribution of the quality to the concept. But there is undoubtedly more to say here. In what follows I will assume that the direct realist view is incorrect, but direct realists are free to hold that what I say about phenomenal properties applies equally to the relevant external properties.

Addendum*: I think the direct realist is correct in some possible worlds, although not in our world. In particular, the direct realist is correct in Eden (chapter 12), where subjects can form direct color concepts, direct spatial concepts, and so on.

This conclusion is apparently revealed by an examination of cases, but it would be preferable not to leave it as a brute conclusion. In particular, it is natural to suggest that the conclusion holds because we bear a special relation to the phenomenal properties instantiated in our experience: a relation that we do not bear to the other instantiated properties in question and a relation that is required in order to form a direct concept of a property in the manner described. This relation would seem to be a peculiarly intimate one that is made possible by the fact that experiences lie at the heart of the mind rather than standing at a distance from it, and it seems to be a relation that carries the potential for conceptual and epistemic consequences. We might call this relation *acquaintance.*

As things stand, acquaintance has been characterized only as that relation between subjects and properties that makes possible the formation of direct phenomenal concepts, so it is not yet doing much explanatory work. Still, having inferred the relation of acquaintance, we can put it to work. As characterized, acquaintance is a relation that makes possible the formation of pure phenomenal concepts, and we have seen that pure phenomenal concepts embody a certain sort of lucid understanding of phenomenal properties. So acquaintance is a relation that makes this sort of lucid understanding possible. As such, it is natural to suppose that the relation can also do work in the epistemic domain. If so, the result will be an attractive picture in which the distinctive conceptual character and the distinctive epistemic character of the phenomenal domain have a common source.

It is independently plausible to hold that phenomenal properties and beliefs have a distinctive epistemic character. Many have held that phenomenal properties can (at least sometimes) be known with a distinctive sort of justification or even with certainty, and many have held that phenomenal beliefs have a special epistemic status. Even those who explicitly deny this often tacitly concede that there is at least a prima facie case for this status. For example, it is striking that those who construct skeptical scenarios almost always ensure that phenomenal properties are preserved. So it is arguable that simply having a phenomenal property provides the potential for a strong sort of phenomenal knowledge. Something similar is suggested by the Mary case: Mary's experience of the phenomenal property R allows her to have not just a distinctive phenomenal belief but also distinctive phenomenal knowledge. Some element of this distinctive epistemic character can be captured in the present framework.

One natural suggestion is the following: direct phenomenal beliefs are always justified. Certainly Mary's belief on leaving her room seems to be justified, and most other examples seem to fit this thesis. This thesis has to be modified slightly. There are presumably subjects who are so irrational or confused that none of their beliefs qualify as justified, so that their direct phenomenal beliefs are not justified, either. In addition, perhaps there could be subjects who are so confused about phenomenology that they accept not just direct phenomenal beliefs but their negations as well, casting doubt on whether either belief is truly justified. To meet this sort of case, we might adjust the thesis to say that all direct phenomenal beliefs have some prima facie justification, where prima facie justification is an element of justification that can sometimes be overridden by other elements, rendering a belief below the threshold for "justification" *simpliciter.* Something similar presumably applies to other features of a belief that might seem to confer justification, such as being inferred from justified beliefs by a justified rule of inference.

Still, it is one thing to make the case that direct phenomenal beliefs are (prima facie) justified and another to give an account of what this justification consists in. It may be tempting to appeal to infallibility, but infallibility alone does not entail justification (as the mathematical case shows), and while certain higher-order accessibility theses might close the gap, it is not obvious that they are satisfied for direct phenomenal beliefs.

A better idea is to appeal to the acquaintance relation, thus unifying the distinctive conceptual and epistemic character of phenomenal beliefs. In particular, one might assert the following:

> **Justification Thesis:** When a subject forms a direct phenomenal belief based on a phenomenal quality, then that belief is prima facie justified in virtue of the subject's acquaintance with that quality.

Certainly many philosophers, including especially sense-datum theorists and more recent foundationalists, have appealed to a relation of acquaintance (or "direct awareness") in supporting the special epistemic status of phenomenal beliefs. The current account offers a more constrained version of such a thesis, suggesting that it holds for a special class of phenomenal beliefs (on which the epistemic content of a predicated concept is required to mirror and be constituted by the acquainted quality, to which it is applied) and on the basis of a relation whose existence we have made an independent case for.

Some philosophers (e.g., Russell 1910; Fumerton 1995) have held that we are "acquainted with acquaintance" and have made the case of its existence that way. I think there is something to the idea that our special epistemic relation to experience is revealed in our experience, but I note that the proponent of acquaintance is not forced to rely on such a thesis. It is equally possible to regard acquaintance as a theoretical notion that is inferred to give a unified account of the distinctive conceptual and epistemic character that we have reason to believe is present in the phenomenal domain.

Acquaintance can be regarded as a basic sort of epistemic relation between a subject and a property. Most fundamentally, it might be seen as a relation between a subject and an *instance* of a property: I am most directly acquainted with *this instance* of phenomenal greenness. This acquaintance with an instance can then be seen to confer a derivative relation to the property itself. Or, in the experience-based framework, one might regard acquaintance as most fundamentally a relation between a subject and an experience that confers a derivative relation between the subject and the phenomenal properties of the experience. I will usually abstract away from these fine details, however. What is central is the shared feature that whenever a subject has a phenomenal property, the subject is acquainted with that phenomenal property.

Even if acquaintance is a theoretical notion, it clearly gains some pretheoretical support from the intuitive view that beliefs can be epistemically grounded in experiences, where experiences are not themselves beliefs but nevertheless have an epistemic status that can help justify a belief. One might view acquaintance as capturing that epistemic status.

In certain respects (though not in all), the justification of a direct phenomenal belief by an experience can be seen as analogous to the justification of an inferred belief by another belief. For an inferred belief to be prima facie justified, there are three central requirements: one concerning the content of the belief in relation to the justifying state, one concerning the natural connection between the belief and the justifying state, and one concerning the epistemic status of the justifying state. First, the epistemic content of the belief must be appropriately related to that of the belief that it is inferred from. Second, the belief must be appropriately caused by the justifying belief. Third, the justifying belief must itself be justified.

In the prima facie justification of a direct phenomenal belief by an experience, there are three factors of the same sort. First, content: the epistemic content of the direct phenomenal belief must mirror the quality of the experience. Second, a natural connection: the phenomenal belief must be appropriately constituted by the experience. And third, epistemic status: the subject must be acquainted with the justifying quality. The details of the requirements are different, as befits the difference between belief and experience, but the basic pattern is very similar.

It is plausible that a subject can have phenomenal properties without having corresponding concepts, corresponding beliefs, or corresponding justification.[4] If so, the same goes for acquaintance. Acquaintance is not itself a conceptual relation: rather, it makes certain sorts of concepts possible. And it is not itself a justificatory relation: rather, it makes certain sorts of justification possible. Phenomenal concepts and phenomenal knowledge require not just acquaintance but also acquaintance in the right cognitive background: a cognitive background that minimally involves a certain sort of attention to the phenomenal quality in question, a cognitive act of concept formation, the absence of certain sorts of confusion and other undermining factors (for full justification), and so on. But it is acquaintance with the quality or the experience itself that does the crucial justifying work.[5]

Some philosophers hold that only a belief can justify another belief. It is unclear why this view should be accepted. The view has no pretheoretical support. Pretheoretically, it is extremely plausible that experiences (e.g., a certain experience of phenomenal greenness) play a role in justifying beliefs (e.g., my belief that there is something green in front of me or my belief that I am having a certain sort of experience), even though experiences are not themselves beliefs. In addition, the view has no obvious theoretical support. Perhaps the central motivation for the view comes from the idea that inference is the only sort of justification that we understand and have a theoretical model for and that we have no model for any other sort of justification. But this is obviously not a strong reason, and the account I have just sketched suggests a theoretical model of how experiences can

---

4. Nothing I have said so far requires that experiences can exist without concepts; at most, it requires that experiences can exist without phenomenal concepts. So what I have said may be compatible with views on which experiences depend on other concepts in turn. Still, I think it is independently plausible that experiences do not require concepts for their existence, and I will occasionally assume this in what follows. This is not to deny that *some* experiences depend on concepts, and it is also not to deny that experiences have representational content.

In chapters 11 and 12, I develop a view on which at least for perceptual experiences (and perhaps for all experiences), experiences have representational content by virtue of their phenomenology. This yields an interesting possibility: the constitutive relation between phenomenal states and phenomenal concepts might be extended to yield a similar constitutive relation between perceptual phenomenal states and a special class of perceptual concepts by virtue of the phenomenal states' representational content. Such an account might yield some insight into the content and epistemology of perceptual belief.

5. *A common objection to acquaintance models (see e.g. Sosa's discussion in BonJour and Sosa 2003) holds that one can have acquaintance without prima facie justification. Suppose that one has phenomenology as of 48 speckles on a hen. If one is acquainted with all one's phenomenal properties, one will be acquainted with the as-of-48-speckles phenomenal property. But if one does not attend to one's phenomenology carefully, one will not be prima facie justified in believing that one has that phenomenal property. On the current model, the need for attention is explained by the observation that attention to the relevant phenomenal property is required to form a direct phenomenal belief about that property. If one wants to give attention a justificatory role and not just an enabling role, however, one can easily adjust the model so that it is acquaintance-based attention and not merely acquaintance that does the justificatory work.

justify beliefs that fits well with our pretheoretical intuitions. So it seems that the cases of justification of beliefs by other beliefs and by experiences are on a par here.

Another motivation for the view comes from the thesis that for a state to justify another state, it must itself be justified (along with the claim that only beliefs can be justified), but again, it is unclear why this thesis should be accepted. Again, it is pretheoretically reasonable to accept that beliefs are justified by experiences and that experiences are not themselves the sort of states that can be justified or unjustified. And there is no obvious theoretical reason to accept the thesis. It may be that for a state to justify, it must have *some* sort of epistemic status, but there is no clear reason why the status of acquaintance should be insufficient.

BonJour (1978) suggests that to deny that justifying states must be justified is to make an ad hoc move aimed at stopping the regress argument against foundationalism, but considerations about foundationalism and about regress arguments have played no role in my claims. The claims are independently supported by observations about the epistemic and conceptual relations between belief and experience. BonJour also claims that a justifying state must involve assertive content, but again, there is no clear pretheoretical or theoretical reason to accept this. Pretheoretically, experiences can justify beliefs without obviously involving assertive content. Theoretically, acquaintance with a property makes the property available to a subject in a manner that makes concepts and assertions involving the property possible and that enables these assertions to be justified. There is no reason why this requires acquaintance to itself involve an assertion.

A number of epistemological issues remain. One concerns the strength of the justification of phenomenal beliefs. It is often held that phenomenal beliefs are (or can be) *certain*, for example. Can the present framework deliver this? It can certainly deliver infallibility, but certainty requires something different. I think that the relevant sense of certainty involves something like *knowledge beyond skepticism*: intuitively, knowledge such that one's epistemic situation enables one to rule out all skeptical counterpossibilities. There is an intuition that phenomenal belief at least sometimes involves this sort of knowledge beyond skepticism, as the standard construction of skeptical scenarios suggests.

This epistemic status might be captured by a claim to the effect that acquaintance with a property enables one to eliminate all (a priori) epistemic possibilities in which the property is absent. If so, then in the right cognitive background (with sufficient attention, concept formation, lack of confusion, and so on), the justification of a direct phenomenal belief in p by acquaintance with a property will sometimes enable a subject not just to know that p by the usual standards of knowledge but also to eliminate all skeptical counterpossibilities in which p is false. This matter requires further exploration, but one can see at least the beginnings of a reasonable picture.[6]

A second further issue is this: can the justification thesis be extended to all pure phenomenal concepts, including standing phenomenal concepts? There is some intuitive appeal in the idea that application of a standing phenomenal concept to an instantiated quality may also carry some justification by virtue of acquaintance with the quality (perhaps under the restriction that the content of the standing concept match the quality and that there be an appropriate natural connection between the quality and the belief). If this belief were justified directly by acquaintance, however, we would need an account of justification by acquaintance that does not give a central role to constitution. Such an account is not out of the question, but it is worth noting that justification for beliefs involving standing phenomenal concepts can also be secured indirectly.

---

6. I argue in *The Conscious Mind* (1996) that something like acquaintance is required to secure certainty and that a mere causal or reliable connection cannot do the job. If the justification of a belief is based solely on a reliable or causal connection, the subject will not be in a position to rule out skeptical scenarios in which the connection is absent and the belief is false, so the belief will not be certain. In response, a number of philosophers, including Bayne (2001a), have argued that acquaintance accounts can be criticized in a similar way. Bayne notes that acquaintance alone is compatible with the absence of certainty (e.g., in conditions of inattention), so certainty requires background factors in addition to acquaintance. But we cannot be certain that these factors obtain, so we cannot rule out skeptical scenarios in which they fail to obtain, so a phenomenal belief cannot be certain.

This argument stems from a natural misreading of my argument against reliabilist accounts. The misreading is as follows: certainty requires certainty about the factors that enable certainty, and a reliabilist account cannot deliver this sort of certainty. That argument would requires a strong version of a CJ thesis, holding that certain justification requires certainty about the basis of certain justification (analogous to the KJ thesis that justification requires knowledge of justification). I think such a thesis should clearly be rejected. The intended argument is rather as follows: certainty about p requires (first-order) "knowledge beyond skepticism" or an epistemic state that enables a subject to rule out all skeptical scenarios in which p is false. Reliabilism by its nature cannot do this: there will always be skeptical scenarios in which the reliable connection fails and in which p is false.

Bayne's argument against acquaintance gives an analogue of the invalid CJ argument. At most this establishes that we cannot rule out scenarios in which the belief is uncertain. Even this is unclear, as it is not obvious that certainty about certainty requires certainty about the factors enabling certainty, But even if this point is granted, the existence of skeptical scenarios in which the belief is uncertain does not entail the existence of skeptical scenarios in which p is false. Acquaintance yields certainty about experiences, not about beliefs. It enables one to directly rule out skeptical scenarios in which p is false, whether or not it enables one to rule out skeptical scenarios in which a belief is uncertain. In cases of justification by a reliable connection, there are separate reasons to hold that skeptical scenarios in which p is false cannot be ruled out, but in the case of acquaintance, these reasons do not apply. (The published version of Bayne's article takes these points into account and offers some further considerations.)

Indirect justification for such beliefs can be secured by virtue of the plausible claim that any belief of the form $S = R$ is (prima facie) justifiable, where S and R are standing and direct phenomenal concepts with the same epistemic content. This is an instance of the more general claim that any belief of the form $A = B$ is justifiable when A and B have the same epistemic content. (This thesis may need some restriction to handle cases of deep hyperintensionality, but it is plausibly applicable in this case.) Such beliefs are plausibly justifiable a priori: experience may enter into a grasp of the concepts involved in such a belief, but it does not enter into the belief's justification. If so, then beliefs involving standing phenomenal concepts can inherit justification by a priori inference from direct phenomenal beliefs, which will be justified in virtue of the justification thesis.

Finally, a note on ontology. Talk of acquaintance often brings sense-datum theories to mind, so it may be worth noting that a commitment to phenomenal realism and to acquaintance does not entail a commitment to sense data. First, the picture is entirely compatible with an "adverbial" subject-property model and with other quality-based ontologies on which there are phenomenal properties but not phenomenal individuals. Second, the picture I have sketched is quite compatible with a model on which phenomenal properties are representational properties: here one will be acquainted with one's representing of a color property or some other appropriate property. Third, even if one accepts the existence of phenomenal individuals such as experiences, one might well reject a sense-datum model of perception, on which one perceives the world by perceiving these entities. It is also worth noting that one need not regard the acquaintance relation that a subject bears to a phenomenal property as something ontologically over and above the subject's instantiation of the property, requiring a subject-relation-quality ontology at the fundamental level. It is arguable that it is a conceptual truth that to have a phenomenal quality is to be acquainted with it (at least insofar as we have a concept of acquaintance that is not wholly theoretical). Certainly it is hard to conceive of a scenario in which a phenomenal quality is instantiated but no one is acquainted with it. If so, then the picture I have sketched is combined with a simple subject-quality ontology, combined with this conceptual truth. The ontological ground of all this might lie in the nature of phenomenal qualities rather than in some ontologically further relation.

3. Epistemological Problems for Phenomenal Realism

Phenomenal realism, especially property dualism, is often thought to face epistemological problems. In particular, it is sometimes held that these views make it hard to see how phenomenal beliefs can be justified or can qualify as knowledge since the views entail that phenomenal beliefs do not stand in the right sort of relationship to experiences. If what I have said so far is right, this cannot be correct. But it is worth looking at the arguments more closely.[7]

The most influential arguments of this sort have been put forward by Sydney Shoemaker (1975). Shoemaker's arguments are intended as arguments against a view that admits the conceptual possibility of "absent qualia": an experience-free functional duplicate of an experiencing being. The view under attack is slightly stronger than phenomenal realism (a phenomenal realist could admit inverted qualia without absent qualia), is slightly weaker than a view on which zombies (experience-free physical duplicates) are conceptually possible, and is weaker than property dualism. But for the purposes of the argument, it will not hurt to assume a property dualist version of the view, according to which zombies are metaphysically possible. This has the effect of making Shoemaker's arguments harder to answer, not easier. The answers can easily be adapted to weaker versions of phenomenal realism.

The starkest version of Shoemaker's epistemological argument runs as follows:

1. If phenomenal realism is true, experiences are causally irrelevant to phenomenal beliefs.
2. If experiences are causally irrelevant to phenomenal beliefs, phenomenal beliefs are not knowledge.

---

3. If phenomenal realism is true, phenomenal beliefs are not knowledge.

Some phenomenal realists might deny the first premise: a type-B materialist could hold that experiences have effects on beliefs by virtue of their identity with physical states, and a property dualist could hold that these effects proceed through a fundamental causal connection between the phenomenal and physical domains or through a fundamental causal

---

7. I discussed these arguments at length in chapter 5 of *The Conscious Mind*, under the label "The Paradox of Phenomenal Judgment." I now think that discussion is at best suboptimal. The final section of the chapter put forward a preliminary and sketchy version of the view of phenomenal concepts I have discussed here, but I did not give it a central epistemological role (except in a tentative suggestion on pp. 207–208). I now think that this view of phenomenal concepts is central to the epistemology. The present discussion can be viewed in part as a replacement for that discussion.

connection among nonphysical mental states. For the purposes of the argument, I will assume the version of phenomenal realism that makes answering the argument as hard as possible, so I will rule out these responses. In particular, I temporarily assume epiphenomenalism, according to which the phenomenal has no effects on the physical domain.

The view I have outlined makes it easy to see why this argument fails even against an epiphenomenalist. Whatever the status of the first premise, the second premise is false. The second premise assumes that a causal connection between experience and phenomenal belief is required for the latter to count as knowledge. If what I have said is correct, the connection between experience and phenomenal belief is tighter than any causal connection: it is constitution. If a causal connection can underwrite knowledge, a constitutive connection can certainly underwrite knowledge, too.

Even without appealing to constitution, the epiphenomenalist can respond reasonably to this argument by appealing to the notion of acquaintance and arguing that a subject's acquaintance with experience can noncausally justify a phenomenal belief. (I use this strategy in *The Conscious Mind*.) But when the role of constitution is made clear, the reply becomes even stronger. Acquaintance and constitution together enable a theoretical model of the justification of phenomenal belief (as in the previous section), a model that is compatible with epiphenomenalism. Any residual worries about the lack of an appropriate connection between the experience and the belief are removed by the presence of a constitutive connection.

This first argument is only a subsidiary argument in Shoemaker's discussion. Shoemaker's main argument specifically concerns the possibility of absent qualia. His argument involves functional duplicates and conceptual possibility, but as before I modify these details to involve physical duplicates and metaphysical possibility, thus making the argument harder to answer. The modified argument runs roughly as follows:

1. If phenomenal realism is true, then every conscious being has a possible zombie twin.
2. If zombies are possible, they have the same phenomenal beliefs as their conscious twins, formed by the same mechanism.
3. If zombies are possible, their phenomenal beliefs are false and unjustified.
4. If it is possible that there are beings with the same phenomenal beliefs as a conscious being, formed by the same mechanism, where

those phenomenal beliefs are false and unjustified, then the conscious being's phenomenal beliefs are unjustified.

---

5. If phenomenal realism is true, every conscious being's phenomenal beliefs are unjustified.

Some phenomenal realists could respond by denying premise 1 and holding that zombies are impossible. But even the conceptual possibility of functional duplicates with absent qualia is arguably enough to make an analogous argument go through if there are no other problems. Premise 3 is relatively unproblematic. Perhaps one could argue that a zombie's phenomenal beliefs have some sort of justification, but the conclusion that our phenomenal beliefs are no more justified than a zombie's would be strong enough for an opponent. Disputing premise 4 holds more promise. If one accepts an acquaintance model of justification, one might hold that the justification of a phenomenal belief does not supervene on its mechanism of formation. (I use this strategy in *The Conscious Mind*.) But given what has gone before, by far the most obvious reply is to dispute premise 2. There is no reason to accept that zombies have the same phenomenal beliefs as their conscious twins and every reason to believe that they do not.

It is by no means obvious that zombies have beliefs at all. The basis of intentionality is poorly understood, and one might plausibly hold that a capacity for consciousness is required for intentional states. Even if we allow that zombies have beliefs, however, it is clear that a zombie cannot share a conscious being's phenomenal beliefs. The content of a conscious being's direct phenomenal beliefs is partly constituted by underlying phenomenal qualities. A zombie lacks those qualities, so it cannot have a phenomenal belief with the same content.

Let us take the case of Zombie Mary, where we recombine thought experiments in the obvious way. Assuming that Zombie Mary has a belief where Mary has a direct phenomenal belief, what sort of content does it have? Mary has a belief with the content $this_E = R$, and Inverted Mary has a belief with the content $this_E = G$. Let us focus on the direct phenomenal concepts R and G and their zombie counterpart. It is obvious that Zombie Mary's concept is neither R nor G. If this concept has content at all, it has a different content entirely. I think that the most plausible view is that the zombie's concept is *empty*: it has no content. On the view I have been outlining, a phenomenal quality can be thought of as filling a slot that is left open in the content of a direct phenomenal concept and thus contributing its content. If there is no phenomenal quality to fill the slot, as in Zombie Mary's case, the concept will have no content at all.[8]

What about Zombie Mary's analogue of Mary's direct phenomenal belief $this_E = R$? It is not obvious that a zombie can possess a demonstrative phenomenal concept. For a start, a concept whose content is that of 'this experience' seems to require a concept of experience, which a zombie may lack. But even if a zombie could possess a demonstrative phenomenal concept, any such concept would fail to refer (like failed demonstratives in other domains). More importantly, the other half of the identity (the zombie's analog of R) would be empty. So Zombie Mary's belief would be entirely different from Mary's belief.

It is natural to wonder about the truth value of Zombie Mary's belief. Clearly, her belief is not true. I would say that it is either false or empty, depending on one's view about beliefs involving empty concepts. The latter view is perhaps the more plausible, since it seems that Zombie Mary's belief has no propositional content to evaluate. As for Zombie Mary's "new knowledge," it is clear that she gains no propositional knowledge (though she may think that she does). One might see her as in the position that type-A materialists (and in particular proponents of the "ability hypothesis") hold that we are in the actual world. When Zombie Mary first sees a flower, she may gain certain abilities to recognize and discriminate, although even these abilities will be severely constrained since they cannot involve experiences.

This is enough to see that the epistemological argument against phenomenal realism does not get off the ground. A zombie clearly does not have the same phenomenal beliefs as its conscious twin in general, and its corresponding beliefs are not even formed by the same mechanism, since constitution by a phenomenal quality plays a central role in forming a direct phenomenal belief. So the second premise is false, and there is no bar to the justification of direct phenomenal beliefs.[9]

8. *Correspondingly, the present proposal can be seen as disjunctivist about introspection in a manner loosely analogous to the familiar disjunctivism about perception. Acquaintance-based introspection of the sort that tends to lead to direct phenomenal beliefs and concepts is loosely analogous to veridical perception here, while its counterpart in a zombie is loosely analogous to hallucinatory cases of perception. The zombie counterpart of acquaintance-based introspection is an entirely different sort of state that leads to an entirely different sort of belief. A similar moral is suggested by the treatment of pseudodirect phenomenal beliefs in section 1 and by other cases in which a subject attempts to introspect a phenomenal property that is not present. The discussion of direct perceptual concepts in section 2 also tends toward the conclusion that disjunctivist proposals about perception are more aptly applicable to introspection. Macpherson (2010) offers a quite different disjunctivist proposal about introspection, one that allows that zombies have the same sort of phenomenal concepts as us but that denies that these concepts can be combined into genuine beliefs. I think that the considerations in this chapter and the last strongly suggest that the disjunctivism should be located at an earlier stage.

9. Conee (1985) and Francescotti (1994) also respond to Shoemaker's argument by denying the equivalent of premise 2, although for somewhat different reasons.

What about other phenomenal beliefs? We have seen that standing phenomenal concepts differ between twins and that their content is plausibly constituted either by phenomenal properties or by dispositions involving those properties. A zombie lacks all phenomenal properties, so it is plausible that its analogs of standing phenomenal concepts will be empty, too. So beliefs involving standing phenomenal concepts are also immune from this argument.

What about the standing concept of *experience* (or *qualia*, or *phenomenal consciousness*) generally? In this case there is no difference in content between conscious twins, but it remains plausible that phenomenal properties and the capacity to have them play a crucial role in constituting its content, just as they do for specific standing phenomenal concepts. And it is equally plausible that the zombie's analog of this standing concept is empty.[10] So beliefs involving the standing concept of experience (such as *I am conscious*) are equally unthreatened by this argument. The same goes for beliefs involving concepts in which the concept *experience* plays a part, such as relational phenomenal concepts and perhaps demonstrative phenomenal concepts.

How are these beliefs justified? For beliefs involving standing phenomenal concepts, such as $this_E = S$, we have seen that one reasonable model involves inference from $this_E = R$ and $R = S$. Here, the former belief is justified by acquaintance and constitution, and the second belief is justified a priori by virtue of its content. These two beliefs combine by virtue of the common element R to justify the belief $this_E = S$. (One can also hold that $this_E = S$ is justified directly by acquaintance, at the cost of losing the special contribution of constitution.) One can justify general beliefs of the form $this_E$ *is a phenomenal property* in much the same way, given that R *is a phenomenal property* is a priori.

From here, beliefs such as *I am conscious* are a short leap away. The leap is nontrivial, as there are distinctive problems about the epistemology of the self: witness Hume's skepticism about the self, and Lichtenberg's point that in the *cogito*, Descartes was entitled only to *there is thought*, not to *I*

10. This is relevant to Balog's (1999) argument against conceivability arguments for property dualism (also discussed in chapters 6 and 10). Balog's argument requires as a premise the claim that a zombie's assertion 'I am phenomenally conscious' (and the like) expresses a truth. The discussion here suggests that it is much more plausible that the assertion is false or truth-valueless.

Balog also discusses "yogis," creatures that make a form of direct reference to brain states without this being mediated by phenomenology. I think it is clear that yogis have at most a sort of demonstrative concept (roughly, "*this* inner state") and do not have the analog of pure phenomenal concepts. For these concepts, no analogous epistemic gap arises. For example, given full physical and indexical information, yogis will be in a position to know all truths involving the concepts in question. See the next chapter for more on this issue.

think. I have nothing special to say about these epistemological problems. But assuming that these problems can be solved, it is not implausible that a belief such as *if this*$_\text{E}$ *exists, I have this*$_\text{E}$ is justified (perhaps a priori). Then the whole range of first-person phenomenal beliefs lies within reach.

(If one takes direct phenomenal beliefs as truly foundational, one might even suggest that the *cogito* should have a three-stage structure: from *this*$_\text{E}$ = R (or some such), to *I have this*$_\text{E}$, to *I exist!*)

As for beliefs involving relational phenomenal concepts: presumably beliefs such as S = *red*$_1$, where S is a standing pure concept of phenomenal redness, will be justified a posteriori, perhaps by inference from the observation that the relevant paradigmatic objects typically cause one to experience instances of S. And beliefs of the form S = *red*$_\text{C}$ will be justified at least insofar as *red*$_1$ = *red*$_\text{C}$ is justified. Of course, for the first sort of belief to be justified, skeptical problems about the external world (and about the self) must be overcome, and for the second sort of belief to be justified, skeptical problems about other minds must be overcome. I have nothing special to say about these problems here. But assuming that these problems can be dealt with, then both general relational phenomenal beliefs (e.g., S = *red*$_\text{C}$) and particular relational phenomenal beliefs (e.g., *this*$_\text{E}$ = *red*$_\text{C}$) will be justified straightforwardly.

It seems, then, that a wide range of phenomenal beliefs can be justified by inference from direct phenomenal beliefs (such as *this*$_\text{E}$ = R), a priori phenomenal beliefs (such as R = S and perhaps *If this*$_\text{E}$ *exists, I have this*$_\text{E}$), and a posteriori phenomenal beliefs such as (S = *red*$_1$ and S = *red*$_\text{C}$). I have given a model for the justification of direct phenomenal beliefs. Phenomenal realism and even epiphenomenalism seem to pose no particular problem for the justification of the a priori phenomenal beliefs (or at least no distinctive problem that does not arise for a priori justification on any view). The same goes for the justification of the a posteriori phenomenal beliefs. Even if experience plays no causal role, this does not matter. Experiences have no special role in justifying the a priori beliefs, and the justification of the a posteriori beliefs can be seen as derivative on beliefs of the form *this*$_\text{E}$ = S (which are already accounted for), plus general methods of external observation and inductive inference.

So all we need to justify all of these beliefs is the justification of direct phenomenal beliefs, the justification of a priori beliefs by virtue of their content, and the justification involved in inference, observation, and induction. There are no special problems in any of these matters for the phenomenal realist. One might think that inference poses a problem for the epiphenomenalist. How do *this*$_\text{E}$ = R and R = S justify *this*$_\text{E}$ = S if the content of R is partly constituted by an epiphenomenal quality and if inference requires causation? But this is no problem: R acts as a middle term, and its content is not required to play any special causal role. We can think of the inference in question as being *this$_E$ is R, which is S, so this$_E$ is S*. Here the content of R is inessential to the validity of the inference: as long as the premises are justified, the conclusion will be justified.

Perhaps the main residual epistemological issue concerns the persistence of standing phenomenal concepts. One might worry if S is partly constituted by an element that is epiphenomenal, then even if one acquires a justified belief—say of the form *roses cause S*—at one time, it is not clear how this justification carries over to instances of a belief with that content at a later time. It is plausible that more than a match in content is required for justification: the later belief must be in some sense the "same" belief or at least a "descendant" belief involving the "same" (or "descendant") concepts. The same sort of issue arises with inference of the sort in the previous paragraph. Whether or not *this$_E$ is S* is wholly distinct from the two premises, we certainly want later beliefs of the form *that was S* to be justified and to play a role in further inferences in turn. But this arguably requires that the later concept be a "descendant" of the earlier concept in a sense that allows beliefs involving the later concept to inherit justification from beliefs involving the earlier concepts.

In response, I have no good account of what it is for one token of a concept to be a "descendant" of another in a manner that allows it to inherit justification.[11] Nor, I think, does anyone. Clearly more than sameness in content is required: if a new concept with the same content were to be formed de novo, no justification would be inherited. So some sort of natural connection between concept tokens is required. But it is plausible that this sort of connection need only require an appropriate causal connection between the physical vehicles of the concept, along with an appropriate match in content: it is not required that the elements constituting the content of the initial concept do any distinctive causal work.

To see this, consider the persistence of concepts on an externalist view, where content is constituted by external factors that may lie in the distant past. Here, the external factors that constitute the content of two tokens of the concept will clearly play no distinctive role in causally connecting the

---

11. This sort of persistence relation among tokens is central to our use of concepts and beliefs, but it has received less discussion than it might have. In effect, it introduces a "typing" of concepts and beliefs that is more fine-grained than a mere typing by content but less fine-grained than a typing by numerical identity of tokens. This sort of typing was already tacit in my earlier discussion, when I said that direct phenomenal concepts do not persist beyond the lifetime of an experience but that standing phenomenal concepts do.

tokens. The persistence will instead be supported by appropriate connections between the tokens' physical vehicles. It is plausible that both the phenomenal realist and the epiphenomenalist can say something similar: conceptual persistence is underwritten by natural connections among vehicles, perhaps along with an appropriate match in content. Of course, it would be desirable to have a full positive account of this sort of conceptual persistence, but it seems that there is no distinctive problem for the phenomenal realist here.

Further questions concern the justification of beliefs about the representational content of experiences and the role phenomenal beliefs might play in justifying beliefs about the external world. I will not say anything about these issues here, but it is plausible that these issues pose mere challenges for the phenomenal realist to answer rather than distinctive arguments against it. If what I have said so far is correct, the distinctive epistemological problems for phenomenal realism have been removed.

4. "The Myth of the Given"

A traditional view in epistemology and the philosophy of mind holds that experiences have a special epistemic status that renders them "given" to a subject. This epistemic status is traditionally held to give phenomenal beliefs a special status and sometimes to allow experiences to act as a foundation for all empirical knowledge. In recent years, this sort of view has often been rejected. The *locus classicus* for this rejection is Wilfrid Sellars's "Empiricism and the Philosophy of Mind" (1956), which criticized such views as involving "the myth of the given." Sellars's (deliberately abusive) term for the view has caught on, and today it is not uncommon for this label to be used in criticizing such views as if no further argument is necessary.

I do not know whether my view is one on which experiences are "given." It does not fit Sellars's official characterization of the given (as we will see), and there are other characterizations that it also does not fit. But the term "given" (along with "myth of the given") often shifts to encompass many different views, and it may well be that my view shares something of the spirit of the views that were originally criticized under this label. So rather than trying to adjudicate the terminological issue, we can simply ask: are any of the arguments that have been put forward against the "given" good arguments against the view I have put forward here?

Here one runs up against the problem that clear arguments against the "given" are surprisingly hard to find. There are many suggestive ideas in

Sellars's article but few explicit arguments. When arguments appear, they
often take the form of suggesting alternative views rather than directly
criticizing an existing view. But there is at least one clear argument against
the "given" in Sellars's article. This is his famous "inconsistent triad." This
was intended as an argument against sense-datum theories, but it clearly
applies to a wider class of views:

> It is clear from the above analysis, therefore, that classical sense-datum
> theories . . . are confronted by an inconsistent triad made up of the
> following three propositions:
>> A. *x senses red sense content s* entails *x non-inferentially knows that s
>> is red.*
>> B. The ability to sense sense contents is unacquired.
>> C. The ability to know facts of the form *x is phi* is acquired.
> A and B together entail not-C; B and C entail not-A; A and C entail
> not-B. (Sellars 1956, section 6)

It is clear how the view I have put forward should deal with this inconsistent triad: by denying A. I have said nothing about just which mental
capacities are acquired or unacquired, but on the view I have proposed, it
is clearly possible to have experiences without having phenomenal beliefs
and therefore without having knowledge of phenomenal facts. On my
view, phenomenal beliefs are formed only rarely, when subjects attend to
their experiences and make judgments about them. The rest of the time,
the experiences pass unaccompanied by any phenomenal beliefs or phenomenal knowledge.

Underlying Sellars's critique is the idea that knowledge requires concepts and that experiences do not require concepts, so that having
experiences cannot entail having knowledge. The view I have put forward is compatible with all of this. On my view, experiences require
little cognitive sophistication and in particular do not require the possession of concepts. There may be some experiences that require concepts (for example, the experience of a spoon as a spoon), but not all
experiences do. No concepts are required to experience phenomenal
redness, for example. Knowledge of facts requires belief, however, and
belief requires the possession of concepts. So experience does not entail
knowledge.

Sellars associated the "given" most strongly with the acceptance of
A, and the denial of A is what he argues for himself. In discussing the
possibility that a sense-datum theorist might deny A, all he says is the
following:

He can abandon A, in which case the sensing of sense contents becomes a non-cognitive fact—a non-cognitive fact, to be sure, which may be a necessary condition, even a logically necessary condition, of non-inferential knowledge, but a fact, nevertheless, which cannot constitute this knowledge.

On my view, all of this is correct. Experiences do not, on their own, constitute knowledge. They play a role in *justifying* knowledge, and they play a role in *partly* constituting the beliefs that qualify as knowledge, in combination with other cognitive elements. But experiences themselves are to be sharply separated from beliefs and items of knowledge. So none of this provides any argument against my view.

(On my reading, a number of the sense-datum theorists also deny A, making clear distinctions between the sort of nonconceptual epistemic relation that one stands in by virtue of having an experience and the sort of conceptual epistemic relation that one has when one knows facts. Such theorists clearly avoid the conflation between experience and knowledge that Sellars accuses sense-datum theorists of making.)

Curiously, Sellars does not discuss the possibility that experiences could justify knowledge without entailing knowledge. It seems clear that he would reject such a view, perhaps because he holds that only conceptual states can enter into justification, but this is never made explicit in his article.[12]

Although Sellars does not argue explicitly against this sort of view, such arguments have been given by a number of later philosophers writing in the same tradition. In particular, there is a popular argument against any view on which experiences are nonconceptual states that play a role in justifying beliefs. This argument, which we might call the *justification dilemma*, has been proposed by BonJour (1969), Davidson (1986), and McDowell (1994), among others. We can represent it as follows:

---

12. The one further part of Sellars's article that may be relevant to the view I have proposed is part VI (sections 26–29), where he addresses the traditional empiricist idea that experience involves awareness of determinate repeatables. This is closely related to my claim that experience involves acquaintance with properties. Sellars does not provide any direct argument against this view, however. He simply notes (sections 26–28) that Locke, Berkeley, and Hume take this thesis as a presupposition rather than a conclusion (they use it to give an account of how we can be aware of determinable repeatables). Then he asserts (section 29) that this awareness must either be mediated by concepts (e.g., through the belief that certain experiences resemble each other or that they are red) or be a purely linguistic matter. He gives no argument for this claim, which I think should be rejected. On my view, our acquaintance with qualities requires neither concepts nor language.

1. There can be no inferential relation between a nonconceptual experience and a belief since inference requires connections within the conceptual domain.
2. But a mere causal relation between experience and belief cannot justify the belief.

_____

3. Nonconceptual experiences cannot justify beliefs.

The first premise is plausible since it is plausible that inference is mediated by concepts. The status of the second premise is much less clear. While it is plausible that the mere existence of a causal connection does not suffice to justify a belief, it is far from clear that the right *sort* of causal connection could not serve to justify a belief. McDowell (1994) says that a causal connection "offers exculpation where we wanted justification." But clearly causal connections do not involve mere exculpation simply by virtue of being causal connections. The case of inference shows that a causal connection of the right kind between states can be seen to justify. So further argument is required to show that no other sort of causal connection (perhaps with subtle constraints on the content of a belief and on the relationship between belief and experience) can provide justification.

In any case, even if the two premises are accepted, the conclusion does not follow. An option has been missed: inference and causation do not exhaust the possible justifying relations between nonconceptual experiences and beliefs. On my view, the relation in question is not inference or causation, nor is it identity or entailment, as on the views that Sellars criticized. Rather, the relation is partial constitution.

I have already given a model of how the justification of a direct phenomenal belief by an experience works, involving three central elements that parallel the three central elements in the case of inference. The analog of the causal element is the constitutive connection between experience and belief; the analog of the content element is the match between epistemic content of belief and quality of experience; and the analog of the epistemic element is the subject's acquaintance with the phenomenal quality. If the model of justification by inference is accepted, there is no clear reason why this model should be rejected.

Some philosophers hold that only a conceptual state can justify another conceptual state. But as with the thesis that only a belief can justify another belief, it is not clear why this thesis should be accepted. It is not supported pretheoretically. Pretheoretically, there is every reason to hold that experiences are nonconceptual and can justify beliefs. There is no clear theoretical support for this claim, either. Proponents sometimes talk of "the space of reasons" in this context, but the slogan alone does not convert easily into an argument. McDowell suggests that justifications for our beliefs should be *articulable*, which requires concepts. But as Peacocke (2001) points out, we can articulate a justification by referring to a justifying experience under a concept whether or not the experience itself involves concepts. Perhaps the central motivation for the thesis lies in the fact that we have a clear theoretical model for conceptual justification but not for other sorts of justification. Again, however, this is a weak argument, and again, the exhibition of a theoretical model (such as the model given earlier in this chapter) ought to remove this sort of worry.

In any case, the view I have proposed avoids Sellars's central version of the given (an entailment from experience to knowledge) and BonJour's, Davidson's, and McDowell's central versions of the given (a mere causal connection), along with the arguments against those views. It may be that the view I have suggested accepts a "given" in some expanded sense. But the substantive question remains: are there good arguments against the given that are good arguments against this view? I have not been able to find such arguments, but I would welcome candidates.

5. Further Questions

I have in effect argued for a sort of limited foundationalism within the phenomenal domain. Direct phenomenal beliefs are in a certain sense foundational: they receive justification directly from experience, and their prima facie justification does not rely on other beliefs. I have also argued that direct phenomenal beliefs can justify at least some other phenomenal beliefs in turn, when aided by various sorts of a priori reasoning. Does this give any support to foundationalism about a broader class of empirical beliefs or about empirical knowledge in general?

Nothing I have said implies this sort of foundationalism. The gap between phenomenal knowledge and knowledge of the external world remains as wide as ever, and I have done nothing to close it. The framework here is compatible with various standard suggestions: that phenomenology might justify external beliefs through inference to the best explanation or through a principle that gives prima facie justification to a belief that endorses an experience's representational content. But so far, the framework outlined here does nothing special to support these suggestions or to answer skeptical objections. Furthermore, the framework is equally compatible with many alternative nonfoundationalist accounts of our knowledge of the external world.[13]

Still, this framework may help to overcome what is sometimes taken to be the largest problem for foundationalism: bridging the gap between experience and belief. I have argued that an independently motivated account of the role of experience in phenomenal belief and of a subject's epistemic relation to phenomenal properties has the resources to solve this problem, by exploiting the paired notions of constitution and acquaintance.

Any plausible epistemological view must find a central role for experience in the justification of both beliefs about experience and beliefs about the world. If what I have said here is correct, then we can at least see how experience gains a foothold in this epistemic network. Many other problems remain, especially regarding the relationship between experience and beliefs about the external world. But here, as in the case of phenomenal belief, a better understanding of the relationship between experience and belief may take us a long way.

13. A particular problem in extending this account to a general foundationalism is that we do not usually form direct phenomenal beliefs associated with a given experience, so such beliefs are not available to help in justifying perceptual beliefs. (Thanks to Alvin Goldman for discussion on this point.) Here there are a few alternatives: (1) deny that perceptual beliefs are usually justified in the strongest sense, but hold that such justification is available; (2) hold that the mere availability of justifying direct phenomenal beliefs confers a sort of justification on perceptual beliefs; or (3) extend the account so that perceptual experiences can justify perceptual beliefs directly through a constitutive connection to perceptual concepts analogous to the connection to phenomenal concepts.

10

PHENOMENAL CONCEPTS AND THE EXPLANATORY GAP

Confronted with the apparent explanatory gap between physical processes and consciousness, philosophers have reacted in many different ways. Some deny that any explanatory gap exists at all. Some hold that there is an explanatory gap for now but that it will eventually be closed. Some hold that the explanatory gap corresponds to an ontological gap in nature.

In this chapter, I explore another reaction to the explanatory gap. Those who react in this way agree that there is an explanatory gap, but they hold that it stems from the way we *think* about consciousness. In particular, this view locates the gap in the relationship between our concepts of physical processes and our concepts of consciousness, rather than in the relationship between physical processes and consciousness themselves.

Following Stoljar (2005), we can call this the *phenomenal concept strategy*. Proponents of this strategy argue that phenomenal concepts—our concepts of conscious states—have a certain special nature. Proponents suggest that given this special nature, it is predictable that we will find an explanatory gap between physical processes conceived under physical concepts and conscious states conceived under phenomenal concepts. At the same time, they argue that our possession of concepts with this special nature can itself be explained in physical terms.

If this is right, then we may not have a straightforward physical explanation of consciousness, but we have the next best thing: a physical explanation of why we find an explanatory gap. From here, proponents infer that the existence of the explanatory gap is entirely compatible with the truth of physicalism. From there, they infer that there can be no sound argument from the existence of the explanatory gap to the falsity of physicalism.

In addition, proponents often use this strategy to deflate other intuitions that lead some to reject physicalism about consciousness: intuitions about conceivability and about knowledge, for example. They suggest that these intuitions are consequences of the special nature of phenomenal concepts (which, again, can itself be explained in physical terms). They conclude that these intuitions cannot give us conclusive reason to reject physicalism.

This extremely interesting strategy is perhaps the most attractive option for a physicalist to take in responding to the problem of consciousness. If it succeeded, the strategy would respect both the reality of consciousness and the epistemic intuitions that generate the puzzle of consciousness while explaining why these phenomena are entirely compatible with physicalism.

I think that the strategy cannot succeed. On close examination, we can see that no account of phenomenal concepts is both powerful enough to explain our epistemic situation with regard to consciousness and tame enough to be explained in physical terms. That is, if the relevant features of phenomenal concepts can be explained in physical terms, the features cannot explain the explanatory gap. And if the features can explain the explanatory gap, they cannot themselves be explained in physical terms. In what follows I explain why.

1. Epistemic Gaps and Ontological Gaps

As in chapter 6, let P be the complete microphysical truth about the universe: a long conjunctive sentence detailing the fundamental microphysical properties of every fundamental microphysical entity across space and time. Let Q be an arbitrary truth about phenomenal consciousness: for example, the truth that somebody is phenomenally conscious (that is, that there is something it is like to be that person) or that I am experiencing a certain shade of phenomenal blueness.

We noted earlier that many puzzles of consciousness start from the observation that there is an apparent *epistemic gap* between P and Q: a gap between knowledge of P and knowledge of Q or between our conception of P and our conception of Q. Frank Jackson's case of Mary in the black-and-white room suggests that the truth of Q is not deducible by a priori reasoning from the truth of P, where Q is a truth about the phenomenal character of seeing red. The zombie scenario suggests that

$P\&\sim Q$ is conceivable, where Q is a truth such as 'Someone is phenomenally conscious.'

Many hold further that these epistemic gaps go along with an explanatory gap between P and Q. The explanatory gap comes from considering the question: why, given that P is the case, is Q the case? (Why, given that P is the case, is there phenomenal consciousness? And why are there the specific conscious states that there are?) The gap is grounded in part in the apparent inability to deduce Q from P: If one cannot deduce that Q is the case from the information that P is the case, then it is hard to see how one could explain the truth of Q *wholly* in terms of the truth of P. It is grounded even more strongly in the conceivability of P without Q. If one can conceive of a world that is physically just like this one but without consciousness, then it seems that one has to add something more to P to explain why there is consciousness in our world. And if one can conceive of a world that is physically just like this one but with different states of consciousness, then it seems that one has to add something more to P to explain why conscious states are the way they are in our world.

From these epistemic gaps, some infer an ontological gap. One may infer this ontological gap directly from the explanatory gap: if we cannot explain consciousness in terms of physical processes, then consciousness cannot be a physical process. Or one may infer it from one of the other epistemic gaps. For example, one may infer from the claim that $P\&\sim Q$ is conceivable that $P\&\sim Q$ is metaphysically possible and conclude that physicalism is false. If there is a possible world physically just like this one but without consciousness, then the existence of consciousness is an ontologically further fact about our world.

At this point, materialists typically respond in one of two ways. Type-A materialists deny the epistemic gap. This is an important view, but proponents of the phenomenal concept strategy reject type-A materialism, so I do not discuss it further here. Type-B materialists accept that there is an epistemic gap but deny the inference to an ontological gap. Paradigmatic type-B materialists hold that Mary lacks knowledge but not of ontologically distinct facts about the world. They hold both that zombies are conceivable but not metaphysically possible and that although there may be no satisfying explanation of consciousness in physical terms, consciousness is a physical process all the same.

Type-B materialists typically embrace *conceptual dualism* combined with *ontological monism*. They hold that phenomenal *concepts* are distinct from any physical or functional concepts. But they hold that phenomenal *properties* are identical to certain physical or functional properties or at least that they are constituted by these properties in such a way that they supervene on them with metaphysical necessity. On this view, conceptual dualism gives rise to the explanatory gap, whereas ontological monism avoids any ontological gap.

Here type-B materialists often appeal to analogies with other cases in which distinct concepts refer to the same property. 'Heat' and 'molecular motion' express distinct concepts, for example, but many hold that they refer to the same property. By analogy, some type-B materialists suggest that a phenomenal term (e.g., 'pain') and a physical term (e.g., 'C-fiber firing') may express distinct concepts but pick out the same property.

However, as we saw in chapter 6, the success of these analogies is widely disputed. Kripke argued that the relation between mental and physical expressions is different in kind from the relation between 'heat' and 'the motion of molecules' or that between 'water' and 'H_2O,' so that the grounds for a posteriori identities or necessities in these standard cases are not present in the mental-physical case. Since then, many opponents and even proponents of type-B materialism have argued that mental and physical properties are not analogous. Some (e.g., White 1986, Loar 1990/1997) argue that in the standard cases, the distinct concepts (e.g., 'heat' and 'the motion of molecules') are associated with distinct properties at least as modes of presentation of their referent, if not as their actual referent. Some argue (as I do in *The Conscious Mind* and chapter 6 of this book) that the standard cases are all compatible with an attenuated link between conceivability and possibility, which is expressible using two-dimensional semantics. Some (e.g., Jackson 1998) argue that the standard cases are all compatible with the thesis that physicalism requires a priori entailment of all truths by physical truths. Some (e.g., Levine 2001) argue that the physical-phenomenal case involves a "thick" explanatory gap that is unlike those present in the standard cases.

These differences strongly suggest that the standard way of reconciling conceptual dualism with ontological monism does not apply to the conceptual dualism between the physical and the phenomenal. If the principles that hold in the standard cases applied here, then the conceptual dualism would lead to an ontological dualism. For example, we would expect distinct properties to serve as modes of presentation for physical and phenomenal concepts, and from here one can reason to an underlying ontological dualism at the level of these properties. Likewise, we would expect there to be some metaphysically possible world in the vicinity of what we conceive when we conceive of zombies and inverts, and from here one can reason to a failure of metaphysical supervenience of everything on the physical. If so, then the epistemic gap will once again lead to an ontological gap.

2. The Phenomenal Concept Strategy

Partly to avoid these problems, many type-B materialists have turned to a different strategy for reconciling conceptual dualism and ontological monism. Instead of focusing on quite general features of a posteriori identities and necessities, this strategy focuses on features that are specific to phenomenal concepts. Proponents of the phenomenal concept strategy typically allow that we are faced with a distinctive epistemic gap in the physical-phenomenal case, one that is in certain respects unlike the epistemic gaps that one finds in the standard cases, but they hold that this distinctive epistemic gap can be explained in term of certain distinctive features of phenomenal concepts. They also hold that these distinctive features are themselves compatible with an underlying ontological monism. There are at least four common versions of this strategy.

Recognitional concepts: The *locus classicus* for the phenomenal concept strategy is Brian Loar's article "Phenomenal States" (1990/1997), in which he suggests that phenomenal concepts are recognitional concepts that pick out their objects via noncontingent modes of presentation. (Related proposals involving recognitional concepts are made by Carruthers 2004, Tye 2003c, and Levin 2007.) Recognitional concepts are concepts deployed when we recognize an object as being one of *those*, without relying on theoretical knowledge or other background knowledge. For example, we may have a recognitional concept of a certain sort of cactus. One may also have a theoretical concept of that sort of cactus, so that there are two concepts referring to the same sort of entity. In standard cases, these two concepts will be associated with distinct properties as modes of presentation (for example, one's recognitional concept of a cactus may be associated with the property *typically causes such-and-such an experience*), so this will not ground a full-scale ontological monism. But Loar suggests that phenomenal concepts are nonstandard recognitional concepts because the property that is the referent also serves as a mode of presentation. He argues that this special character of phenomenal concepts explains the distinctive epistemic gap in a manner that is compatible with ontological monism.

Distinct conceptual roles: Developing a suggestion by Nagel (1974), Hill (1997; see also Hill and McLaughlin 1999) suggests that phenomenal concepts and physical concepts are associated with distinct faculties and modes of reasoning and that they play very different conceptual roles. Hill argues that the distinctive epistemic gaps between the physical and phenomenal are explained by this distinctness in conceptual roles, and he suggests that we should expect the epistemic gaps to be present even if the distinct concepts refer to the same property.

Indexical concepts: A number of philosophers (including Ismael 1999, O'Dea 2002, and Perry 2001) have suggested that phenomenal concepts are a sort of indexical concept analogous to *I* and *now*. There are familiar epistemic gaps between objective and indexical concepts, noted by Perry (1979) and many others. For example, even given complete objective knowledge of the world, one might not be able to know what time it is now or where one is located. Proponents of the indexical concept strategy suggest that the epistemic gap between the physical and the phenomenal has a similar character. On this view, just as 'now' picks out a certain objective time under an indexical mode of presentation, phenomenal concepts pick out states of the brain under an indexical mode of presentation.

Quotational concepts: Finally, some philosophers have suggested that phenomenal concepts are special because their referents—phenomenal states—serve as constituents of the concepts themselves (or as constituents of the corresponding mental representations). Sometimes this view of phenomenal concepts is proposed without any associated ambition to support type-B materialism, as I did in chapter 8. But some, such as Papineau (2002, 2007) and Block (2007), suggest that this view of phenomenal concepts can explain the epistemic gap in terms acceptable to a materialist. For example, Papineau sees phenomenal concepts as *quotational concepts*, which represent their referent as *that state:—*, where the blank space is filled by an embedded phenomenal state in a way loosely analogous to the way that a word might be embedded between quotation marks. Papineau suggests that even if the embedded state is a neural state, this quotational structure will still give rise to the familiar epistemic gaps.

Other proponents of the phenomenal concept strategy include Sturgeon (1994), who proposes that the explanatory gap is grounded in the fact that phenomenal states serve as their own canonical evidence; Levine (2001), who suggests that phenomenal concepts may crucially involve a nonascriptive mode of presentation of their referent; and Aydede and Güzeldere (2005), who give an information-theoretic analysis of the special relation between phenomenal concepts and perceptual concepts.

I have discussed many of these specific views earlier in this book (see chapter 6 for the first two views and chapter 8 for the third and fourth). Here I focus instead on what is common to all of the views, arguing on quite general grounds that no instance of the phenomenal concept strategy can succeed in grounding a type-B materialist view of the phenomenal. Later I apply this general argument to some specific views.

The general structure of the phenomenal concept strategy can be represented as follows. Proponents put forward a thesis *C* attributing certain psychological features—call these the key features—to human beings.

They argue (1) that C is true (humans actually have the key features); (2) that C explains our epistemic situation with regard to consciousness (C explains why we are confronted with the relevant distinctive epistemic gaps); and (3) that C itself can be explained in physical terms (one can at least in principle give a materialistically acceptable explanation of how it is that humans have the key features).

This is a powerful strategy. If it is successful, we may not have a direct physical explanation of consciousness, but we will have the next best thing: a physical explanation of the explanatory gap. One might plausibly hold that if we have a physical explanation of all the epistemic data that generate arguments for dualism, then the force of these arguments will be undercut. This matter is not completely obvious—one might hold that the residual first-order explanatory gap still poses a problem for physicalism—but I concede the point for the purposes of this chapter. There is no question that a physical explanation of the relevant epistemic gaps would at least carry considerable force in favor of physicalism.

For the strategy to work, all three components are essential. If (1) or (2) fails, then the presence of the relevant epistemic gaps in us will not be explained. If (3) fails, on the other hand, then although thesis C may help us understand the conceptual structure of the epistemic gap, it will carry no weight in deflating the gap. If the epistemic gap is grounded in special features of phenomenal concepts that are not physically explainable, then these features will generate a gap of their own. Opponents of the strategy will then argue that the special features themselves require nonphysical explanation and may plausibly suggest that the special features themselves reflect the presence of irreducible phenomenal experience. If so, the phenomenal concept strategy will do little to support physicalism.

Not all proponents of the phenomenal concept strategy are explicitly committed to (3), the thesis that the relevant features of phenomenal concepts must be physically explicable. Some proponents, such as Loar and Sturgeon, are silent on the matter. Almost all of them, however, use the phenomenal concept strategy to resist the inference from the epistemic gap to an ontological gap. I argue later that without (3), the phenomenal concept strategy has no force in resisting this inference.

There is a related strategy that I will not discuss here. This is the type-A materialist strategy of appealing to psychological features to explain why we have false beliefs or mistaken epistemic intuitions about consciousness (see, for example, Dennett 1979; and Jackson 2003). In its most extreme form, this strategy may involve an attempted psychological explanation of why we think we are conscious when in fact we are not. In a less extreme form, the strategy may involve an attempted psychological explanation of why we think there is an epistemic gap between physical and phenomenal truths when in fact there is not. For example, it may attempt to explain why we think Mary gains new knowledge when in fact she does not, or why we think zombies are conceivable when in fact they are not. This is an important and interesting strategy, but it is not my target here. My target is, rather, a type-B materialist who accepts that we are phenomenally conscious and that there is an epistemic gap between physical and phenomenal truths and who aims to give a psychological explanation of the existence of this epistemic gap.

3. A Master Argument

I will argue that no account can simultaneously satisfy (2) and (3). For any candidate thesis C about psychological features of human beings, then either:

1. C is not physically explicable

or

2. C does not explain our epistemic situation with regard to consciousness.

To choose between these two options, the key diagnostic question is this: is $P\&\sim C$ conceivable? That is, can we conceive of beings physically identical to us (in physically identical environments, if necessary) that do not have the psychological features attributed by thesis C?

One might approach this question by asking: would zombies have the key features attributed by thesis C? Or at least by asking: is it conceivable that zombies lack the key features? Note that neither question assumes that zombies are metaphysically possible. We simply need the assumption that zombies are conceivable, an assumption that type-B materialists typically grant.

One can also approach the question by considering a scenario closer to home. Instead of considering physically identical zombies, we can consider functionally identical zombies: say, functionally identical creatures that have silicon chips where we have neurons and that lack consciousness. Most type-B materialists allow that it is at least an open epistemic possibility that silicon functional isomorphs in the actual world would lack consciousness. We can then ask: assuming that these functional isomorphs lack consciousness, do they also lack the key features attributed by thesis C? If it is conceivable that a functional isomorph lacks these features, then it will almost certainly be conceivable that a physical isomorph lacks these features.

In any case, either physical duplicates that lack the key features are conceivable or they are not. This allows us to set up a master argument against the phenomenal concept strategy in the form of a dilemma:

1. If $P\&\sim C$ is conceivable, then C is not physically explicable.
2. If $P\&\sim C$ is not conceivable, then C cannot explain our epistemic situation.

_____

3. Either C is not physically explicable, or C cannot explain our epistemic situation.

The argument is valid. It has the form of a dilemma, with each premise representing one of the horns. In what follows I discuss each horn in turn, arguing for the corresponding premise.

(i) First Horn: $P\&\sim C$ Is Conceivable

Premise 1 says that if $P\&\sim C$ is conceivable, then C is not physically explicable. The argument for this premise is straightforward. It parallels the original reasoning from the claim that $P\&\sim Q$ is conceivable to the claim that Q is not physically explicable. If one can conceive of physical duplicates that lack the key features attributed by thesis C, then there will be an explanatory gap between P and C. That is, there will be no wholly physical explanation that makes transparent why thesis C is true. To explain why, in the actual world, creatures with the relevant physical structure satisfy thesis C, we need additional explanatory materials, just as we need such principles to explain why actual creatures with this physical structure are conscious.

Here, again, we are assuming nothing about the relationship between conceivability and possibility. It may be that creatures satisfying $P\&\sim C$ are metaphysically impossible. We are simply assuming a connection between conceivability and explanation. More precisely, we are assuming a connection between conceivability and a certain sort of reductive explanation, the sort that is relevant here: explanation that makes transparent why some high-level truth obtains, given that certain low-level truths obtain. If it is conceivable that the low-level truths obtain without the high-level truths obtaining, then this sort of transparent explanation will fail. The original explanatory gap between consciousness and the physical turns on the absence of just this sort of transparent explanation. If it is conceivable that *P* obtains without *C* obtaining, then we will have just the same sort of explanatory gap between physical processes and the relevant features of phenomenal concepts.

Type-B materialists typically accept this connection between conceivability and transparent explanation even though they reject the connection between conceivability and possibility. So for now, I take the connection between conceivability and explanation for granted. Later I will argue that even rejecting the connection will not remove the dilemma for the type-B materialist.

One might think that a proponent of the phenomenal concept strategy *must* take this first horn of the dilemma, as thesis *C* will be a thesis about *phenomenal* concepts. If thesis *C* explicitly requires the existence of phenomenal concepts, and if phenomenal concepts require the existence of phenomenal states, then it is out of the question that zombies could have the features attributed by thesis *C*. If *C* builds in the truth of *Q*, and $P\&\sim Q$ is conceivable, then $P\&\sim C$ will automatically be conceivable. A physical explanation of the truth of thesis *C* would then be ruled out.

We can avoid this problem by stipulating that thesis *C* should be cast in *topic-neutral* terms: terms that do not explicitly attribute phenomenal states or concepts that refer to them. The restriction to topic-neutral terms allows that thesis *C* may include psychological or epistemological vocabulary, but phenomenal vocabulary is barred. For example, instead of casting thesis *C* as a thesis explicitly about phenomenal concepts, one can cast it as a thesis about *quasi-phenomenal* concepts, where these can be understood as concepts deployed in certain circumstances that are associated with certain sorts of perceptual and introspective processes and so on. Phenomenal concepts will be quasi-phenomenal concepts, but now it is not out of the question that zombies might have quasi-phenomenal concepts, too.

Formulated this way, thesis *C* will then say that quasi-phenomenal concepts have certain properties such as being recognitional concepts without contingent modes of presentation. We can likewise appeal to quasi-phenomenal concepts in characterizing our epistemic situation with regard to consciousness. This allows the possibility that even if consciousness cannot be physically explained, we might be able to physically explain the key psychological features and our epistemic situation. If we could physically explain why we are in such an epistemic situation, we would have done the crucial work in physically explaining the existence of an explanatory gap.

Henceforth, I take it for granted that thesis *C* should be cast in topic-neutral terms. The same goes for the characterization of our epistemic situation. Understood this way, it is by no means out of the question that zombies would have quasi-phenomenal concepts with the properties in question and that $P\&\sim C$ is not conceivable, leading to the second horn of the dilemma. That question is no longer prejudiced by building in theses about phenomenology. Rather, the question will turn on the character of the psychological features themselves.[1]

Of course, it remains possible that even when thesis C is understood in topic-neutral terms, the character of the psychological features involved in C is such that $P\&\sim C$ is conceivable. If so, then the first horn of the dilemma is raised as strongly as ever. On this horn, the relevant psychological features will raise just as much of an explanatory gap as consciousness itself, and an appeal to these features can do little to deflate the explanatory gap.

(ii) Second Horn: $P\&\sim C$ Is Not Conceivable

Premise 2 says that if $P\&\sim C$ is not conceivable, then C cannot explain our epistemic situation. The case for this premise is not quite as straightforward as the case for premise 1. One can put the case informally as follows:

4. If $P\&\sim C$ is not conceivable, then zombies satisfy C.
5. Zombies do not share our epistemic situation.
6. If zombies satisfy C but do not share our epistemic situation, then C cannot explain our epistemic situation.

   _____

7. If $P\&\sim C$ is not conceivable, then C cannot explain our epistemic situation.

Strictly speaking, the references to zombies should be put within the scope of a conceivability operator. One can formalize the argument in this fashion, but for now I use the informal version for ease of discussion.[2]

_____

1. This point is relevant to a response to the current argument by David Papineau (2007), who suggests that he might take both horns of the dilemma. Once one stipulates that C is cast in topic-neutral terms, it is clear that Papineau takes the second horn. Papineau is not the only commentator to have missed the importance of the crucial stipulation that C (and E) are cast in topic-neutral terms. Without this stipulation, one would end up trivially on the first horn, but not much of interest would follow.

2. A formalized version might run as follows, where c is a conceivability operator and E represents our epistemic situation: (4) If $\sim c(P\&\sim C)$ & $c(P\&\sim E)$, then $c(P\&C\&\sim E)$; (5) $c(P\&\sim E)$; (6) If $c(P\&C\&\sim E)$, then C cannot explain E; so (7) If $\sim c(P\&\sim C)$, then C cannot explain E. Premise 4 is slightly more complicated in this version than in the informal version in order to capture the crucial claim that the specific zombie relevant to premise 5 satisfies C. This formalization does not play a central role as its force can be captured by the simpler formalization of the overall argument summarized in the next section.

Here, premise 6 is simply another application of the connection between conceivability and explanation. Premise 4 might be derived from a principle of completeness about the conceivable (if R is conceivable, then for arbitrary S, either $R\&S$ is conceivable, or $R\&\sim S$ is conceivable). But in this context, one can also defend premise 4 more straightforwardly by noting that if the truth of C is transparently explained by P, as the first horn requires, then if we specify that P holds in a conceivable situation, it will follow transparently that C holds in that situation.

The real work in this argument is done by premise 5. This premise amounts to the claim that $P\&\sim E$ is conceivable, where E characterizes our epistemic situation. To clarify this premise further, one needs to clarify the notion of our epistemic situation.

I will take it that the epistemic situation of an individual includes the truth values of their beliefs and the epistemic status of their beliefs (as justified or unjustified and as cognitively significant or insignificant). As before, an epistemic situation (and a sentence E characterizing it) should be understood in topic-neutral terms, so that it does not build in claims about the presence of phenomenal states or phenomenal concepts. We can say that two individuals share their epistemic situation when they have corresponding beliefs, all of which have corresponding truth values and epistemic status.

A zombie will share the epistemic situation of a conscious being if the zombie and the conscious being have corresponding beliefs, all of which have corresponding truth values and epistemic status. Here, I assume an intuitive notion of correspondence between the beliefs of a conscious being and the beliefs (if any) of its zombie twin. For example, corresponding utterances by a conscious being and its zombie twin will express corresponding beliefs. It is important to note that this notion of correspondence does not require that corresponding beliefs have the same *content*. It is plausible that a nonconscious being such as a zombie cannot have beliefs with exactly the same content as our beliefs about consciousness. We can nevertheless talk of the zombie's *corresponding* beliefs. So the claim that a zombie and a conscious being share their epistemic situation does not require that their beliefs have the same content. This mirrors the general requirement that epistemic situations be understood in topic-neutral terms.

I assume here, at least for the sake of argument, that zombies can have beliefs (that is, that it is conceivable that zombies have beliefs). This is by no means obvious. But if zombies cannot have beliefs, then the phenomenal concept strategy cannot get off the ground. If zombies cannot have beliefs, then presumably they cannot possess concepts either, so there will be an explanatory gap between physical processes and the possession of concepts. If so, then there will be an explanatory gap between physical processes and the key features of phenomenal concepts, leading to the first horn of the dilemma. And even if zombies can have concepts with the key features, then as long as they cannot have beliefs, the key features cannot explain our epistemic situation, leading to the second horn of the dilemma. So the assumption that zombies can have beliefs should be seen as a concession to the type-B materialist for the sake of argument.

For a given conscious being with a given epistemic situation as understood here, E will be a sentence asserting the existence of a being with that epistemic situation. This sentence will be made true by that being in its original epistemic situation, and it will be made true by any being that shares this epistemic situation in the current sense. Premise 5, the claim that zombies do not share our epistemic situation, can be understood as the claim that $P\&\sim E$ is conceivable, where E characterizes the epistemic situation of an actual conscious being. That is, it is the claim that (it is conceivable that) zombies' beliefs differ in their truth value or their epistemic status from the corresponding beliefs of their actual conscious twins.

Why think that zombies do not share our epistemic situation? The first reason for this is intuitive. On the face of it, zombies have a much less accurate self-conception than conscious beings do. I believe that I am conscious, that I have states with remarkable qualitative character available to introspection, that these states resist transparent reductive explanation, and so on. My zombie twin has corresponding beliefs. It is not straightforward to determine just what content these beliefs might possess. But there is a strong intuition that these beliefs are false or at least that they are less justified than my beliefs.

One can develop this intuitive consideration by considering a zombie's utterances of sentences such as 'I am phenomenally conscious.' It is not clear exactly what a zombie asserts in asserting this sentence, but it is plausible that the zombie does not assert a truth.

Balog (1999) suggests that the zombie does assert a truth as its term 'phenomenal consciousness' will refer to a brain state. This seems to give implausible results, however. We can imagine a debate in a zombie world between a zombie eliminativist and a zombie realist:

Zombie Eliminativist: "There's no such thing as phenomenal consciousness."
Zombie Realist: "Yes, there is."

Zombie Eliminativist: "We are conscious insofar as 'consciousness' is a functional concept, but we are not conscious in any further sense."

Zombie Realist: "No, we are conscious in a sense that is not functionally analyzable."

When such a debate is held among ordinary humans in the actual world, the type-B materialist and the property dualist agree that the realist is right and the eliminativist is wrong. But it is plausible that in a zombie scenario, the zombie realist would be wrong, and the zombie eliminativist would be right. If so, then where we have true beliefs about consciousness, some corresponding beliefs of our zombie twins are false, so that zombies do not share our epistemic situation.

Still, because judgments about the truth value of a zombie's judgments are disputed, we can also appeal to a different strategy, one that focuses on the nature of our knowledge compared to a zombie's knowledge. Let us focus on the epistemic situation of Mary upon seeing red for the first time. Here, Mary gains cognitively significant knowledge of what it is like to see red, knowledge that could not be inferred from physical knowledge. What about Mary's zombie twin, Zombie Mary? What sort of knowledge does Zombie Mary gain when she emerges from the black-and-white room?

It is plausible that Zombie Mary at least gains certain abilities. For example, upon seeing a red thing, she will gain the ability to perceptually classify red things under a perceptual concept. It is also reasonable to suppose that Zombie Mary will gain certain *indexical* knowledge of the form *I am in this state now*, where *this state* functions indexically to pick out whatever state she is in. But this knowledge is analogous to trivial indexical knowledge of the form *it is this time now* and is equally cognitively insignificant. There is no reason to believe that Zombie Mary will gain cognitively significant introspective knowledge analogous to the cognitively significant knowledge that Mary gains. On the face of it, there is nothing for Zombie Mary to gain knowledge of. For Zombie Mary, all is dark inside, so even confronting her with a new sort of stimulus will not bring about new significant introspective knowledge.

If this is right, then Zombie Mary does not share Mary's epistemic situation. In addition to Mary's abilities and her indexical beliefs, she has significant knowledge of what it is like to see red, knowledge not inferable from her physical knowledge. But Zombie Mary does not have significant nonindexical knowledge that corresponds to Mary's knowledge. If so, then Zombie Mary does not share Mary's epistemic situation.

One can also bring out the contrast by considering a case somewhat closer to home. Balog (1999) appeals to hypothetical conscious humans called "yogis," who have the ability to refer directly to their brain states by deploying direct recognitional concepts of those states even when those states have no associated phenomenal quality. She suggests that zombies likewise might have direct recognitional knowledge of their brain states by deploying a recognitional concept analogous to a yogi's.

Even if yogi concepts like this are possible, however, it is clear that they are nothing like phenomenal concepts. A yogi going into a new brain state for the first time *might* sometimes acquire a new recognitional concept associated with that state. But a yogi will not acquire new, cognitively significant knowledge that is analogous to Mary's phenomenal knowledge. At best, a yogi will acquire trivial knowledge, which we might express roughly as 'that sort of brain state is that sort of brain state.' So even if Zombie Mary can have a recognitional concept like this, she will still not have an epistemic situation like Mary's. (I think a yogi's concept is probably best understood as a response-dependent concept: if the concept is *flurg*, it is a priori for the yogi that a flurg is whatever brain state normally triggers flurg judgments. Once a yogi discovers that brain state B triggers these judgments, he will know that a flurg is an instance of B, and there will be no further question about flurgs. This contrasts with a phenomenal concept: once we discover that our phenomenal redness judgments are typically triggered by brain state B, we will still regard the question of the nature of phenomenal redness as wide open. This difference between response-dependent concepts and phenomenal concepts tends to further undercut Balog's suggestion that yogis' concepts are just like phenomenal concepts.)

If the foregoing is correct, then $P\&\sim E$ is conceivable, and premise 5 is correct. When this is combined with premises 4 and 6, the conclusion follows: if $P\&\sim C$ is not conceivable, then Zombie Mary has the psychological features attributed by C, but she does not share Mary's epistemic situation. So the psychological features attributed by C cannot explain Mary's epistemic situation and, more generally, cannot explain our epistemic situation with respect to consciousness.

(iii) Summary

We can summarize these arguments more briefly as follows:

1. $P\&\sim E$ is conceivable.
2. If $P\&\sim E$ is conceivable, then $P\&\sim C$ is conceivable or $C\&\sim E$ is conceivable.

3. If $P\&\sim C$ is conceivable, P cannot explain C.
4. If $C\&\sim E$ is conceivable, C cannot explain E.

———————————

5. P cannot explain C or C cannot explain E.

Premise 1 is supported by the earlier considerations about Zombie Mary. Premise 2 is a plausible consequence of the logic of conceivability. Premises 3 and 4 are applications of the connection between conceivability and explanation. The conclusion says that C cannot satisfy the constraints laid out in the general requirements for the phenomenal concept strategy. The argument here is general, applying to any candidate for C. It follows that the phenomenal concept strategy cannot succeed. No psychological features are simultaneously physically explicable and able to explain the distinctive epistemic gaps in the phenomenal domain.

4. Reactions

Proponents of the phenomenal concept strategy may react to this argument in one of four ways. First, they may accept that P cannot explain C but hold that the phenomenal concept strategy still has force. Second, they may accept that C cannot explain E (at least as I have construed E) but hold that the phenomenal concept strategy still has force. Third, they may deny that $P\&\sim E$ is conceivable and hold that Zombie Mary shares the same epistemic situation as Mary. Fourth, they may deny the connection between conceivability and explanation. (Each of these reactions has been suggested in discussions I have had with type-B materialists, with the first and third reactions being somewhat more common than the second and fourth.) In what follows, I discuss each of the reactions in turn.

(i) Option 1: Accept That P Cannot Explain C

The first response adopts what we might call the "thick phenomenal concept" strategy. On this approach, proponents appeal to features of phenomenal concepts that are thick enough to explain our distinctive epistemic situation with respect to consciousness but are too thick to be physically explained.

An example of such an approach may be the proposal that phenomenal concepts involve a direct acquaintance with their referent of a sort that discloses an aspect of their referent's intrinsic nature. Such a proposal may well help to explain the distinctive epistemic progress that Mary makes and that Zombie Mary does not make: Mary has concepts that involve direct acquaintance with their referents, whereas Zombie Mary does not. But the very fact that Mary has such concepts and that Zombie Mary does not suggests that this feature of phenomenal concepts cannot be physically explained. The proposal requires a special psychological feature (acquaintance) whose existence one would not predict from just the physical/functional structure of the brain.

The obvious problem here is the problem mentioned before. On this account, even if there is a sort of explanation of the explanatory gap in terms of features of phenomenal concepts, the explanatory gap recurs just as strongly in the explanation of phenomenal concepts themselves. Because of this, the strategy may make some progress in *diagnosing* the explanatory gap, but it will do little to deflate it.

A proponent may suggest that just as the first-order explanatory gap can be explained in terms of second-order features of phenomenal concepts, the second-order explanatory gap concerning phenomenal concepts can be explained in terms of third-order features of our concepts of phenomenal concepts, and so on. Alternatively, an opponent may suggest that the second-order explanatory gap can be explained in terms of the same second-order features of phenomenal concepts that explain the first-order explanatory gap. The first move here obviously leads to a regress of explanation, and the second move leads to a circular explanation. Explanatory structures of this sort can be informative, but again they will do nothing to deflate the explanatory gap unless the chain of explanation is at some point grounded in physical explanation.

A proponent may also suggest that to require that the key psychological features be physically explicable is to set the bar too high. On this view, all that is needed is a psychological explanation of the epistemic gap that is *compatible* with the truth of physicalism, not one that is itself transparently explainable in physical terms. However, an opponent will now question the compatibility of the account with the truth of physicalism. Just as the original explanatory gap gave reason to think that consciousness is not wholly physical, the new explanatory gap gives reason to think that phenomenal concepts are not wholly physical.

At this point, the proponent may respond by saying that ontological physicalism is compatible with the existence of explanatory gaps. But now we are back where we started, before the phenomenal concept strategy came in. Antiphysicalists argue from an epistemic gap to an ontological gap. The phenomenal concept strategy as outlined earlier was supposed to ground the rejection of this inference by showing how such epistemic gaps can arise in a purely physical system. If successful, the strategy would help to *justify* the claim that the epistemic gap is compatible with ontological physicalism and so would lend significant support to type-B materialism. But the weaker version of the strategy outlined here can give no such support. On this version, the proponent needs *independent* grounds to reject the inference from an explanatory gap to an ontological gap. If the proponent has no such grounds, then the phenomenal concept strategy does nothing to provide them. An opponent will simply say that the explanatory gap between physical processes and phenomenal concepts provides all the more reason to reject physicalism. If the proponent already has such grounds, on the other hand, then the phenomenal concept strategy is rendered redundant. Either way, the strategy will play no role in supporting type-B materialism against the antiphysicalist.[3]

This limitation does not entail that the limited version of the phenomenal concept strategy is without interest. Even if it does not *support* a type-B materialist view, we can see this sort of account of phenomenal concepts as helping to *flesh out* a type-B materialist view by giving an account of what phenomenal concepts might be like under the assumption that type-B materialism is true. If we have independent reasons to be type-B materialists, we may then have reason to suppose that phenomenal concepts work as the account suggests. Furthermore, if we have some independent method of deflating the original explanatory gap, then presumably this method may also apply to the new explanatory gap. For example, if a type-B materialist accepts an explanatorily primitive identity between certain physical/functional properties and phenomenal properties, she may also accept an explanatorily primitive identity between certain physical/functional properties and the properties of phenomenal concepts. Still, insofar as one has reasons to reject type-B materialism, the phenomenal concept strategy will do nothing to undermine these reasons.

(Note that I am not arguing in this chapter that type-B materialism is false. I do that elsewhere—in chapters 5 and 6. Here I am simply arguing that the phenomenal concept strategy provides no support for type-B materialism and provides no grounds for rejecting arguments from the epistemic gap to an ontological gap.)

---

3. *Balog (forthcoming) takes a version of the current option, and says that what I overlook here is that the strategy "provides a conceivable physicalistic explanation of the conceptual/epistemic gaps". But the phenomenological explanation is a "physicalistic explanation" only if we assume as part of the explanation the key claim that phenomenal states are physical states. If we do, then the explanation cannot add support to the key claim. If we do not, then likewise the explanation cannot add support to the key claim.

Overall, I think that accepting an explanatory gap between physical processes and phenomenal concepts is the type-B materialist's most reasonable reaction to the current arguments. To accept such a gap does not immediately rule out the truth of type-B materialism, and the account of phenomenal concepts may help in elaborating the position. But now, the phenomenal concept strategy does nothing to *support* type-B materialism against the anti-materialist. To resist anti-materialist arguments and to deflate the significance of the explanatory gap, the type-B materialist must look elsewhere.

(ii) Option 2: Accept That *C* Does Not Explain *E* but Hold That It Explains a Reconstructed *E*

The second possible reaction for a type-B materialist is to embrace the second horn of the dilemma, accepting that the key psychological features that it appeals to do not explain our epistemic situation, at least as I have construed that epistemic situation. We might think of this as a "thin phenomenal concept" strategy. Here, the psychological features in question are tame enough to be physically explained, but they are not powerful enough to explain the full-blown epistemic gaps associated with consciousness.

The problem with this strategy is the same as the problem for the first strategy. Because it leaves a residual explanatory gap, the strategy does little to close the original explanatory gap. The issues that come up here are similar to those under the first reaction, so I will not go over them again. If anything, this reaction is less attractive than the first one because an account of phenomenal concepts that cannot explain our epistemic situation with regard to consciousness would seem to have very little to recommend it.

There is a version of this reaction that is worth considering, however. This version concedes that the key psychological features in question cannot explain our full epistemic situation *as I have defined it* but asserts that the features can explain our epistemic situation in a narrower sense that is crucial to explaining away the explanatory gap. In particular, a proponent may suggest that I raised the bar unnecessarily high by stipulating that our epistemic situation includes the *truth values* of our beliefs and by including their status as *knowledge.* It may be suggested that there is a sense in which truth value is external to our epistemic situation and that the phenomenal concept strategy needs only to explain our epistemic situation more narrowly construed.

I can think of three main versions of this strategy. A proponent may suggest: (1) that a physically explicable account of phenomenal concepts can explain the *justification* of our phenomenal beliefs; or (2) that such an account can explain the *inferential disconnection* between our physical and phenomenal beliefs, including the fact that the latter are not deducible from the former, for example (this suggestion meshes especially well with Hill's account of phenomenal concepts in terms of dual conceptual roles); or (3) that such an account can explain the *existence* of our phenomenal beliefs and of associated beliefs, such as the belief in an explanatory gap. In each of these cases, proponents may claim that corresponding features will be present in zombies, so that there is no obstacle to a physical explanation.

Each of these strategies is interesting, but each suffers from the same problem. To restrict the ambition of the phenomenal concept strategy in this way undercuts its force in supporting type-B materialism. Recall that the strategy is intended to resist the antiphysicalist's inference from an epistemic gap to an ontological gap by showing how the relevant epistemic gap may exist even if physicalism is true. In the antiphysicalist's arguments, the relevant epistemic gap (from which an ontological gap is inferred) is characterized in such a way that truth and knowledge are essential. For example, it is crucial to the knowledge argument that Mary gains new factual *knowledge* or at least new true beliefs. It is crucial to the conceivability argument that one can conceive beings that lack phenomenal states that one actually has. And it is crucial to the explanatory gap that one has cognitively significant knowledge of the states that we cannot explain. If one characterized these gaps in a way that were neutral on the truth of phenomenal beliefs, the arguments would not get off the ground. So truth value is essential to the relevant epistemic gaps. If so, then to undercut the inference from these gaps to an ontological gap, the phenomenal concept strategy needs to show how the relevant truth-involving epistemic gaps are consistent with physicalism. The earlier strategies do not do this, so they do nothing to undercut the inference from the epistemic gap to an ontological gap.

Perhaps proponents could augment their explanation of the narrow epistemic situation with an additional element that explains why the relevant beliefs are true and qualify as knowledge. For example, one might augment it with an explanation (perhaps via a causal theory of reference?) of why phenomenal beliefs refer to physical states and an explanation (perhaps via a reliabilist theory of knowledge?) of why such beliefs constitute knowledge. However, the augmented explanation is now subject to the original dilemma. If such an account applies equally to a zombie (as might be the case for simple causal and reliabilist theories, for example), then it cannot account for the crucial epistemic differences between conscious beings and zombies. And if it does not apply equally to a zombie (if it relies on a notion of acquaintance, for example), then crucial explanatory elements in the account will not be physically explainable.

So I think that none of these strategies gives any support to type-B materialism. Each of them deserves brief discussion in its own right, however. For example, strategy (1), which involves justification, has a further problem in that it is plausible that Mary's introspective beliefs have a sort of justification that Zombie Mary's corresponding beliefs do not share. One could make this case by appealing to the widely accepted view that conscious experience makes a difference to the justification of our perceptual and introspective beliefs. Or one could make it by considering the scenario directly: whereas Mary's belief that she is currently conscious and having a color experience is plausibly justified with something approaching Cartesian certainty, there is a strong intuition that Zombie Mary's corresponding belief is not justified to the same extent, if it is justified at all. If so, then a physically explicable account of phenomenal concepts cannot explain even the justificatory status of Mary's phenomenal knowledge.

The second strategy, involving inferential disconnection, does not have this sort of problem, since it is plausible that a zombie's physical and quasi-phenomenal beliefs are no more inferentially connected than a conscious being's beliefs. Here, the main problem is that given earlier. Whereas the inferential disconnection strategy may physically explain an inferential disconnection between physical and phenomenal *beliefs*, the antiphysicalist's crucial epistemic gap involves a disconnection between physical and phenomenal *knowledge*. This strategy does not help to reconcile this crucial epistemic gap with physicalism, so it lends no support to type-B materialism. At best, it shows that zombie-style analogs of phenomenal beliefs (inferentially disconnected from physical beliefs) are compatible with physicalism, but this is something that we knew already.[4]

The most interesting version of strategy (3) is the one that appeals to phenomenal concepts to explain our belief in an epistemic gap (including our belief that Mary gains new knowledge, that zombies are conceivable, and that there is an explanatory gap). For the reasons given earlier, this strategy cannot

---

4. *Diaz Leon (forthcoming a) takes a version of this strategy. She responds to the line I take here by saying that if we characterize the epistemic gap as requiring the truth of phenomenal beliefs, then we will illegitimately build phenomenology into the epistemic gap by definition. However, as before, the epistemic gap can be characterized topic neutrally, perhaps along the following lines: we possess a quasi-phenomenal concept q, such that our quasi-phenomenal belief *someone has q* is true [and constitutes knowledge] and *if P, then someone has q* is not a priori. This characterization of the epistemic gap requires truth of the relevant belief and does not build in any claims about phenomenology. If the existence of an epistemic gap so construed could be physically explained, this could reasonably be taken to undermine arguments from an epistemic gap to an ontological gap. But if the epistemic gap is construed without requiring truth of the relevant quasi-phenomenal belief, then physically explaining it will not undermine the relevant arguments, as those arguments take the truth of our phenomenal beliefs as a key premise.

help the type-B materialist undermine the *inference* from an epistemic gap to an ontological gap. However, one might think that it helps undermine the premise of that inference by explaining why the belief in such a gap is to be predicted even if no such gap exists. This is an important strategy, but it is one more suited to a type-A materialist than to a type-B materialist. The type-B materialist agrees with the antiphysicalist, against the type-A materialist, on the datum that there *is* an epistemic gap (e.g., that zombies are conceivable, that Mary gains new phenomenal knowledge, and that there is an explanatory gap). Given this datum and given that the inference from an epistemic gap to an ontological gap is unchallenged by this strategy, then the strategy does nothing to support type-B materialism against the antiphysicalist.

(iii) Option 3: Assert That Zombies Share Our Epistemic Situation

The third reaction is to assert that zombies share our epistemic situation. Where we have beliefs about consciousness, zombies have corresponding beliefs with the same truth values and the same epistemic status. And where Mary acquires new phenomenal knowledge on seeing red for the first time, Zombie Mary acquires new knowledge of a precisely analogous sort. If this is right, then the crucial features of phenomenal concepts might simultaneously be physically explicable and able to explain our epistemic situation.

Of course, a zombie's crucial beliefs will not be *phenomenal* beliefs, and Zombie Mary's crucial knowledge will not be *phenomenal* knowledge. Zombies have no phenomenal states, so they cannot have true beliefs that attribute phenomenal states to themselves, and they cannot have first-person phenomenal knowledge. Instead, the proponent of this strategy must conceive of zombies as attributing some *other* sort of state to itself. We might think of these states as "schmenomenal states" and the corresponding beliefs as "schmenomenal beliefs." Schmenomenal states stand to phenomenal states roughly as "twater," the superficially identical liquid on Twin Earth, stands to water: schmenomenal states are not phenomenal states, but they play a role in zombies' lives that is analogous to the role that phenomenal states play in ours. In particular, on this proposal, a zombie's schmenomenal beliefs have the same truth value and epistemic status as a nonzombie's phenomenal beliefs.

One might worry that on a type-B materialist view, schmenomenal states must be the same as phenomenal states, since both are identical to the same underlying physical states. In reply, one can note that the discussion of zombies falls within the scope of a conceivability operator, and the type-B materialist allows that although physical states are identical to phenomenal states, it is at least conceivable that they are not so identical. The zombie scenario will presumably be understood in terms of conceiving that the same physical states are identical to nonphenomenal (schmenomenal) states instead. To avoid this complication, one might also conduct this discussion in terms of a functionally identical silicon zombie rather than in terms of a physically identical zombie. Then the type-B materialist can simply say that ordinary humans have neural states that are identical to phenomenal states, whereas silicon zombies have silicon states that are identical to schmenomenal states. On the current view, silicon zombies will have schmenomenal knowledge that is epistemically analogous to humans' phenomenal knowledge.

This proposal might be developed in two different ways: either by deflating the phenomenal knowledge of conscious beings or by inflating the corresponding knowledge of zombies. That is, a proponent may argue either that Mary gains *less* new knowledge than I suggested earlier or that Zombie Mary gains *more* new knowledge than I suggested earlier. Earlier I argued that Mary gains new, cognitively significant nonindexical knowledge, whereas Zombie Mary does not. The deflationary strategy proposes that Mary gains no such knowledge; the inflationary strategy proposes that Zombie Mary gains such knowledge, too.

The deflationary strategy will presumably involve the claim that the only new factual knowledge that Mary gains upon seeing red for the first time is *indexical* knowledge. That is, Mary gains knowledge of the form 'I am in *this* state now,' where '*this* state' picks out the state that she happens to be in: presumably some sort of neural state. According to this proposal, Zombie Mary gains analogous knowledge, also of the form 'I am in *this* state now,' where '*this* state' picks out the state she happens to be in: presumably a neural or silicon state. There seems to be no problem in principle with the idea that Zombie Mary could gain indexical knowledge of this sort, at least if a zombie can have knowledge at all. This strategy meshes particularly well with the proposal that phenomenal concepts are a species of indexical concept.

In response, I think there is good reason to accept that Mary gains more than indexical knowledge. I have made this case earlier in this book, so I just summarize it briefly here. The key points are first, that indexical knowledge is perspective dependent and evaporates from an objective perspective (see chapter 6), while Mary's new knowledge does not, and second, that the connection between indexical concepts and the key phenomenal concepts in Mary's new knowledge is cognitively significant (see chapter 8). These points strongly suggest that Mary's new knowledge is not merely indexical knowledge.

The inflationary strategy involves the proposal that just as Mary gains cognitively significant nonindexical knowledge involving phenomenal concepts, Zombie Mary gains analogous, cognitively significant nonin-dexical knowledge involving schmenomenal concepts. So where Mary gains significant knowledge of the form *tomatoes cause such-and-such phe-nomenal state*, *I am in such-and-such phenomenal state*, and *this state is such-and-such phenomenal state*, Zombie Mary gains significant knowledge of the form *tomatoes cause such-and-such schmenomenal state*, *I am in such-and-such schmenomenal state*, and *this state is such-and-such schmenomenal state*. Zombie Mary's new beliefs have the same truth value, the same epistemic status, and the same epistemic connections as Mary's corre-sponding beliefs.[5]

Here, the natural response is that this scenario is simply not what we are conceiving when we conceive of a zombie. *Perhaps* it is possible to conceive of a being with another sort of state—call it 'schmonsciousness'—to which it stands in the same sort of epistemic relation that we stand in to con-sciousness. Schmonsciousness would not be consciousness, but it would be epistemically just as good. It is by no means obvious that a state such as schmonsciousness is conceivable, but it is also not obviously inconceivable. However, when we ordinarily conceive of zombies, we are not conceiving of beings with something analogous to consciousness that is epistemically just as good. Rather, we are conceiving of beings with nothing epistemi-cally analogous to consciousness at all.

Put differently, when we conceive of zombies, we are not conceiving of beings whose inner life is as rich as ours but different in character. We are conceiving of beings whose inner life is dramatically poorer than our own. And this difference in inner lives makes for dramatic difference in the richness of our introspective knowledge. Where we have substantial knowl-edge of our phenomenal inner lives, zombies have no analogous introspec-tive knowledge: there is nothing analogous for them to have introspective knowledge of.

Perhaps a zombie can have a sort of introspective knowledge of some of its states: its beliefs and desires, say, or its representations of external stimuli, but this sort of introspective knowledge is not analogous to our phenomenal introspective knowledge. Rather, it is analogous to our non-phenomenal introspective knowledge. Phenomenology is not all that is available to introspection, and it is not out of the question that zombies could have the sort of nonphenomenal introspective knowledge that we

---

5. *In a response to this article, Carruthers and Veillet (2007) take just this line. Papineau (2007) also appears to take a version of this line, although it is not entirely clear (see http://consc.net/papineau.html for clarification). Neither article addresses the claim that zombies without this epistemic situation are at least conceivable.

have. But none of this knowledge will have the character of our introspective knowledge of phenomenal states because there is nothing analogous for zombies to introspect.

At this point a proponent might appeal to certain naturalistic theories of the mind: perhaps a functionalist theory of belief, a causal theory of mental content, and/or a reliabilist theory of knowledge. Zombies have the same functional organization as conscious beings and the same reliable causal connections among their physical states, so a proponent could suggest that these theories entail that zombies will have corresponding beliefs with the same epistemic status as ours. It is not obvious that the theories will make this prediction: that depends on whether they are a priori theories that apply to all conceivable scenarios. If they do not, then they do not undermine the conception of zombies whose epistemic status differs from ours. But in any case, to appeal to these theories in this context is to beg the question. Consideration of the Mary situation and related matters gives us good reason to believe that consciousness is relevant to matters such as mental content and epistemic status. It follows that if consciousness is not itself explainable in physical/functional terms, then any entirely physical/functional theory of content or knowledge will be incomplete. If a theory predicts that a nonconscious zombie would have the same sort of introspective knowledge that we do, then this is reason to reject the theory.

The upshot of all this is that the inflationary strategy does not adequately reflect what we are conceiving when we conceive of a zombie. It is arguably conceivable that a nonconscious duplicate could have some analogous state, schmonsciousness, of which they have analogous introspective knowledge. But it is also conceivable that a nonconscious duplicate would have no such analogous introspective knowledge. And this latter conceivability claim is all that the argument against the phenomenal concept strategy needs.

(iv) Option 4: Reject the Link between Conceivability and Explanation

The fourth possible reaction for proponents of the phenomenal concept strategy is to deny the connection between conceivability and explanation. Such proponents might allow that $P\&\sim C$ is conceivable but hold that, nevertheless, P explains C. Alternatively, they might allow that $C\&\sim E$ is conceivable but hold that, nevertheless, C explains E.

Of course, everyone should allow that there are *some* sorts of explanation such that explaining B in terms of A is consistent with the conceivability of B without A. For causal explanation, for example, this is precisely what one expects. The crucial claim is that there is a *sort* of explanation that is tied to conceivability in this way and that this sort of explanation is relevant to the explanatory gap. This is the sort of micro-macro explanation that I earlier called transparent explanation: explanation that makes transparent why relevant high-level truths obtain, given that low-level truths obtain. If it is conceivable that the low-level truths obtain without the high-level obtaining, the explanation will not be transparent in the relevant way. Instead, one will need to appeal to substantive further principles to bridge the divide between the low-level and the high-level domains. It is just this sort of transparent explanation that is absent in the original explanatory gap.

Opponents may deny that this sort of transparent explanation is required for a good reductive explanation or that it is present in typical reductive explanations. Or they may at least deny this for a notion of transparent explanation that is strongly tied to conceivability. For example, Block and Stalnaker (1999), Levine (2001), and Yablo (2002) all argue that typical cases of micro-macro explanation—the explanation of water in terms of H_2O, for example—are not associated with an a priori entailment of macro truths by micro truths. If they are right about this, then insofar as the notion of transparent explanation is tied to a priori entailment, it is not required for ordinary micro-macro explanation. I have argued elsewhere (chapter 7) that they are not right about this: even in cases such as the relation between microphysics and water, there is a sort of associated a priori entailment, and this sort of entailment is crucial for a good reductive explanation.

It is also worth noting that even if these theorists are right, this will at best undermine a link between one sort of conceivability and explanation. As in chapter 6, let us say that S is *negatively* conceivable when the truth of S cannot be ruled out a priori. Then the claim that A entails B a priori is equivalent to the claim that $A\&{\sim}B$ is negatively conceivable. If these theorists are right, then even 'zombie H_2O' (Levine's 2001 term for a microphysically identical substance that is not water) will be negatively conceivable, so that ordinary micro-macro explanation of B by A cannot require that $A\&{\sim}B$ is negatively conceivable. However, Levine himself notes that there is a different sort of "thick" conceivability such that zombies are conceivable in this sense and zombie H_2O is not, and he notes that this sort of conceivability is tied to explanation: $A\&{\sim}B$ is thickly conceivable if and only if there is an explanatory gap between A and B. If so, we can use this sort of thick conceivability in the previous arguments.

I think that Levine's thick conceivability corresponds closely to what I earlier called *positive* conceivability, which requires a clear and distinct positive conception of a situation that one is imagining. Positive conceivability is arguably the central philosophical notion of conceivability, and it is highly plausible that in cases of ordinary reductive explanations of B by A, $A\&\sim B$ is not positively conceivable. We can form a positive conception of a zombie in a way that we cannot form a positive conception of zombie H_2O. Furthermore, this positive conceivability seems to be particularly strongly associated with the sense of apparent contingency that goes along with the explanatory gap. So it remains plausible that for the sort of explanation that is relevant here, positive conceivability of $A\&\sim B$ entails an explanatory gap between A and B.

Opponents may insist more strongly that no sort of conceivability is tied in this way to micro-macro explanation. They may hold that this sort of explanation simply requires a relevant correlation or a relevant identity between the low-level and the high-level domain, where this correlation or identity does not require any strong conceptual connection between low-level truths and high-level truths. I think this gets the character of micro-macro explanation wrong by failing to account for the sense of transparency in a good micro-macro explanation. In any case, an opponent of this sort is unlikely to be too worried by the explanatory gap in the first place. If this sort of move works to dissolve the explanatory gap between physical processes and phenomenal concepts, say, then it will work equally well to dissolve the original explanatory gap between physical processes and consciousness. If so, then once again the phenomenal concept strategy is rendered redundant in explaining the explanatory gap.

Of course, such a theorist may still appeal to the phenomenal concept strategy to explain the remaining epistemic gaps (such as the conceivability of zombies) in their own right, independent of any connection to the explanatory gap. Here the general idea will be as before: there is no valid inference from these epistemic gaps to an ontological gap because the existence of these epistemic gaps is compatible with physicalism. Still, as before, an opponent will question the strategy on the grounds that there is as much of an epistemic gap between physical processes and phenomenal concepts (as characterized by the proponent's account), or between phenomenal concepts and our epistemic situation, as there was between physical processes and consciousness. To respond, the opponent must either deny this epistemic gap (which will raise all of the previous issues) or give independent reasons to think that the epistemic gap is compatible with physicalism (which will render the phenomenal concept strategy redundant). Either way, the theoretical landscape will be much as before.

(Strictly speaking, there may be one version of this strategy on which the theoretical landscape will differ. A proponent might appeal to phenomenal concepts solely to explain Mary's new knowledge without using it to explain either the conceivability of zombies or the explanatory gap. If so, then the conceivability of zombies who do not satisfy this account of phenomenal concepts will not raise the usual regress worry. To avoid a residual epistemic gap with the same character as the original epistemic gap, the proponent would simply need to make the case that Mary could know all about the relevant structural features of phenomenal concepts from inside her black-and-white room. Of course, this proponent will then need some other means to deal with the conceivability argument and with the explanatory gaps posed both by consciousness and by the account of phenomenal concepts.)

In any case, many of the central points of this chapter can also be made directly in terms of explanation without proceeding first through conceivability. The analysis in terms of conceivability is useful in providing a tool for fine-grained analyses and arguments and for getting a sense of the options in the theoretical landscape. But with these options laid out, one can also make the case directly that any given account of phenomenal concepts will generate either an explanatory gap between physical processes and phenomenal concepts or between phenomenal concepts and our epistemic situation. I make this sort of case in the next section.

5. Applications

I now look at some specific accounts of phenomenal concepts in light of the preceding discussion. If what has gone before is correct, then any fully specific account of phenomenal concepts will fall into one of two classes. It will be either a "thick" account, in which the relevant features of phenomenal concepts are not physically explainable (although they may explain our epistemic situation), or a "thin" account, in which the relevant features of phenomenal concepts do not explain our epistemic situation (although they may be physically explainable).

I have already discussed the indexical account of phenomenal concepts (of Ismael, O'Dea, Perry, and others) under option 3 above. For the reasons given there, I think that this account is clearly a thin account; for example, it does not adequately explain the character of Mary's new cognitively significant knowledge. So there is reason to believe that phenomenal concepts are not indexical concepts.

I have also discussed the dual-conceptual-role account (of Nagel, Hill, McLaughlin, and others) under option 2 above. If this account is understood in wholly functional terms, involving the distinctness in functional role of certain representations in the brain, then it is clearly a thin account. For reasons discussed earlier, this account may help to explain an inferential disconnection between physical and phenomenal beliefs, but it cannot explain the character of phenomenal *knowledge*. Perhaps the account could be supplemented by some further element to explain this character (for example, postulating a special faculty of sympathetic knowledge), but then the original dilemma will arise once again for the new account.

The quotational account (of Block, Chalmers, Papineau, and others) might be understood either as a thin or a thick account, depending on how it is specified. One may understand this either in a "bottom-up" way, in which we start with purely physical/functional materials and make no assumptions about consciousness, or in a "top-down" way, in which we build consciousness into the account from the start. I examine each of these versions in turn.

The bottom-up version of the quotational account is specified in purely physical/functional terms without building in any assumptions about consciousness. The basic idea is that there are some neural states N (those that correspond to phenomenal states, though we do not assume that) that can come to be embedded in more complex neural representations by a sort of "quotation" process, which allows the original state to be incorporated as a constituent. Perhaps this will go along with some sort of demonstrative reference to the original neural state, so that the complex state has the form 'That state: N.' Of course, it is not obvious that one can explain any sort of demonstrative reference in physical/functional terms, but I leave that point aside.

At this point, we can think of the account as an engineer might. If we designed a system to meet the specifications, what sort of results would we expect? In particular, what sort of knowledge of state N would one expect? I think the answer is reasonably clear. One would expect a sort of indexical knowledge of the state, of the form 'I am in this state now.' But one would not expect any sort of cognitively significant knowledge of the state's intrinsic character. To see this, note that one might design an identical system where state N is replaced by a different state M (perhaps another neural state or a silicon state) with different intrinsic properties. From a bottom-up perspective, we would not expect this change to affect the epistemic situation of the subject in the slightest. States N and M may make a difference to the subject's knowledge by virtue of their functional role, but from an engineering perspective there is no reason to think that the subject has access to their intrinsic character.

So the bottom-up version of the quotational account is best understood as a thin account of phenomenal concepts. It may ground a sort of indexical or demonstrative knowledge of neural states, but it cannot ground the sort of significant nonindexical knowledge of internal states that Mary gains on leaving her black-and-white room. In this respect, the bottom-up version of the quotational account seems to be no better off than the indexical account.

On the top-down version of the quotational account, we build consciousness into the account from the start. In particular, we assume that our initial state Q is a *phenomenal* state. (It does not matter to what follows whether we take a stand on whether Q is a neural state or whether we stay silent on the matter.) We then stipulate a concept-forming process that incorporates phenomenal states as constituents. Perhaps this process will involve a sort of demonstrative reference to the original phenomenal state, so the resulting concept has the form 'That state: Q.' What sort of results will we then expect?

We *might* then reasonably expect the subject to have some sort of cognitively significant knowledge of the character of Q. In general, when we make demonstrative reference to phenomenal states, we can have cognitively significant knowledge of their character. We could also imagine a functionally identical subject who, in place of Q, has a different phenomenal state R. In this case, one might expect the substitution to affect the subject's epistemic situation: the new subject will have cognitively significant nonindexical knowledge that it is in phenomenal state R, which is quite different from the first subject's knowledge.

This top-down version of the quotational account is quite clearly a thick account of phenomenal concepts. By building phenomenal states into the account, it has the capacity to help explain features of our epistemic situation that the bottom-up account cannot. But precisely because the account builds in phenomenal states from the start, it cannot be transparently explained in physical terms. This version of the account presupposes the special epistemic features of phenomenal states rather than explaining them.

(Papineau's version of the quotational account appears to be a thin version. Papineau discusses a silicon zombie (2002, 125–27) and suggests that it will have semantic and epistemic features analogous to those of a conscious being. His account seems to point in a direction in which the relevant phenomenal knowledge is all a kind of indexical or demonstrative knowledge, although he does not explicitly make this claim or address the objections to it. By contrast, my own version of this sort of account in chapter 8 is certainly intended as a thick account.)

The recognitional-concept account (of Loar, Carruthers, Tye, and others) can be handled in a similar way. If we understand the concept in a bottom-up way, involving recognitional processes triggered by neural states, what sort of knowledge will we expect? Here, we would once again expect a sort of indexical or demonstrative knowledge of the neural states in question without any cognitively significant knowledge of their intrinsic character. Once again, we would expect that substituting one neural state for another would make no significant difference to a subject's epistemic situation. So this version of the account can be understood as a thin account.

On the other hand, if we understand the account in a top-down way as involving recognitional concepts triggered by phenomenal states, then one might well expect it to lead to significant knowledge of the character of these states. It is plausible that merely having a phenomenal state enables us to have a conception of its character, by which we can recognize it (or at least recognize states reasonably similar to it) when it reoccurs and such that substituting a different phenomenal state will make a difference to our epistemic situation. This top-down account might well capture something about the difference between a conscious being's epistemic situation and a zombie's situation. But again, this account presupposes the existence of consciousness, along with some of its special epistemic features, so the account is clearly a thick account.

(Loar's own account appears to be a thick account. His discussion of phenomenal concepts presupposes both the existence of consciousness and some of its special epistemic features. In particular, his account crucially relies on the thesis that phenomenal states are presented to us under non-contingent modes of presentation, thus enabling significant knowledge of their character. He defends this assumption by saying that the nonphysicalist accepts the thesis, so the physicalist is entitled to it as well. Of course, the thesis poses a special explanatory burden on the physicalist. How can a neural state of a physical system be presented to a subject under a noncontingent mode of presentation, thus enabling significant knowledge of its character? Loar does not say.)

What about Sturgeon's account of phenomenal concepts, according to which phenomenal states constitute their own canonical evidence? I think that this is probably best understood as a thick account. From a bottom-up perspective, would we expect neural states to constitute their own canonical evidence? When zombies deploy their analogs of phenomenal concepts, do they have analogous states that constitute their own canonical evidence? The answer is not entirely obvious, but on the face of it, the more plausible answer is no. If so, then Sturgeon's account can be seen as a thick account, one that rests on a special epistemic feature of phenomenal concepts.

What do the thick accounts of phenomenal concepts have in common? All of them implicitly or explicitly build in special epistemic features of phenomenal concepts: the idea that phenomenal states present themselves to subjects in especially direct ways, or the idea that simply having a phenomenal state enables a certain sort of knowledge of the state, or the idea that the state itself constitutes evidence for the state. If we build in such features, then we may be able to explain many aspects of our distinctive epistemic situation with respect to consciousness. But the cost is that such features themselves pose an explanatory problem. If these features are powerful enough to distinguish our epistemic situation from that of a zombie, then they will themselves pose as much of an explanatory gap as does consciousness itself.

If one rejects physicalism, there is no obvious problem in accommodating these epistemic features of consciousness. Dualists sometimes postulate an epistemic relation of acquaintance that holds between subjects and their phenomenal states and that affords knowledge of these states. If necessary, a dualist can simply take this relation as primitive. The dualist is already committed to positing primitive mental features, and this relation may reasonably be taken to be part of the primitive structure of consciousness. However, this move is not available to a physicalist, who must either explain the features or accept a further explanatory gap.

Our examination of specific accounts of phenomenal concepts reaches a conclusion very much compatible with that of Levine (2007). It appears that such accounts build in either strong epistemic relations such as acquaintance, which themselves pose problems for physical explanation or weak epistemic relations such as indexical or demonstrative reference, which cannot explain our epistemic situation with regard to consciousness. The arguments earlier in the chapter suggest that this is not a mere accident of these specific accounts that a better account may evade. Any account of phenomenal concepts can be expected to have one problem or the other. For this reason, the phenomenal concept strategy cannot reconcile ontological physicalism with the explanatory gap.

Part V

THE CONTENTS OF CONSCIOUSNESS

11

THE REPRESENTATIONAL CHARACTER OF EXPERIENCE

1. Introduction

Consciousness and intentionality are perhaps the two central phenomena in the philosophy of mind. Human beings are conscious beings: there is something it is like to be us. Human beings are intentional beings: we represent what is going on in the world. Correspondingly, our specific mental states, such as perceptions and thoughts, often have a phenomenal character: there is something it is like to be in them. These mental states also often have intentional content: they serve to represent the world.

On the face of it, consciousness and intentionality are intimately connected. Our most important conscious mental states are intentional states: conscious experiences often inform us about the state of the world. Our most important intentional mental states are conscious states: there is often something it is like to represent the external world. It is natural to think that a satisfactory account of consciousness must respect its intentional structure and that a satisfactory account of intentionality must respect its phenomenological character.

With this in mind, it is surprising that in the last few decades the philosophical study of consciousness and intentionality has often proceeded in two independent streams. This was not always the case. In the work of philosophers from Descartes and Locke to Brentano and Husserl, consciousness and intentionality were typically analyzed in a single package. But in the second half of the twentieth century, the dominant tendency was to concentrate on one topic or the other and to offer quite separate analyses of the two. On this approach, the connections between consciousness and intentionality receded into the background.

In the last few years, this has begun to change. The interface between consciousness and intentionality has received increasing attention on a number of fronts. This attention has focused on topics such as the representational content of perceptual experience, the higher-order representation of conscious states, and the phenomenology of thinking. Two distinct philosophical groups have begun to emerge. One focuses on ways in which consciousness might be grounded in intentionality. The other focuses on ways in which intentionality might be grounded in consciousness.

Grounding consciousness in intentionality. Those who take this approach typically try to analyze consciousness in terms of intentionality, without remainder. Some (such as David Rosenthal and Peter Carruthers) analyze conscious states in terms of higher-order states that represent them. Perhaps the most popular approach (taken by Michael Tye and Fred Dretske, among others) focuses on the first-order intentional content of conscious states and advocates *representationalism*, analyzing conscious states as a certain sort of first-order intentional state. This approach is often combined with the view that intentionality can be explained in physical terms to motivate a physically acceptable explanation of consciousness.[1]

Grounding intentionality in consciousness. Those who take this approach argue that phenomenology plays a crucial role in grounding representational content. Some (such as John Searle) argue that consciousness is the ground of all true intentional content. Others (such as Terence Horgan and John Tienson, Colin McGinn, and Charles Siewert) argue that there is at least a distinctive and crucial sort of intentional content that accrues in virtue of the phenomenal character of mental states. These theorists do not typically offer reductive analysis of intentionality in terms of consciousness, but they typically hold that consciousness has a certain priority in the constitution of intentionality.[2]

My own sympathies lie more with the second group, but the ideas of both groups deserve close attention. In particular, I think that there is significant promise in representationalism. Representationalism is often understood as taking a reductive view of consciousness, but this association is inessential. The insights of representationalism cohere equally well

---

1. See Rosenthal (1997), Carruthers (2000), Tye (1995), and Dretske (1995). Others who take this sort of approach include Harman (1990) and Lycan (1996).

2. See Searle (1990), Horgan and Tienson (2002), McGinn (1988), and Siewert (1998). Others who take this sort of approach include Strawson (1994) and Loar (2003).

with a view on which consciousness cannot be reduced to anything more basic than itself.

In what follows I proceed largely from first principles in analyzing aspects of the relationship between consciousness and intentionality, while leaning on the analyses of others along the way. I focus on the phenomenal character and the intentional content of perceptual states, canvassing various possible relations among them. I argue that there is a good case for a sort of representationalism, although this may not take the form that its advocates often suggest. By mapping out some of the landscape, I try to open up territory for different and promising forms of representationalism to be explored in the future. In particular, I argue for a nonreductive, narrow, and Fregean variety of representationalism, which contrasts strongly with more widely explored varieties. I conclude with some words about the fundamental relationship between consciousness and intentionality.

2. Phenomenal Properties and Representational Properties

Consciousness involves the instantiation of *phenomenal properties*. These properties characterize aspects of what it is like to be a subject (what it is like to be me right now, for example, or what it is like to be a bat), or what it is like to be in a mental state (what it is like to see a certain shade of green, for example, or what it is like to feel a certain sharp pain). Whenever there is something it is like to be a subject, that subject has specific phenomenal properties. Whenever there is something it is like to be in a mental state, that state has specific phenomenal properties. For many purposes it does not make much difference whether one focuses on the phenomenal properties of subjects or of mental states (it is easy to translate between the two ways of talking), and in what follows I move back and forth between them.

Intentionality involves the instantiation of *representational properties*. We can say that a *pure representational property* is the property of representing a certain intentional content (or the property of having a certain intentional content; I will not usually pay much attention to this grammatical distinction). Intuitively, this involves representing things as being a certain way in the world. A perceptual state might have the content that there is a green object in front of me, and a belief might have the content that javelinas live in the desert. We can be neutral on just what sort of content this is: it might involve a set of possible worlds, a complex of objects and properties, a complex of Fregean senses, or something else again. What is most important is that intentional contents have *conditions of satisfaction*: they are the sort of thing that can be satisfied or can fail to be satisfied by states of the world. As with phenomenal properties, we can regard representational properties as being instantiated by either subjects or mental states.

An *impure representational property* is the property of representing a certain intentional content in a certain manner. This involves representing such-and-such as being the case in such-and-such a way. Here the "way" is a *manner of representation*, which involves a mental characterization of the state of representing. There are many different manners of representation. For example, one can represent a content perceptually, and one can represent a content doxastically (in belief): these correspond to different manners of representation. At a more fine-grained level, one can represent a content visually or auditorily. Manners of representation may also involve functional characterizations of the representing state. For example, one can represent a certain content in such a way that the content either is or is not available for verbal report.[3]

Whenever an impure representational property is instantiated, the corresponding pure representational property will also be instantiated (whenever a content is represented in a certain way, it is represented). And whenever a pure representational property is instantiated, numerous corresponding impure representational properties will be instantiated (whenever a content is represented, it is represented in certain ways).

I take *representationalism* to be the thesis that phenomenal properties are identical to certain representational properties (or that they are equivalent to certain representational properties; see later). We can say that *pure representationalism* is the thesis that phenomenal properties are identical to pure representational properties, while *impure representationalism* is the thesis that phenomenal properties are identical to impure representational properties. In practice, almost all representationalists are impure representationalists, for reasons discussed shortly.

Some representationalists, such as Dretske and Tye, put their view by saying that phenomenal properties are identical to certain *represented* external properties, such as physical redness. As I am putting things, that would be a category mistake. Phenomenal properties are by definition properties of subjects or of mental states, and physical redness is not (or need not be) such a property. This is simply a terminological difference, however. For example, Dretske defines phenomenal properties (qualia) as the properties we are directly aware of in perception and concludes these are properties such as colors. This is quite compatible with the claim that phenomenal properties

---

3. Manners of representation are closely related to what Crane (2003) calls "intentional modes." I do not use this way of speaking as it invites confusion with the quite distinct notion of modes of presentation (which are contents rather than psychological properties), used later in this chapter.

in my sense are representational properties, as long as one holds that one is directly aware of the represented property rather than the representational property. Once we make the relevant translation, these representationalists' most important claims can be put in the terms used here without loss.

3. Relationships

What are the relationships between phenomenal and representational properties? Do phenomenal properties *entail* (pure or impure) representational properties, or vice versa? Are phenomenal properties *identical* to representational properties? Are phenomenal properties *reducible* to representational properties, or vice versa?

We can say that one property entails another property when it is necessarily the case that whatever has the first property has the second property. We can say that two properties are equivalent when each entails the other: that is, if it is necessarily the case that whatever has one of the properties has the other. I take it in what follows that the equivalence of two properties suffices for them to be identical. Not much rests on this: if one thinks properties are finer grained than this, one can simply replace talk of identity throughout this chapter with talk of equivalence.[4]

This approach yields the following more detailed characterization of representationalism. Representationalism (about a class of phenomenal properties) is the thesis that for every phenomenal property (in that class), there is some representational property such that, necessarily, a mental state (or a subject) has that representational property if and only if it has that phenomenal property.

I will concentrate on the class of perceptual phenomenal properties and in some places more specifically on the class of visual phenomenal properties. So in the first instance, I am interested in the relationship between visual phenomenal properties and (pure or impure) representational properties, though it is natural to hope that this relationship will generalize to other phenomenal properties. In what follows, I consider various possible relations among these properties, one step at a time.

Do pure representational properties entail phenomenal properties? That is, is it necessarily the case that any subject (mental state) that represents a certain content also has a certain phenomenal character? Here, it is most

---

4. *One might respond that the issue is not just verbal because in order for representationalism to tell us about the *nature* of phenomenal states, it must be cast in terms of property identity and not just property equivalence. For what it is worth, I am inclined to accept that phenomenal properties are identical to representational properties even if one adopts a fine-grained view of properties, although this takes somewhat more argument than is given in this chapter.

natural to answer no. The reason is that it seems that most or all representational contents can be represented *unconsciously*, without any associated phenomenal character at all. There can be unconscious beliefs and subconscious perception, and it seems that in principle these unconscious states can represent a very wide range of intentional contents. One could preserve the entailment thesis by denying that there are unconscious representational states, but that view is now almost universally rejected.

There are some weaker theses that may be left on the table here. First, one could hold that there are some special intentional contents (perhaps concerning phenomenal properties themselves or intimately related to phenomenal properties) that cannot be represented unconsciously. If so, the corresponding pure representational properties would entail phenomenal properties. Second, one could hold (with Searle 1990) that representing an intentional content requires that one (at least potentially) have some corresponding conscious state at some time or other. If so, there could be an entailment from pure representational properties to certain diachronic or dispositional phenomenal properties (the property of having certain phenomenal properties in the past or the future, or potentially), if not to phenomenal properties in the strict sense. Finally, one could hold that there is an entailment from certain *impure* representational properties to phenomenal properties. I will return to this possibility later.

Do phenomenal properties entail pure representational properties? That is, is it necessarily the case that any subject with a certain phenomenal character thereby represents the world as being a certain way? Here the answer is quite plausibly yes, at least in the case of perceptual phenomenal properties. It seems intuitively clear that perceptual phenomenology, by its very nature, involves the representation of the external world. For example, my visual phenomenology right now involves the representation of a computer on a desk in front of me, with various books and papers scattered on the desk.

The claim that phenomenal experiences (in a given class) always have representational content is sometimes called *weak representationalism*. Weak representationalism (at least about visual experiences) is extremely plausible and rarely denied.[5] A stronger thesis also seems plausible: that any two phenomenally identical states will share some aspect of their representational content. As Colin McGinn (1988) has put it, there is a strong intuition that something about representational content is *internal* to phenomenology. That is, given a specific phenomenology, it seems that if a

5. Weak representationalism is characterized in roughly this way by Crane (2003), Levine (2003), and Lycan (2000). Even the views of antirepresentationalists such as Block and Peacocke appear to be compatible with weak representationalism. Travis (2004) appears to reject even weak representationalism.

mental state has this phenomenology, it must also have a certain specific representational content. If this is right, then phenomenal properties entail certain pure representational properties.

This line of thought has been developed into an argument at greatest length by Charles Siewert (1998). I will not recapitulate Siewert's extensive arguments here, but the basic idea is that visual experiences are *assessable for accuracy* in virtue of their phenomenal character. For example, when I have a visual experience as of something X-shaped in front of me, this experience may be either accurate or inaccurate, depending on what is really in front of me. Further, it seems that any visual experience with the same phenomenal character would be assessable for accuracy in the same sort of way. Roughly, it would be correct if and only if there is an object with an appropriate shape in front of the subject. If this is right, then a phenomenal property (having an experience with the phenomenal character as of seeing something X shaped) entails a pure representational property (roughly, representing that there is an object with a certain shape in the world).

Something similar plausibly applies to other visual experiences, such as experiences of position and color, and to other perceptual experiences, such as auditory and tactile experiences. Siewert argues that this reasoning can be extended to the phenomenology and intentionality of thought, as well as perception, but this raises complications that I will not go into here. For now, what matters is that there is plausibly an entailment from perceptual phenomenal properties to pure representational properties.

A similar point can be made for subjects of experience, as well as for mental states. Terence Horgan and John Tienson (2002) have argued that necessarily, any two subjects that are phenomenal duplicates will share significant representational content.[6] Even a brain in a vat that has experiences that are phenomenally identical to mine will represent its environment as being in significant respects just as I represent my environment as being. This suggests that the phenomenal properties of a subject entail pure representational properties for that subject.

Just what sort of representational properties are entailed by phenomenal properties? Some tricky questions arise here. If phenomenal properties are intrinsic properties of an individual, then presumably the corresponding representational properties must be intrinsic, too. One might reasonably

6. Loar (2003) makes a related argument from phenomenal duplicates, although his conception of phenomenal intentionality (unlike Horgan and Tienson's) is shorn of the connection to conditions of satisfaction, so it is arguable that Loar's account delivers intentionality only in a watered-down sense.

wonder just how to characterize these properties, given the apparent extrinsicness of many representational properties. I look more closely at these questions later. For now, I will take it that there is at least a strong prima facie case that phenomenal properties entail pure representational properties.

Are phenomenal properties identical to pure representational properties? That is, for a given phenomenal property, is there some representational content that is represented if and only if that phenomenal property is instantiated? The answer to this question is plausibly no, for reasons given earlier. Identity requires entailment, and it is plausible that phenomenal properties are not entailed by pure representational properties. If any given representational content can be represented unconsciously, then pure representational properties cannot be identical to phenomenal properties, and pure representationalism is false.

The only hope for pure representationalism is to deny that any given representational content can be represented unconsciously. The pure representationalist might deny that unconscious representation is possible, or might hold that there are some special representational contents that cannot be represented unconsciously and can be represented only by a specific sort of phenomenal state.[7] If such contents exist, the property of representing one of them might be identical to a phenomenal property. In the absence of strong reasons for thinking that such contents exist, however, I pass over this option in what follows.

Are phenomenal properties identical to impure representational properties? We have seen that pure representational properties are plausibly entailed by phenomenal properties but that the reverse is not the case because of the possibility of unconscious representation. This rules out an identity between phenomenal properties and pure representational properties. However, it leaves open the possibility of an identity between phenomenal properties and *impure* representational properties, where the latter require an appropriate manner of representation. If we stipulate the right manner of representation, the possibility of unconscious representation might be ruled out, removing at least one obstacle to an identity.

The obvious suggestion is to require a *phenomenal* manner of representation. Representational contents can be represented either phenomenally (as in conscious vision, for example) or nonphenomenally (as in unconscious

---

7. Something like pure representationalism is advocated by Lloyd (1991), who takes the first strategy, and by Thau (2002), who takes the second strategy.

thought). For any given content, we can define a corresponding impure representational property: the property of phenomenally representing that content. It is natural to wonder whether phenomenal properties might be identical to impure representational properties of this sort.

For a given phenomenal property, one can find a corresponding impure representational property of this sort. If the phenomenal property entails some representational properties (as at least perceptual phenomenal properties plausibly do), then it will entail some maximally specific representational property that involves a specific representational content. We can then define the impure representational property of phenomenally representing that content. The original phenomenal property will clearly entail this impure representational property. If the impure representational property itself entails the original phenomenal property, then the two properties are identical.

The only obstacle to this identification is the possibility that two distinct phenomenal properties might correspond to the same impure representational property. This will happen if two distinct phenomenal states can have exactly the same representational content. This would happen if a perceptual state and a nonperceptual state (a visual experience and a conscious belief, for example) could phenomenally represent the same content. It would also happen if two perceptual experiences in different modalities (a visual experience and an auditory experience) could have the same content. Finally, it would happen if two phenomenally distinct perceptual experiences in the same modality (two visual experiences, for example) could have the same content.

It is not clear whether any of these cases can arise, but if they arise, there is a natural strategy for dealing with them: one can add more specificity to the manner of representation. Taking the first sort of case, one might argue that an experience of color and a belief about color could in principle have the same content, perhaps representing an object as having a certain specific shade of red. If this sort of case can arise, the perceptual phenomenal property will not be identical to the property of phenomenally representing the content in question. But one can handle the case by moving to a more specific impure representational property, such as the property of *perceptually* phenomenally representing the content in question.[8]

---

8. *One might suggest that the property of *phenomenally* representing such-and-such is a *semipure* representational property in contrast to those involving more specific manners of representationalism. Then *semipure representationalism* identifies phenomenal states with semipure representational properties. If one is moved to reject pure representationalism by the objection from unconscious representation but not by the objection that different experiences could have the same content, semipure representationalism is the natural result.

Likewise, one might argue that a visual experience and an auditory experience might have the same content, perhaps representing that there is an object on one's left. In this case, it is far from clear that such states can have the same *specific* representational content, which is what is needed for a counterexample to equivalence. In most of the cases one might introduce, even if there is an equivalence in unspecific content (that there is an object on one's left), there is usually a difference in specific content (say, that there is a red spherical object on one's left or that there is an object making a certain sound on one's left). So it is far from clear that this sort of case can arise. But if it can arise, one need only move once again to a more specific impure representational property, such as the property of *visually* (or auditorily) phenomenally representing the content in question.

Finally, one might argue that two phenomenally distinct visual experiences might have the same content. It is not easy to see how this could happen. Byrne (2001) has argued that this could not happen on the grounds that any phenomenal difference between visual experiences is a difference in how things seem, and any difference between how things seem is a difference in representational content. Even if one resists this argument (on the grounds, perhaps, that it involves an equivocation on "how things seem"), it is not easy to come up with specific cases of phenomenally distinct visual experiences with the same content. When we conceive of phenomenally distinct visual experiences, it seems that we almost always conceive of experiences that differ in aspects of their representational content.

Peacocke (1983) has argued that there are such cases. For example, he suggests that images of two trees at different distances might represent them as having the same height, while the images take up differently sized portions of the visual field. In response, representationalists (e.g., Tye 1995) have plausibly replied that these images differ in certain representational properties, such as their representation of distance or visual angle. Block (1990) has argued that subjects with phenomenally distinct color experiences in different environments might represent the same external colors. In response, one can argue along lines developed later in this chapter that such experiences always differ in certain key aspects of their representational content. Other purported examples involving cases of blurry vision, double images, and the like have received reasonably plausible replies (e.g., Tye 2003a) from representationalists.

To my mind, the most plausible potential cases of phenomenally distinct visual experiences with the same representational content involve differences in attention. Shifts in attention clearly make a phenomenal difference to visual experiences. In typical cases, they also make a representational difference. For example, shifting attention to a word may lead one to represent the shapes of its letters with greater specificity. But there are cases that are less clear. For example, one might look at two red pinpoint lights against a black background and shift attention from one to the other. Here it is not obvious that there is a representational difference between the cases. There are various suggestions one might make in response, however. One might argue that the position or color of the light to which one is attending is represented with greater specificity than that of the light to which one is not attending. Or one might argue that the light to which one is attending is represented as being more salient than the other light. It is not completely clear what sort of property "salience" is, but it is plausible that there is such a property (though it may be relative to a subject at a time), and the suggestion that it is represented in attention seems reasonably apt to the phenomenology.

If there are any cases of phenomenally different visual experiences with the same representational content, one will have to build further differences into the manners of representation in impure representational states (so one might have the property of attentively representing a certain content, and so on). But it is not clear that such cases exist. My own view is that the claim that phenomenal differences between visual experiences always correspond to representational differences has some prima facie plausibility and serves as a sort of null hypothesis that should be rejected only if there is strong evidence against it. If the view is correct, then visual phenomenal properties are identical to impure representational properties of the form involving the (visual) phenomenal representation of a certain content.

Is representationalism correct? If what has gone before is correct, then there is a strong prima facie case for the truth of impure representationalism, at least about visual phenomenal properties. These properties are plausibly equivalent to certain impure representational properties. These impure representational properties have the character: *phenomenally representing such-and-such content*, or (if nonperceptual phenomenal states can have the same content) *perceptually phenomenally representing such-and-such content*, or (if experiences in a different perceptual modality can have the same content) *visually phenomenally representing such-and-such content*.

4. Reductive and Nonreductive Representationalism

I have argued that phenomenal properties are plausibly identical to certain impure representational properties. In the characterization of these impure representational properties, however, the concept of the *phenomenal* itself plays an important role. So the analysis I have given certainly does not offer any sort of reductive analysis of phenomenal properties in terms of nonphenomenal notions.

Here, it is useful to distinguish *reductive* from *nonreductive* representationalism. Representationalism is the thesis that phenomenal properties are identical to certain pure or impure representational properties. Reductive representationalism holds that phenomenal properties are identical to certain pure or impure representational properties that can be understood without appeal to phenomenal notions. Nonreductive representationalism holds that phenomenal properties are identical to certain pure or impure representational properties, where these cannot be understood without appeal to phenomenal notions.

In a little more detail: representationalism holds that any given phenomenal property is identical to the property of representing a certain content in a certain manner (or in the case of pure representationalism, to the property of representing a certain content). Here, the right-hand side invokes a number of notions: the notion of representation, the notion of a certain content, and the notion of a certain manner of representation. If all of these notions can be understood without appeal to phenomenal notions, then the right-hand side offers a reductive account of phenomenal properties. If any of these notions can be understood only in terms of phenomenal notions, then the right-hand side offers a nonreductive account of phenomenal properties.[9]

The analysis I have given is clearly not a reductive analysis. The manner of representation invoked in this analysis makes explicit appeal to the notion of the phenomenal. It may also be, for all I have said so far, that the contents involved in characterizing the representational properties must themselves be understood in terms of phenomenal notions (for example, if they involve the attribution of phenomenal properties to objects, or if they involve the attribution of certain dispositions to cause phenomenal properties). It might even be that the notion of representation cannot be understood in wholly nonphenomenal terms. The status of the last two claims is unclear, but certainly the first claim makes it clear that this is not a reductive analysis.

Proponents of reductive representationalism need to do three things. First, they need to argue that an account of representation can be given in

---

9. One can also distinguish *epistemically* reductive representationalism from *metaphysically* reductive representationalism depending on whether the identity between phenomenal properties and nonphenomenally-specified representational properties is held to be a priori (or conceptually true) or simply to be true. Epistemically reductive representationalism entails metaphysically reductive representationalism but not vice versa. For example, Tye's representationalism is metaphysically but not epistemically reductive.

nonphenomenal terms. Second, they need to argue that the relevant contents can be specified in a manner that is independent of phenomenal notions (this is a version of what Peacocke 1983 calls the "adequacy constraint"). Third, they need to argue that the appeal to a phenomenal manner of representation can be replaced by some nonphenomenally characterized manner of representation.

In practice, this is just what reductive representationalists (such as Tye 1995 and Dretske 1995) try to do.[10] They appeal to an independently motivated account of representation in causal, informational, and teleological terms. They argue that the relevant representational contents can be understood as involving the attributions of ordinary physical properties (such as surface reflectance properties in the case of color experiences) to physical objects in the world without any need for phenomenal notions. They also argue that the relevant manner of representation can be understood in wholly functional terms.

I will set aside the first two points for now and focus on the third. For the reasons given earlier, it seems that a manner of representation is needed to distinguish phenomenal from nonphenomenal representation of a given content. At this point, Tye introduces the constraint that the representing state must be *poised* to play a certain role in the control of speech and action. This constraint is introduced precisely to distinguish phenomenal from nonphenomenal representation in cases such as blindsight. Dretske's account is less explicit about how to handle unconscious representation, but at some places he appeals to the constraint that the representational states must play an appropriate role in the formation of beliefs.

These accounts involve broadly *functional* accounts of the manner of representation: they require that the relevant representational states play the right sort of functional role within the cognitive system. In effect, this functional constraint is offered as an account of the difference between phenomenal and nonphenomenal representations (of the content in question). To this extent, then, the accounts involve functionalism about the phenomenal/nonphenomenal distinction. We might say these accounts are a species of *functionalist representationalism*. They are not functionalist across the board (both Dretske and Tye lean on nonfunctionalist teleological accounts of what it is to represent the contents in question), but they involve functionalism about the crucial distinction between phenomenal and nonphenomenal representation of the relevant contents.

---

10. Reductive representationalists include Clark (2000), Dretske (1995), Droege (2003), Harman (1990), Jackson (2003), Lycan (1996), and Tye (1995).

Functionalist representationalism might be seen as the result of *conjoining* the relatively neutral version of representationalism given earlier with functionalism about the phenomenal/nonphenomenal distinction. If we grant that phenomenal properties are identical to the property of phenomenally representing a certain content, and if we grant that what it is to phenomenally represent a content is to represent the content with a state that plays an appropriate functional role, the result is just this sort of account. So if functionalism about the phenomenal/nonphenomenal distinction can be justified, then functionalist representationalism can be justified.

Conversely, however, if there is reason to doubt functionalism about the phenomenal/nonphenomenal distinction, then there is reason to doubt functionalist representationalism. And there are many reasons to doubt functionalism about the phenomenal/nonphenomenal distinction. While there is some reason to believe that phenomenology is *correlated* with certain functional properties (such as the property of global availability), there are familiar reasons to doubt that it is reducible to these properties. For example, it seems coherent to suppose that any such functional property can be instantiated without any associated phenomenology at all. Many have argued that such a situation is metaphysically possible, and some (e.g., Block 1978 and Searle 1980) have even argued that it is nomologically possible. Others (e.g., Levine 1983) have argued that there is an explanatory gap between a functional characterization of a state and a phenomenal characterization: there is no clear reason why the fact that a state plays a certain functional role should somehow make it the case that there is something it is like to be in that state.[11]

I will not try to adjudicate these arguments here. I simply note that the functionalism in these varieties of representationalism is entirely optional. It is also worth noting that this functionalism is largely unargued in the work of Dretske and Tye. Tye's defense consists mostly in noting that the functional criterion handles cases such as blindsight, but clearly this falls well short of establishing any sort of reduction. Dretske is not explicit about the matter at all. In arguing for their views, both spend by far the greatest portion of their time arguing for representationalism, and the crucial functionalism is left mostly in the background.

---

11. A teleological representationalist such as Dretske allows that any narrow functional property can be instantiated without phenomenology since phenomenology requires the relevant sort of environment. However, the central antifunctionalist arguments (by Block, Searle, etc.) also tend to suggest that any given functional property could in principle be instantiated in any given environment without phenomenology. So "teleofunctionalist" views are vulnerable to the same sort of arguments as functionalist views.

This leaves the following situation. There are good arguments for representationalism, but these are not good arguments for reductive representationalism. There is good reason to believe that phenomenal properties are identical to impure representational properties involving the phenomenal representation of certain contents. Both the reductive and the nonreductive representationalist can accept this. The reductive representationalist must conjoin this with a reductive account of the phenomenal/nonphenomenal distinction. But there are familiar reasons to doubt that such an account is possible, and the arguments for representationalism give no special reason to think that such an account exists.[12]

For my part, I think that nonreductive representationalism is a much more plausible view.[13] This view articulates an internal connection between phenomenal properties and representational properties without trying to reduce the phenomenal to a wholly nonphenomenal domain. At the very least, the nonreductive style of analysis presented here provides a reasonably neutral starting point for further representationalist analyses. Representationalists of many different stripes can agree that visual phenomenal properties are equivalent to impure representational properties of the form: phenomenally (or visually phenomenally or whatever) representing such-and-such a content.

The questions for further debate concern: (i) the specificity in the manner of representation (e.g., phenomenal, perceptual phenomenal, or visual phenomenal?); (ii) whether the phenomenal manner of representation can itself be reductively analyzed; and (iii) the nature of the represented contents. So far, I have addressed the first two questions. In what follows I address the third.

5. Narrow and Wide Representationalism

It is widely believed that phenomenal properties depend only on the internal state of the subject. It is also widely believed (following the arguments of

12. Versions of this point are made by Chalmers (1996, 377), Kriegel (2002a), Vinueza (2000), and Warfield (1999). The point that representationalism on its own does not close the explanatory gap is also made in a slightly different way (focusing on the represented contents rather than the manner of representation) by Stoljar (2007). Similar objections can be mounted to related views such as higher-order representationalism (Rosenthal 1997) and self-representationalism (Kriegel 2009).

13. To my knowledge, nonreductive representationalism has not (at the time of writing the article on which this chapter is based) been discussed explicitly as such in the literature, but Byrne (2001) notes the possibility of representationalism without reduction, and Crane (2003) and Levine (2003) indicate sympathy for this combination. The views suggested by Horgan and Tienson (2002), Searle (1983), and Siewert (1998) seem broadly compatible with the same combination.

Putnam 1975 and Burge 1979) that most representational properties depend not only on the internal state of the subject but also on the subject's environment. For example, it is widely accepted that if two physically identical subjects have relevantly different environments (e.g., an "Earth" environment containing H_2O or a "Twin Earth" environment containing XYZ), the contents of their mental states may be relevantly different (e.g., one has beliefs about H_2O, while the other has beliefs about XYZ).

This poses a prima facie problem for representationalism. Let us say that a property is *narrow* when necessarily, for any individual who has the property, an intrinsic duplicate of that individual has the property (regardless of environment). Let us say that a property is *wide* when it is possible for an individual to have the property while an intrinsic duplicate lacks that property. Then the following three propositions form an inconsistent triad:

   i. Phenomenal properties are equivalent to representational properties.
  ii. Phenomenal properties are narrow.
 iii. Representational properties are wide.

One can react to this inconsistent triad in three different ways: one could deny (i), (ii), or (iii). The first strategy leads to *antirepresentationalism*. Block (1990) takes this strategy, in effect using the plausibility of (ii) and (iii) as an argument against representationalism.

The second strategy leads to *wide representationalism*, on which both phenomenal properties and the representational properties that they are equivalent to are taken to depend on a subject's environment. This strategy is taken by Dretske (1995), Tye (1995), and Lycan (1996), who in effect use the plausibility of (i) and (iii) to argue against the narrowness of phenomenal properties.

Both of these strategies have significant costs. The antirepresentationalist strategy has trouble doing justice to the persistent intuition that phenomenal duplicates are deeply similar in certain representational respects. The wide representationalist strategy is even more counterintuitive, entailing that what it is like to be a subject depends constitutively on factors that may be far away from the subject and in the distant past. Some wide representationalists (especially Lycan 2001) have tried to defend this view, but it has many odd consequences. To pick just one: a change in environment can often yield a gradual change from one wide representational content to another quite different content (e.g., from representing red to representing green), with a period of indeterminate representation of both contents (or divided reference) in the middle. But it is hard to know what an indeterminate phenomenal state involving both phenomenal red and phenomenal green could be like (striped? superimposed?), and it is hard to believe that a subject going through this change in environment would pass through such a state. Lycan suggests that there may be much less indeterminacy in perceptual representation than in cognitive representation, but it is hard to believe that indeterminacy can be eliminated entirely. If there is even a brief period of indeterminacy, then the puzzle arises.

I think that by far the best-motivated strategy is the third. This is the strategy of *narrow representationalism*, which holds that both phenomenal properties and the representational properties they are equivalent to depend only on a subject's internal state. The arguments by Putnam, Burge, and the like give good reason to think that *many* representational properties are wide, but they give little reason to think that *all* representational properties are wide. If we accept that some representational properties are narrow, the inconsistent triad disappears. The natural strategy is then to exploit narrow representational properties in developing a narrow representationalism.[14]

Narrow representational properties can most naturally be developed by an appeal to *narrow contents*: contents of the sort that, if they are represented by a subject, they are represented by any intrinsic duplicate of that subject (regardless of the environment). The arguments of Putnam and Burge suggest that many contents are wide, especially the contents of beliefs about natural kinds and individuals and those involving deference to a linguistic community. But these arguments are consistent with the view that many other contents are narrow.

For example, it is widely accepted that many logical and mathematical beliefs have narrow content. More generally, Horgan and Tienson (2002) have argued that the existence of rich narrow content is a consequence of the plausible view that phenomenal duplicates share rich representational content. It is also possible to hold on quite general grounds that all mental states have a sort of narrow content in addition to any wide content they might have. On the latter sort of view, although two corresponding "water" beliefs of subjects on Earth and Twin Earth may differ in that one is about H_2O and the other is about XYZ (wide content), the beliefs will also have significant narrow content in common, perhaps characterizing the relevant liquids in qualitative terms.

I have argued elsewhere (Chalmers 2002a) for a view of the latter sort, holding that the narrow content of beliefs can be understood as a sort of

14. Versions of narrow representationalism are advocated by Rey (1998), Kriegel (2002b), and Levine (2003).

Fregean epistemic content. This sort of account can naturally be extended to give an account of the narrow content of perceptual states. But first it is useful to examine different ways of characterizing representational content.

6. Russellian Representationalism

One natural way of characterizing the content of mental states involves objects and properties in the world. A belief, such as the belief that Hesperus is bright, can be regarded as composed of concepts (which I regard here as mental items of some sort). One can naturally say that concepts have *extensions*: objects and properties that are picked out by these concepts. The extension of the concept *Hesperus* is the planet Venus, and the extension of the concept *bright* is the property of brightness. One can then characterize the content of a belief in terms of the extensions of the concepts that are involved in the belief. For example, a belief that Hesperus is bright might have the following content: [*Venus, brightness*]. Contents of this sort, involving complexes of specific objects and/or properties in the world, may be thought of as Russellian contents (following Russell, who thought all contents are like this).

Let us say that a Russellian representational property is the property of representing a certain Russellian content or the property of representing a certain Russellian content in a certain way. Then *Russellian representationalism* holds that phenomenal properties are identical to Russellian representational properties. Most contemporary representationalists are Russellian representationalists.[15]

It is natural to think that perceptual experiences have Russellian content. They involve the attribution of properties to objects. For example, when I have a veridical experience of a green ball B, it is natural to think that I represent the ball as being green and that my experience has an *object-involving* Russellian content roughly as follows: [*B, greenness*]. It is also natural to think that my experience has a sort of *existential* (or merely *property-involving*) Russellian content to the effect that there is an object in front of me that is green.

To develop a Russellian representationalism, most Russellian representationalists invoke something like the property-involving Russellian content mentioned earlier rather than an object-involving Russellian content. The

---

15. Thompson (2003) also distinguishes Fregean and Russellian representationalism. McLaughlin (2003) uses "denotational intentionalism" for something like Russellian representationalism.

reason is that it seems that phenomenology can be dissociated from the object-involving content. My visual experience when I look at a green ball has a certain object-involving content, but it seems that a phenomenally identical experience could lack that content if I were looking at a different object, for example, or if I were hallucinating. (Some direct realists will deny this claim, but most contemporary representationalists accept it.) However, in these cases, the property-involving content of the original experience is still plausibly present: my visual experience still represents that there is a green object in front of me.

To go into more detail, it is useful to focus on the case of phenomenal properties associated with colors (though I think the discussion that follows generalizes). Let us say that *phenomenal redness* is the phenomenal property typically associated in our community with seeing red things. (Phenomenal redness should be distinguished from ordinary redness. The first is a property of experiences or of subjects; the second is a property of objects in one's environment.) It is natural to think that instances of phenomenal redness have the content that certain objects in the environment are *red*. That is, these instances have contents that attribute the property of redness.

This line of thought naturally leads to the most common Russellian representationalist view, which holds that phenomenal redness is equivalent to the impure representational property of (visually) phenomenally representing a certain Russellian content involving the attribution of redness. For this view to be made more specific, one needs to specify just what sort of property redness is.[16]

Most commonly, Russellian representationalists of this sort take the view that redness is a physical property, such as a certain surface spectral reflectance. Then phenomenal redness is equivalent to a certain sort of attribution of this physical property to objects. Something analogous is usually said about other perceptual phenomenal properties: all are equivalent to representational properties involving the attribution of physical properties. The resulting view might be called *physical Russellian representationalism*. This strategy has the advantage of being reductive, at least where the content is concerned: there is no need to use phenomenal notions in characterizing the relevant contents.

---

16. The distinctions that follow between physical, projectivist, primitivist, and dispositionalist versions of representationalism are also made by Stoljar (2007). Stoljar calls the first of these the "physicalist" interpretation of representationalism, but I avoid this usage to avoid a natural confusion. Stoljar suggests that projectivism is not really a form of representationalism because it appeals directly to qualia, but once we acknowledge the possibility of nonreductive representationalism, this problem falls away.

Physical Russellian representationalism is plausibly a sort of wide representationalism. To have the relevant representational property, the subject must represent the relevant physical property, which plausibly requires the subject to have inhabited an appropriate environment. This leads to numerous counterintuitive consequences. For example, it seems possible that a subject might have experiences phenomenally identical to my experiences of redness even though her experiences have been caused by objects that are not physically red (i.e., objects that have a different surface spectral reflectance), and it seems possible that these color experiences in such a subject might nevertheless be veridical. But physical Russellian representationalism must deny this possibility. I do not pursue this matter here, as it has been explored at length by others (e.g., Block 1990; Shoemaker 2002).

If we are interested in the prospects for narrow representationalism, it seems that other forms of Russellian representationalism are more compatible with this view. For example, *projectivism* about colors holds that colors are phenomenal properties or perhaps that they are qualitative properties of a visual field. *Projectivist Russellian representationalism* holds that color experiences attribute these properties to objects and that phenomenal color properties are equivalent to corresponding representational properties.[17] (One might embrace projectivist Russellian representationalism without embracing projectivism about colors if one holds that the relevant contents do not involve attribution of colors.) This is most naturally seen as a sort of narrow and nonreductive representationalism: two intrinsic duplicates will share the relevant representational properties, given that they share their phenomenal properties.

A related view, *primitivism* about colors, holds that colors are certain primitive intrinsic properties that are not phenomenal properties or properties of a visual field but are nevertheless constitutively connected to such properties. On this view colors have an intrinsic "qualitative" nature that is revealed in some fashion by color experiences. *Primitivist Russellian representationalism* holds that color experiences attribute these primitive properties to objects and that phenomenal color properties are equivalent to corresponding representational properties.[18] (One might embrace primitivist Russellian representationalism without embracing primitivism about colors if one holds that the relevant contents do not involve attribution of

17. Boghossian and Velleman (1989) have a view that seems compatible with projectivist Russellian representationalism. They advocate projectivism about colors and hold that properties of this sort are represented in color experience.

18. The "figurative projectivism" of Shoemaker (1990) is a sort of primitivism, while projectivism corresponds to his "literal projectivism." Advocates of (something like) primitivist Russellian representationalism include Maund (1995), Holman (2002), Jakab (2003), and Wright (2003) (who are also primitivists about colors) and Thau (2002) (who is not). See also the closely related view in the next chapter.

colors.) This is again naturally seen as a sort of narrow representationalism, given that phenomenal duplicates represent the same primitive properties and given that phenomenal properties are narrow. It is also plausibly seen as nonreductive, given that colors are taken to be irreducible properties that are constitutively tied to phenomenal properties.

There is a certain phenomenological plausibility in both projectivist and primitivist Russellian representationalism. Both involve the attribution of intrinsic properties to objects, properties with a qualitative nature that is closely connected to the qualities of experience itself, but these views seem to have the counterintuitive consequence that color experience is massively illusory. When we have an experience as of a red apple, it seems unlikely that the apple itself instantiates phenomenal redness or that it instantiates a corresponding property of our visual field. It also seems unlikely that it instantiates a simple intrinsic property with a qualitative nature that is constitutively connected to the quality of my visual experience. Further, it seems plausible (as above) that two subjects in different environments might have phenomenally red experiences that are caused by objects that share no relevant intrinsic properties without either subject being in a privileged position with respect to veridicality. If both experiences attribute the same intrinsic properties, then both cannot be correct, so neither is correct. Generalizing, it seems that projectivist or primitivist representationalism leads to the consequence that all color experiences are illusory. Some have accepted this consequence, but it seems a high price to pay.[19]

Finally, *dispositionalism* about color holds that colors are dispositional properties, involving the disposition to cause certain sorts of experiences. For example, redness might be the disposition to cause phenomenally red experiences in a certain class of subjects in normal conditions. *Dispositionalist Russellian representationalism* holds that color experiences attribute these dispositional properties to objects and that phenomenal color properties are equivalent to corresponding representational properties. (As before, one might embrace dispositionalist Russellian representationalism without embracing dispositionalism about colors if one holds that the relevant contents attribute properties other than colors.) This sort of view is most closely associated with Shoemaker (1994, 2001).

Dispositionalist representationalism characterizes the relevant representational contents in partly phenomenal terms, so it can easily be seen as a sort of nonreductive representationalism. Shoemaker does not see it this way. He conjoins the basic view with the view that phenomenal properties

---

19. Boghossian and Velleman, Holman, Jakab, Maund, and Wright all accept that color experiences are illusory. Thau is not explicit about the matter.

are identical to certain neurophysiological properties and so holds that the relevant dispositional properties can be identified nonphenomenally. So his version of the view is a sort of reductive representationalism. Nonetheless, the reductive aspect of his view is largely independent of the representationalist aspect, and one might well embrace the basic shape of the representationalist view without embracing the reductive claim. If so, the result is a nonreductive version of representationalism.[20]

Dispositionalist representationalism can also easily be seen as a sort of narrow representationalism. It seems plausible to think that two intrinsic duplicates will share their representational contents: both will have phenomenally red experiences, attributing the disposition to cause red experiences to their objects. However (as Egan 2006 and Thompson 2003 have pointed out), it is not clear just how this dispositional property should be characterized. If it is the disposition to cause phenomenally red experiences in a specific subject (the subject of the experience), the phenomenally red experiences in different subjects will attribute *different* dispositional properties to their objects and will differ in the relevant content. This content will not be narrow (the attributed properties will differ between duplicate subjects); and worse, the corresponding representational property will not be entailed by the phenomenal property. An appeal to dispositions to cause the experience in a specific community has the same problem.

Partly to deal with this sort of problem, Shoemaker's version of dispositionalist representationalism appeals to the "higher-order" disposition to cause the experience in one or more sorts of creature in some circumstance, but this view has the consequence that illusory representation is impossible (every object will have the relevant disposition). Egan suggests that the experience attributes an *indexical* disposition: something like the disposition to cause phenomenally red experiences in *me*, where this disposition is attributed equally by both subjects. But it is not clear that this indexical disposition is a legitimate property or that it could be shared by objects of veridical perception by different subjects in different environments. Alternatively, one might hold that one is attributing to *oneself* the property of being confronted by an object with the disposition to cause certain experiences in one, but it is counterintuitive to hold that experience involves the attribution of properties to oneself and not to an external object.

This is one difficulty with the view. Another difficulty is that it seems implausible for various reasons that colors are dispositions. It seems

---

20. Kriegel (2002b) and Levine (2003) embrace the basic shape of Shoemaker's dispositionalist representationalism without Shoemaker's reductive claim.

possible that in counterfactual circumstances, red objects might be disposed to cause phenomenally green experiences in normal observers or in me. If this is right, redness is distinct from the disposition to cause phenomenally red experiences. It seems more compatible with our judgments about the cases that redness is an intrinsic property, such as surface spectral reflectance. But then the dispositional representationalist must say (as Shoemaker does) that the relevant contents attribute properties other than colors to objects. This is at least a counterintuitive thing to say.

We can sum up the problems for Russellian representationalism as follows. The following three claims are plausible: (i) color experiences attribute colors to objects; (ii) colors are intrinsic properties; (iii) there can be veridical phenomenally identical color experiences (in different subjects) of objects with relevantly different intrinsic properties. But these claims entail that phenomenally identical color experiences can attribute different properties to objects. So these claims are inconsistent with Russellian representationalism about color experience.

Denying any of these claims has significant costs. It is possible that some of these costs might be worth paying, if Russellian representationalism were the only way to get a viable representationalism off the ground. However, one can avoid these costs. The problems arise only if we assume that the relevant contents must be Russellian contents. If we appeal to a quite different sort of content, the problems may be avoided.

7. Fregean Content

Frege distinguished between the sense and the reference of linguistic expressions. The referent of an expression such as 'Hesperus' is the planet Venus, but its sense is a *mode of presentation* of that planet. Two distinct terms such as 'Hesperus' and 'Phosphorus' may have the same referent but different senses. Something similar goes for a property term such as 'bright.' Here one might say that the referent of the term is the property of brightness, while its sense is a mode of presentation of that property. Frege held that the sense of an expression determines the expression's referent in some fashion.

One can make a similar distinction for mental states. A belief such as *Hesperus is bright* is composed of concepts such as *Hesperus* and *bright*. The concepts can be said to have extensions: the planet Venus and the property of brightness, respectively. The concepts can also be said to have *modes of presentation* of those extensions. These modes of presentation can be thought of as an aspect of the content of the concepts. Two different concepts such as *Hesperus* and *Phosphorus* may have the same extension but different modes of presentation. The belief as a whole may have a complex content that is at least partly composed of these modes of presentation.

What is a mode of presentation? Frege was not entirely clear on this, but one natural approach characterizes a mode of presentation as a *condition on extension*. The idea is that every concept is associated with some *condition*, such that an entity in the world must satisfy this condition to qualify as the extension of the concept. For example, the concept *Hesperus* might be associated with a condition something like *the object usually visible at a certain point in the evening sky*. (Strictly speaking, the condition is *being the object . . .* , but I usually use the simpler form.) In the actual world, Venus satisfies this condition, so Venus is the extension of *Hesperus*. The concept *Phosphorus* might be associated with a different condition (involving the morning sky). Venus also satisfies this condition, so Venus is the extension of *Phosphorus*. On this analysis, *Hesperus* and *Phosphorus* have the same extensions but different modes of presentation, just as desired.

We can think of these modes of presentation as the *Fregean contents* of concepts. We can also speak of the Fregean contents of entire thoughts by composing the Fregean contents of the concepts involved. For example, the Fregean content of the thought *Hesperus is Phosphorus* might be something like the condition *the object usually visible at a certain point in the evening sky is usually visible at a certain point in the morning sky*. This is a condition on the state of the world, reflecting what it takes for the thought to be true. That is, it is a sort of truth condition.

To determine the condition of extension associated with a concept or a thought, one can consider different hypothetical possibilities concerning the way one's world might turn out to be and determine what the concept's extension (or the thought's truth value) would be under those possibilities. For example, if it turned out that star A was the bright object in the evening sky, and a different star B was the bright object in the morning sky, we would say that *Hesperus* picks out A and *Phosphorus* picks out B, and we would say that *Hesperus is Phosphorus* is false. Formally, one can say that the Fregean content of a concept is a mapping from scenarios to extensions and that the Fregean content of a thought is a mapping from scenarios to truth values, where scenarios are maximal epistemic possibilities, or centered possible worlds. I develop this sort of approach in the appendix, but for the most part the informal understanding will suffice here.

(Note that modes of presentation are quite distinct from the manners of representation invoked earlier. Manners of representation are psychological features of an individual. By contrast, modes of presentation are a sort of *content*. Unlike manners of representation, modes of presentation have built-in conditions of satisfaction. Rather than being psychological entities, they are abstract entities to which psychological states may be related by having them as their content.)

One can extend this approach to the content of perceptual experiences. Perceptual experiences attribute properties to objects: for example, my visual experience might attribute greenness to a ball. As with beliefs and concepts, we can hold that a perceptual experience involves some *modes of presentation* of these properties and objects. As before, these modes of presentation can be seen as conditions on extension. For example, there is a condition that an object must satisfy in order to be the object represented by my experience. The ball satisfies this condition, so it is the object represented by my experience. There is also a condition that a property must satisfy in order to be the property attributed by my experience. Greenness satisfies this condition, so greenness is the property represented by my experience.

What are the modes of presentation associated with a given perceptual experience? To determine these, one considers scenarios involving different ways the world might turn out and considers what the objects and properties represented by the experience will then be. Take a visual experience as of a green sphere. At a very rough first approximation, one might say that for an object to be represented by an experience, it must cause the experience in the appropriate way. So the mode of presentation of the object will be something like *the object that is causing this experience in the appropriate way*. Likewise, one might say that for a property (say, greenness) to be attributed by the experience, it must be the property that has usually caused that sort of color experience in normal conditions in the past. So the mode of presentation of the property will be something like *the property that usually causes phenomenally green experiences in normal conditions*.[21]

Overall (if we abstract from all other features of the experience, such as its spatial features), the experience will be associated with a Fregean content such as *the object causing this experience has the property that usually causes experiences of phenomenal greenness*. This is very roughly compatible with our intuitive judgments about cases. If it turns out that no object is causing the experience in the appropriate way (e.g., if we are hallucinating the object), then we will judge that the experience is not veridical. If it turns out that the object has a property that normally causes phenomenally red experiences but

---

21. The suggestion that color experiences have dispositional modes of presentation of this sort, fixing reference to intrinsic properties in the external world, can be seen as analogous to a corresponding claim about color expressions: for example, that 'red' refers to an intrinsic property, with a mode of presentation that picks out whatever normally causes phenomenally red experiences.

is now causing a phenomenally green experience due to abnormal conditions, we will judge that the experience is not veridical, and so on.

(One could also make a case for dropping the "object causing this experience" aspect of the content, yielding a "pure existential" Fregean content along the lines of "there exists an object [at such-and-such location] with the property that usually causes experiences of phenomenal greenness." This turns on subtle issues about whether alleged cases of "veridical hallucination"—e.g., when one hallucinates a red square in front of one, and by coincidence there is a red square in front of one—should be classified as veridical or nonveridical. If veridical, one should go with the pure existential Fregean content. If nonveridical, one should go with the more complex causal Fregean content.)

One can formalize this approach to Fregean content by using the two-dimensional framework for analyzing mental and linguistic content. I develop this sort of analysis in the afterword to this chapter.[22] However, the informal understanding above suffices for most present purposes.

8. Fregean Representationalism

This leads to a natural proposal. Let us say that a *Fregean representational property* is the property of having a certain Fregean content (in a certain way). Let us say that *Fregean representationalism* is the thesis that phenomenal properties are equivalent to certain (pure or impure) Fregean representational properties. Then one might use the Fregean contents of the sort described earlier to put forward a version of Fregean representationalism.[23]

For example, one might propose that phenomenal redness is equivalent to the property of having a certain Fregean content (in the appropriate phenomenal way), where this Fregean content involves a mode of presentation such as *the property that normally causes experiences of phenomenal redness*. On this view, the relevant representational content does not directly involve the property attributed by the experience. It may well be that the experience attributes the property of redness to an object and that redness is a surface spectral reflectance property. This attributed property may enter into the Russellian content of the experience, but it does not enter

22. On this approach, the Fregean content of an experience can be analyzed as a primary intension mapping epistemic possibilities to extensions. In the next chapter I develop a more refined view of the Fregean content of experience in a way that respects some of the phenomenological insight of primitivism.

23. Thompson (2003) also defends Fregean representationalism.

into the Fregean content. Rather, the Fregean content involves a mode of presentation of this property.

It is highly plausible that two phenomenally identical experiences will have the same Fregean content. This will certainly be the case if the Fregean content of perceptual experiences works as described in the previous section, by requiring a certain relation to the relevant phenomenal property. For example, any two phenomenally red experiences will involve the mode of presentation *the property that normally causes phenomenally red experience.* Of course, this mode of presentation may pick out different properties in different environments or in creatures with different perceptual systems. In me, it might pick out a certain surface spectral reflectance; in a subject in a different environment or with a different perceptual system, it might pick out a different property entirely. But this is just what one would expect. One might worry about the reference to the perceiver: if the condition is characterized using different individuals in different cases, it will yield different Fregean contents. We can handle this by specifying that the content involves an indexical mode of presentation of the perceiver, one that can be shared between two different perceivers but is satisfied by different individuals in different contexts. (See the appendix for a way to model this using centered worlds.)

If this is correct, then a phenomenal property entails the corresponding Fregean representational property. For example, phenomenal redness entails visually phenomenally attributing a property under the Fregean mode of presentation *the property that normally causes phenomenally red experiences.* As for the converse, it seems plausible that any mental state that visually phenomenally attributes a property under this mode of presentation will itself be phenomenally red. One might be able to replace "visually" with "perceptually" as it is implausible that a nonvisual perceptual experience could attribute a property under this mode of presentation. It may well be that a *belief* could attribute a property under this mode of presentation, however, so one needs to at least specify a perceptual manner of presentation. As a result, it seems plausible that phenomenal redness is equivalent to the representational property of perceptually phenomenally representing the relevant Fregean content.

This view handles the central problems for Russellian representationalism straightforwardly. These views arose because Russellian representationalism is inconsistent with the plausible claims that (i) color experiences attribute colors to objects, (ii) color is an intrinsic property, and (iii) there can be veridical phenomenally identical experiences (in different subjects) of objects with relevantly different intrinsic properties.

By contrast, Fregean representationalism is clearly compatible with these claims, for the reasons given here.

The view is plausibly a sort of narrow representationalism. I have argued elsewhere that the Fregean content of thoughts (understood appropriately) is always a sort of narrow content. It can equally be argued that the Fregean content of perception is always a sort of narrow content. Given that the Fregean contents of a subject's experiences are determined by the subject's phenomenal properties and that the phenomenal properties are intrinsic properties of a subject, this conclusion follows automatically. So as long as the relevant manners of representation are also narrow, the resulting Fregean representational properties will be narrow, and we will have a sort of narrow representationalism.

The view is also naturally seen as a sort of nonreductive representationalism, as phenomenal notions are used in specifying the relevant Fregean contents. If one holds that the relevant manners of representation are also phenomenally specified (as I do), the result is a *doubly nonreductive* representationalism, involving phenomenal elements in both the manner of representation and the content.

This view has the potential to accommodate most of the problems mentioned so far. It is compatible with the narrowness of phenomenology, while also being compatible with the view that experience attributes intrinsic properties to objects. It is also compatible with our intuitions about the veridicality or nonveridicality of experiences in specific cases. Fregean content is defined in such a way that most of these intuitions are accommodated automatically. If one judges that a certain experience in a certain environment will be nonveridical, this requires only that the Fregean content of the experience be a condition that maps this environment to "false." The overall Fregean content of the experience will be a condition that mirrors our judgments about the veridicality of an experience under arbitrary hypotheses about the state of the external world.

Of course, this means that the Fregean content may need to be refined beyond the very crude first characterization given earlier (involving *the property that normally causes phenomenally red experiences*). But this was only a rough approximation. The real content will be a condition (or mapping) that reflects our specific judgments about cases. So if there are cases that the crude characterization of the content misclassifies as veridical or nonveridical (as there certainly will be), one may want to refine the characterization, but in any case the problem concerns only the characterization, not the content. The general thesis that phenomenal properties are Fregean representational properties will be unthreatened by any such case.

This Fregean representationalism is closely related to Shoemaker's dispositional Russellian representationalism, discussed earlier. Both views give a key role to dispositional notions such as *normally causes phenomenally red experiences*. The difference is that where Shoemaker's view holds that color experiences attribute these dispositions to objects, my view holds that color experience attributes intrinsic properties (colors) to objects, with the dispositional notions serving as a mode of presentation of these intrinsic properties. That is, a dispositional relation to experience is used to *determine* the property attributed by the experience, but the property attributed is not itself dispositional. This avoids one major difficulty for Shoemaker's view: the claim that the primary properties attributed by color experiences are not colors.

The other major difficulty for Shoemaker's view was the problem of specifying the relevant dispositions. This problem is easily handled here. The mode of presentation, spelled out more fully, will be something like *the property that normally causes phenomenally red experiences in me*, where the last part involves an indexical mode of presentation of oneself, a shared mode of presentation that different individuals can use to refer to themselves.[24] Indexical modes of presentation are already required for many other purposes in this sort of account of Fregean content, for example in specifying the Fregean content of indexical concepts such as *I* and *here*. Formally, they can be modeled using functions from centered possible worlds (worlds marked with an individual and a time) to extensions. So the Fregean content of *I* can be seen as a mapping that takes a centered world to the individual at the center of that world, and the Fregean content of a phenomenally red experience can be seen as a mapping that takes a centered world to whatever property normally causes red experiences in the individual at the center. (See the appendix for more on this approach.) While the notion of an indexical *property* is problematic, there is no such problem with the notion of an indexical mode of presentation. When a perceptual experience (embedded in an environment) has this sort of indexical mode of presentation, it will usually determine a perfectly objective property as its extension.

Another advantage of the Fregean view is that it accommodates the strong intuition that things could have been as they perceptually seem to be even had there been no observers. Counterfactual judgments of this sort generally reflect Russellian content rather than Fregean contents. (More

---

24. One might be tempted to replace *normally causes phenomenally red experiences in me* with *normally causes phenomenally red experiences in my community*. This would have the odd consequence that those who are spectrally inverted with respect to their community will have mostly illusory experiences.

generally, they reflect the second dimension in the two-dimensional framework rather than the first.) A view on which Russellian contents are dispositional has trouble respecting these judgments. In a world without observers, objects plausibly lack the relevant dispositional properties, so that the
Russellian content is not satisfied. By contrast, by allowing that Russellian
contents involve physical properties (picked out under a dispositional
mode of presentation), the Fregean view allows that the content can be
satisfied even in a world without observers.

One might wonder whether the Fregean view is compatible with the
oft-noted *transparency* of experiences. As I construe it, the central datum
of transparency is that when we attempt to introspect the qualities of our
experiences (e.g., phenomenal redness), we do so by attending to the
qualities of external objects (e.g., redness). In effect, we look "through"
the phenomenal property. But this is just what one would expect where
modes of presentation are involved. When one introspects the content of
a belief such as *Hesperus is bright,* one does so by thinking about Hesperus; one looks right through the mode of presentation. Nevertheless,
the mode of presentation exists, and one can become introspectively
aware of it. The same goes for manners of representation, such as visual-
ness. One looks "through" this manner of representation when introspecting an experience of phenomenal greenness, but the manner is nevertheless there, and one can obviously become introspectively aware of it.
(This case shows especially clearly that there is no inference from the
datum of transparency to the absence of introspective awareness). So if
phenomenal properties are associated with having certain modes of presentation of represented properties under certain manners of representation, it is to be expected that these properties will be transparent.

One might object that the sort of modes of presentation I have been
discussing overintellectualize the contents of experience. When one
attends to a red ball, one does not usually conceive of it as the cause of
one's experience or as possessing properties that normally cause that sort
of experience. This point is compatible with what I have said, however.
The Fregean contents I have appealed to may very often be *nonconceptual*
contents: to have a state with these contents, a subject need not deploy a
concept with those contents. So a subject's visual experience can have a
mode of presentation along the lines of *the object causing this experience*
without the subject's deploying the concept of causation or a concept of
the experience. It should be kept in mind that modes of presentation are
fundamentally *conditions*, which can be seen as mappings from scenarios
to extensions. The descriptive characterizations such as *the object causing
this experience* are only rough ways of characterizing these conditions. We

have to use linguistic expressions and concepts to formulate these characterizations, but the conditions themselves may be entirely nonlinguistic and nonconceptual.

Further, it seems clear that there is some psychological reality to these modes of presentation. When a subject has a perceptual experience, the subject is usually capable of judging whether the experience is veridical or not, depending on further information about the state of the world. For example, if a rational subject discovers that there is no object causing the experience, the subject will conclude that the experience is nonveridical. Speaking broadly, one might think of this pattern of judgments as part of the *inferential role* of the experience. The Fregean content of an experience reflects this sort of inferential role directly, and it is plausible that the (rational) inferential role of an experience is grounded in some fashion in the representational content of the experience. So there is good reason to think that Fregean representational properties play an important psychological role.

I have outlined how this account works for the case of a simple color experience. The account can be generalized to other visual experiences, though some tricky issues arise. Thompson (2003) argues that one can handle spatial experiences in a similar way. These function by attributing properties (or relations) to objects, where these properties are picked out under a mode of presentation that characterized them as being those properties that stand in the relevant causal relation to spatial phenomenal properties. Other aspects of visual experience might be handled similarly.

It is natural to extend the account to other perceptual experiences and to bodily sensations. It is easy enough to see how this will go: in every case, there will be a mode of presentation that picks out a property as something like the normal cause of the sort of experience in question. Here I do not address the issue of whether this extension would be appropriate. There are some difficult questions, not least about whether (for example) olfactory or pain experiences can be veridical or nonveridical. I am inclined to say that *if* these experiences can be veridical or nonveridical, then an extension of the current approach will give a reasonable analysis of their content.

9. Summary

It may be useful to sum up the various distinctions that have been introduced and to indicate where the view I have advocated falls.

Representationalism holds that phenomenal properties are equivalent to pure or impure representational properties: properties of representing a certain content (in a certain manner).

Pure representationalism holds that phenomenal properties are equivalent to pure representational properties: properties of representing a certain content. *Impure representationalism* holds that phenomenal properties are equivalent to impure representational properties: properties of representing a certain content in a certain manner.

Reductive representationalism holds that phenomenal properties are equivalent to representational properties that can be fully characterized in nonphenomenal terms. *Nonreductive representationalism* holds that phenomenal properties are equivalent to representational properties that cannot be fully characterized in nonphenomenal terms. Nonreductive representationalism might be nonreductive about the manner of representation or about the representational content or both.

Narrow representationalism holds that phenomenal properties are equivalent to narrow representational properties, depending only on a subject's intrinsic properties. *Wide representationalism* holds that phenomenal properties are equivalent to wide representational properties, depending partly on the subject's environment.

Russellian representationalism holds that phenomenal properties are equivalent to Russellian representational properties, with contents involving objects and/or properties in the world. (One can further distinguish *physical, projectivist, primitivist,* and *dispositionalist* Russellian representationalism, depending on what properties are held to be represented.) *Fregean representationalism* holds that phenomenal properties are equivalent to Fregean representational properties, with contents involving modes of presentation of objects and properties in the world.

The view I have advocated is a form of impure, nonreductive, narrow, Fregean representationalism. The view is in fact doubly nonreductive, with phenomenal elements involved in both the manner of representation and the representational content. In the case of a phenomenal color property, the associated manner of representation is required to be a perceptual phenomenal manner of representation. The associated representational content is a Fregean mode of presentation, one that picks out whatever property normally causes that sort of color experience in the subject. This view contrasts sharply with the most common versions of representationalism, which are reductive, wide, and Russellian.

10. Conclusion

I expect that the interface between consciousness and intentionality will be the central topic in the next few years of the philosophy of mind. I hope that the analysis I have given here helps to clarify some crucial issues in exploring this interface and opens up some underexplored possibilities for making progress.

What of the issues mentioned at the start of the chapter? Is consciousness grounded in intentionality, or is intentionality grounded in consciousness? I have argued for a necessary equivalence between phenomenal and representational properties, but which of the phenomenal and the representational is more fundamental?

The nonreductive approach I have taken offers little prospect for grounding consciousness wholly in intentionality, where the latter is construed independently of consciousness. The representational analyses I have given all make unreduced appeal to phenomenal notions, and I think there is little hope of giving analyses that do without such notions altogether. So a reduction of the phenomenal to the representational is not on the cards.

One might think that this approach offers more hope of grounding intentionality in consciousness. It is not implausible that there is something about consciousness that by its very nature yields representation of the world. One might hold that at least with perceptual experiences, representational content accrues *in virtue* of the phenomenology. One might further hold that something similar holds for beliefs: their representational content accrues either in virtue of their phenomenal character or in virtue of their connections to other beliefs and experiences whose content is grounded in phenomenal character.

Still, for this approach to provide a reductive grounding of the intentional, we would need to characterize the underlying phenomenal domain in nonintentional terms, and it is far from clear that this is possible. On the face of things, a characterization of my phenomenology that avoids intentional notions entirely would be quite inadequate. Rather, intentional content appears to be part and parcel of phenomenology: it is part of the essential nature of phenomenology that it is directed outward at a world. If so, we cannot reduce intentionality to something more fundamental. At best, we can locate its roots in the intentionality of the phenomenal.

I think, then, that the most attractive view is one on which neither consciousness nor intentionality is more fundamental than the other. Rather, consciousness and intentionality are intertwined, all the way down to the ground.

Afterword: The Two-Dimensional Content of Perception

The Fregean and Russellian content of perceptual experience can be modeled using the two-dimensional framework for the analysis of content. This analysis is not required in order to make use of the notions of Fregean and Russellian content (which can be understood intuitively as in the text), but it helps in order to make the use of these notions more precise and in order to analyze certain subtleties that arise. It can also help us to shed light on the relationship between the content of perception and belief.

In the linguistic version of the two-dimensional framework, expression tokens are associated with two intensions, or functions from possible worlds to extensions. The Fregean content of an expression is associated with a primary intension: a function from centered worlds to extensions, where a centered world is a world marked with a designated individual and a designated time (intuitively, these represent the perspective of the subject who utters the expression). The Russellian content of an expression is simply its extension. For more complex expressions, their Fregean and Russellian contents will be complex structures determined by the Fregean and Russellian contents of their parts.

For example, the Fregean content of 'Hesperus' can be seen as a primary intension that, in a given centered world, picks out (roughly) the bright object that has been visible in the appropriate location in the evening sky around the center of that world, while the Fregean content of 'Phosphorus' is an analogous intension involving the morning sky. The Russellian content associated with 'Hesperus' is the planet Venus. Likewise, the Fregean content of 'Hesperus is Phosphorus' is a structured intension involving both the morning-sky and evening-sky intensions, and will be true in a centered world (roughly) iff the bright objects that have been visible at certain positions in the evening and morning skies around the center of that world are identical. The Russellian content associated with 'Hesperus is Phosphorus' is the structured object-involving proposition that Venus is Venus.

This framework can be extended to the contents of mental states such as beliefs (Chalmers 2002a), and the preceding discussion suggests that it can also be extended to the contents of perceptual experiences. The Fregean content of a perceptual experience can be seen as a structured primary intension. The Russellian content is a structured Russellian proposition involving objects and properties.

Suppose I see a red object in front of me. The Russellian content of this experience might be the Russellian proposition composed from the object O, its color C, and its location L: roughly, the proposition that O is at L

and has *C*. The Fregean content of this proposition will be a structured primary intension composed from the primary intensions related to the objectual, spatial, and color aspects of the experience. The objectual primary intension might be an intension picking out the object that is causing a certain experience (in the right sort of way) in the subject at the center of the world. The spatial primary intension might be an intension picking out the location that stands in a certain spatial relation to the subject at the center (strictly speaking, this may need to be complicated to invoke spatial relations that typically bring about certain experiences, for reasons I discuss in the next two chapters, but for now I stay with the simpler account). The color primary intension might be an intension picking out the property that normally causes phenomenally red experiences in the subject at the center. Putting these together, the Fregean content of the experience will be a structured primary intension that is satisfied at a centered world iff the object causing the relevant experience stands in the relevant spatial relation to the center and has a property that typically causes phenomenally red experiences there.

The Fregean content of an experience, along with the environment, determines its Russellian content. For example, in the preceding case, object *O* is precisely the object that meets the condition laid down by the Fregean content: the condition of being the object that appropriately causes the experience. Something similar applies to *C* and *L*. Of course, if one has a phenomenally identical experience that involves a different object *O′*, the Fregean content will be the same, but the Russellian content will involve *O′* instead of *O*. If one has a phenomenally identical hallucination, then no object will meet the criterion of appropriately causing the experience. In this case, the Fregean content of the experience will be as before, but where the previous Russellian contents involved objects *O* and *O′*, the Russellian content of the hallucinatory experience will involve no object at all.[25]

Likewise, in different environments, one can have two phenomenally identical experiences of objects at different locations. These experiences will have the same Fregean content, representing the objects to be at a location that stands in the right spatial relation to the location at the center of a centered world.[26] But the two experiences will occur at the

25. *Here it is most natural to model the Russellian content as a so-called gappy proposition. For other approaches that use gappy propositions to model the contents of hallucinations, see Schellenberg (forthcoming) and Tye (2009).

26. *Schroeder and Caplan (2007) argue that phenomenally identical veridical experiences of objects at different locations pose a problem for representationalism. The problem is removed if one embraces centered-world contents, as on the current account. See Brogaard (forthcoming) for more on this.

center of two different centered worlds, so different locations will stand in the spatial relation to the location at the center. This will result in different Russellian contents involving different locations. Something similar can happen with color, at least in the inversion cases discussed previously.

Strictly speaking, we might say that the Fregean content of an experience *determines* a primary intension rather than that it *is* a primary intension. This allows these contents to have a finer-grained structure than functions from worlds to extensions. For example, following Peacocke (1992), one might argue that when one sees an object as a square and then as a regular diamond, there is a phenomenological difference that corresponds to a difference in content (representing something as a square or a regular diamond) that cannot easily be modeled as a function from worlds to extensions. In these cases one might appeal to conditions on extension that are finer-grained than functions from worlds to extensions. Still, as before, these contents will at least determine associated intensions. In what follows the differences do not play a large role, so it will be useful to use primary intensions to analyze Fregean contents.

Can we define the Fregean content of a perceptual experience more precisely, so that it is grounded in antecedently understood notions? In the two-dimensional analysis of belief and language, as I understand it, primary intensions correspond to the evaluation of epistemic possibilities: ways the world might actually be, for all we know a priori. The same goes for the analysis of perceptual experience.

Intuitively, a perceptual experience places a constraint on epistemically possible states of the world. For all I know a priori, there are many ways that the world could turn out to be. We can think of these ways as epistemic possibilities (in a broad sense), and we can model them using centered worlds. The same goes for the epistemic possibilities that confront a perceiver. For example, when I have a phenomenally red experience, it is epistemically possible that the object I am looking at has property P_1 and that P_1 normally causes phenomenally red experiences, and it is epistemically possible that the object I am looking at has property P_2 and that P_2 normally causes phenomenally red experiences. These two hypotheses correspond to different centered worlds w_1 and w_2. Intuitively, whether w_1 or w_2 turns out to be actual, my experience will be veridical. So we can say that w_1 and w_2 both verify the experience. On the other hand, there are worlds w_3 and w_4, where the object that the subject at the center is looking at has P_1 and P_2 (respectively) but in which that property normally causes phenomenally green experiences. Intuitively, if w_3 or w_4 turn out to be actual, my experience will be falsidical. So we can say that w_3 and w_4 both falsify the experience. These intuitions can be encapsulated in the claim that the primary intension of the experience is true in w_1 and w_2 but false in w_3 and w_4.

We can likewise evaluate perceptual experiences with respect to counterfactual circumstances considered via subjunctive conditionals. If I have a phenomenally red experience directed at a red book B, then I can ask: if my eyes had been closed, but the book had still been present, would things have been as I (actually) perceive them to be? The intuitive answer is yes. Or I can ask: if the book had been present with the same intrinsic properties, but if I had been such that the book normally caused phenomenally green experiences in me, would things have been as I (actually) perceive them to be? The intuitions about this case are a bit less clear, but there is at least some intuition that the answer is yes. Intuitions of this sort suggest that with respect to counterfactual circumstances, the perceptual experience will be veridical (at least with respect to color) roughly iff the book B is (physically) red in those circumstances. This can be encapsulated by saying that the secondary intension of the experience is true in a world iff book B is red in that world.

One might even define the secondary intension of a perceptual experience in terms of these subjunctive conditionals. One can say that the secondary intension of an experience E is true at a world w iff, had w obtained, things would have been the way that they appear to be to the subject (actually) undergoing E. To the extent that our judgments about these subjunctive conditionals are not fully determinate, the corresponding secondary intension may not be fully determinate, but the intension may nevertheless capture some of our intuitions about content. In any case, secondary intensions for experiences play little role in the current framework as the corresponding work can be done by Russellian content instead.

Defining the primary intension of a perceptual experience is not as straightforward. So far I have talked in an intuitive way of a condition on extension and about the evaluation of epistemic possibilities, but this falls short of a definition. One could simply leave a notion here as basic, but it would be nice to do more. One thought is to appeal to indicative conditionals. For example, one could hold that the primary intension of an experience E is true in a centered world w iff: given that the actual world is qualitatively like w (and if I am in the position of the person at the center of w at the time of w), then E is veridical. The trouble is that one may want to evaluate the experience at worlds where the experience is not itself present. It is not obviously part of the content of an experience E that E itself obtains: one may want to hold that the content constrains only the external world. Furthermore, in the case of beliefs and utterances, there are good reasons not to define primary intensions in terms of conditionals that make explicit reference to whether a belief or utterance would be true as it occurs in some circumstance (see Chalmers 2004b), and these reasons plausibly extend to the case of perceptual experience. So it would be useful to have a definition that applies more broadly than this.

In the case of beliefs, one can define a primary intension in terms of the belief's inferential connections. In particular, one can say that the primary intension of belief B is true at a centered world w if there is an appropriate inferential connection between the hypothesis that w is actual and B. (The hypothesis that w is actual can be understood more strictly as the hypothesis that D is the case, where D is an appropriate canonical specification of w.) One way of understanding the inferential connection is in terms of rational inference: if a subject were to accept that w is actual, ought the subject rationally accept B? Another arguably better way is to understand it in terms of a priori entailment: if the subject accepts that w is actual, ought (idealized) a priori reasoning from there lead the subject to accept B?

A definition along these lines is not as straightforward in the case of perceptual experiences, as the notion of an inferential connection from an arbitrary hypothesis to a perceptual experience is not entirely clear. However, one can give such a definition by relying on certain inferential connections between perceptual experiences and beliefs that are somewhat clearer. In particular, we have a reasonable grip on what it is for a subject to *take an experience at face value*, yielding a perceptual belief. In such a case, we can say that the perceptual belief *endorses* the perceptual experience. Note that a belief that endorses a perceptual experience should be distinguished from a belief that the perceptual experience is true. The latter is a belief directed at the experience, but the former is a belief directed at the world.

The notion of endorsement is a primitive in the current account, but one can say some things to characterize it. Endorsement is a sort of truth-preserving inference between perception and belief: when a belief endorses a veridical experience, the belief will be true. This need not be true in reverse: that is, it can happen that a belief endorses a falsidical experience without being false itself. This can happen for a complex experience, for example, when intuitively the belief takes certain aspects of the experience at face value and abstracts away from others. For example, a belief might endorse my current visual experience where color is concerned and abstract away from shape. If my experience is veridical with respect to color but not to shape, the experience will be overall falsidical, but the endorsing belief will be veridical. On this conception, an endorsing belief may make fewer commitments than the experience that it endorses, but it cannot make any commitments that are not made by the experience that it endorses.

One can also introduce a notion of *complete endorsement*. A belief completely endorses an experience when it endorses that experience in all its aspects. Complete endorsement preserves both truth and falsity: when a belief endorses a falsidical experience, the belief will be false. For experiences of any complexity, it is not clear that we have the capacity to completely endorse them (as it is not clear that we can have beliefs with the relevant detail and complexity), but it seems that the notion is reasonable at least for simple experiences and as an idealization in the case of complex experiences.

With these notions in place, we can use them in conjunction with the already defined notion of the primary intension of a belief to characterize the primary intension of a perceptual experience. One can say that the primary intension of an experience E is true at a centered world w iff the primary intension of any possible belief that endorses E is true at w. One could also appeal to complete endorsement here by simply equating the primary intension of a perceptual experience with that of a belief that completely endorses it, but the definition in terms of endorsement has fewer commitments. It does not require that complete endorsements exist for all perceptual experiences. Intuitively, it simply requires that for any aspect of a perceptual experience, there is some belief that endorses that aspect.

The picture needs to be complicated slightly to handle the two-stage view in the next chapter (knowledge of which is presupposed by the following two paragraphs). We could say that just as there are two standards of veridicality for perceptual experiences, there are two standards of truth for perceptual beliefs: perfect and imperfect truth, say. On this model, endorsing a perfectly veridical experience will produce a perfectly true perceptual belief, and endorsing an imperfectly veridical experience will produce an imperfectly true belief. One could then associate a perceptual belief with two different primary intensions that correspond to the standards of perfect and imperfect truth. These intensions will then ground two different primary intensions for an experience, corresponding to perfect and imperfect veridicality.

Alternatively, and perhaps more plausibly, one could say that there is just one standard of truth for beliefs and two sorts of endorsement: perfect and imperfect endorsement, say. Intuitively, perfectly endorsing an experience requires holding that experience to the standard of perfect veridicality, while imperfectly endorsing it requires holding it only to the standard of imperfect veridicality. On this model, imperfectly endorsing an imperfectly (or perfectly) veridical experience will produce a true belief, and perfectly endorsing a perfectly veridical experience will produce a true belief, but perfectly endorsing an imperfectly veridical experience may produce a false belief. In this model a belief will be associated with just one primary intension, but the two different endorsement relations will yield two different primary intensions for an experience. I will not choose between the two models here.

One might argue that there are representational aspects of perceptual experience that cannot be endorsed by any possible belief. For example, one might hold that extremely fleeting experiences or experiences that are far outside attention cannot be endorsed. Or one might argue that experiences in animals that lack concepts cannot be endorsed. In these cases one could make a case that it is at least *possible* for the experiences to be endorsed, perhaps assuming some idealization of the subject's actual cognitive capacity, but this is clearly a substantive issue, and the answer is unclear. For this reason, the earlier characterization is probably best not regarded as a definition but it is at least a useful characterization that gives reasonably precise results for a wide range of ordinary experiences.

So far I have characterized an unstructured primary intension for an experience rather than a structured primary intension. To do the latter, one needs to associate primary intensions with experiential qualities such as experiences as of color, space, and objects. The story here is a natural development of the story already given. A subtlety arises concerning the object-oriented aspect of the experience. If one holds that the Russellian content of a nonhallucinatory experience involves the object of the experience, then there should be a corresponding element of the Fregean content of the experience that picks the object out. Here the natural suggestion is that Fregean content picks out the object as the object that is causing (or that is appropriately perceptually connected to) the current experience. This suggests a primary intension that maps a centered world to the object causing (or perceptually connected to) the relevant experience of the subject at the center of the centered world. To model this, one may need to build in a marked experience to the center of the relevant centered worlds since the subject at the center may have many experiences (this is something that one has to do in any case; see the objection from demonstratives in chapter 6). One can then say that the primary intension of a phenomenally red experience is true in a centered world if the object that causes (or is appropriately connected to) the marked experience at the center of that world stands in the relevant spatial relation to the subject at the center and has the property that normally causes phenomenally red experiences.

There is no requirement that either Russellian content or Fregean content be *conceptual* content. That is, it is not required that to have an experience with a given Russellian or Fregean content, a subject must have concepts with corresponding content. Frege's own favored variety of content was a sort of conceptual content: Fregean senses were always grasped through the possession of corresponding concepts. But the Fregean contents discussed here need not be Fregean in that respect. Rather, they are Fregean in the sense that they involve modes of presentation of objects and properties in the world, whether or not these modes of presentation involve concepts.

My own view is that a subject can have perceptual experiences with quite determinate content even without possessing corresponding concepts. For example, one can have a color experience that represents a given shade even without possessing a concept of that shade. It is nevertheless plausible that such an experience possesses a Russellian content (attributing that shade to an object), and it also possesses a Fregean content (one that is true if the object appropriately related to the perceiver has the property that normally causes the relevant sort of experience). If so, these contents are nonconceptual contents. An experience can have such contents even if the subject lacks a concept of the relevant shade, lacks a concept of the relevant experience, and lacks a concept of "normally causes." I will not argue for this claim here, however, and it is inessential for the other claims in this chapter.

These nonconceptual Fregean contents need not themselves be a different sort of object from conceptual Fregean contents. For example, it could be that an experience as of a red object and a belief that completely endorses it have the same Fregean content. Instead, one might say that the Fregean content of perception involves a nonconceptual content *relation*: the relation that associates perceptual states with their Fregean contents is such that subjects need not possess the relevant concepts in order for their states to have the relevant content.[27] A pluralist about content can hold that there are both conceptual and nonconceptual content relations, but nonconceptual content relations are likely to be particularly useful in the analysis of perception.

---

27. Heck (2000) distinguishes the "content view" of nonconceptual content (on which nonconceptual contents are objects quite distinct from conceptual contents) from the "state view" (on which nonconceptual contents are contents of nonconceptual states). One might call the conception suggested here the "relational view" of nonconceptual content. It is somewhat closer to the state view than to the content view, but it need not invoke the idea of a "conceptual state."

12

PERCEPTION AND THE FALL FROM EDEN

1. Eden

In the Garden of Eden, we had unmediated contact with the world. We were directly acquainted with objects in the world and with their properties. Objects were presented to us without causal mediation, and properties were revealed to us in their true intrinsic glory.

When an apple in Eden looked red to us, the apple was gloriously, perfectly, and primitively *red*. There was no need for a long causal chain from the microphysics of the surface through air and brain to a contingently connected visual experience. Rather, the perfect redness of the apple was simply revealed to us. The qualitative redness in our experience derived entirely from the presentation of perfect redness in the world.

Eden was a world of perfect color. But then there was a Fall.

First, we ate from the Tree of Illusion. After this, objects sometimes seemed to have different colors and shapes at different times, even though there was reason to believe that the object itself had not changed. So the connection between visual experience and the world became contingent: we could no longer accept that visual experience always revealed the world exactly as it is.

Second, we ate from the Tree of Science. After this, we found that when we see an object, there is always a causal chain involving the transmission of light from the object to the retina and the transmission of electrical activity from the retina to the brain. This chain was triggered by microphysical properties whose connection to the qualities of our experience seemed entirely contingent. So there was no longer reason to believe in acquaintance with the glorious primitive properties of Eden, and there was no good reason to believe that objects in the world had these properties at all.

We no longer live in Eden. Perhaps Eden never existed, and perhaps it could not have existed. But Eden still plays a powerful role in our perceptual experience of the world. At some level, perception represents our world as an Edenic world, populated by perfect colors and shapes, with objects and properties that are revealed to us directly. And even though we have fallen from Eden, Eden still acts as a sort of ideal that regulates the content of our perceptual experience. Or so I will argue.

2. Phenomenal Content

My project in this chapter concerns the *phenomenal content* of perceptual experience. This notion can be defined in terms of the notions of *phenomenal character* and *representational content*.

The phenomenal character of a perceptual experience is what it is like to have that experience. Two perceptual experiences share their phenomenal character if what it is like to have one is the same as what it is like to have the other. We can say that in such a case, the experiences instantiate the same phenomenal properties. As I use the term "perceptual experience," it is true by definition that any perceptual experience has phenomenal character. As I use the term, it is not true by definition that every perceptual experience has an object in the external world: hallucinatory experiences count as perceptual experiences.

A representational content of a perceptual experience is a condition of satisfaction of the experience. I take it for granted that perceptual experiences can be veridical or falsidical: they can represent the world correctly or incorrectly. Intuitively, perceptual illusions and hallucinations are falsidical, while nonillusory perceptual experiences of objects in the external world are veridical. And intuitively, a given experience will be either veridical or falsidical, depending on what the world is like. If so, we can say that an experience is associated with a condition of satisfaction. If and only if the world satisfies the condition, then an experience will be veridical. For example, one might plausibly hold that an ordinary experience of a red square in front of one will be veridical roughly when there is a red square in front of one.

A *phenomenal content* of a perceptual experience is a representational content that is determined by the experience's phenomenal character. More precisely, a representational content C of a perceptual experience E is a phenomenal content if and only if, necessarily, any experience with the phenomenal character of E has representational content C.

Put this way, it is a substantive thesis that perceptual experiences have phenomenal content. But there is good reason to believe that they do. As I discuss in the previous chapter (and see Siewert 1998), it is plausible that perceptual experiences are assessable for accuracy in virtue of their phenomenal character. Intuitively, by virtue of their phenomenal character, experiences present the world as being a certain way. My experience of a red square in front of me has a certain phenomenal character, and by virtue of this phenomenal character, the experience places a constraint on the world. The world can be such as to satisfy the constraint imposed by the phenomenal character of the experience or such as to fail to satisfy the constraint. This is to say that the phenomenal character determines a condition of satisfaction for the experience, one that is shared by any experience with the same phenomenal character. This condition of satisfaction will be a phenomenal content.

The plausible thesis that perceptual experiences have phenomenal content leaves many other questions open. For example, the thesis is neutral on whether phenomenal character is prior to representational content or vice versa. The thesis is compatible with the claim that phenomenal character is grounded in representational content and with the claim that representational content is grounded in phenomenal character.

The thesis also leaves open the nature of phenomenal content. On the face of it, there are many ways to associate representational contents with perceptual experience. For example, one might associate a perceptual experience with an object-involving content (the content that O is F, where O is the object of the experience), an existential property-involving content (for example, the content that there exists something in location L that is F), a content involving modes of presentation of these objects and properties (more on this shortly), and perhaps others.

My own view is that one should be a pluralist about representational content. It may be that experiences can be associated with contents of many different sorts by different relations: we can call such relations *content relations*. For example, there may be one content relation that associates experiences with object-involving contents and another that associates experiences with existential contents. Each of the different sorts of content and the corresponding content relations may have a role to play for different explanatory purposes. On this view, there may not be such a thing as *the* representational content of a perceptual experience. Instead, a given experience may be associated with multiple representational contents via different content relations.

On the other hand, not all of these contents are equally plausible candidates to be *phenomenal* contents. Some of these contents seem to be such that they can vary independently of the phenomenal character of an experience. If so, they may be representational contents of the experience, but they are not phenomenal contents. More precisely, we can say that a given content relation is a *phenomenal content relation* when any two experiences with the same phenomenal character are related by the content relation to the same content. A phenomenal content relation relates a given experience to a phenomenal content of the experience. For ease of usage, I will speak of *the* phenomenal content of an experience, but we should leave open the possibility that there is more than one phenomenal content relation so that a given experience can be associated with phenomenal contents of more than one sort. Later in the chapter I explore this possibility in detail.

In this chapter I focus on the following question: what is the phenomenal content of a perceptual experience? This is a more constrained question than the corresponding question simply about representational content, but it is an important question to answer. On the face of it, the phenomenal content of an experience is an extremely important aspect of its representational content: it captures a way in which the world is presented in the *phenomenology* of the experience. One can reasonably expect that if we can understand phenomenal content, this will help us to understand the relationship between phenomenal character and representational content, and it may well help us to understand the nature of phenomenology itself.

In the previous chapter, I discussed two hypotheses about phenomenal content. There I argued (in effect) that phenomenal content is a sort of Fregean content rather than a sort of Russellian content. In what follows, I briefly recapitulate that discussion in a way that brings the question of phenomenal content to center stage. I then raise some further problems for the Fregean hypothesis, involving its phenomenological adequacy. I will argue that these problems are best handled by moving to a more refined view of phenomenal content, one that gives Edenic representation a key role.

3. Russellian Content

I will focus on the phenomenal content of visual experiences and especially of experiences of color. I take the canonical sort of color experience to be an experience as of an object having a certain color at a certain location. Our experiences typically present objects to us as having a certain distribution of colors at different locations on their surfaces. A book might be

presented to me as being certain shades of blue at some points on its surface and as being certain shades of red at other points. For simplicity, I
focus just on the experience of color at a specific point: for example, the
experience of a book's being a specific shade of blue at a specific location
on its surface. The conclusions generalize, however, and I will discuss the
generalization later in the chapter.

What is the phenomenal content of such a color experience? That is,
what sort of representational content is shared by all experiences with the
same phenomenal character as the original experience?

A first attempt to answer this question might be the following: the experience represents object O (the book) as having color C (a specific shade of blue)
at location L (a particular point in space). So one can associate the experience
with the following condition of satisfaction: the experience is satisfied iff object
O has color C at location L. This is an *object-involving* content: it involves a
specific object O, and its satisfaction depends on the properties of O. We can
say that in this case, the experience attributes a certain sort of color property to
the object O.

It is plausible that experiences have contents of this sort. When a
certain book appears red to us, there is a quite reasonable sense in which
the experience will be satisfied iff the book in question is red at the relevant location. That is, satisfaction conditions for experiences can often
be understood in terms of the instantiation of certain properties (such
as redness) by certain objects (such as the book). In these cases, we can
say that the experience *attributes* the property to the object.

It is implausible that this object-involving content is a phenomenal content, however. On the face of it, there might be an experience with the
same phenomenal character as the original experience but directed at a
quite different object O' (perhaps an experience that I could have when
looking at a different copy of the same book, for example). And plausibly,
there might be an experience with the same phenomenal character as the
original experience but directed at no object at all (a hallucinatory experience, for example). These experiences could not have an object-involving
content involving the original object O. The former experience will at best
have a content involving a different object O', and the latter experience
may have no object-involving content at all. If so, the object-involving
content is not phenomenal content.[1]

---

1. One sort of disjunctivism about perceptual experience (disjunctivism about phenomenology)
denies both that experiences directed at different objects could have the same phenomenology and that
a hallucinatory experience could have the same phenomenology as an experience of an external object.
According to this view, phenomenal content might be object-involving. I assume that this view is false
in what follows. Another variety of disjunctivism (disjunctivism about metaphysics) allows that a hal-

A somewhat more plausible candidate for the phenomenal content of the experience is the following: the experience represents that there is an object that has color C at location L. This content is not object involving: in effect it is existentially quantified, so it does not build in any specific object. Unlike the object-involving content, this content can be possessed by experiences that are directed at different objects or at no object at all. The content is property-involving, however: in effect, it has a color property and a location property as its constituents. For the content to be a remotely viable candidate for phenomenal content, the location property cannot be an *absolute* location property. A phenomenally identical experience might be instantiated in a quite different location, and it is not plausible that this experience could attribute the same absolute location property as the original experience. Rather, the location property must be a *relative* location property: the property of being a certain distance in front of the perceiver at a certain angle, for example.

The contents discussed above are all Russellian contents in that they are composed of objects and properties. The object-involving content can be seen as a certain structured complex of an object, a location property, and a color property, while the existential content can be seen as a structured complex involving an existential quantifier, a location property, and a color property. We can say that both of these contents involve the attribution of certain specific properties, although in one case the properties are attributed to specific objects, and in the other case to an unspecified object under an existential quantifier. Contents of this sort contrast with Fregean contents, composed of modes of presentation of objects and properties in the world, to be discussed shortly.

Let us say that the *Russellian hypothesis* holds that the phenomenal content of a perceptual experience is a sort of Russellian content. To assess this hypothesis, I henceforth abstract away from issues involving the representation of objects and focus on the representation of properties. In

---

lucinatory experience and an ordinary perceptual experience may share phenomenal character but holds that they have a fundamentally distinct underlying metaphysical nature: one experience involves an object, and one does not. I am neutral about this view in what follows. A third variety (disjunctivism about content) allows that these experiences have the same phenomenology but holds that they have different representational contents: for example, experiences of different objects will have different object-involving contents. Proponents of this view will agree that these object-involving contents are not phenomenal contents. They may deny that there is any phenomenal content, holding that the relevant experiences share no content, or they may accept that there is phenomenal content while holding that it is less fundamental than object-involving content. I am inclined to reject both varieties of disjunctivism about content, but I will not assume that they are false. In what follows I in effect argue against the former view, but some of what I say may be compatible with the latter view.

particular, I will focus on the representation of color properties—or at least on the representation of properties by color experience. Later I will discuss the representation of other properties.

According to the Russellian hypothesis, the phenomenal content that is distinctively associated with color experience will be a Russellian property-involving content, involving the attribution of a property C. The Russellian hypothesis requires the *Russellian constraint*: all phenomenally identical color experiences attribute the same property to their object.

Strictly speaking, the Russellian hypothesis requires only that *globally* identical experiences attribute the same property to their objects, so that the property attributed may depend on the holistic character of a visual experience, including its spatial phenomenal character and its overall pattern of color phenomenal character. For simplicity, I usually assume a view on which the property attributed depends on the *local* phenomenal character of the experience, so that any two experiences with the same local phenomenal character in respect of color will attribute the same property. Nothing important depends on this assumption, however.

We can say two experiences that share their local phenomenal character instantiate the same local phenomenal properties. Local phenomenal properties include properties such as *phenomenal redness*. This is a property instantiated by all experiences that share a certain specific and determinate local phenomenal character, one that is often caused (in us) by seeing things with a certain specific shade of red. ("Phenomenal red$_{31}$-ness" might be a more apt label for a determinate property than "phenomenal redness," but I use expressions of the latter sort for ease of presentation.) Note that phenomenal redness (a property of experiences) will plausibly be distinct from ordinary redness and from the property attributed by phenomenally red experiences.

If the phenomenal content of color experience is Russellian, what sort of properties does it attribute? Intuitively, these properties are color properties. A phenomenally red experience plausibly attributes redness, for example. I do not assume this in what follows, so that room is left open for views on which color experiences represent properties other than color properties. However, as in chapter 11, the natural hypotheses concerning the nature of the attributed properties correspond fairly closely to the standard range of options concerning the nature of color properties.

As before, one might hold that the properties attributed are *physical* properties: something along the lines of a surface spectral reflectance. One might hold that the properties attributed are *dispositional* properties, involving the disposition to cause a certain sort of experience in appropriate conditions. One might hold that the properties attributed are *mental* properties of some sort: perhaps properties that are actually instantiated by one's experiences or by one's visual fields. Or one might hold that the properties attributed are *primitive* properties: simple intrinsic qualities of the sort that might have been instantiated in Eden.

Each of these views is a version of the Russellian hypothesis. We might call them *physicalist, dispositionalist, projectivist,* and *primitivist* versions of Russellianism concerning phenomenal content. Each of these views is held by some philosophers. For example, the physicalist view is held by Tye (1995); the dispositionalist view is held by Shoemaker (2001); the projectivist view is held by Boghossian and Velleman (1989); and the primitivist view is held by Maund (1995).[2]

Each of these views has well-known problems, discussed in the previous chapter. The physicalist view is incompatible with intuitions about spectrum inversion, according to which phenomenally identical color experiences could have represented quite different physical properties in different environments, and it also seems to be incompatible with the internalist intuition that phenomenal character does not constitutively depend on an individual's environment. The dispositionalist view is incompatible with the intuition that color experience attributes nonrelational properties and also has serious difficulties in individuating the relevant dispositions so that phenomenally identical experiences always attribute the same dispositions. The projectivist and primitivist views suffer from the problem that it seems that the relevant properties are not actually instantiated by external objects, with the consequence that all color experience is illusory.

One can summarize the problems with the following general argument against a Russellian view:

1. Some phenomenally red experiences of ordinary objects are veridical.
2. Necessarily, a phenomenally red experience of an object is veridical iff its object instantiates the property attributed by the experience.
3. The properties attributed by color experiences are nonrelational properties.
4. For any veridical phenomenally red experience of an ordinary object, it is possible that there is a falsidical phenomenally red

---

2. The physicalist view is also held by Byrne and Hilbert (2003), Dretske (1995), and Lycan (1996). Versions of the dispositionalist view are also held by Egan (2006) and Kriegel (2002b). Versions of the primitivist view are also held by Campbell (1993), Holman (2002), Johnston (forthcoming), McGinn (1996), Thau (2002), and Wright (2003). See Stoljar (2007) and chapter 11 for more discussion of these alternatives.

experience of an object with the same nonrelational properties as
the original object.

_____

5. There is no property that is attributed by all possible phenomenally
red experiences.

Here, premise 1 has obvious plausibility, and premise 2 is a natural part
of any view on which experiences attribute properties. Premise 3 is grounded
in the phenomenology of color experience, and premise 4 corresponds to
a fairly weak inversion claim. In fact, a version of premise 4 with a mere
existential quantifier instead of a universal quantifier would suffice for the
conclusion. But, the universally quantified claim seems no less plausible.
Take any veridical phenomenally red experience of an ordinary object such
as an apple. Then it is plausible that there could be a community (one with
a somewhat different visual apparatus or with a somewhat different environment) in which apples of that sort normally cause phenomenally green
experiences rather than phenomenally red experiences and in which phenomenally red experiences are caused by objects of a quite different sort. In
such a community, it might happen that on one occasion in unusual conditions, such an apple causes a phenomenally red experience. It is plausible
that such an experience would not be veridical.

The conclusion follows straightforwardly from the premises. Premises 1
and 4 entail that there are possible veridical and nonveridical phenomenally red experiences of objects with the same nonrelational properties.
Conjoined with premises 2 and 3, one can conclude that there is no property attributed by both experiences. The conclusion entails that that there
is no Russellian content that is shared by all phenomenally red experiences
(given the natural assumption that if an experience has Russellian content,
the property attributed by the experience is attributed by its Russellian
content). The argument generalizes straightforwardly from phenomenal
redness to any phenomenal property that can be possessed by veridical
color experiences, including global phenomenal properties and local phenomenal properties. It follows that no veridical experience of an ordinary
object has a Russellian phenomenal content. Given that there are veridical
experiences of ordinary objects (premise 1), it follows that the Russellian
hypothesis about color experience is false.

One can strengthen the argument by noting that there is no requirement that the original and inverted communities perceive distinct apples.
If we replace premises 1 and 4 by the premise that there can be phenomenally identical veridical and nonveridical experiences of the same object,
then even without premise 3, it follows that there is no property that is

attributed by all phenomenally red experiences. For there is no property that the apple simultaneously possesses and lacks: not even a relational or dispositional property.

(A possibility left open is that what is attributed is what we might call a "relational property radical": perhaps something like *normally causes phenomenally red experiences in_*, where the open place is to be filled by the subject of the experience (see Egan 2006 for a view in this vicinity). We could say that different subjects attribute the same relational property radical, which determine different relational properties for different subjects. Of course, relational property radicals are not really properties, and this proposal is also subject to the usual phenomenological objections.)

Proponents of Russellian views will respond by denying one of the premises of the argument. Depending on the view, they might deny premise 1, 3, or 4 of the original argument. This leads to a well-worn dialectic that I do not want to get into here. For now I will just note that each of the premises enjoys strong intuitive support, and I take this as strong prima facie reason to believe that the Russellian hypothesis is false.

If we accept premises 1–4, we are left with something like the following view. Color experiences attribute nonrelational properties, and these properties are sometimes instantiated by ordinary objects. The most plausible candidates for such properties are intrinsic physical properties, such as surface reflectance properties,[3] so our phenomenally red experiences might attribute a specific physical property, which we can call physical redness. On this view, color experiences have Russellian content that involves the attribution of these properties. However, it is possible that experiences with the same phenomenal character (perhaps in a different community) can have different Russellian contents of this sort due to differences in the perceivers' environment. It follows that Russellian content is not phenomenal content.

4. Fregean Content

If one thought that all content were Russellian content, one might conclude from the foregoing that experiences (or at least color experiences) do not have phenomenal content. This would require denying the strong

---

3. One might understand a surface reflectance property as a sort of dispositional property, involving dispositions to reflect certain sorts of light. If so, then the physical properties attributed by color experiences should probably be understood to be the categorical bases of surface reflectance properties rather than reflectance properties themselves. I usually simply talk of reflectance properties in what follows, however.

intuition that experiences are assessable for accuracy in virtue of their phenomenal character. The alternative is to hold that phenomenal content is something other than Russellian content.

In the previous chapter I suggested that perceptual experiences (like linguistic expressions) have both Russellian and Fregean content. Where the Russellian content of a color experience involves a property attributed by the experience (such as a reflectance property), the Fregean content will be a mode of presentation of that property. On the face of it, color experiences attribute colors under a distinctive mode of presentation, one quite distinct from a physical mode of presentation of a reflectance property. It is natural to suggest that this distinctive mode of presentation corresponds to a distinctive sort of Fregean content.

On the model suggested in the last chapter, where Russellian content involves extensions (objects and properties), Fregean content involves conditions on extensions. In particular, the Fregean content associated with a color experience involves a condition that a property must satisfy in order to be the property attributed by the experience. For a phenomenally red experience, the condition is something like the following: the attributed property must be the property that normally causes phenomenally red experiences (in normal conditions for the perceiver). This Fregean content is a natural candidate for the phenomenal content associated with phenomenal redness.

Fregean content accommodates inversion scenarios quite straightforwardly. We have seen that two phenomenally red experiences in different environments can have different Russellian contents: one might attribute physical redness, while the other attributes physical greenness. But their Fregean contents will be exactly the same: both are the condition that picks the property that normally causes phenomenally red experiences in the perceiver. (As in chapter 11, the perceiver will be picked out under an indexical mode of presentation that can be shared between two different perceivers.) Due to differences in the environment, this common Fregean content yields distinct Russellian contents: the condition picks out physical redness in an ordinary environment and physical greenness in the alternative environment. All of this suggests that Fregean content is a plausible candidate to be phenomenal content.

The Fregean content of a given color experience can itself be seen as a condition of satisfaction. To a first approximation, the Fregean content of a phenomenally red experience will be satisfied when there is an object at the appropriate location relative to the perceiver that instantiates the property that normally causes phenomenally red experiences in the perceiver. To a second approximation, one might want to give a corresponding

Fregean treatment to the attributed location property (as I discuss later), and one might want to give a Fregean treatment to the object of the experience (for example, holding that the Russellian content of the experience is the specific object and that the corresponding Fregean content is the condition that picks out the object that is causing the current experience). For now, I abstract away from these matters and concentrate on that aspect of the content that is associated with color. Still, however we flesh out the details, this Fregean content will be a condition of satisfaction for the experience. If the perceiver's environment meets the condition, then the experience will be veridical; if it does not, the experience will be non-veridical.

The arguments in the previous chapter suggest that Fregean content is a much more plausible candidate to be phenomenal content than either physicalist or dispositionalist Russellian content. Compared to physicalist Russellian content, it accommodates inversion scenarios much better and also accommodates the intuition that phenomenology is internally determined. Compared to dispositional Russellian content, it accommodates the claim that the properties attributed by color experiences are nonrelational, it avoids problems associated with indexical individuation of dispositional properties, and it more easily accommodates the claim that things could have been as they perceptually seem to be even had there been no observers. So there is good reason to think that phenomenal content may be Fregean content.

5. Phenomenological Adequacy

The hypothesis that phenomenal content is Fregean content has many virtues. In particular, it seems to capture our intuitions about the environments in which an experience with a given phenomenal character will be veridical, yielding a condition of satisfaction that is determined by phenomenal character. Still, there remains a cluster of worries about the view.

This cluster of worries concerns what we might call the *phenomenological adequacy* of the view. Simply put, the worry is that Fregean content does not seem to adequately reflect the phenomenal character of an experience. In particular, one can argue that when we introspect and reflect on the way that the world is presented in the phenomenology of perceptual experience, the phenomenology seems to have properties that are in tension with the Fregean view of phenomenal content. These properties include the following:

Relationality. Intuitively, it seems to us that when we have an experience as of a colored object, there is a certain property (intuitively, a color property) that the object seems to have. And intuitively, it is natural to hold that the phenomenology of the experience alone suffices for it to seem that there is an object with that very property. That is, reflection on phenomenology suggests that there is an internal connection between phenomenology and certain properties that objects seem to have. One could summarize this by saying that the phenomenology of color experience seems to be *relational*: in virtue of its phenomenology, a specific color experience seems to relate us to a specific color property. If this point is correct, it suggests that color experiences have Russellian phenomenal content.

In a critical discussion of the Fregean view, Shoemaker (2006) brings this point out by an appeal to the Moorean "transparency" intuition. According to this intuition, we attend to the phenomenal character of an experience by attending to the properties that objects in the world appear to have. An extension of this intuition suggests that we discern similarities and differences in phenomenal character by discerning similarities and differences in the properties that objects in the world seem to have. This suggests a strong connection between phenomenal character and Russellian content. Shoemaker says:

> The phenomenal character of veridical experiences of a given color can be different in different circumstances (e.g., different lighting conditions), and for creatures with different sorts of perceptual systems. So the same color will have to have a number of distinct modes of presentation associated with it. To say that this variation is only a variation in the *how* of perceptual representation and in no way a variation in *what* is represented seems to me at odds with the phenomenology. When the light-brown object in shadow and the dark-brown object not in shadow look the same to me, the sameness is experienced as being *out there*—and in such a case the perception can be perfectly veridical. Similarity in the presenting manifests itself in represented similarity in what is represented and in the absence of perceptual illusion requires that there is similarity in what is represented. More generally, the best gloss on the Moorean transparency intuition is that the qualitative character that figures in the perception of the color of an object is experienced as in or on the perceived object. (Shoemaker 2006, 475).

One can also bring out the point by appealing to an inversion scenario. Jack and Jill are phenomenal duplicates but live in different environments.

Jack's phenomenally green experiences are normally caused by objects with property X, while Jill's experiences are normally caused by objects with property Y. Shoemaker's point suggests that even if Jack's and Jill's experiences are associated with distinct properties (X and Y), there is a strong intuitive sense in which the objects look to be the same to Jack and to Jill. That is, the phenomenal similarity suggests that there is a common property (intuitively, a sort of greenness) such that the relevant objects look to have that property both to Jack and to Jill.

This intuitive point stands in tension with the Fregean view. The Fregean view entails that Jack's and Jill's experiences share a mode of presentation, but it does not entail that the experiences represent a common property. In fact, it suggests that Jack's and Jill's experiences represent distinct properties, X and Y. So it is difficult for the Fregean view to accommodate any internal connection between an experience's phenomenal character and the properties that it represents.

A related point is that phenomenologically, a color experience appears to represent an object as having a certain *specific* and *determinate* property. Intuitively, the specificity and determinacy are tied very closely to the specific and determinate phenomenal character of the experience. According to the Fregean view, while an experience may represent a specific and determinate property, its phenomenal character leaves the nature of this property wide open. The determinate property represented may depend on matters quite extrinsic to the phenomenology. This seems to conflict with a strong phenomenological intuition.

Simplicity. A second objection is that Fregean contents seem to be overly complex. One might say that they "overintellectualize" the content of an experience. According to this objection, the phenomenological structure of a visual experience is relatively simple. The experience represents certain objects as having color and shape properties and so on, and one cannot find anything like "the normal cause of such-and-such an experience" in the visual phenomenology. On the face of it, the "normal cause" relation is not phenomenologically present at all. It is something imposed after the fact by theorists rather than directly reflecting the experience's phenomenology.

A related objection turns on the fact that Fregean contents require reference to *experiences*. Properties are picked out as the normal cause of a certain type of experience, and objects might be picked out as the cause of a certain token experience. Here one can object that the perceptual phenomenology does not (or at least need not) involve representation of experiences: it need only involve representation of the world. This is another often-invoked aspect of the "transparency" of experiences. The phenomenology of perception usually seems to present the world directly, not in virtue of representation of any experiential intermediaries. Again, to invoke the representation of experience seems to overintellectualize the experience by introducing complexity that is not apparent in the experience's phenomenology.

Internal unity. A final objection is that it seems that there can be internal unity among the contents of experiences that have quite different phenomenal character. For example, one can argue that there is an internal unity between the representation of space in visual and tactile experience in virtue of which these are constrained to represent a common set of spatial properties. Phenomenologically, it seems that when an object looks flat and when it feels flat, it looks and feels to have the same property (flatness). This commonality seems to hold in virtue of an internal relationship between the phenomenology of visual and tactile experiences. It is arguable that something similar applies to experiences as of the same color in quite different lighting conditions. For example, experiences of a white object both in shadow and out of shadow may have quite different phenomenal characters, but it is arguable that the experiences are internally related in a way so that both represent the object as being white.

This internal unity is not straightforwardly accommodated by a Fregean view (assuming that the Fregean view might also apply to experiences of space). One might think that because visual and tactile experiences of space are phenomenally quite different, they will be associated with quite different Fregean modes of presentation. One will represent the normal cause of certain visual experiences, and another will represent the normal cause of certain tactile experiences. It might turn out that as a matter of contingent fact these normal causes coincide, so that the properties represented coincide, but nothing in the experiences themselves guarantees this. This stands in tension with the intuition that there is an internal phenomenological connection between tactile and visual representations of space, according to which these have common contents in virtue of their phenomenology. The same goes for the case of phenomenally different experiences as of the same color. The Fregean view suggests that these will have distinct modes of presentation that at best contingently pick out a common property, which stands in tension with the intuition that these experiences have common representational content by virtue of their phenomenology.

I do not think that any of these three objections—from relationality, simplicity, and internal unity—are knockdown objections to the Fregean view. For a start, all of them rest on phenomenological intuitions that could be disputed. I will not dispute them, however. I am inclined to give each of the intuitions some prima facie weight. But even if one takes the intuitions at face value, it is not clear that any of them entail that the Fregean view is false. Rather, all of them can be seen as pointing to a certain *incompleteness* in the Fregean view: the Fregean account so far is not a full story about the phenomenal content of experience. For a full story, the Fregean view needs to be supplemented.

The relationality objection, for example, suggests that there is a Russellian aspect to the phenomenal content of perceptual experience, in that phenomenally identical experiences involve representation of some common property. The intuitions here are somewhat equivocal. In the Jack and Jill case, for example, at the same time as we have the intuition that some common property is phenomenologically represented (as a Russellian view of phenomenal content would suggest), we also have the intuition that different properties might be represented by virtue of distinct environmental connections (as a Fregean view of phenomenal content would suggest). If we are pluralists about content, these two intuitions need not contradict each other. Rather, they might be reconciled if we adopt a view that posits both a Russellian and a Fregean aspect to the phenomenal content of experiences. The intuition here does not entail that Fregean content is not phenomenal content. Rather, it suggests that Fregean content is not all there is to phenomenal content.

The force of the simplicity objection is somewhat unclear. Construed as an argument against Fregean phenomenal content, it turns on the tacit premise that the phenomenal content of an experience must have a structure that directly mirrors the phenomenological structure of the experience (or perhaps that it directly mirrors the way it seems to us on introspection that the world is perceptually presented). We might call this somewhat elusive idea the "mirroring constraint." A proponent of the Fregean view might reply simply that the mirroring constraint is an unreasonable constraint on an account of the phenomenal content of experience. As I have defined it, phenomenal content is content that supervenes on the phenomenal character of an experience. There is nothing in this definition that requires a tighter connection than mere supervenience, and the simplicity objection does not give any reason to deny supervenience. So the Fregean may hold that unless one has an argument that supervenience of content on phenomenal character requires mirroring (or unless we redefine the notion of phenomenal content to build in the mirroring constraint), there is no objection to the claim that Fregean content is phenomenal content.

Still, the simplicity objection once again suggests a certain incompleteness in the Fregean view. One might reasonably hold that the supervenience of content on phenomenal character requires some sort of explanation. If there were a direct correspondence between the elements of the content and the elements of phenomenal character, this explanation would be much easier to give. As it is, the extra complexity of Fregean content (such as the invocation of causation and experience) raises the question of how this complex content is connected to the simple experience. In particular, if one adopts a view on which phenomenal content is somehow grounded in the phenomenology of an experience, then one will need to tell a story about how a complex Fregean content can be grounded in a simple experience. And if one thinks that the phenomenology of an experience is grounded in its phenomenal content, then the same applies in reverse. So there is at least a significant explanatory question here.

Finally, the Fregean view could handle the internal unity objection by saying that visual and tactile experiences of space share a common phenomenal type (in effect, a cross-modal type), and it is this phenomenal type that is relevant to the Fregean mode of presentation of these experiences ("the property that normally causes experiences of type T"). If so, then the different experiences will be constrained to represent a common class of properties. One could likewise suggest that phenomenally distinct experiences of the same color (shadowed and unshadowed, for example) share a phenomenal type and draw the same conclusion. This raises the question, however, of just how we assign the relevant phenomenal types. Any given experience belongs to many different phenomenal types, and the selection of the cross-modal phenomenal type (in the spatial case) or the phenomenal type shared by shadowed and unshadowed experiences (in the color case) may seem suspiciously ad hoc. At least, we need to fill in the Fregean view with an account of how the mode of presentation associated with a given experience is determined, by specifying a principled basis for the choice of a phenomenal type.

One can summarize all these worries by saying that as it stands, the Fregean view does not seem to fully reflect the *presentational phenomenology* of perceptual experience: the way that it seems to directly and immediately present certain objects and properties in the world. It is natural to hold that this presentational phenomenology is closely connected to the phenomenal content of experience. So, to make progress, we need to attend more closely to this presentational phenomenology and to how it might be connected to phenomenal content.

6. Back to Primitivism

It is useful at this point to ask: what view of the content of perceptual experience is the most phenomenologically adequate? That is, if we were simply to aim to take the phenomenology of perceptual experience at face value, what account of content would we come up with? In particular, what view of the content of color experience best mirrors its presentational phenomenology?

Here, I think the answer is clear. The view of content that most directly mirrors the phenomenology of color experience is primitivism. Phenomenologically, it seems to us as if visual experience presents simple intrinsic qualities of objects in the world, spread out over the surface of the object. When I have a phenomenally red experience of an object, the object seems to be simply, primitively, *red*. The apparent redness does not seem to be a microphysical property, or a mental property, or a disposition, or an unspecified property that plays an appropriate causal role. Rather, it seems to be a simple qualitative property with a distinctive sensuous nature. We might call this property perfect redness: the sort of property that might have been instantiated in Eden.

One might say: phenomenologically, it seems that visual experience presents the world to us as an Edenic world. Taking the phenomenology completely at face value, visual experience presents a world where perfect redness and perfect blueness are instantiated on the surface of objects, as they were in Eden. These are simple intrinsic qualities whose nature we seem to grasp fully in perceptual experience. For the world to be *exactly* the way that my phenomenology seems to present it as being, the world would have to be an Edenic world in which these properties are instantiated.

This suggests a view on which color experiences attribute primitive properties such as perfect redness and perfect blueness to objects. According to this view, color experiences have a Russellian content involving the attribution of these primitive properties. Furthermore, this content is naturally taken to be phenomenal content. Intuitively, the nature of the primitive properties that are presented to one is fully determined by the phenomenology of the experience. If an experience attributes a primitive property, any phenomenally identical experience will attribute the same primitive property. So this view is a sort of Russellian primitivism about phenomenal content.

For all its virtues with respect to phenomenological adequacy, the Russellian primitivist view has a familiar problem. There is good reason to believe that the relevant primitive properties are not instantiated in our world. That is, there is good reason to believe that none of the objects we perceive are perfectly red or perfectly green. If this is correct, then the primitivist view entails that all color experiences are illusory.[4]

---

4. In practice, primitivists are divided on this issue. For example, Holman, Maund, and Wright hold that the primitive properties are uninstantiated and that color experiences are illusory, while Campbell, Johnston, and McGinn hold that primitive properties are instantiated and that color experiences can be veridical.

A first reason for doubting that these properties exist surfaced when we ate from the Tree of Illusion. This made it clear that there is no necessary connection between primitive properties and perceptual experiences and strongly suggested that, if there is a connection, it is merely causal and contingent. Once we have accepted that one sometimes has phenomenally red experiences in the absence of perfect redness, it is natural to start to wonder whether the same goes for all of our phenomenally red experiences. This is a relatively weak reason as the existence of illusions is compatible with the existence of veridical perception, but it is enough to generate initial doubts.

A second and stronger reason came when we ate from the Tree of Science. Science suggests that when we see a red object, our perception of the object is mediated by the reflection or radiation of light from the surface of the object to our eyes and then to our brains. The properties of the object that are responsible for the reflection or radiation of the light appear to be complex physical properties such as surface spectral reflectances, ultimately grounded in microphysical configurations. Science does not reveal any primitive properties in the object, and furthermore, the hypothesis that objects have the relevant primitive properties seems quite unnecessary in order to explain color perception.

Still, someone might suggest that objects have the primitive properties all the same, perhaps supervening in some fashion on the microphysical properties of the object. In response, one might suggest that this picture will metaphysically complicate the world. It seems at least conceivable that objects with the relevant microphysical properties could fail to instantiate the relevant primitive properties. So it looks as if the relevant primitive properties are a significant addition to the world over and above the microphysical supervenience base. A primitivist might respond in turn by denying that any metaphysical addition is involved (perhaps denying an inference from conceivability to metaphysical possibility) or by accepting that physicalism about ordinary objects is false.[5] But even if so, there is a remaining problem.

The third and strongest reason for doubting that primitive properties are instantiated stems from an elaboration of the inversion argument given earlier.[6] Take an ordinary object such as a red apple. It is familiar from

5. Among the primitivists who think that the primitive properties are instantiated, Campbell and McGinn suggest that they metaphysically supervene on microphysical or dispositional properties, so that they are not a metaphysical addition in the strong sense, while Johnston seems willing to accept that they are a strong metaphysical addition.

6. A version of this sort of argument is deployed by Edwards (1998) against Campbell's version of primitivism.

everyday experience that such an object can cause phenomenally red experiences of the apple and (in some circumstances) can cause phenomenally green experiences of the apple without any change in its intrinsic properties. It then seems that there is no obstacle to the existence of a community in which objects with the intrinsic properties of this apple *normally* cause phenomenally green experiences.[7] We can even imagine that the very same apple normally causes phenomenally red experiences in one community and normally causes phenomenally green experiences in the other.

We can now ask: when a subject in the first community has a phenomenally red experience of the apple, and a subject in the second community has a phenomenally green experience of the apple, which of these experiences is veridical?

Intuitively, there is a case for saying that both experiences are veridical. But this is an unhappy answer for the primitivist. On the primitivist view, any phenomenally red experience attributes perfect redness, and any phenomenally green experience attributes perfect greenness. If both experiences are veridical, it follows that the apple instantiates both perfect redness and perfect greenness. The argument generalizes. For any phenomenal color, it seems that there is a community in which the apple normally causes experiences with that phenomenal color. Taking the current line, it follows that the apple instantiates every perfect color! The choice of an apple was unimportant here, so it seems to follow that every object instantiates every perfect color. It follows that no color experience of an object can be illusory with respect to color. Whatever the phenomenal color of the experience, the object will have the corresponding primitive property, so the experience will be veridical. This conclusion is perhaps even more counterintuitive than the conclusion that all color experiences are illusory.

A primitivist might suggest that one of the experiences is veridical and one of them is not. But this imposes an asymmetry on what otherwise seems to be a quite symmetrical situation. When a subject in one community has a phenomenally red experience of the apple and a subject in the other community has a phenomenally green experience of the apple, both subjects' perceptual mechanisms are functioning in the way that is normal

7. *A primitivist (such as Campbell) who is also an externalist about phenomenology may deny this claim by holding that phenomenal greenness is constituted by a normal causal connection to instances of primitive greenness in the environment. On such a view, while it may be possible for a single instance of phenomenal greenness to be caused by an apple that is not primitively green, it will not be possible for this to be the normal state of affairs. I reject phenomenal externalism for reasons discussed in the previous chapter. One could also argue for the possibility of the relevant state of affairs by noting that it is hard to deny that it is at least conceivable, and by arguing for a connection between conceivability and possibility as in chapter 6.

in those communities. Furthermore, the perceptual mechanisms themselves, involving light and brain, seem to be symmetrically well-functioning in both communities. A primitivist may hold the line and assert that one of the experiences is veridical and one is falsidical simply because the apple is perfectly red and it is not perfectly green. But this line leads to the conclusion that color experiences in one of the communities are *normally* falsidical (after all, objects like the apple normally cause phenomenally green experiences in that community) where corresponding experiences in the other community are normally veridical.

Apart from the unappealing asymmetry, this view yields a serious skeptical worry. It seems that we have little reason to believe that we are in a community that normally perceives veridically as opposed to falsidically. After all, nature and evolution will be indifferent between these two communities. Evolutionary processes will be indifferent among perceivers in which apples produce phenomenally red experiences, perceivers in which apples produce phenomenally green experiences, and perceivers in which apples produce phenomenally blue experiences. Any such perceiver could easily come to exist through minor differences in environmental conditions or brain wiring.[8] If we accept the earlier reasoning, only a very small subset of the class of such possible perceivers will normally have veridical experiences, and there is no particular reason to think that we are among them.

Once these options are ruled out, the reasonable conclusion is that neither experience is veridical: the apple is neither perfectly red nor perfectly green. Generalizing from this case, the reasoning suggests that primitive properties are not instantiated at all. I think that this is clearly the most reasonable view for a primitivist to take: on this view, experiences attribute primitive properties, but their objects never possess these properties.

Still, this view has the consequence that all color experiences are illusory. This is a counterintuitive conclusion and runs counter to our usual judgments about the veridicality of experience. On the face of it, there is a significant difference between a phenomenally red experience of a red wall and a phenomenally red experience of a white wall that looks red because (unknown to the subject) it is illuminated by red light. As we ordinarily classify

---

8. *Byrne and Hilbert (2007) respond to this argument on behalf on the primitivist by noting that it is far from obvious that there could easily have been "inversion mutations" producing genes for spectrum inversions. But genetic mutations are not required here, and nor is a perfect inversion of color space: a difference in environmental conditions so that the same brain structures are causally connected to different distal properties will suffice. A relatively superficial difference in properties of the retina may also suffice. Of course these arguments presuppose that phenomenal externalism of the sort discussed in the previous footnote is false.

experiences, the former is veridical and the latter is not. In classifying both experiences as falsidical, primitivism cannot respect this distinction.

7. Perfect and Imperfect Veridicality

Here is where things stand. The Fregean view of phenomenal content seems to most accurately capture our judgments about veridicality, but it is not especially phenomenologically adequate. The primitivist view of phenomenal content is the most phenomenologically adequate view, but it yields implausible consequences about veridicality. For a way forward, what we need is an account that captures both the phenomenological virtues of the primitivist view and the truth-conditional virtues of the Fregean view. In what follows I argue that such an account is available.

One can begin to motivate such a view with the following pair of intuitions:

1. For a color experience to be *perfectly veridical*—for it to be as veridical as it could be—its object would have to have perfect colors. The perfect veridicality of color experience would require that our world be an Edenic world, in which objects instantiate primitive color properties.

2. Even if the object of an experience lacks perfect colors, a color experience can be *imperfectly veridical*: veridical according to our ordinary standard of veridicality. Even after the fall from Eden, our imperfect world has objects with properties that suffice to make our experiences veridical by our ordinary standards.

This pair of intuitions has strong support. The first is supported by the phenomenological observations in the previous section. If we were to take our experience *completely* at face value, we would accept that we were in a world where primitive properties such as perfect redness and perfect blueness are spread over the surface of objects. The second is supported by our ordinary judgments about veridicality. When an ordinary white wall looks white to us, then even if it merely instantiates physical properties and not perfect whiteness, it is good enough to qualify as veridical by our ordinary standards.

These two intuitions need not contradict each other. Instead, they suggest that we possess two notions of satisfaction for an experience: perfect and imperfect veridicality. An experience can be imperfectly veridical, or veridical in the ordinary sense, without being perfectly veridical.

The terminology should not be taken to suggest that when an experience is imperfectly veridical, it is not really veridical. In fact, it is plausible that imperfect veridicality is the property that our ordinary term "veridicality" denotes. We speak truly when we say that a phenomenally red experience of an ordinary red object is veridical. It is just that the experience is not perfectly veridical. To capture this, one could also call imperfect veridicality "ordinary veridicality" or "veridicality simpliciter." Or one could use "veridical" for imperfect veridicality and "ultraveridical" for perfect veridicality. But I will usually stick to the terminology above.

Corresponding to these distinct notions of satisfaction, one will have distinct associated conditions of satisfaction. Imperfect veridicality will be associated with something like the Fregean condition of satisfaction discussed earlier: a phenomenally red experience will be imperfectly veridical iff its object has the property that normally causes phenomenally red experiences. Perfect veridicality will be associated with the primitivist condition of satisfaction: a phenomenally red experience will be perfectly veridical iff its object instantiates perfect redness.

Imperfect and perfect veridicality can therefore be seen as associated with distinct *contents* of an experience. We might call the content associated with perfect veridicality the *Edenic content* of an experience and the content associated with imperfect veridicality the *ordinary content* of the experience.

As we have already seen, our ordinary assessments of veridicality can be seen as associated with two contents in turn. For example, a phenomenally red experience has a Fregean content (satisfied iff its object has the property that normally causes a phenomenally red experience) and a Russellian content (satisfied iff its object has physical redness). We might call these contents the *ordinary Fregean content* and the *ordinary Russellian content* of the experience.

One could also, in principle, associate assessments of perfect veridicality with both a Fregean and a Russellian content, but here the Fregean content is much the same as the Russellian content. The Russellian content involves the attribution of perfect redness: it is satisfied in a world iff the relevant object is perfectly red there. Unlike the ordinary Russellian content mentioned previously, this content does not depend on how the subject's environment turns out. Regardless of how the environment turns out, the experience in question will attribute perfect redness. So there is no nontrivial dependence of the property attributed on the way the subject's environment turns out. It follows that the Edenic Fregean content of the experience (which captures the way that the perfect veridicality of the experience depends on the way the environment turns out) is satisfied iff the object of the experience has perfect redness. There may be some differences between the Edenic Fregean and Russellian contents here in the treatment of objects (as opposed to properties) and in the formal modeling (with worlds and centered worlds), but where the color-property aspect of the content is concerned, the contents behave in very similar ways. So for most purposes one can simply speak of the Edenic content of the experience, one that is satisfied iff a relevant object has perfect redness.[9]

So we have found three distinctive sorts of content associated with an experience: an Edenic content, an ordinary Fregean content, and an ordinary Russellian content. We have seen already that the ordinary Russellian content is not plausibly a phenomenal content: phenomenally identical experiences can have distinct (ordinary) Russellian contents. However, for all we have said, both Edenic contents and ordinary Fregean contents are phenomenal contents. It is plausible that any phenomenally red experience will have the ordinary Fregean condition of satisfaction (where satisfaction is understood as imperfect veridicality) and will also have the primitivist condition of satisfaction (where satisfaction is understood as perfect veridicality). So we have more than one phenomenal content for an experience depending on the associated notion of satisfaction.

8. A Two-Stage View of Phenomenal Content

Perfect and imperfect veridicality are not independent of each other. It is plausible to suggest that there is an intimate relation between the two and that there is an intimate relation between the associated sorts of phenomenal content.

A natural picture of this relation suggests itself. A phenomenally red experience is perfectly veridical iff its object instantiates perfect redness. A phenomenally red experience is imperfectly veridical iff its object instantiates a property that *matches* perfect redness. Here, to match perfect redness is (roughly) to play the role that perfect redness plays in Eden. The key role played by perfect redness in Eden is that it brings about phenomenally red experiences. So a property matches perfect redness if it causes phenomenally red experiences. This yields a condition of satisfaction that mirrors the ordinary Fregean content discussed earlier.

9. In terms of the two-dimensional framework, one can say that phenomenal color properties (at the standard of perfect veridicality) are associated with the same primary and secondary intension. In this way they are reminiscent of expressions such as "consciousness," "philosopher," and "two," which also arguably have the same primary and secondary intensions. These terms can be seen as semantically neutral (see chapter 6), as witnessed by the fact that their content does not seem to have the same sort of dependence on empirical discoveries about the environment as terms such as "water" and "Hesperus." One might say that perceptual representations of perfect redness are semantically neutral in an analogous way.

The notion of matching is what links imperfect veridicality to perfect veridicality. I will say more about this notion later, but one can motivate the idea as follows. For our experiences to be perfectly veridical, we would have to live in Eden. But we have undergone the fall from Eden: no primitive color properties are instantiated by objects in our world. So the best that objects in our world can do is to have properties that can play the role that primitive properties play in Eden. Of course, no property instantiated in our world can play that role perfectly, but some can play it well enough by virtue of normally bringing about phenomenally red experiences. Such a property might be called *imperfect redness*. In our world, imperfect redness is plausibly some sort of physical property such as a surface spectral reflectance.

More generally, the following is a plausible thesis. If an experience is such that its perfect veridicality conditions require the instantiation of primitive property X, then the experience's imperfect veridicality conditions will require the instantiation of a property that matches X. As before, a property matches X (roughly) if it plays the role that X plays in Eden. The key role is causing experiences of the appropriate phenomenal type. In our world, these properties will typically be physical properties: the imperfect counterparts of X.

This relation suggests the following *two-stage* picture of the phenomenal content of experience. On this picture, the most fundamental sort of content of an experience is its Edenic content, which requires the instantiation of appropriate primitive properties. This content then determines the ordinary Fregean content of the experience: the experience is imperfectly veridical if its object has properties that match the properties attributed by the experience's Edenic content.[10]

On the two-stage view, the ordinary Fregean content of a phenomenally red experience will be satisfied (in an environment) iff a relevant object instantiates a property that matches perfect redness (in that environment). This ordinary Fregean content will itself be associated with an ordinary Russellian content: one that is satisfied iff the (actual) object of the experience has P, where P is the property that matches perfect redness in the

---

10. Aaron Zimmerman (in a conference commentary) suggested that instead of associating an experience with two contents, we could associate an experience with a single graded content that has degrees of satisfaction. The content might be perfectly satisfied, imperfectly satisfied, and so on depending on how the world turns out. A pluralist can allow that we can associate experiences with graded contents like these. However, this single graded content will lose some of the structure present in the dual contents. In particular, we cannot easily analyze it in terms of attribution of a property to objects in the environment, and the matching relation between Edenic and ordinary content will not easily be reflected in this account. So this picture will lose some of the explanatory structure that is present in the two-stage view.

environment of the original experience. On this view, all phenomenally red experiences will have the same Fregean content, but they may have different Russellian contents depending on their environment.

Of course, this Fregean content gives exactly the same results as the Fregean content discussed earlier: an object will instantiate a property that matches perfect redness iff it instantiates a property that normally causes phenomenally red experiences. But the two-stage view gives a more refined account of how this Fregean content is grounded, one that more clearly shows its roots in the phenomenology of the experience. The view also has the promise of being more phenomenologically adequate than the original Fregean view seemed to be, by giving a major role to the Edenic content that directly reflects the experience's phenomenology. The resulting view is a sort of semiprimitivist Fregeanism: a version of the Fregean view on which the Fregean content is grounded in a primitivist Edenic content.

On this view, Eden acts as a sort of regulative ideal in determining the content of our color experiences. Our world is not Eden, but our perceptual experience requires our world to match Eden as well as possible. Eden is central to the content of our experience: it is directly reflected in the perfect veridicality conditions of the experience, and it plays a key role in determining the ordinary veridicality conditions of our experiences.

One might put the two-stage view as follows. Our experience *presents* an Edenic world and thereby *represents* an ordinary world. We might say that the perfect veridicality conditions of the experience are its *presentational content*, and the imperfect veridicality conditions of the experience are its *representational content*. As pluralists we can allow that experiences have both sorts of content, with an intimate relation between them. Presentational content most directly reflects the phenomenology of an experience; representational content most directly reflects its intuitive conditions of satisfaction.

Because of this, the two-stage view yields natural answers to the objections to the Fregean view that were grounded in phenomenological adequacy. On the relationality objection, the two-stage view accommodates relationality by noting that there are certain specific and determinate properties—the perfect color properties—that are presented in virtue of the phenomenology of color experience. When Jack and Jill both have phenomenally green experiences in different environments, the two experiences have a common Edenic content, and so both are presented with perfect greenness. This captures the intuitive sense in which objects look to be the same to both Jack and Jill. At the same time, the level of ordinary Fregean and Russellian content captures the intuitive sense in which objects look to be different to Jack and Jill. By acknowledging Edenic phenomenal content in addition to Fregean phenomenal content, we capture the sense in which perceptual phenomenology seems to be Russellian and relational.

On the simplicity objection: in the two-stage view, the simplicity of phenomenological structure is directly mirrored at the level of Edenic content. In Edenic content, there need be no reference to normal causes and no reference to experiences. Instead, simple properties are attributed directly. The residual question for the Fregean view concerned how a complex Fregean content might be grounded in simple phenomenology. The two-stage view begins to answer this question. A given experience is most directly associated with a simple Edenic content, and this Edenic content is then associated with a Fregean content by the matching relation. There is still an explanatory question about just where the matching relation comes from and how it might be grounded: I address this question later in the chapter. But the two-stage view already gives us a skeleton around which we can build an explanatory connection between phenomenology and Fregean content.

On the internal unity objection: the two-stage view can accommodate the internal unity between visual and tactile experience of space by holding that the Edenic content of both visual and tactile experiences involves the attribution of perfect spatial properties (although the other perfect properties attributed by the experiences may differ). If so, then internal unity is present at the level of Edenic content. Further, the Fregean content of each will invoke the properties that match perfect spatial properties (in effect, the common typing of visual and spatial experiences is induced by the commonality in their Edenic content), and this common Fregean content will entail a common, ordinary Russellian content. So the unity at the level of Edenic content will lead to unity at the level of ordinary content. Something similar applies to the case of representing the same color under different illumination; I will discuss this case in some detail shortly.

The two-stage view respects the insights of both the primitivist and the Fregean views in obvious ways. Like the original Fregean view, it can also respect certain key elements of dispositionalist and physicalist views. On the two-stage view, dispositions to cause relevant sorts of experiences still play a key role, not as the properties that are represented by experiences but as a sort of reference fixer for those properties. The properties that are represented by the experience (at the standard of imperfect veridicality) are themselves plausibly physical properties at least in the actual world. We might say that the view generates a broadly dispositionalist ordinary Fregean content and a broadly physicalist ordinary Russellian content.

9. Eden and Edenic Content

What Constraints Are Imposed by Edenic Content?

The view I have proposed raises many questions. In the remainder of this chapter I address some of these questions and in doing so flesh out a number of aspects of the view. These include questions about Eden and Edenic content; about colors and color constancy; about matching and Fregean content; and about generalizing the model beyond the case of color. The order of these topics is arbitrary to some extent, so it is possible to skip to the topics that seem the most pressing.

A world with respect to which our visual experience is perfectly veridical is an *Edenic world*. (I defer until later the question of whether Edenic worlds are metaphysically possible.) It is natural to ask: what is the character of an Edenic world? A full answer to this question depends on a full analysis of the phenomenology of visual experience, which cannot be given here, but we can say a few things. As before, I will concentrate mostly on the aspects of phenomenology and representation associated with color and leave other aspects until later.

For any given experience, there will be many worlds with respect to which it is perfectly veridical. A visual experience—even a total visual experience corresponding to an entire visual field—typically makes quite limited claims on the world and is neutral about the rest. For example, a visual experience typically presents things as being a certain way in a certain location and is neutral about how things are outside that location. So, strictly speaking, in order to make an experience perfectly veridical, a world need merely be Edenic in certain relevant respects in a certain relatively limited area and may be quite non-Edenic outside that area. Correspondingly, there will be a very large range of worlds that satisfy the relevant Edenic content. Here we can focus on what is *required* in order to satisfy the content.

In a world that satisfies a typical Edenic content, primitive color properties such as perfect redness and perfect blueness are instantiated. Most often, visual phenomenology presents color as instantiated on the surface of objects, so an Edenic world will contain objects with perfect colors instantiated at certain locations on their surfaces. Strictly speaking, it will contain objects with certain perfect location-color properties: properties of having certain perfect colors at certain locations. Occasionally we have the phenomenology of volumes of color, as with certain transparent colored objects or perhaps with smoke and flames. In these cases, the corresponding Edenic world will have objects in which the relevant perfect colors are instantiated at locations throughout the relevant volume. It may be that sometimes we have the phenomenology of color not associated with objects at all: perhaps our experience of the sky is like this, just representing blueness at a certain distance in front of us. If so, then a corresponding Edenic world will simply have perfect color qualities instantiated (by the world?) at relevant locations.[11]

From the fable at the beginning of the chapter, one might infer that Edenic worlds must meet a number of further constraints: perceivers must be directly acquainted with objects and properties in those worlds, illusion must be impossible, and there must be no microphysical structure. On my view this is not quite right, however. Edenic content puts relatively simple constraints on the world that involve the instantiation of perfect properties by objects in the environment, and the further constraints above are not part of Edenic content itself. Their relation to Edenic content is somewhat more subtle than this.

Perfect color properties are plausibly *intrinsic* color properties. By virtue of presenting an object as having a perfect color at a certain location, an experience does not seem to make claims about how things are outside that location. So, when an object is perfectly red in Eden, it is this way by virtue of its intrinsic nature. In particular, it seems that an object can be perfectly red without anyone experiencing the object as perfectly red. The phenomenology of color does not seem to be the phenomenology of properties that require a perceiver in order to be instantiated. (The phenomenology of pain is arguably different in this respect, as I will discuss later.) It seems coherent to suppose that there is a world in which perfect colors are instantiated but in which there are no perceivers at all.

One *could* hold a view on which, for an experience to be perfectly veridical, a subject must perceive the relevant perfect colors. According to such a view, the character of visual experience is such that in addition to representing the presence of colors, visual experiences also represent the *perception* of colors. If one held this view, one would hold that no such experience is perfectly veridical unless the relevant perfect colors are perceived by a subject (the subject at the center of the relevant centered world), perhaps by direct acquaintance.

I am inclined to think that the character of visual experience is not like this, however. The phenomenology of color vision clearly makes claims

11. Austen Clark (2000) suggests that visual experience always involves the mere attribution of colors to locations rather than to objects. I find this suggestion phenomenologically implausible, but if it is correct, one could accommodate it by saying that Edenic worlds involve the instantiation of perfect color qualities by locations (or the instantiation of perfect color-location properties by the world) without requiring any special relationship between these qualities and objects.

about objects in the world, but it does not obviously make claims about us and our perceptual relation to these objects. As theorists who introspectively reflect on our phenomenology, we can say that it seems (introspectively) as if we are acquainted with objects and properties in the world. But it is not obvious that perceptual phenomenology itself makes such a claim. To suggest that it does is arguably to overintellectualize perceptual experience. If perceptual experience does not make such claims, then the Edenic content of a visual experience will require the relevant perfect properties to be instantiated, but it will not require that we stand in any particular perceptual relation to those properties.

If this is correct, then in order to satisfy the Edenic content of an experience, a world must be Edenic in that perfect properties are instantiated within it, but it need not be a world in which we have not yet eaten from the Tree of Illusion. If an experience does not represent itself, it cannot represent that it is nonillusory.

Likewise, a world that satisfies the Edenic content of an experience need not be one in which we have not yet eaten from the Tree of Science. The phenomenology of vision is arguably quite neutral on whether the world has the relevant scientific structure as long as it also has primitive properties, and there is no obvious reason why a possible world could not have both.

To reinforce this view, we can note that the argument from the existence of illusions and scientific structure to the nonexistence of perfect colors in our world was not a deductive argument. Rather, it was a sort of abductive argument: it undercut our reasons for accepting (instantiated) perfect colors by suggesting that they are not needed to explain our visual experience. It remained *coherent* to suppose that primitive properties are instantiated in our world, but there was now good reason to reject the hypothesis as unnecessarily complex. On this view, eating from the Trees (by discovering the existence of illusions and scientific structure) did not directly contradict the Edenic contents of our experience, but it gave us good reason to believe that our world is not an Edenic world.

A more complete account of the Edenic content of color experience would require careful attention to all sorts of phenomenological details that I have largely ignored so far, such as the phenomenal representation of the distribution of colors in space, the fineness of grain of color representation, the different levels of detail of color experience in the foreground and background of a visual field, and so on. I cannot deal with all of this here, but as a case study I will shortly pay attention to one such detail, the phenomenon of color constancy.

What Is the Character of Edenic Perception?

Even if perceivers are not presented in the Edenic content of an experience, it is natural to speculate about how perception might work in an Edenic world. One way to put this is to ask: what sort of world maximally reflects how things seem to us *both perceptually and introspectively*? Even if perception makes no claims about our perceptual experiences and our perceptual relation to the world, introspection does. It seems to us, introspectively and perceptually, as if we stand in certain sorts of relations to the world. For this seeming to be maximally veridical, an Edenic world must contain subjects who stand in certain intimate relations to perfect properties in the world. We can call a world in which these seemings are maximally veridical a *pure Edenic world*.

Of course, there are (possibly impure) Edenic worlds in which subjects perceive perfect colors via a mediated causal mechanism, at least to the extent that we perceive imperfect colors via such a mechanism in our world. But it is natural to think that this is not the best they could do. It seems reasonable to hold that in Eden, subjects could have a sort of direct acquaintance with perfect colors. Perfect colors seem to be the sort of properties that are particularly apt for direct acquaintance, after all. And phenomenologically, there is something to be said for the claim that we seem to perceive colors directly. Certainly there does not seem to be a mediating causal mechanism, and one could suggest more strongly that at least introspectively, there seems not to be a mediating causal mechanism.

It is natural to suggest that in the purest Edenic worlds, subjects do not perceive instances of perfect color by virtue of having color experiences that are distinct from but related to those instances. That would seem to require a contingent mediating connection. Instead, Edenic subjects perceive instances of perfect colors by standing in a direct perceptual relation to them: perhaps the relation of acquaintance. Edenic subjects still have color experiences: there is something it is like to be them. But their color experiences have their phenomenal character precisely in virtue of the perfect colors that the subject is acquainted with. It is natural to say that the experiences themselves are constituted by a direct perceptual relation to the relevant instances of perfect color in the environment.[12] We might say that in Eden, if not in our world, perceptual experience extends outside the head.

---

12. Is Edenic perception causal? Given that a perceptual experience consists of a relation of acquaintance with a perfect color property, is its character causally related to the perfect color property? This depends on subtle questions about the causation of relational properties by their relata. Consider this: when a boy's first sibling is born, does this sibling cause the boy to be a brother? I am inclined to say yes and to say the same thing about Edenic perception, holding that it involves a sort of unmediated

In the purest Edenic worlds, there are no illusions (if we take both intro-spection and perception to be maximally veridical, we conclude that things are just as they seem). In such a world, all color experience involves direct acquaintance with instances of perfect color in the environment. As soon as we eat from the Tree of Illusion, we have good reason to believe that we are not in such a world. But this need not cast us out of Eden entirely. There are somewhat less pure Edenic worlds in which there are illusions and hallucinations: perceivers sometimes have experiences as of perfect redness when the perceived object is perfectly blue or when there is no object to be perceived. In these cases, the color experience cannot consist of a direct perceptual relation to an instance of perfect redness, because the subject stands in no such relation. Instead, it seems that the character of the experience is constituted independently of the properties of the per-ceived object.

In these impure Edenic worlds, an illusory or hallucinatory color experi-ence involves a relevant relation to the property of perfect redness that is not mediated by a relation to an instance of this property. (Something like this view is suggested as an account of hallucination in the actual world by Johnston 2004.) If so, then in such a world there may be phenomenally identical experiences (say, veridical and falsidical phenomenally red experi-ences) whose underlying metaphysical nature is quite distinct: one is con-stituted by a perceptual relation to a property instance in the subject's environment, and one is not. This picture is reminiscent of that held by some disjunctivists about perceptual experience in our world. We might say that in Eden, if not in our world, a disjunctive view of the metaphysics of perceptual experience is correct.

Is Eden a Possible World?

Eden does not exist, but could it have existed? That is, is there a possible world in which there are perfect colors? Could God have created such a world, if he had so chosen? I am not certain of the answer to this question, but I am inclined to say yes: there are Edenic possible worlds.

To start with, it seems that perceptual experience gives us some grip on what it would be for an object to be perfectly red or perfectly blue. It would have to be exactly like *that*, precisely as that object is pre-sented to us as being in experience. It seems that we can use this grip

---

causal relation. One could also say no, saying that this is a constitutive relation that is stronger than any causal relation. Even if so, however, there will at least be a counterfactual dependence of perceptual experience on perfect color properties in the world by virtue of the constitutive relation.

to form concepts of qualities such as perfect redness and perfect blue-ness (I have been deploying these concepts throughout this chapter). Furthermore, there is no obvious incoherence in the idea that an object could be perfectly red or perfectly blue. On the face of it we can con-ceive of such an object, so there is a prima facie case for believing that such an object is possible.

One can also reason as follows. There are good reasons to think that perfect redness is not instantiated in our world, but these reasons are empirical reasons, not a priori reasons. It was eating from the Tree of Illu-sion and the Tree of Science that led us to doubt that we live in an Edenic world. Moreover, eating from these trees was an empirical process based on empirical discoveries about the world. Before eating from these trees, there was no special reason to doubt that our experience was perfectly veridical. In particular, it is hard to see how one could be led to the conclusion that perfect redness is not instantiated by a priori reasoning alone (although see below). So the hypothesis that our world is Edenic seems at least to be conceivable, and it is reasonable to suggest that it cannot be ruled out a priori.

I have argued earlier (chapter 6) that this sort of conceivability is a good guide to metaphysical possibility. In particular, there is good rea-son to believe that if a hypothesis is ideally negatively conceivable in that it cannot be ruled out by idealized a priori reasoning, then there is a metaphysically possible world that verifies the hypothesis. There is even better reason to believe that if a hypothesis is ideally positively conceivable, in that one can imagine a situation in which the hypoth-esis actually obtains (in a way that holds up on idealized a priori reflec-tion), then there is a metaphysically possible world that verifies the hypothesis.

The hypothesis that our world is Edenic (that is, that perfect colors are instantiated in our world) seems to be at least prima facie negatively con-ceivable (it cannot easily be ruled out a priori) and prima facie positively conceivable (we can imagine that it actually obtains). Furthermore, it is not clear how this hypothesis could be undercut by further a priori reason-ing. If it cannot, then the hypothesis is ideally (negatively and positively) conceivable. If so, and if the conceivability-possibility thesis is correct, then there is a metaphysically possible world that verifies the hypothesis. Verifi-cation is a technical notion from two-dimensional semantics (verification goes with primary intensions, satisfaction with secondary intensions), but the technicalities do not matter too much in this case (the primary and secondary intensions of perfect color concepts are plausibly identical, so that if a world verifies the hypothesis that perfect colors are instantiated, it also satisfies the hypothesis). So, if this reasoning is correct, one can simply say that it is metaphysically possible that perfect colors are instantiated.

One could resist the conclusion either by denying that the Edenic hypothesis is conceivable in the relevant senses or by denying the connection between conceivability in the relevant senses and possibility. Speaking for myself, I am reasonably confident about the latter, but I am not certain about the former. I do not see any obvious way of ruling out the Edenic hypothesis a priori, but I cannot be sure that there is no such way. We will see that in the case of perfect pains, discussed later, there is arguably such a way. These considerations do not generalize to colors, but they make salient the possibility that other considerations might. For now, I am inclined to think that an Edenic world is metaphysically possible, but I am not certain of this.

Is There a Property of Perfect Redness?

If what I have said so far is right, there is no *instantiated* property of perfect redness, but it is natural to hold that perfect redness may be an uninstantiated property. It seems that we have a grip on such a property in experience: we grasp what it would be for an object to have the property of perfect redness. Certainly, if an Edenic world is metaphysically possible, then objects in those worlds will be perfectly red, and it seems reasonable to conclude that they have the property of perfect redness. Even if an Edenic world is metaphysically impossible, one might still hold that there is such a property, albeit a necessarily uninstantiated property (like the property of being a round square). These issues will interact with one's views on the metaphysics of properties to some extent. For example, if one thinks that properties are just sets of possible objects, or if one thinks that properties are very sparse relative to predicates, one might resist some of the reasoning here. But overall I think there is a good prima facie case for thinking that there is a property of perfect redness.

If there is no such property or if there is no metaphysically possible Edenic world, then some of the details in this chapter might have to change. If there is no metaphysically possible Edenic world, one cannot model the conditions of satisfaction associated with perfect veridicality using sets of (or functions over) metaphysically possible worlds. If there is no property of perfect redness, one cannot say that there is a content that attributes this property to an object. Even if so, however, one could understand the contents in other terms. For example, one could understand Edenic contents in terms of sets of epistemically possible scenarios rather than metaphysically possible worlds, or one could understand Edenic conditions of satisfaction using something like Fregean concepts rather than properties. One could also regard Eden as some sort of mere world model, not yet a possible world. Such a world model might still play a key role in determining the ordinary Fregean contents of perception via the requirement that the actual world must match the world model in various respects. In this fashion numerous key elements of the two-stage model of perceptual content could be preserved.

If there is a property of perfect redness, what sort of property is it? It is most natural to conceive of perfect redness as a sort of simple, irreducible quality, one that might be instantiated on the surface of objects in some possible world. Perfect color properties might not all be maximally simple. For example, they might be seen as a sort of composition from simpler perfect properties, such as certain perfect unique hues (so that a particular shade of perfect orange may be a composite of perfect redness and perfect yellowness to certain degrees and a certain amount of perfect brightness). But the underlying properties are naturally held to be irreducible.

In particular, it is natural to hold that perfect colors are not reducible to physical properties. If one accepts the earlier arguments that perfect color properties are not instantiated in our world, this consequence follows naturally. Even if one thought that perfect color properties are instantiated in our world, one could still argue that they are irreducible to physical properties, by analogs of familiar arguments concerning phenomenal properties.[13] For example, one could argue that one can conceive of a physically identical world in which they are not instantiated and infer that such a world is metaphysically possible. Alternatively, one could argue that someone without color vision could know all about the physical properties of objects without knowing about their perfect colors.

Still, it is at least coherent to hold a view on which experiences have Edenic content that represents the instantiation of perfect color properties and to hold that as a matter of empirical fact, perfect color properties are identical to certain physical properties (such as surface reflectances). On this view, our *concepts* of perfect color properties may be simple and irreducible concepts, but they pick out the same properties as those picked out by certain physical properties. Such a view would be analogous to certain "type-B" materialist views about phenomenal properties, according to which phenomenal properties are empirically identical to certain physical properties because simple phenomenal concepts pick out the same properties as certain physical concepts. On the resulting view, experiences could be seen to

13. Analog arguments of this sort are discussed in detail by Byrne (2006). Byrne conceives these arguments as arguments for the irreducibility of color properties. I think the arguments work best as arguments for the irreducibility of perfect color properties.

have a Russellian phenomenal content that represents the instantiation of certain physical properties (although the experience does not represent these properties *as* physical properties). On this sort of view, our experiences might be perfectly veridical even in a purely physical world. I do not find this view plausible myself: it is vulnerable to the usual objections to Russellian physicalist views based on inversion scenarios, for example (requiring either strong externalism about phenomenology or arbitrary asymmetries among inverted communities), and it is also subject to the conceivability arguments presented earlier. But there is at least an interesting variety of Russellian physicalism regarding phenomenal content in the vicinity.[14]

One could likewise hold a view on which perfect color properties are empirically identical to certain dispositional properties, or one could hold a view on which perfect color properties are distinct from physical and dispositional properties but on which they metaphysically supervene on such properties.[15] These views will be confronted with familiar problems: for example, the question of how to individuate the properties while still retaining plausible results about veridicality and illusion (for the view on which perfect colors are identical to or supervene on dispositional properties) and the questions of inversion and conceivability (for the view on which perfect colors supervene on intrinsic physical properties). But again, views of this sort are at least worth close consideration.

Finally, it is possible to hold that perfect color properties are identical to certain mental properties, such as those instantiated by one's visual field. This view agrees with the ordinary Edenic view that perfect colors are not instantiated by ordinary external objects but holds that they are instantiated by certain mental objects (though they need not be represented *as* mental properties). The resulting view, a version of projectivism, does not suffer from the problems for the physicalist and dispositionalist views outlined above.[16] I am inclined to reject this view myself because of familiar problems with holding that mental objects instantiate color properties or their analogs (Chisholm's 1942 "speckled hen" problem, for example) and because the view becomes particularly hard to accept when extending beyond the case of color (it is hard to accept that mental objects instantiate perfect height, for example, of the sort that we represent in spatial experience). But the question of whether perfect properties might be instantiated

14. The version of Russellian physicalism about phenomenal content advocated by Byrne and Hilbert (2003) may be particularly close to this view.

15. The views of Campbell (1993) and McGinn (1996) are at least closely related to the views in which perfect color properties supervene on intrinsic physical properties (for Campbell) and on dispositional properties (for McGinn).

16. The projectivist view of color defended by Boghossian and Velleman (1989) seems to be compatible with an Edenic view on which the perfect color properties are instantiated by a visual field.

in mental objects is at least well worth considering, and the corresponding version of projectivism might be able to accommodate many of the features of the two-stage view that I have been advocating.

For the remainder of this chapter I assume that perfect color properties are irreducible properties that are not instantiated in our world. But at least some aspects of the discussion may generalize to the other views I have outlined.

How Can We Represent Perfect Redness?

If perfect redness is never instantiated in our world, then we have never had contact with any instances of it. If so, one might wonder how perfect redness can be represented in the content of our experiences.

Construed as an objection, this point turns on the tacit premise that representing a property requires contact with instances of it. In reply, one can observe that we can certainly represent other uninstantiated properties (the property of being phlogistonated, Hume's missing shade of blue) and can even represent uninstantiable properties (being a round square). An opponent might suggest that these are complex properties whose representation derives from the representation of simpler properties and so might propose the modified premise that representing a *simple* property requires contact with instances of it. It is far from clear why we should accept this, however. For example, there seem to be perfectly coherent Humean views of causation on which we represent the simple property (or relation) of causation in our experience and in our thought but on which no causation is present in the world.

Certainly, there are cases in which representing a property crucially depends on contact with instances of it, but there also many cases of representation that do not work like this. One can plausibly represent the property of being a philosopher without being acquainted with any philosophers. On the Humean view just discussed, the same goes for causation. One might divide representations into those that are subject to Twin Earth thought experiments (so that twins in a different environment would represent different properties) and those that are not. Representations in the first class (including especially the representation of natural kinds such as water) may have content that depends on instantiation of the relevant property in the environment. But representations in the second class (including perhaps representations of philosophers and causation, at least if this representation does not involve deference to a surrounding linguistic community) do not depend on instances of the property in this way. In these cases, representation of a property comes not from instances of that property in the environment but rather from some sort of internal grasp of what it would take for something to instantiate the property. It is plausible that representation of perfect redness falls into this second class.

To say this much is just to respond to the objection and not to fully answer the question. The residual question concerns just *how* our mental states get to have a given Edenic content. I will not answer this question here. We do not yet have a good theory of how our mental states represent any properties at all, and the cases of "narrow" representation, such as the representation of philosophers and causation, are particularly ill understood. To properly answer these questions and the analogous question about Edenic content requires a theory of the roots of intentionality.

I would speculate, however, that the roots of Edenic content lie deep in the heart of phenomenology itself. Horgan and Tienson (2002) have suggested that there is a distinctive sort of "phenomenal intentionality" that is grounded in phenomenology rather than in extrinsic causal connections. It is not unreasonable to suppose that Edenic content is a basic sort of phenomenal intentionality—perhaps even the most basic sort. This could be combined with a variety of views about the metaphysics of phenomenal intentionality. For example, one could hold that such intentionality is grounded in the projection of properties of certain mental objects, as on the projectivist view. Or one could hold that the representation of Edenic content is even more primitive than this. If one is inclined to think that there is something irreducible about phenomenology, one might naturally hold that perceptual phenomenology simply consists in certain primitive relations to certain primitive properties: the presentation of perfect redness, for example. In any case, it is likely that understanding the roots of Edenic content will be closely tied to understanding the metaphysics of phenomenology.

10. Colors and Color Constancy

What about Color Constancy?

Color constancy is the phenomenon wherein instances of the same color in the environment, when illuminated by quite different sorts of lighting so that they reflect different sorts of light, nevertheless seem to have the same color. A paradigmatic example is a shadow. When we see a surface that is partly in shadow, although there is something different about the appearance of the shadowed portion of the surface, it often does not seem to us as if the object has a different color in the shadowed portion. One might say that although there is a sense in which the shadowed and unshadowed portions look different, there is also a sense in which they look the same. Certainly, the shadowed and unshadowed portions produce phenomenally distinct experiences, but we often do not judge the object to have a different color in those areas.

To say this much is to stay neutral on the representational content of the relevant experience. But it is natural to wonder just how the content of such experiences should be analyzed. In particular, it is natural to wonder how the two-stage model can handle such contents. To address this question, one can ask as before: how would the world have to be in order for experiences of this sort to be perfectly veridical? A definite answer to this question requires a close phenomenological analysis. I will not give a full analysis here, but I will outline some options.

It is useful to focus on the case of shadows. As an example, we can take a white floor on which an object casts a crisp dark shadow. I will take it that there are visual cues indicating that a shadow is being cast, so that we judge that the floor is still white in the relevant area, though we also judge that it is in shadow. What is the content of this experience? How would the world have to be in order for the experience to be perfectly veridical?

The answer depends on how we analyze the phenomenology of the experience. To start, one might take either a *simple* or a *complex* view of the phenomenology. On the simple view, the apparent sameness in color between the shadowed and the unshadowed areas is not present in visual phenomenology at all. Rather, the sameness is detected only at the level of visual judgment or perhaps at the level of other perceptual mechanisms whose contents are not reflected in phenomenology. For simplicity, let us say it is at the level of visual judgment. On this view, the phenomenal character of the experience of the floor may be the same as the phenomenal character of a floor where the relevant portion of the floor is painted the relevant shade of gray and in which the floor is under constant illumination; it might also be the same as in a case where the floor is in shadow in the relevant portion but where there are no cues. (We can stipulate that the last two cases involve exactly the same retinal stimulation, so that there is not much doubt that the resulting experiences are phenomenally identical.) On the simple view, the original shadow case will differ merely in that relevant cues lead to a judgment of sameness in that case but not in the others. The simple view will say something similar about all cases of color constancy: the constancy is present at the level of judgment, not at the level of perceptual experience.

The simple view is naturally associated with a view on which the local phenomenology of color experience is three-dimensional: the relevant experiences can be arranged in a three-dimensional color solid that exhausts the relevant dimensions of variation. At least, the view will hold that if there are further dimensions of variation, then variations due to shadows, illumination, and so on are not among them. On this view, the local phenomenology of perceiving the shadow will be the same as the local phenomenology of veridically perceiving an unshadowed object that is the relevant shade of gray. It is natural to hold that the Edenic content of such an experience involves the attribution of perfect grayness. It follows that on this view, the perfect veridicality of a shadow experience will require the instantiation of the relevant shade of perfect grayness in the object of perception. If we accept the simple view, then if a shadow is cast in a pure Edenic world (one without illusion), the color of the object will change.

On the simple view, what are the imperfect veridicality conditions of such an experience? An experience of the shadow will be correct iff the floor instantiates a property that matches perfect grayness. A property matches perfect grayness, to a first approximation, if it normally causes phenomenally gray experiences. If we take it that there is a canonical normal condition that involves unshadowed light, then this property will be something like a certain specific surface reflectance that the shadowed area of the floor does not instantiate, so the experience will be (imperfectly) falsidical. If we allow that there is a wide range of normal conditions that includes both shadowed and unshadowed light, things are more complicated. I discuss this complication further in the next section.

One other position compatible with the simple view holds that while the *local* phenomenology of seeing the partially shadowed floor is the same as the *local* phenomenology of seeing a partially gray floor without cues, the *global* phenomenology of the two cases is different (because of the difference in cues), and this difference in global phenomenology makes for a difference in conditions of veridicality. This view requires a certain antiatomism about perceptual content: the veridicality conditions of an experience of a color at a location are not determined just by the local phenomenology associated with the location but also by the phenomenology of the entire visual experience. That is, two experiences can have the same local phenomenology but different local content due to different global phenomenology. This view leads to a complicated further range of options about perceptual content, on some of which the shadow experience may end up being (imperfectly) veridical. These options end up roughly mirroring the options for the complex view that follows (which also postulates differences in local content, this time associated with differences in local phenomenology), so I will not discuss them further here.

The alternative to the simple view is the *complex* view, on which the apparent sameness in color between the shadowed and unshadowed areas is present in some fashion in the visual phenomenology of seeing the floor. On this view, the experience of seeing the partially shadowed floor is phenomenally different from the experience of seeing a partially gray floor under uniform lighting, and the phenomenal difference is present in the visual phenomenology associated with the floor itself (and not merely in the experience of background cues). On this view, the presence or absence of cues makes a difference to the visual experience of the floor itself: one might say that the cues play a pre-experiential role and not just a pre-judgmental role.

This view is naturally associated with a view on which the local phenomenology of color experience is more than three-dimensional. For the sameness to be accommodated in visual phenomenology, it is natural to hold that the color contents associated with the shadowed and unshadowed areas are in some respect the same. If local phenomenology three-dimensional and if differences in local content went along with differences in local phenomenology (the alternative that rejects this second thesis collapses into the antiatomistic version of the simple view presented earlier), then this sameness in local content would entail that the local phenomenology of seeing the shadowed and unshadowed white regions is exactly the same. That claim is not phenomenologically plausible. So the complex view suggests that the local phenomenology of seeing color has more than three relevant dimensions of variation, with correspondingly more dimensions of variation in representational content.

On this view, the shadowed and unshadowed areas will be represented as being the same in some respect: intuitively, both will be represented as white. They will also be represented as being different in some respect: intuitively, one will be represented as being in shadow and one will not. These respects of sameness and difference will both be present in the phenomenology. One can argue that this view is more phenomenologically attractive than the simple view in allowing phenomenological and representational differences between seeing something as shadowed white and as unshadowed white, on the one hand, and between seeing something as shadowed white and as unshadowed gray, on the other. I am inclined to favor the complex view over the simple view for this reason, although the correct characterization of the phenomenology is far from obvious, and neither view is obviously correct or incorrect.

If the complex view is correct, what should we say about the Edenic content of an experience of shadowed white? Phenomenologically, such an experience seems to characterize the intrinsic properties of a surface: if one takes the experience completely at face value, there seems to be an intrinsic (although perhaps temporary) difference between the shadowed and unshadowed parts of the floor. So it is natural to say that the Edenic content of the experience attributes a complex intrinsic property to the floor. One might see this property as the conjunction of two intrinsic properties: roughly, perfect whiteness and perfect shadow. That is, the Edenic content presents the floor as being perfectly white, infused in the relevant areas with a perfect shadow. This conjunctive treatment of perfect shadowed white is not mandatory: one could see the property as a certain mode of perfect white rather than as a conjunction of perfect white with an independent perfect shadow property. The conjunctive proposal has a certain phenomenological plausibility, however, insofar as one can see differently colored areas as subject to the same sort of shadow.

On this view, perfect shadows are things that can come and go in Eden, while the perfect color of an object stays the same. When a perfect shadow is cast on a perfectly white object, the shadow is *on* the object in the sense that it affects the intrinsic nature of the object's surface. Of course there are different sorts of shadows corresponding to different degrees of shadowing, each of which can come and go while an object's perfect color stays the same. Strictly speaking, it is best to talk of shadow properties instantiated at locations on objects rather than talking of shadows. While we sometimes have the phenomenology of seeing shadows as objects, it is arguable that more often we do not.

One might worry that this view cannot adequately capture the dimension of sameness between shadowed white and unshadowed gray. There is a clear respect in which these experiences are phenomenally similar, and one might argue that this respect corresponds to a representational similarity: perhaps one could say that the objects of such experience seem the same with respect to superficial color or something along those lines. The representational claim is not obviously mandatory here, but if one accepts it, one might elaborate the Edenic model by saying that there is a respect in which any objects with perfect shadowed white and perfect unshadowed gray are similar to each other. One might say that both of these perfect properties entail perfect superficial grayness, for example. This might either be seen as a composite property or simply as corresponding to another way of carving up the underlying multidimensional space.

What are the imperfect veridicality conditions of such an experience? Presumably an experience as of shadowed white is veridical iff its object has a property that matches perfect shadowed white, or, on the conjunctive treatment of shadowed white, iff it has a property that matches perfect white and a property that matches perfect shadow. The former is plausibly a physical property such as a certain surface reflectance (although see below). As for the latter, it will be a property that normally causes experiences as of the appropriate sort of shadow. It seems that no intrinsic property of surfaces is a good candidate here. Rather, the reasonable candidates are all relational: for example, the property of being subject to the occlusion of a light source to a relevant degree in the relevant area. This is a relational property rather than an intrinsic property, so it does not match the property of perfect shadow as well as it could. But with no intrinsic property being even a candidate, it seems that this property may match well enough. If so, then we can say the experience is imperfectly veridical iff the object has the relevant physical property (imperfect whiteness) and the relevant relational property (imperfect shadow). If it has one but not the other, one can say that the experience is imperfectly veridical in one respect but not the other.

One can extend something like this treatment to other cases of color constancy and to cases of variation in illumination in general. One might hold that whenever there are relevant cues about illumination, these make a difference to the complex phenomenology of an experience with a corresponding difference in content. If the perceptual system is doing its job, then the object will be represented as having the same color, but it will also be represented as being different in some relevant respect, analogous to the presence or absence of shadows earlier. The difference in phenomenology seems to involve a difference in intrinsic (if temporary) properties, so the associated Edenic properties are intrinsic: one might call them perfect illumination properties (with the recognition that perfect illumination is intrinsic rather than extrinsic). There will plausibly be a complex space of such perfect illumination properties, perhaps a three-dimensional space, and a corresponding space of matching imperfect properties (which may once again be relational properties, such as the property of being illuminated by certain sorts of light. Once we consider color and illumination together, we will plausibly have at least a six-dimensional space of complex Edenic properties in the vicinity and a corresponding space of imperfect physical/relational properties.

One might wonder about the experience of darkness. What happens in Eden when darkness falls? I am inclined to say that darkness is in some respects like the experience of shadow, but more pervasive. As darkness falls, darkness seems to pervade the environment, present at every location. The whole space appears to become dark. Objects do not seem to change their colors, exactly, although the representation of their colors may become much less specific, and it eventually becomes absent altogether (as does the representation of objects, in pitch blackness). So it is natural to say that in

Eden, when things become dark, perfect darkness is present throughout the relevant volume of space, intrinsically altering that volume, although it need not alter objects' colors. In Eden, when darkness falls, perfect darkness pervades.

What Are Imperfect Colors?

The imperfect colors are the properties that match the perfect colors (in our world) and whose instantiation or noninstantiation makes our color experiences veridical or falsidical. Just which properties are these? So far, I have said that these are the intrinsic physical properties that serve as the normal cause of experiences with the corresponding phenomenal properties. A first approximation suggests that these may be certain surface reflectance properties or, better, the categorical bases of the relevant surface reflectance dispositions. But there are some tricky issues.

One tricky issue, stressed by Hardin (1987), arises from the fact that there is no such thing as a canonical normal condition for the perception of colors. Instead, there is a wide range of normal conditions, including bright sunlight, muted cloudy light, shaded light, and so on. For a given subject, the same object may cause experiences with different phenomenal characters in each of these conditions. So it is not obvious that there will be any specific physical property that can be singled out as the "normal cause" of a given phenomenal character property.[17]

How we handle this issue depends on whether we take the simple view or the complex view of color constancy. On the complex view, as long as the mechanisms of color constancy work reasonably well, then the same object may cause experiences that are the same in certain key respects while differing in others. For example, a white object will cause an experience of shadowed white in shadowed conditions and an experience of unshadowed white in unshadowed conditions. On the complex view, the Edenic contents of these experiences attribute the same perfect color property (perfect whiteness) but different perfect illumination properties (perfect shadow and perfect unshadow). We can put this by saying that the experiences have the same phenomenal color property and different phenomenal illumination properties. On this view, while a given object may trigger

17. Hardin (1987) also stresses variations between normal perceivers, as well as variations in normal conditions. Variations between normal perceivers are no problem for the two-stage view, as matching is always relative to a subject, and it is the normal cause for a given subject that determines the Russellian content of a color experience. At worst, this sort of variation has the consequence that the Russellian content of phenomenally identical color experiences in different subjects may represent different physical properties.

experiences with different phenomenal character in different conditions, these experiences will usually attribute the same phenomenal color (though different phenomenal illuminations), associated with the same perfect color property. So on this view, the wide range of normal conditions is not incompatible with the existence of a reasonably specific property that typically causes experiences with the relevant phenomenal color (that is, experiences that attribute the relevant perfect color) across the range of normal conditions.

If we take the simple view of color constancy, the issue is more difficult. According to this view, a white object may cause quite different experiences under bright and shadowed light: let us call them phenomenally white and phenomenally gray experiences. On this view, there is no relevant phenomenal property that is shared by such experiences: any sameness in content enters only at the level of judgment. A phenomenally gray experience may be caused by a white object in one condition and by a gray object in another condition, where both conditions are equally normal. So it appears that on the simple view, there is no fine-grained intrinsic property that can serve as "the normal cause" of a phenomenally gray experience. (A similar issue could arise on the complex view if it turns out that the mechanisms of color constancy are sufficiently unreliable.) Appealing to dispositional properties will not help as the fine-grained dispositional properties of a white and a gray object differ as much as their intrinsic properties.

Here a number of reactions are possible. One could hold that one condition (e.g., bright midday sunlight) is singled out as normal. One could hold that the matching imperfect property is not an intrinsic or a dispositional property of the object but a (transient) relational property, such as the property of (currently) causing phenomenally gray experiences or the property of reflecting a certain sort of light or the disjunction of being white under shadowed light, gray under unshadowed light, and so on. Alternatively, one could hold that it turns out empirically that no imperfect property matches perfect grayness, so that the (imperfect) Fregean content of such an experience determines no nontrivial Russellian content in the actual world (it is akin in certain respects to a sentence containing an empty description).

In my view the most plausible line for a proponent of the simple view to take is to hold that the normal cause of phenomenally gray experiences is a disjunctive or coarse-grained intrinsic property: one whose instances include white objects, gray objects, and any objects that cause phenomenally gray objects in some normal condition. On this view, a phenomenally gray experience of any such object will be veridical. This view has the advantage of capturing our intuitions that no such experience in reasonably normal conditions should be privileged over others and that at least some of these experiences are veridical. The disadvantage of this view is that it suggests that the (imperfect) color properties attributed by color experiences are less fine grained than one might have thought, so that a phenomenally gray and a phenomenally white experience do not attribute incompatible (imperfect) properties even when they occur simultaneously. On reflection, however, this consequence does not seem too bad. The incompatibility is still captured at the level of Edenic content, and if one takes the simple view and thinks of shadowed cases, it is reasonably intuitive that phenomenally gray and phenomenally white experiences might be compatible (for example, that both might veridically represent a white floor).[18]

Properties such as imperfect redness will be disjunctive in other respects. Color experience is most often caused by the reflection of light from objects, but it is also caused by the radiation of light from light sources, by the transmission of light from semitransparent sources, and so on. The relevant cause of phenomenal color experiences in the first case will be something like a surface reflectance (or its categorical basis), but in other cases it will be something like a radiation profile (or its categorical basis). It seems reasonable to hold that color experiences of radiating objects and the like can be just as (imperfectly) veridical as those of reflecting objects. So imperfect redness is best seen as a disjunction of a range of reflectance properties, radiation properties, and other properties that can serve as the relevant basis.

What Are Colors?

What does this view say about the nature of colors? Philosophers argue about whether colors (such as redness) are best seen as physical properties, dispositional properties, mental properties, primitive properties, or something else. So far I have taken no stand on this matter. What view of colors does the two-stage view suggest?

It is reasonable to hold that much of the issue here is terminological. We can acknowledge a role for properties of each of these sorts. Once we understand the precise role that each plays, we understand the substantive

18. It might be objected that on this view, a phenomenally gray and white "striped" experience of an unstriped floor will be counterintuitively classified as veridical. This could be handled by saying that such an experience represents that the relevant areas are *differently* colored, a sort of relational color property. One could then say that the imperfect relation that best matches the relevant Edenic relation here is that of having different fine-grained surface reflectances or something along those lines. Then the ordinary content of the experience will require that different fine-grained intrinsic properties are present in the relevant areas, but it will not take a precise stand on which fine-grained properties these are.

issues in the vicinity, whichever of them we choose to call "color." That being said, the terminological issue is not wholly without content. There are certain core roles that we expect colors to play, and different properties are differently suited for the label "color" to the extent that they play more or fewer of these core roles.

On the two-stage view, the natural candidates to be called "colors" are perfect colors and imperfect colors. Both of these can be seen as playing one crucial role associated with colors: they are properties attributed in color experiences. Perfect colors are attributed in Edenic contents, and imperfect colors are attributed in ordinary contents. Perfect colors play certain further core roles that imperfect colors do not. We seem to be acquainted with their intrinsic nature in color experience, and the perfect colors arguably stand in relevant intrinsic structural relations to each other in a way that imperfect colors do not.

Still, perhaps the core role of colors is that they are the properties whose instantiation is relevant to the truth of ordinary color attributions. That is, an utterance of 'that apple is red' will be true if and only if the apple instantiates redness. Furthermore, it is natural to hold that some apples really are red. The two-stage view is partly driven by the thesis that some ordinary color experiences are veridical (even if they are not perfectly veridical). It seems equally reasonable to hold that apples really are red (even if they are not perfectly red). If so, this suggests that redness is not perfect redness but imperfect redness.

So I am inclined to say that color terms, in their ordinary uses, designate imperfect color properties. Just which properties these are depends on how matching is understood. To the extent that matching is somewhat indeterminate, the designation of color terms may be somewhat indeterminate. But I am inclined to think that our ordinary uses of color terms designate certain disjunctive physical properties, with properties such as surface reflectance properties among the disjuncts. The physical properties designated by ordinary color terms will be relatively coarse grained, but there will be more fine-grained physical properties in the vicinity, which we might regard as the different shades of these colors.[19]

Of course, one can also reasonably use color terms to refer to Edenic properties ("perfect redness"), phenomenal properties ("phenomenal redness"), and maybe other properties as well. On this view, there are multiply interlocked families of properties: the perfect colors, the imperfect colors,

19. If an advocate of the simple view of color constancy takes the line I suggest, according to which experiences with specific phenomenal shades attribute relatively coarse-grained physical properties, then we will have three relevant sorts of physical properties. There will be highly coarse-grained properties (with some indeterminacy at the edges) that are the referents of terms such as "red"; there will be some-

possibly further families of imperfect colors associated with different notions of matching, and the phenomenal colors. As long as we understand the complex relationships between these families, as well as the roles that each can play, not much of real substance rests on which of these families we deem to be the true family of colors.

There is nothing especially original or distinctive about the view of the ontology of color that emerges from the two-stage view. In identifying colors (in the core sense) with physical properties, the resulting ontology of colors may be very similar to that of the physicalist about color. The various families of color properties that are introduced may also be acknowledged by the primitivist. Although primitivists about color identify perfect color properties with the colors, they may also recognize that physical and dispositional properties play some of the roles of the colors. For example, Maund (1995) says that terms such as "red" refer in their core sense to the perfect colors (which he calls "virtual colors") but also in an extended or metonymic sense to the physical properties that I have called imperfect colors. So the ontology recognized by this sort of primitivist view is not dissimilar to that recognized by the two-stage view.

What is distinctive about the two-stage view is not its associated ontology of colors but rather its view of perceptual content. On the primitivist view, experiences have a single content (an Edenic content) that determines their veridicality. On the two-stage view, experiences have two layers of content, an Edenic content, which reflects their phenomenology, and a Fregean content, which determines their veridicality. It is this two-layered view of content that is responsible for most of the explanatory power of the two-stage view.

Is This Indirect Realism?

One might worry that this view is a form of indirect realism about color perception. According to standard indirect realism, we perceive objects in the world only indirectly, in virtue of directly perceiving certain intermediate objects such as sense data, which opponents see as a "veil of perception" that cuts off perceivers from the external world. The two-stage view I have outlined is certainly not a variety of standard indirect realism, as it does

---

what coarse-grained properties that are attributed by specific color experiences; and there will be fine-grained physical properties of which these coarse-grained properties can be seen as ranges or disjunctions. Probably the fine-grained properties are the best candidates to be called the "shades." The main costs are that we lose a tight correspondence between physical shades and phenomenal shades and that there will not turn out to be a specific physical shade that qualifies as "unique red" (though there may still be unique phenomenal red and unique perfect red). If we take the complex view of color constancy (and if the mechanisms of color constancy are sufficiently reliable), then these problems are avoided.

not invoke any intermediate objects as objects of perception. But one might worry that it is a form of indirect realism about the perception of *properties*. In particular, one might suggest that, on this view, instantiated color properties (that is, imperfect color properties) are perceived only indirectly, in virtue of directly perceiving perfect color properties.

This objection invokes the relation of *perception* between subjects and properties. This relation is analogous to the relation of perception between subjects and objects. It is natural to say that when I veridically perceive a green square in the environment, I perceive both the square and its greenness. So far in this chapter, I have focused on the relation of perceptual representation but not on the relation of perception. These seem to be different relations: one can perceptually represent an object or a property without perceiving it (in a hallucination, for example).

The standard view of the perceptual relation between subjects and objects holds that it is a *causal* relation. To perceive an object is roughly to have a perceptual experience that is appropriately caused by the object (and perhaps that has a phenomenal character that is appropriately related to the character of the object). The standard view of the perceptual relation between subjects and properties is presumably something similar. To perceive a property is roughly to have a perceptual experience whose phenomenal character is appropriately causally related to an instance of that property (and perhaps whose phenomenal character represents the instantiation of the property or otherwise "matches" the property in some fashion).

If we adopt this standard view of the perceptual relation, there is no threat of indirect realism. In a typical veridical experience of a green object, the phenomenal character of my experience is causally related to the relevant instance of physical greenness and represents the instantiation of physical greenness in its Russellian content. By contrast, the phenomenal character of my experience is not causally related to any instance of perfect greenness, as there are no such instances. So it seems that on the two-stage view, as much as on other views of perceptual experience, we perceive imperfect colors directly and not in virtue of perceiving any other property.

It is true that on the two-stage view, perception is not as "direct" as perception could be. There is a sense in which perception in Eden is more direct than it is in our non-Edenic world. In Eden, perception works by direct acquaintance, and there need be no mediation between objects and properties perceived and a perceptual experience. In our world, there is complex causal mediation. This does not entail that our perception is *perceptually* mediated, though, as on the indirect realist view.

We might say that, in Eden, an especially strong perceptual relation obtains, one that we might call *perfect perception*. Perfect perception of an object or property requires unmediated acquaintance with the object or the property and perhaps also that the object or the property itself be a constituent of one's perceptual experience. By contrast, *imperfect perception* requires only the appropriate sort of causal connection to an object or a property. As before, it is plausible to suggest that if we took the deliverances of both perception and introspection fully at face value, we would conclude that we live in an Edenic world in which we perfectly perceive objects and properties in that world. But after the fall from Eden, there is no perfect perception; there is just imperfect perception.

We might call this view not *indirect realism* but *imperfect realism*. Our acquaintance with the world is not as direct as it would be in Eden, and perception does not reveal the intrinsic nature of things in the way that it does in Eden. But this is so for any causal theory of perception. Perception on the view I have outlined is no more and no less imperfect than on most causal theories. The idea of Eden just brings out the contrast, for all these theories, with the kind of perfect perception that we cannot have in our non-Edenic world. One might yearn for the kind of perfect contact with the world that we had in Eden, but after the fall, we have learned to live with the imperfection of perception.

11. Matching and Fregean Content

What Is Matching?

The notion of matching serves as a bridge between Edenic content and ordinary content. An experience is imperfectly veridical when its object has properties that match the perfect properties attributed by the experience. But what is it for a property to match a perfect property? To a first approximation, we can say that a property matches a given perfect property (for a given subject) if the property is the normal cause of the associated phenomenal property (in that subject). But this is clearly just a first approximation.

A basic constraint is that at most one imperfect property can match a given perfect property. Or at least, at most one imperfect property can match a perfect property for a subject at a time. Different imperfect properties can match the same perfect properties for different subjects and probably for the same subject at widely separated times. (Strictly speaking, matching is a three- or four-place relation involving subjects and times, but I usually leave the subject and the time in the background.) But we need at most one matching property for a subject at a time so that the ordinary Russellian content of an experience can attribute a property to its object. Of course it could be, for all we have said, that matching imperfect properties are often disjunctive properties or determinable properties with many different determinates. It may also be that sometimes there is no imperfect property that matches a given perfect property.

Matching is best understood as a holistic relation. Rather than saying that imperfect redness is the property that normally causes phenomenal redness, one can say that the set of imperfect color properties is that three-dimensional manifold of properties that serves as the normal causal basis for the associated three-dimensional manifold of phenomenal color properties. This requires that there is a mapping from imperfect properties to phenomenal properties such that in many or most cases a given imperfect property will normally cause the associated phenomenal property, but this relation need not hold in all cases. If there are exceptions associated with certain imperfect properties in the manifold (such as Kripke's "killer yellow," a shade of yellow that always kills the perceiver if observed, or perhaps a Humean missing shade of blue that is never instantiated in our world for a lawful reason), this will not stop the manifold as a whole from matching, and the imperfect property will still be associated with a corresponding phenomenal property. When this mapping associates an imperfect property with a phenomenal property that attributes a given perfect property, we can say that the imperfect property matches the perfect property.

Clearly, the notion of matching is a vague and messy one. One source of messiness arises from the issue discussed earlier: there is no precise delineation of the class of normal conditions. Even if there were such a delineation, there is no precise criterion for when a property causes an experience often enough in these conditions to count as its normal cause. Further, there is more to matching than normally causing an associated phenomenal property. We have seen that there are structural constraints, such as the constraint that imperfect color properties fall into the same sort of three-dimensional manifold as perfect color properties. There are also categorical constraints, such as the constraint that imperfect color properties be intrinsic properties if possible. It is presumably also desirable that (imperfect) color properties be properties that can stand in the sort of relations to (imperfect) spatial properties that perfect color properties stand in to perfect spatial properties.

One could attempt to encapsulate all these constraints and others in a full and precise definition of matching, but I am not optimistic about the prospects for such a definition any more than I am for definitions of other philosophically important notions such as perception and knowledge. An alternative approach is simply to say: matching is that relation M such that, necessarily, an experience is imperfectly veridical iff its objects have properties that bear M to the properties attributed by its Edenic content. In effect, this notion exploits our relatively pretheoretical grip on imperfect veridicality, along with an independently grounded notion of Edenic content (explained in terms of perfect veridicality, say), to explicate the notion of matching.

Of course, this explication does not say anything substantive about what matching involves. For a substantive characterization, we have to rely on judgments about the (imperfect) veridicality and falsidicality of experiences. We do have quite clear judgments in many cases. And it is plausible that we judge experiences to be veridical precisely when objects in the world instantiate certain properties, properties that correspond in some fashion to the perfect properties in the Edenic content of our experiences. Even if we cannot give a full account antecedently of what this correspondence consists in, there is good reason to believe that it is present, and one can say quite a lot about what it involves in specific cases, as we have already done. For example, it usually seems to require normal causation of an associated phenomenal property, and there are other constraints as suggested by various cases. As in the case of analyzing knowledge, there will probably be no straightforward articulation of necessary and sufficient constraints; nevertheless, the consideration of cases can help us to flesh out the constraints in the vicinity.

One might worry that this characterization taken together with the two-stage view will be circular. The two-stage view says that an experience is imperfectly veridical iff its objects have properties that match the relevant perfect properties. The characterization here says that matching is that relation M such that an experience is imperfectly veridical iff its objects have properties that bear M to the relevant perfect properties. There is no circularity, however. In the project of explication, we have a prior grip on the notion of imperfect veridicality, and we use this prior grip in order to explicate the notion of matching. Via this explication, we theoretically characterize a relation M. One can then use relation M for certain theoretical purposes, if one likes. At the very least, we can appeal to it in analyzing the relationship between imperfect and perfect conditions of veridicality. One might go further and hold that, metaphysically, for an experience to be imperfectly veridical is for its objects to bear M to the relevant perfect properties. Or one might hold that epistemically, our intuitive judgments about imperfect veridicality are mediated by a tacit prior grasp of M. I am cautious about making such further claims here, although I think there is something to them. In any case, there is no more circularity here than in any other case where one uses a pretheoretical notion to help characterize a theoretical notion, which one then may use to help give a theoretical account of the pretheoretical notion.

Of course, our judgments about (imperfect) veridicality are not always clear. There are many cases in which we are not sure what to say or in which we are tugged in two different directions. Sometimes these judgments are cleared up on a certain amount of rational reflection, but sometimes they are not. When they cannot be cleared up in this way, the natural thing to say is that the relevant case is a vague case of imperfect veridicality. The vagueness of imperfect veridicality will give rise to a corresponding vagueness of matching: it will be vague whether the object in question instantiates a property that matches the relevant perfect property. There may be different ways of precisifying the notion of imperfect veridicality, which will give rise to corresponding precisifications of the notion of matching. But some vagueness and messiness in the notion of matching is just what we should expect, given the vagueness and messiness of imperfect veridicality.

Is Fregean Content Phenomenologically Adequate?

Although the two-stage view has a clearer grounding in phenomenological structure than the original Fregean view, one might still worry about its phenomenological adequacy. The Edenic content of an experience (in which the two-stage content is grounded) seems to nicely mirror the structure of the phenomenology. But the imperfect Fregean content does not. In particular, there is nothing discernible in the phenomenology of visual experience that obviously corresponds to matching. Certainly, it is hard to see that there is any clear phenomenology of "normal causation" in a typical visual experience. And to the extent that matching is messier and more complex than a notion based on normal causation, it seems all the more distant from the phenomenology. For example, we have seen that matching can often be vague, as can the associated Fregean content, but the phenomenology itself need not be vague, or, if it is vague in some respects, it need not be vague in relevant respects. For example, it is plausibly vague in some cases whether an object has a property that matches perfect redness. But the associated phenomenally red experience may be quite precise, with the phenomenology of precisely presenting a specific property of the object. So one may ask, as we did before, whether this Fregean view is phenomenologically adequate.

I think one should concede that matching does not correspond directly to any element of the visual phenomenology. The phenomenology of visual experience is the same in our world and in Eden. The presentation of an Edenic world does not (or need not) involve attribution of normal causation and the like. So the phenomenology of ordinary visual experience does not (or need not) involve this, either. Perhaps there are some experiences that present causal and dispositional relations, but it seems wrong to say that every ordinary color experience does this.

Where does matching come from then? I think the answer is clear: it comes from the *inferential role* of visual experience. The content of a mental state need not be something that one can read off the intrinsic properties of its vehicles. There is good reason to believe that quite generally, mental content is tied to inferential role. This is especially so in the case of Fregean content, which was introduced by Frege to mirror the cognitive and inferential significance of thought and language. A belief expressed by 'Hesperus is Phosphorus' has a very different inferential role from a belief expressed by 'Hesperus is Hesperus,' and this difference in inferential role is reflected in a difference in their inferential content. It is even possible to define the Fregean conditions of satisfaction of a belief partly in terms of the belief's inferential role, such as the conditions under which a subject will rationally accept or reject the belief, given information about the world (see Chalmers 2002a for such an account).

Beliefs are not the only mental states that have inferential roles. Perceptual experiences also have an inferential role, broadly understood. Just as one belief can serve as grounds for accepting or rejecting another belief, a perceptual experience can likewise serve as grounds for accepting or rejecting beliefs and, more generally, for guiding our knowledge about the world. Most obviously (as discussed in the afterword to the previous chapter), one can *endorse* a perceptual experience, yielding a perceptual belief about the character of one's environment, and that belief can be used to accept or reject other beliefs in turn. For example, when one has a phenomenally red experience as of an object in one's environment, this can be used as grounds for accepting a belief that there is a red object in front of one. One would not normally call this relation between experience and belief an "inference," but it can be seen as a sort of quasi-inferential relation.

Just as with belief, the inferential role of a perceptual experience can be analyzed in part by asking: when given information about how things are in the world, will a subject accept or reject the perceptual experience? That is, will the subject accept or reject the belief that things are as they perceptually seem to be? If one takes an example, such as a subject having a phenomenally red experience as of an object in front of her, one finds a specific pattern of judgments. If the subject discovers that there is really no object in front of her, she will reject the experience: things are not as they seem. If she discovers that there is an object in front of her but it has the sort of physical makeup that usually causes phenomenally green experiences (causing phenomenally red experiences this time only due to unusual lighting), then she will reject the experience: again, things are not as they seem. But if she discovers that the object in front of her has the sort of makeup that usually causes phenomenally red experiences, then she will accept the experience: at least in the relevant respects, things are as they seem.

In effect, the core inferential role of a perceptual experience is reflected in the pattern of judgments about veridicality and falsidicality that the subject of such an experience makes or, more strictly, in the pattern of judgments that should be rationally made. We have already seen that this pattern of judgments closely corresponds to the Fregean content presented earlier. The pattern of judgments does not require that objects in the environment have any specific property such as a surface reflectance or even perfect redness. It requires only that the property be the property that plays the appropriate causal role. So as in the case of beliefs, this Fregean content closely mirrors the experience's inferential role.[20]

Here we can respond to the charge of phenomenological adequacy by rejecting the claim that phenomenal content must precisely mirror phenomenological structure. Phenomenal content can equally be grounded in inferential role.

Of course, a proponent of the original Fregean view could have made the same response (as I did in response to a similar worry in the last chapter). So how is the two-stage view any better in this respect? To see the difference, recall where things stood at the end of section 5. It was not clear that the objections from phenomenological adequacy had knockdown force, but they raised the issue of a serious explanatory incompleteness in the Fregean view. Fregean content is supposed to be a sort of phenomenal content, such that necessarily, an experience with the same phenomenology has the same Fregean content. But the presentational phenomenology of visual experience does not simply wear its Fregean content on its sleeve. So there needs to be some explanatory story about how Fregean content is related to the phenomenology of the experience and why it is that any experience with that phenomenology will have this Fregean content.

---

20. If someone is doubtful that experiences have Fregean content (perhaps holding that there is only Edenic phenomenal content and ordinary Russellian nonphenomenal content), it is this pattern of judgments about veridicality, as well as the corresponding inferential role, that gives the best reason to believe in it. There is no doubt that experiences are associated with this sort of pattern of judgments of veridicality, and there is no obstacle to our using this pattern to ground a notion of experiential content.

It is this explanatory story that the two-stage view provides. The presentational phenomenology of an experience immediately grounds an Edenic content. The Fregean content is grounded in the Edenic content in virtue of inferential role. The subject is immediately presented, in visual phenomenology, with an Edenic world. But a rational subject need not hold the world to an Edenic standard. In effect, a rational subject will use the Edenic phenomenology of a phenomenally red experience to ground the claim that the object in front of her is *red*, but she need not make strong claims about the intrinsic nature of redness. That is left open: if the subject discovers that objects with property P typically cause red experiences, then she will decide that those objects are red and that if the original object has property P, then the original experience was veridical. In effect, the presentational phenomenology of the experience serves as direct ground for the first stage of the two-stage view (the Edenic content) and as indirect ground for the second stage (matching the Edenic content) by virtue of inferential role.

Is Fregean Content Phenomenal Content?

Once we observe that ordinary Fregean content derives from inferential role, this may raise another worry: is Fregean content really *phenomenal* content? The mere fact that Fregean content does not completely mirror phenomenological structure here is no objection since the definition of phenomenal content does not require this sort of mirroring. However, the definition does require that any experience with the same phenomenology has the same phenomenal content. One may then worry: if inferential role is extrinsic to phenomenology, could not two phenomenally identical experiences have different inferential roles, yielding distinct Fregean contents?

Of course, there is an obvious sense in which phenomenally identical experiences can have different inferential roles. For example, if I believe that red snakes are poisonous and you do not, then relevantly similar visual experiences in the two of us might produce quite different beliefs. But this difference in inferential role need not be a difference in the core aspect of inferential role that is relevant to defining Fregean content. This core aspect involves the subject's pattern of judgments of veridicality and falsidicality associated with the experience. More precisely, it turns on whether the subject should rationally accept or reject the experience (that is, judge that things are or are not as they perceptually seem to be) when given relevantly complete information about the world. Two subjects may have the same pattern of judgments here despite different beliefs. For example, in the preceding case, both subjects may well have the same rational dispositions to accept or reject the experience, given full information.

Fregean content will be phenomenal content as long as the same experience rationalizes the same pattern of judgments, given relevant information, in all subjects. (Of course, there may be differences in an associated *actual* pattern of judgments due to cognitive limitations, but a rational inferential role idealizes away from such limitations.) This will be the case as long as (i) every phenomenally identical experience has the same Edenic content; (ii) every subject should rationally accept an experience, given relevant information, iff (according to that information) the relevant object has properties that match the properties attributed in the Edenic content; and (iii) the matching relation is the same for all subjects.

I think there is good reason to accept (i) and (ii). We have already seen that Edenic content is a sort of phenomenal content. Further, the match-involving inferential role is rational for any subject with a perceptual experience. Such an experience presents a world with a certain distribution of Edenic properties, and rational judgments of veridicality should turn on whether objects in the world have properties that match those Edenic properties. What is not so clear is whether one should accept (iii). We have already seen that the notion of matching is somewhat vague and imprecise. Could there not be subjects whose equally rational judgments invoke somewhat different matching relations, perhaps held to somewhat different standards in each case?

For example, one might suggest that before the fall from Eden, the inferential role of our experiences required a strict standard of matching. Perhaps an Edenic subject would judge an experience falsidical if they discovered that its object merely has an imperfect property that serves as its normal cause. However, there is good reason to hold that even our Edenic counterparts have dispositions such that *if* they were to discover that their world is non-Edenic, they would still judge their experiences to be (imperfectly) veridical when their objects have the relevant imperfect properties. After all, when we discovered that our world was non-Edenic, these were the judgments that we made. So there is reason to believe that the Fregean inferential role is present even in Eden.

Still, one can ask whether there *could* be rational subjects (whether in Eden or outside) who have such a strict standard of matching that they will accept a phenomenally red experience only if the relevant object is perfectly red? If such subjects discover that the world is non-Edenic, they will reject all of their color experiences as falsidical. For such subjects, the relevant standard of matching would be the strict standard of identity: a property matches perfect redness iff it is perfect redness. Certainly there could be a subject that has an actual pattern of judgments like this. The relevant question is: could this pattern of judgments be as rational as the pattern of judgments that we have been discussing? The answer is not obvious.

Likewise, we can imagine subjects who make different judgments in difficult cases. For example, let us assume the simple view of color constancy. Then one subject might judge a phenomenally red experience to be veridical iff the relevant object has the property that causes such experiences in bright sunlight. Another subject might judge such an experience to be veridical iff the relevant object has any property in the range that might cause the experience in some normal condition. Still another subject might judge that no such experience is veridical as there is no single specific property that plays the right role. The question then is: could these patterns of judgment be equally rational?

Finally, we can consider a possible difference between visual and olfactory experience. We do not usually judge olfactory experiences to be veridical or falsidical. We do not say that a rotten egg smell is veridical iff there is sulfur dioxide nearby and falsidical iff there is not, for example. This is not because the phenomenology of smell is not representational: intuitively, it seems to represent that certain smells are present in the world. It is just that we are not inclined to make judgments of veridicality and falsidicality; at best, we make judgments of misleadingness or otherwise. On the other hand, perhaps there could be subjects who make judgments of veridicality or falsidicality for phenomenally identical olfactory experiences. For example, one can imagine that if dogs could make judgments, this is what they would do! One could diagnose this by saying that for those subjects (but not for us), there are properties in the environment that match perfect smells. The question is whether both patterns of judgment are equally rational.

It is possible to say no in all of these cases. One might hold that one pattern of judgments in these cases is rational and that the others are not. For example, one could argue that in the first case there is some irrationality in holding the world to an Edenic standard and that in the second case it is irrational to reject a color experience when its object has a property that normally causes that sort of experience.

One could also hold that in at least some of these cases, insofar as it is possible for corresponding experiences to rationalize different patterns of judgment, there will be a corresponding difference in the phenomenology. For example, in case of olfactory experience, one could suggest that the phenomenology of smell in dogs and humans differs: perhaps dogs have a more strongly presentational phenomenology, for example. More generally, one might hold that certain differences in the character of presentational phenomenology might go along with differences in the associated standard of matching. In such cases, the existence of different rationalized patterns of judgment will be no obstacle to Fregean content serving as a sort of phenomenal content.

My own view is that it is not obvious that phenomenology underdetermines the standard of matching, but it is not obvious that it does not. Whether it does or not depends on difficult questions about the rational role of perception and also about its presentational phenomenology, which I cannot adjudicate here. But I think that it is at least a live possibility that the standard of matching is underdetermined and that there could be distinct, equally rational patterns of judgment associated with the same sort of experience in different subjects.

If this is so, then what follows? One could say that the phenomenally identical experiences have distinct Fregean contents (in which case Fregean content is not phenomenal content), or one could say that they have the same highly indeterminate Fregean content (in which case imperfect veridicality is highly indeterminate). Perhaps the best thing to say in this event, however, is that these experiences have the same *unsaturated* Fregean content. This content is one that is satisfied iff the relevant object has properties that match the relevant primitive properties. However, the standard of matching is left unspecified by this unsaturated content, so the condition of satisfaction is in a certain sense incomplete. To yield a complete condition of satisfaction, the unsaturated content needs to be saturated by specifying a standard of matching. The resulting saturated Fregean content will yield a reasonably determinate condition of imperfect veridicality.

According to this view, only unsaturated Fregean content and not saturated Fregean content will be phenomenal content.[21] This is a step back from the original view of Fregean content as phenomenal content, as an unsaturated Fregean content is not a complete condition of satisfaction. That is, it is not the sort of thing that is true or false absolutely in a scenario.

---

21. Gideon Rosen (in a conference commentary) suggested that for our counterparts on Psychedelic Earth, where experiences drift in a way that is completely unrelated to the environment (and where subjects know this), the experiences will have no inferential role at all and so will not even have unsaturated Fregean content. Biggs (2009) has used a similar case (the Scrambler, which scrambles experiences) to argue against all versions of representationalism. However, it seems that if these subjects were to discover that the environment contains drifting properties that match the drifting experiences, or scrambled properties that match the scrambled experiences, they would then judge their experiences to be veridical. (It is precisely because they have discovered that there is no such match with the environment that they reject their experiences as a guide to the external world.) So it seems that these subjects still have the inferential disposition to endorse their experiences if they discover that the matching relation obtains. If so, this suggests that their experiences have Fregean content.

Correspondingly, the unsaturated Fregean content of an experience does not determine whether or not the experience is imperfectly veridical in its environment. What determines imperfect veridicality is a saturated Fregean content, which is not fully determined by phenomenal character.

What determines saturated Fregean content, if not phenomenology? One natural answer is inferential role, here conceived as something that might vary independently of phenomenology. In the different subjects discussed earlier, phenomenally identical experiences play different inferential roles, yielding different saturated Fregean contents. In effect, the different inferential roles in different subjects (as reflected in a pattern of veridicality judgments) determine different standards of matching. In this way phenomenology and inferential role together determine a saturated Fregean content and a condition of imperfect veridicality.

An alternative suggestion is that saturated Fregean content is determined not by inferential role but by a *standard of assessment* that is extrinsic to the subject. On this view, in effect, one could evaluate the same experience as either veridical or falsidical at different standards of assessment. I have already introduced dual standards of perfect and imperfect veridicality; on this view, there will be a range of different standards in the vicinity of imperfect veridicality. This range of standards will correspond to a range of different standards of matching. To evaluate an experience with an unsaturated Fregean content, we must tacitly introduce a standard of matching. This standard will determine a saturated Fregean content, and according to this standard the experience will qualify as veridical or falsidical.

One can then say that our ordinary notion of veridicality tacitly invokes a certain standard of matching, one that is reasonably although not completely determinate. With this standard fixed, phenomenally identical experiences will have the same saturated Fregean contents. However, there might have been different evaluators with a slightly different notion of veridicality, corresponding to a different standard of matching. With that standard fixed, phenomenally identical experiences will also have the same saturated Fregean contents, but these contents will differ from those associated with our standard. One might say that on this view, any given experience is associated with a whole range of (saturated) Fregean contents, depending on the corresponding notion of veridicality. Each of these Fregean contents could be seen as a sort of phenomenal content.

The two suggestions—according to which saturated content is determined by inferential role or by an external standard—yield a somewhat different treatment of cases. Take a subject whose inferential role holds her experiences to the Edenic standard: upon discovering that the world is non-Edenic, she rationally rejects her perceptual experiences. On the former view, we will say that her experience is nonveridical: it is her own rational inferential role that determines ordinary veridicality. On the latter view, we will say that her experience is veridical: it is our standards that determine the veridicality of an experience (according to the meaning of our term "veridical"). However, if she or someone sharing a similar standard were to say that her experience is "nonveridical," they would also be correct: they express a slightly different notion of satisfaction with their term "veridical." On reflection I find the second suggestion somewhat more plausible and intuitive than the first, although the matter is far from obvious.

In any case, whichever view we take, one can say the following. The phenomenal character of an experience determines an Edenic phenomenal content, and it determines an unsaturated Fregean phenomenal content. According to the unsaturated phenomenal content, an experience is veridical iff the relevant object has properties that match the relevant Edenic properties. Once combined with a standard of matching, this unsaturated content determines a saturated Fregean content. This saturated Fregean content may or may not be phenomenal content, depending on what view one takes on the foregoing questions. If one thinks that there is only one rational standard of matching associated with the phenomenal character of the experience, then the saturated Fregean content will be a phenomenal content. If one thinks that the associated standard of matching depends on a contingently associated inferential role in the subject, then the saturated Fregean content will not be a phenomenal content. If one thinks that the standard of matching is determined by an external standard of assessment, then the Fregean content will be a phenomenal content, but there will be a range of other Fregean contents associated with different standards of veridicality.

The choice among these three alternatives turns on difficult and subtle issues that I will not try to resolve here. In any case, we can be confident that phenomenal character determines Edenic content and unsaturated Fregean content. The status of saturated Fregean content as phenomenal content remains an open question.

12. Beyond Color

I have concentrated on the content of color experience, but I think the two-stage model has much broader application. Here I will much more briefly discuss the extension to other aspects of perceptual experience.

Spatial Experience

Apart from colors, the most salient properties attributed in visual experience are spatial properties. Does the two-stage model of phenomenal content generalize to these? I am inclined to think that it does.

One might think that spatial experience is more amenable to a straightforward Russellian treatment than color experience. But as Thompson
(forthcoming) argues, many of the same problems arise. A natural candidate for the Russellian content of spatial experiences involves the attribution of spatial properties such as that of being in a certain (absolute)
location. However, this content obviously cannot be phenomenal content
since a phenomenally identical experience could be had by a subject light-
years away from that location. A natural next suggestion is a Russellian
content involving the attribution of relative spatial properties (or relations
or relational property radicals) such as being six feet in front of the perceiver. But this cannot be phenomenal content either. In principle, a phenomenally identical experience could be had by a perceiver who is (and has
always been) twice as big and in an environment where everything is twice
as distant. Such an experience would not plausibly attribute the same relative spatial property; it would more plausibly attribute the relative property of being twelve feet away.

One might then move to more relativized spatial properties, such as the
property of being twice as distant or twice as big as some other object. Or
one might suggest that phenomenal content can at least attribute shape
properties, such as being square or circular. But as Thompson argues, similar problems arise. There could conceivably be an "El Greco" world in
which everything is stretched ten times in one direction compared with
our world but in which structure and dynamics are otherwise isomorphic.
In such an environment, phenomenally square experiences would normally be caused by (what we call) long and thin rectangles. Further, there
is good reason to think that such experiences would be veridical. Certainly,
if we found that we inhabit a corner of the universe that is locally stretched
in this fashion relative to the rest of the universe, we would not conclude
that our spatial experiences are falsidical. Rather, the natural thing to say is
that phenomenally square experiences attribute different properties in
these environments: (what we call) squareness in one environment and a
certain sort of rectangularity in another.

A more extreme case along these lines is given by a Matrix scenario, in
which phenomenally identical subjects have been hooked up for their lifetime to a computer simulation of the world. I argue in the next chapter
that such subjects are not massively deluded about the world. Their beliefs

such as "there are tables," "I have hands," and "that is square" are true; it is just that the underlying metaphysics of their environment is not what they expect (in effect, it is an underlying computational metaphysics). The same can be argued for their perceptual experiences: their experiences as of red square objects are as veridical as ours. However, such experiences need not be of (what we would call) square objects: there need be nothing square inside the computer. At best, there are objects with some very different property, which we might call "virtual squareness." If phenomenally identical spatial experiences can be veridical in an environment that is spatially utterly unlike our own, this suggests that the phenomenal content of these experiences does not involve the attribution of ordinary spatial properties.

In this way, one can argue against Russellian views of spatial phenomenal content in ways that directly parallel our earlier arguments in the case of color experience. The natural alternative is a Fregean view of spatial phenomenal content. On this view, spatial experiences have Russellian content, attributing spatial properties and relations, but this content is not phenomenal content. Rather, phenomenal content involves a Fregean mode of presentation of spatial properties and relations: roughly, these are determined as that manifold of properties and relations that serves as the normal causal basis for the corresponding manifold of spatial experiences. On this view, the Fregean content of a spatial experience is one that will be satisfied if the object has a property that normally causes the relevant sort of spatial experience (or if it has a complex of properties each of which normally causes the relevant sort of spatial aspect of the experience). One can then raise concerns about the phenomenological adequacy of this view, motivating a two-stage view of spatial phenomenal content.

On the two-stage view, spatial experiences have an Edenic content that attributes perfect spatial properties: perfect squareness, perfect rectangularity, and so on. Arguably, even an Edenic content does not attribute absolute spatial properties but just relative properties. It is not clear that we have the phenomenology of being presented with absolute spatial properties, and one can make a case that even in Eden, there could be phenomenally identical veridical experiences at different locations. But we do have the phenomenology of being presented at least with absolute shapes and relative distances. So the Edenic contents of our experience will attribute perfect properties of this sort. It is plausible that these properties are not instantiated in our world (though arguing this takes a bit more work than in the case of color). If not, then our spatial experiences are not perfectly veridical.

Our spatial experiences may nevertheless be imperfectly veridical in virtue of their objects instantiating imperfect spatial properties: those that match perfect spatial properties. These will be the properties that serve as the normal causal basis for our spatial experiences. Imperfect veridicality will be associated with a corresponding ordinary Fregean content, one that is satisfied iff relevant objects have properties that match the relevant perfect spatial properties. Phenomenally identical experiences will have the same Edenic contents and the same ordinary Fregean contents (setting aside issues about standards of matching), but they may have different ordinary Russellian contents, because different properties may match the relevant perfect properties in different environments.

The Matrix provides a good illustration. The subjects here do not have perfectly veridical experiences, but they have imperfectly veridical experiences in virtue of the fact that relevant matching properties (virtual squareness and the like) are instantiated in their environment. So subjects in the Matrix may share Edenic spatial contents with us, and may share ordinary Fregean contents also, but they will have different ordinary Russellian contents.

Of course, the two-stage model of spatial experience needs to be elaborated in numerous respects to handle all sorts of aspects of spatial content: for example, perspective, angle, size constancy, and mirror reflections. But there is reason to think it can help explain certain phenomena. For example, it is better suited than the original Fregean view to accommodate internal connections between spatial representation in visual and tactile experience. On the original Fregean view, it might seem that there can be no internal connection since the normal causes of visual spatial experience are not constrained to be the normal causes of tactile spatial experience. On the two-stage model, however, one can argue that the phenomenology entails that tactile and spatial experiences involve the attribution of common, perfect spatial properties in their Edenic content. If so, then the matching imperfect properties will be constrained to be the same, thus grounding an internal connection between tactile and spatial experience.

It is a further question how this model should be extended to the representation of time and motion. I am inclined to say that the two-stage model can be extended to time, as well as to space, though this turns on subtle issues about the metaphysics of time. A natural suggestion is that the Edenic content of temporal experience requires A-theoretic time, with some sort of true flow or passage. Our own universe may not instantiate these perfect temporal properties, but it may nevertheless instantiate matching B-theoretic properties (involving relative location in a four-dimensional "block universe"), which are sufficient to make our temporal experiences imperfectly veridical, if not perfectly veridical. The representation of motion could be treated in a similar way.

One might go so far as to suggest that Eden is a world with classical Euclidean space and an independent dimension of time, in which there is true passage and true change. Our own world is non-Euclidean, with time and space interdependent and with pale shadows of perfect passage and change. On this view, Einstein's theory of space-time was one more bite from the Tree of Science and one more step in our fall from Eden.

The Experience of Objects

Our initial characterization of the Russellian contents of visual experience characterized them as having the following form: object O has color C at location L. In the case of color and location I have argued that this Russellian content is not phenomenal content and have proposed a two-stage Fregean treatment instead. In the case of color, we have seen that the relevant Russellian content is also not plausibly phenomenal content. Does this mean that we should also give a two-stage Fregean treatment of the representation of objects?

A natural first suggestion is that experiences of objects have an Edenic content involving the representation of certain specific perfect objects (as discussed below): for example, perfect object O has perfect color C at perfect location L. However, this suggestion is implausible on reflection. In particular, it is implausible that the perfect veridicality of an experience of an object requires any particular Edenic object to be present. It seems that even in Eden there could be two phenomenally identical experiences of different objects. The phenomenology of object experience seems to present us directly with objects, but it does not seem to acquaint us with their intrinsic nature in a sense over and above acquainting us with their colors, shapes, and so on. If it did, then the phenomenology of object experience would be quite different from what it is: experiences of different tennis balls would typically have quite different phenomenal characters, for example. But the experience of objects does not seem to be this way.[22]

Because of this, it is more natural to hold that even the Edenic content of object experience is existential. For example, one might hold that the Edenic

22. As in note 1, a disjunctivist view about phenomenology may hold that the phenomenology of experiences of different objects differs in precisely this way. Such a disjunctivist view might hold that the Edenic content (and perhaps the non-Edenic phenomenal content) of an experience is object involving. On my view, however, reflection on Eden suggests that a "naive realist" view of perception does not require disjunctivism about phenomenology. In Eden, a sort of naive realism about perception is correct, but this entails only disjunctivism about the metaphysics of experience (as discussed in section 9), not disjunctivism about phenomenology.

content of an experience of a red sphere is satisfied iff there is a perfect sphere at the relevant location that is perfectly red. No specific object is required for the satisfaction of this content. On this view, Edenic content is not especially different from ordinary content in the representation of objects, so the two-stage model has no special role to play.

Still, there may be a further role for the two-stage model. One might hold that a merely existential characterization of phenomenal content does not fully respect the directness of an experience of an object.[23] According to this objection, experience does not merely present that there *is* an object at a certain location with a certain color. Rather, it presents that *that* object is at a certain location with a certain color.

One might accommodate this suggestion without moving all the way to object-involving phenomenal contents, however. The phenomenology of perception does not seem to reveal the intrinsic haecceitistic natures of objects, but it does seem to present us with objects directly. To account for this, one can suggest that the experience of objects involves demonstrative modes of presentation.

In Eden, one is directly acquainted with objects, and no mediation is involved. One can simply demonstrate an object as *this* object, and acquaintance does the rest. This sort of reference is analogous to the unmediated way we refer to ourselves in our world, with 'I,' or perhaps to the unmediated way in which we ostend our conscious experiences. An Edenic content might correspondingly have the form [that is C at L], where 'that' is a primitive demonstrative, C is a perfect color, and L is a perfect location. The demonstrative here does not build in the identity of the object any more than the notion of 'I' builds in a specific person: the same demonstrative could in principle refer to different objects, just as 'I' can refer to different people. But neither is it associated with a substantive criterion of application. When the demonstrative has an object, it simply picks out the object directly as *that* object. In the two-dimensional model, one could say that in Eden, one can refer directly to perceived objects as entities at the center of a centered world.

This Edenic content respects the direct presentational phenomenology of our experience of objects, but it is not clear that it has application outside Eden. In our world, we are not directly acquainted with objects outside ourselves: mediation is always involved. So our epistemic grip on objects is not as direct as it is in Eden, and the primitively demonstrative

23. This sort of concern about the existential characterizations of perceptual content is discussed by Campbell (2002) and Martin (2002). A demonstrative view of perceptual content is suggested by Burge (1991).

aspects of Edenic content are arguably not satisfied. Nevertheless, we stand in a weaker relevant relation to objects in our world: the relation of perception. One might say that in virtue of standing in this relation, the objectual aspects of our experience are *imperfectly satisfied.* There will be an associated condition of imperfect satisfaction. An object imperfectly satisfies the experience iff it is the object perceived with the experience: that is, if it is connected to the experience via an appropriate causal chain. One can think of this as a nonprimitive demonstrative condition of satisfaction. It comes with substantive requirements but is grounded in a primitive connection to the experience itself. So, in effect, the objectual phenomenology of the experience can be perfectly or imperfectly satisfied. Perfect satisfaction turns on primitive acquaintance, and imperfect satisfaction requires at least a mediated perceptual connection.

The imperfect satisfaction conditions of an experience can be seen as a sort of (ordinary) Fregean mode of presentation, picking out the object that the experience is appropriately connected to. The experience as a whole will be imperfectly veridical iff the object that is appropriately connected to the experience has properties that match the relevant perfect properties. According to this view, the ordinary Fregean content of the experience will involve a connectedness condition of this sort, and it will determine in turn a Russellian content involving the relevant objects and its imperfect properties. Of course, the ordinary Fregean content is not a perfect mirror of the phenomenology. As usual, the phenomenology does not seem to involve reference to a causal condition or reference to the subject's experience. But this is just what we expect: Edenic contents mirror the phenomenology, and associated Fregean contents capture veridicality conditions after the fall.

If one takes this view, one will class so-called veridical hallucinations (hallucinations that happen to mirror the environment in front of one) as not really veridical at all. In these cases there is no object that one is perceiving, so the Fregean content is not satisfied, and an object-involving Russellian content is not determined. An alternative route to this result (Searle 1983; Siegel 2005) is to suggest that experiences have existential contents that attribute the relational property of being perceived with the relevant experience to the relevant object. Arguably, however, suggesting that this relational property is attributed along with color and location does not respect the subjunctive intuition that things could have been as they perceptually seem to be, even had there been no perceivers in the vicinity. By contrast, putting the perceptual requirement in the mode of presentation of the object allows this subjunctive intuition to be respected.

There is perhaps one other role for the two-stage model in the representation of objects. The phenomenology of vision seems to present a world that is carved into objects at its joints. One does not simply perceive a distribution of mass and color. One perceives objects on top of other objects, each of which may be articulated into objectual parts. Depending on one's metaphysical views, one may think that the world does not respect this articulation into objects. One might think that macroscopic objects do not exist in the world's basic ontology, or one might give their existence some highly deflationary treatment on which their individuation is a matter of convention or conceptual scheme, or on which there is no deep fact of the matter about when there is an object or when there is not. But even if one's metaphysics is deflationary about objects, one's phenomenology is not. So perhaps, for our visual experiences to be perfectly veridical, there would have to be real, first-class, nonrelative objects in the world. One might say that in Eden, there are perfect objects. If our world's ontology does not have perfect objects, or at least if it does not have perfect objects corresponding to the apparent objects of ordinary perception, then our experiences are not perfectly veridical in this respect. Still, they may be imperfectly veridical, by virtue of there being appropriately arranged matter in the environment, or by virtue of the environment's satisfying some other deflationary condition. Once again, Eden sets the standard, and our imperfect world can only match it.

Other Sensory Modalities

The two-stage model can naturally be extended from visual experience to auditory and tactile experience. The details of these extensions depend on a careful analysis of the phenomenology of these experiences, combined with analysis of judgments about veridicality, but there is reason to believe that the model outlined in the case of vision will apply.

The phenomenology of auditory experience, at a first approximation, seems to represent certain sounds as being present at certain locations. For example, in a musical experience, the phenomenology might suggest that a sound with a certain pitch, timbre, volume, and so on is being produced at a certain approximate location in front of me. As in the case of color, there are physical properties that one might plausibly identify with various pitch, timbre, and volume properties and that one might hold to be attributed in an ordinary Russellian content. But these properties depend on the environment of the experience, and it seems that phenomenally identical experiences could have different Russellian contents of this sort. So one can move to a Fregean phenomenal content in these cases and then, to respect phenomenological adequacy, hold that this content is grounded in the matching of an Edenic phenomenal content.

In Eden, one may hold, there are perfect sounds, with perfect middle-C pitch, perfect loudness, and so on. We grasp these simple intrinsic properties in our experience, but they are not instantiated in our world. Instead, in our world there are simply physical events such as air disturbances with associated physical properties that match the Edenic properties. This is enough to make our auditory experiences imperfectly veridical, if not perfectly veridical.

Something similar goes for tactile experience. In Eden, objects may be perfectly smooth or perfectly slimy or perfectly velvety. These are intrinsic properties of objects or their surfaces, and we seem to be acquainted with these properties in our experience. But in our world there are just complex physical substitutes for these properties, such as imperfect sliminess and imperfect velvetiness. This is enough to satisfy the ordinary Fregean content of our tactile experiences, if not the Edenic content, and enough to make our tactile experiences imperfectly veridical.

Olfactory and gustatory experiences are trickier. The phenomenology of smell and taste seems to be representational. Intuitively, an olfactory experience represents that a certain smell is present in one's environment, perhaps in a certain broad location. A gustatory experience represents that something with a certain taste is in one's mouth or throat or on one's lips. But at the same time, we do not usually assess experiences of smell and taste for veridicality, and the notion of an illusory olfactory or gustatory experience does not get a strong grip on us. Certainly, there can be smell experiences that are caused by properties that do not normally produce such experiences, and the same applies to taste experiences (imagine a rewiring of the connection between receptors and the brain, for example), but it does not seem natural to describe such experiences as illusions. It is slightly more natural to speak of olfactory and gustatory hallucinations, when an experience is generated for reasons quite independent of external objects, but the intuition is not strong.

Taste and smell differ in this way from hearing and touch. We certainly assess auditory experiences for veridicality and speak of auditory illusions if there is not a sound being produced where there seems to be. This way of speaking is less common in the case of touch, as touch seems to be the most reliable of the sensory modalities, but we can nevertheless make good sense of the idea of a tactile illusion or hallucination. An object might feel smooth although it is not really smooth, or one might feel that an object is present when there is no object at all. In these cases we have no hesitation in classifying a tactile experience as falsidical. In the case of taste and smell, by contrast, one hesitates. I suspect that this is partly because we use taste and smell much less to gather information about our environment than we do hearing and touch and partly (perhaps correspondingly) because the presentational element of their phenomenology is less striking.

Still, there is some presentational phenomenology in the experience of smell and taste. We seem to have some grip on intrinsic qualitative properties that are presented, although it is somewhat less obvious than in the case of vision that the phenomenology presents intrinsic properties of objects or of the environment as opposed to intrinsic qualities of experiences (or corresponding relational properties of objects and environment). Overall, though, I am inclined to say that olfactory and gustatory experiences have Edenic contents: the former present perfect smells as being present in one's environment, and the latter present perfect tastes as being instantiated in one's mouth.

It is the ordinary content of these experiences that is problematic. It is plausible that there are physical properties that normally cause the relevant olfactory and gustatory aspects of experiences, so one might think these would be the imperfect smells and tastes attributed in the ordinary content of these experiences. But because our assessments of veridicality are very unclear in these cases, it is likewise unclear whether these physical properties count as matching the relevant Edenic properties. In these cases, the standard for matching seems somewhat different from the case of vision and hearing perhaps because of a difference in presentational phenomenology or perhaps just because we apply a different standard because of different pragmatic purposes. So the status of ordinary Fregean and Russellian content in these cases is unclear. But we can nevertheless invoke Edenic content to help characterize the phenomenology.

Bodily Sensations

What about bodily sensations, such as the pain experiences, itches, hunger, and orgasms? On the face of it, these have a strong presentational phenomenology. The experience of pain, for example, seems to present a certain painful quality as being instantiated in part of one's body, such as one's ankle. The experience of an itch seems to present a certain itchy quality as being presented on one's skin. In the phenomenology, these qualities seem to have a highly distinctive intrinsic qualitative nature. So it is natural to hold that bodily sensations have an associated Edenic content, attributing Edenic properties such as perfect painfulness and perfect itchiness to locations in one's body.

There are two complications in this case. The first resembles the complication in the case of smell and taste. We do not generally assess bodily sensations for veridicality or falsidicality. Perhaps in an extreme case such as phantom limb pain, we are somewhat inclined to say there is some sort of falsidical pain hallucination, but we are not really inclined to speak of pain illusions or of illusory itch experiences. If we did, we would probably be talking of a case where we mistake the phenomenal character of an experience, not where we mistake its object. As in the case of smell and taste, it seems that there are physical properties (such as tissue damage and the like) that normally cause the relevant experiences. But we are not especially inclined to say that when these properties are absent, an experience as of pain or as of an itch is falsidical. Even if there is no associated tissue damage, for example, we are not inclined to say that an intense pain experience is illusory. So the ordinary Fregean and Russellian content of these experiences seems somewhat unclear in the same way as in the case of smell and taste.

A related complication concerns the Edenic content of bodily sensations. What are perfect pains like in Eden? That is, what sort of properties need to be instantiated in one's body in order for a painful experience to be perfectly veridical? Here there are conflicting requirements. First, the properties seem to be intrinsic properties whose nature we grasp in experience. The phenomenology of pain in one's ankle seems to attribute a quality that is intrinsic to one's ankle. But second, the properties seem to have a strong connection to experience itself. Can one conceive of one's ankle being in perfect pain without anyone experiencing the pain? It is not clear that we can. In this respect the phenomenology of pain is quite different from the phenomenology of color, where we have no trouble conceiving of an object being perfectly colored even though no one ever experiences its color. But, this seems strongly to suggest that perfect pain is a relational property because its instantiation places requirements on how things are outside the object in which it is instantiated.

Is the property of perfect pain intrinsic or relational? Neither answer is entirely comfortable. If perfect pain is an intrinsic property of an ankle, it seems that its instantiation should be independent of whether an experience is present. But it is not clear that unexperienced perfect pain is conceivable. If perfect pain is a relational property, on the other hand, what relational property could it be: the property of causing a painful experience, or of having such-and-such intrinsic quality perceived in a painful experience? Neither of these seems apt to the phenomenology. Furthermore, the former seems to claim too little about what is going on in one's ankle, and the latter seems vulnerable to the objection that came up in the intrinsic case: we do not seem to have a grip on any relevant intrinsic quality here that we can conceive instantiated in the absence of a painful experience.

Perhaps the best answer is the following: perfect pain is an intrinsic property, but one whose instantiation entails the existence of an associated painful experience or of associated phenomenal pain. We might think of it as an intrinsic property that, if instantiated, necessarily "broadcasts" further constraints on the world. In effect, it is an intrinsic property that stands in a necessary connection to distinct intrinsic properties of experience. It is a property whose instantiation brings about necessary connections between distinct existences.

If this property could be instantiated, problems would follow. It is not clear that there can be necessary connections between distinct existences of this sort. It seems plausible that for any conceivable or possible situation in which an intrinsic property is instantiated in one's ankle, it should be conceivable or possible that the property is instantiated in an arbitrarily different context. But it is not conceivable or possible that there is perfect pain without pain experience. The natural conclusion is that perfect pain cannot be instantiated: there is no possible world in which there is perfect pain, and on reflection it is not even conceivable that there is perfect pain. In effect, the instantiation of perfect pain places incoherent requirements on the world.

This does not entail that there is no property of perfect pain. There are other properties whose instantiation is impossible and inconceivable: that of being a round square, for example. One might hold that perfect pain is like this. On this view, one has a grip on the property of perfect pain based on one's experience. But one does not need to eat from the Tree of Illusion or the Tree of Science to know that perfect pain is not instantiated: one can know this simply on sufficient reflection. Perhaps there can be matching intrinsic properties (without the relational constraint) or matching relational properties (without the intrinsic constraint), but no property can play both roles. Still, one may hold that the property exists, and one can hold that it is attributed in the Edenic content of our pain experiences.[24]

In effect, the Edenic content of pain sets a standard that is not just hard but impossible to meet. There are related instantiated properties, to be sure: that of causing painful experiences, for example, or that of having a certain sort of tissue damage. But because these fall so far short of playing the role of perfect pain (the former is not intrinsic, and the second has no strong connection to experience), one might suggest that they fail to match perfect pain. It is arguably because of this that we do not judge that the instantiation of these properties yields veridicality or falsidicality of pain experiences. The standard set by Eden is sufficiently high that there is little point in holding the world to it.

24. Adam Pautz explores an idea like this in forthcoming work.

What goes for pain also goes for other bodily sensations, such as the experience of itches, hunger, and orgasms. One finds the same combination in these cases. Phenomenology seems to present an intrinsic property, but one that cannot be instantiated without a corresponding experience. The natural conclusion is that the perfect properties cannot be instantiated at all. One might suggest that this model applies in some other domains: for example, one might suggest that gustatory experiences present properties that cannot be instantiated except while being tasted, so to speak. If this were so, it could help to explain our reluctance to assess such experiences as veridical or falsidical. The phenomenology here is less clear than in the case of pain, and it is not obvious whether the claim of a necessary connection to experience is correct, but the analogy between the cases at least deserves attention.

It may be that some other Edenic properties that we have considered are not just uninstantiated but uninstantiable. For example, one might hold that perfect time (involving the flow of time or a moving now) is incoherent, perhaps for McTaggartian reasons. Or if one is sufficiently deflationary about objects, one might hold that perfect objects cannot exist in any possible world. Nevertheless, the impossibility of satisfying these contents does not automatically stop them from acting as a regulative ideal. Here, the impossible might serve to regulate our experience of the actual.

High-Level Properties

One might try to extend this model beyond the representation of simple properties such as color and shape in experience to the representation of high-level properties such as that of being a duck or being happy. It is plausible that representing such properties can make a difference to the phenomenology of experience (Siegel 2006). It is not clear that the phenomenal content of this sort of experience is easily analyzed using the two-stage model. One difficulty is that the deployment of *concepts* often plays a key role in such experiences, where the content of the experience is inherited from that of an associated concept rather than being determined by the two-stage model. When we see something as a book or as a duck, for example, it is plausible that the associated phenomenal content is inherited from the content of our concept of a book or of a duck. In these cases, we do not seem to have any grip on distinct perfect and imperfect veridicality conditions.

Still, there are a few cases where the two-stage model is at least tempting. For example, there is a phenomenology of moral experience, and it is arguable that moral properties such as being good or bad can be represented in perception. One might naturally suggest that for moral experiences to be perfectly veridical, relevant objects would have to have perfect moral properties: the sort that are objective, intrinsically motivating, and so on. But it is arguable that in our world (and perhaps in every possible world) no such properties are instantiated. If so, our moral experiences cannot be perfectly veridical. But there are various properties (including response-dependent properties, community-relative properties, and so on) that arguably match these properties well enough. If so, our moral experiences can be imperfectly veridical. There has been no perfect goodness since the fall from Eden, but we can at least be consoled by imperfect goodness in the world.

13. Conclusion

On the view I have presented, the most fundamental content of perceptual experience is its Edenic content. Other aspects of content such as ordinary Fregean and Russellian content can be seen as deriving from Edenic content with the aid of the matching relation and the contribution of the environment. To understand the role of perceptual experience in representing the world, one needs to understand all of these levels of content. But to understand the phenomenology of perceptual experience in its own right, understanding Edenic content is the key.

We have seen that the Edenic approach yields a very useful tool in doing phenomenology. To characterize the phenomenology of an experience, it is often helpful to characterize the sort of world in which that experience would be perfectly veridical. To do this, one sketches relevant aspects of the character of Eden. Doing this does not eliminate the need for thorough phenomenological investigation, and it does not solve the many associated hard methodological problems, but it at least provides an analytic tool that gives us some purchase in characterizing the contents of consciousness.

I am inclined to think that Edenic content may also give us an entry point for understanding the metaphysics of experience. I have said little in this chapter about how it is possible for experiences to have Edenic contents or about which of Edenic content or phenomenal character is the more fundamental. My suspicion is that neither is more fundamental than the other. It may be that perceptual experience is fundamentally equivalent to the presentation of an Edenic world. If so, then if we can understand how the presentation of an Edenic world is possible, we will understand perceptual phenomenology.

13

THE MATRIX AS METAPHYSICS

1. Brains in Vats

The Matrix presents a version of an old philosophical fable: the brain in a vat. A disembodied brain is floating in a vat inside a scientist's laboratory. The scientist has arranged for the brain to be stimulated with the same sort of inputs that a normal embodied brain receives. To do this, the brain is connected to a giant computer simulation of a world. The simulation determines which inputs the brain receives. When the brain produces outputs, these are fed back into the simulation. The internal state of the brain is just like that of a normal brain despite the fact that it lacks a body. From the brain's point of view, things seem very much as they seem to you and me.

The brain is massively deluded, it seems. It has all sorts of false beliefs about the world. It believes that it has a body, but in fact it has no body. It believes that it is walking outside in the sunlight, but in fact it is inside a dark lab. It believes it is one place, when in fact it may be somewhere quite different. Perhaps it thinks it is in Tucson, when it is actually in Australia or even in outer space.

Neo's situation at the beginning of *The Matrix* is something like this. He thinks that he lives in a city; he thinks that he has hair; he thinks it is 1999; and he thinks that it is sunny outside. In reality, he is floating in a pod in space; he has no hair; the year is around 2199; and the world has been darkened by war. There are a few small differences from the paradigmatic vat scenario: Neo's brain is located in a body, and the computer simulation is

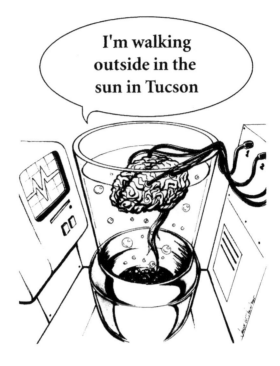

controlled by machines rather than by a scientist. But the essential details are much the same. In effect, Neo is a brain in a vat.

Let's say that a *matrix* (lowercase *m*) is an artificially designed computer simulation of a world. So the Matrix in the movie is one example of a matrix. Let's also say that someone is *envatted*, or is *in a matrix*, if he or she has a cognitive system that receives its inputs from and sends its outputs to a matrix. Then the brain at the beginning is envatted, and so is Neo.

We can imagine that a matrix simulates the entire physics of a world, keeping track of every last particle throughout space and time. (Later we will look at ways in which this setup might be varied.) An envatted being will be associated with a particular simulated body. A connection is arranged so that whenever this body receives sensory inputs inside the simulation, the envatted cognitive system will receive sensory inputs of the same sort. When the envatted cognitive system produces motor outputs, corresponding outputs will be fed to the motor organs of the simulated body.

When the possibility of a matrix is raised, a question immediately follows. How do I know that I am not in a matrix? After all, there could be a brain in a vat structured exactly like my brain, hooked up to a matrix, with experiences indistinguishable from those I am having now. From the inside, there is no way to tell for sure that I am not in the situation of the brain in a vat. So it seems that there is no way to know for sure that I am not in a matrix.

Let us call the hypothesis that I am in a matrix and have always been in a matrix the *Matrix Hypothesis*. Equivalently, the Matrix Hypothesis says that I am envatted and have always been envatted. This is not quite equivalent to the hypothesis that I am in the Matrix, as the Matrix is just one specific version of a matrix. For now I ignore some complications that are specific to the Matrix in the movie, such as the fact that people sometimes travel back and forth between the Matrix and the external world. These issues aside, we can think of the Matrix Hypothesis informally as saying that I am in the same sort of situation as people who have always been in the Matrix.

The Matrix Hypothesis is one that we should take seriously. As Nick Bostrom (2003) has suggested, it is not out of the question that, in the history of the universe, technology will evolve that will allow beings to create computer simulations of entire worlds. There may well be vast numbers of such computer simulations, compared to just one real world. If so, there may well be many more beings who are in a matrix than beings who are not. Given all this, one might even infer that it is more likely that we are in a matrix than that we are not. Whether this is right or not, it certainly seems that we cannot be *certain* that we are not in a matrix.

Serious consequences seem to follow. My envatted counterpart seems to be massively deluded. It thinks it is in Tucson; it thinks it is sitting at a desk writing an article; it thinks it has a body. On the face of it, all of these beliefs are false. Likewise, it seems that if *I* am envatted, my own corresponding beliefs are false. If I am envatted, I am not really in Tucson; I am not really sitting at a desk; and I may not even have a body. So if I do not know that I am not envatted, then I do not know that I am in Tucson; I do not know that I am sitting at a desk; and I do not know that I have a body.

The Matrix Hypothesis threatens to undercut almost everything I know. It seems to be a *skeptical hypothesis*: a hypothesis that I cannot rule out and one that would falsify most of my beliefs if it were true. Where there is a skeptical hypothesis, it looks like none of these beliefs count as genuine knowledge. Of course, the beliefs *might* be true—I might be lucky and not be envatted—but I cannot rule out the possibility that they are false. So a skeptical hypothesis leads to *skepticism* about these beliefs: I believe these things, but I do not know them.

To sum up the reasoning: I do not know that I am not in a matrix. If I am in a matrix, I am probably not in Tucson. So if I do not know that I am not in a matrix, then I do not know that I am in Tucson. The same goes for almost everything else I think I know about the external world.

2. Envatment Reconsidered

This is a standard way of thinking about the vat scenario. It seems that this view is also endorsed by the people who created *The Matrix*. On the DVD case for the movie, one sees the following:

Perception: Our day-in, day-out world is real.

Reality: That world is a hoax, an elaborate deception spun by all-powerful machines that control us. Whoa.

I think this view is not right. Even if I am in a matrix, my world is perfectly real. A brain in a vat is not massively deluded (at least if it has always been in the vat). Neo does not have massively false beliefs about the external world. Instead, envatted beings have largely *correct* beliefs about their world. If so, the Matrix Hypothesis is not a skeptical hypothesis, and its possibility does not undercut everything that I think I know.

Philosophers have held this sort of view before. The eighteenth-century philosopher George Berkeley held, in effect, that appearance is reality. (Recall Morpheus: "What is 'real'? How do you define 'real'? If you're talking about what you can feel, what you can smell, what you can taste and see, then real is simply electrical signals interpreted by your brain.") If this is right, then the world perceived by envatted beings is perfectly real: these beings experience all the right appearances, and appearance is reality. So on this view, even envatted beings have true beliefs about the world.

I have recently found myself embracing a similar conclusion, though for quite different reasons. I do not find the view that appearance is reality plausible, so I do not endorse Berkeley's reasoning. Until recently it has seemed quite obvious to me that brains in vats would have massively false beliefs. But I now think there is a line of reasoning that shows that this is wrong.

I still think I cannot rule out the hypothesis that I am in a matrix. But I think that even if I am in a matrix, I am still in Tucson; I am still sitting at my desk; and so on. So the hypothesis that I am in a matrix is not a skeptical hypothesis. The same goes for Neo. At the beginning of the film, if he thinks, "I have hair," he is correct. If he thinks, "It is sunny outside," he is correct. The same goes, of course, for the original brain in a vat. When it thinks, "I have a body," it is correct. When it thinks, "I am walking," it is correct.

This view may seem counterintuitive at first. Initially, it seemed quite counterintuitive to me. So I will now present the line of reasoning that has convinced me that it is correct.

3. The Metaphysical Hypothesis

I will argue that the hypothesis that I am envatted is not a skeptical hypothesis but a *metaphysical hypothesis*. That is, it is a hypothesis about the underlying nature of reality.

Where physics is concerned with the microscopic processes that underlie macroscopic reality, metaphysics is concerned with the fundamental nature of reality. A metaphysical hypothesis might make a claim about the reality that underlies physics itself. Alternatively, it might say something about the nature of our minds or the creation of our world.

My view is that the Matrix Hypothesis should be regarded as a metaphysical hypothesis with all three of these elements. It makes a claim about the reality underlying physics, about the nature of our minds, and about the creation of the world.

In particular, I think the Matrix Hypothesis is equivalent to a version of the following three-part metaphysical hypothesis. First, physical processes are fundamentally computational. Second, our cognitive systems are separate from physical processes but interact with them. Third, physical reality was created by beings outside physical space-time.

Importantly, nothing about this metaphysical hypothesis is skeptical. The metaphysical hypothesis here tells us about the processes underlying our ordinary reality, but it does not entail that this reality does not exist. We still have bodies, and there are still chairs and tables: it is just that their fundamental nature is a bit different from what we may have thought. In this manner, the metaphysical hypothesis is analogous to a physical hypothesis, such as one involving quantum mechanics. Both the physical hypothesis and the metaphysical hypothesis tell us about the processes underlying chairs. They do not entail that there are no chairs. Rather, they tell us what chairs are really like.

I will make the case by introducing each of the three parts of the metaphysical hypothesis separately. I will suggest that each of them is coherent and cannot be conclusively ruled out. I will also suggest that none of them is a skeptical hypothesis: even if they are true, most of our ordinary beliefs are still correct. The same goes for a combination of all three hypotheses. I will then argue that the Matrix Hypothesis is equivalent to this combination.

(1) The Computational Hypothesis

The Computational Hypothesis says: microphysical processes throughout space-time are constituted by underlying computational processes.

The Computational Hypothesis says that physics as we know it is not the fundamental level of reality. Just as chemical processes underlie biological processes, and microphysical processes underlie chemical processes, something underlies microphysical processes. Underneath the level of quarks, electrons, and photons is a further level: the level of bits. These bits are governed by a computational algorithm, which at a higher level produces the processes that we think of as fundamental particles, forces, and so on.

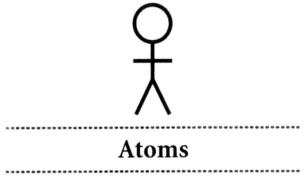

The Computational Hypothesis

The Computational Hypothesis is highly speculative, but some people take it seriously. Most famously, Edward Fredkin has postulated that the universe is at bottom some sort of computer. More recently, Stephen Wolfram (2002) has taken up the idea in his book *A New Kind of Science*, suggesting that at the fundamental level, physical reality may be a sort of cellular automata with interacting bits governed by simple rules. Furthermore, some physicists have looked into the possibility that the laws of physics might be formulated computationally or seen as the consequence of certain computational principles.

One might worry that pure bits could not be the fundamental level of reality: a bit is just a zero or a one, and reality cannot really be zeroes and ones. Or perhaps a bit is just a "pure difference" between two basic states, and there cannot be a reality made up of pure differences. Rather, bits always have to be implemented by more basic states such as voltages in a normal computer.

I do not know whether this objection is right. I do not think it is completely out of the question that there could be a universe of pure bits, but this does not matter for present purposes. We can suppose that the computational level is itself constituted by an even more fundamental level at which the computational processes are implemented. It does not matter what that more fundamental level is. All that matters is that microphysical processes are constituted by computational processes, which may themselves be constituted by more basic processes. From now on I will regard the Computational Hypothesis as saying this.

I do not know whether the Computational Hypothesis is correct, but I do not know that it is false. The hypothesis is coherent, if speculative, and I cannot conclusively rule it out.

The Computational Hypothesis is not a skeptical hypothesis. If it is true, there are still electrons and protons. On this picture, electrons and protons will be analogous to molecules: they are made up of something more basic, but they still exist. Similarly, if the Computational Hypothesis is true, there are still tables and chairs, and macroscopic reality still exists. It just turns out that their fundamental reality is a little different from what we thought.

The situation here is analogous to quantum mechanics or relativity. These may lead us to revise a few metaphysical beliefs about the external world: that the world is made of classical particles or that there is absolute time. However, most of our ordinary beliefs are left intact. Likewise, accepting the Computational Hypothesis may lead us to revise a few metaphysical beliefs: that electrons and protons are fundamental, for example. But most of our ordinary beliefs are unaffected.

(2) The Creation Hypothesis

The Creation Hypothesis says: physical space-time and its contents were created by beings outside physical space-time.

This is a familiar hypothesis. A version of it is believed by many people in our society and perhaps by the majority of the people in the world. If one believes that God created the world, and if one believes that God is outside physical space-time, then one believes the Creation Hypothesis. One need not believe in God to believe the Creation Hypothesis, though. Perhaps our world was created by a relatively ordinary being in the "next universe up," using the latest world-making technology in that universe. If so, the Creation Hypothesis is true.

I do not know whether the Creation Hypothesis is true, but I do not know for certain that it is false. The hypothesis is clearly coherent, and I cannot conclusively rule it out.

The Creation Hypothesis is not a skeptical hypothesis. Even if it is true, most of my ordinary beliefs are still true. I still have hands; I am still in Tucson; and so on. Perhaps a few of my beliefs will turn out to be false, for example if I am an atheist, or if I believe all reality started with the big bang. But most of my everyday beliefs about the external world will remain intact.

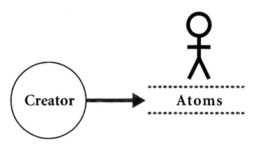

The Creation Hypothesis

If we combine the Creation Hypothesis with the Computational Hypothesis, we obtain the hypothesis that the computational processes constituting our space-time were created by beings outside space-time. Here, one might already discern a certain kinship with the Matrix Hypothesis.

(3) The Mind-Body Hypothesis

The Mind-Body Hypothesis says: my mind is (and has always been) constituted by processes outside physical space-time and receives its perceptual inputs from and sends its outputs to processes in physical space-time.

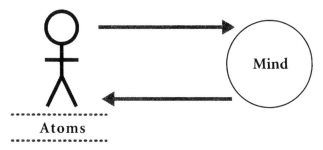

The Mind-Body Hypothesis

The Mind-Body Hypothesis is also quite familiar and quite widely believed. Descartes believed something like this: on his view, we have non-physical minds that interact with our physical bodies. The hypothesis is less widely believed today than in Descartes' time, but there are still many people who accept the Mind-Body Hypothesis.

Whether or not the Mind-Body Hypothesis is true, it is certainly coherent. Even if contemporary science tends to suggest that the hypothesis is false, we cannot rule it out conclusively.

The Mind-Body Hypothesis is not a skeptical hypothesis. Even if my mind is outside physical space-time, I still have a body; I am still in Tucson; and so on. At most, accepting this hypothesis would make us revise a few meta-physical beliefs about our minds. Our ordinary beliefs about external reality will remain largely intact.

(4) The Metaphysical Hypothesis

We can now put these hypotheses together. First we can consider the Combination Hypothesis, which combines all three. It says that physical space-time and its contents were created by beings outside physical space-time, that microphysical processes are constituted by computational processes, and that our minds are outside physical space-time but interact with it.

As with the hypotheses taken individually, the Combination Hypothesis is coherent, and we cannot conclusively rule it out. Also, like the hypotheses taken individually, it is not a skeptical hypothesis. Accepting it might lead us to revise a few of our beliefs, but it would leave most of them intact.

Finally, we can consider the Metaphysical Hypothesis (with a capital M). Like the Combination Hypothesis, this combines the Creation Hypothesis, the Computational Hypothesis, and the Mind-Body Hypothesis. It also adds the following more specific claim: the computational processes underlying physical space-time were designed by the creators as a computer simulation of a world.

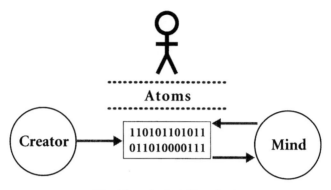

The Metaphysical Hypothesis

(It may also be useful to think of the Metaphysical Hypothesis as saying that the computational processes constituting physical space-time are part of a broader domain and that the creators and my cognitive system are also located within this domain. This addition is not strictly necessary for what follows, but it matches up with the most common way of thinking about the Matrix Hypothesis.)

The Metaphysical Hypothesis is a slightly more specific version of the Combination Hypothesis in that it specifies some relations among the various parts of the hypothesis. Again, the Metaphysical Hypothesis is a coherent hypothesis, and we cannot conclusively rule it out. And again, it is not a skeptical hypothesis. Even if we accept it, most of our ordinary beliefs about the external world will be left intact.

4. The Matrix Hypothesis as a Metaphysical Hypothesis

Recall that the Matrix Hypothesis says that I have (and have always had) a cognitive system that receives its inputs from and sends its outputs to an artificially designed computer simulation of a world.

I will argue that the Matrix Hypothesis is equivalent to the Metaphysical Hypothesis in the following sense: if I accept the Metaphysical Hypothesis, I should accept the Matrix Hypothesis, and if I accept the Matrix Hypothesis, I should accept the Metaphysical Hypothesis. That is, the two hypotheses *imply* each other, where this means that if I accept one, I should accept the other.

Take the first direction first, from the Metaphysical Hypothesis to the Matrix Hypothesis. The Mind-Body Hypothesis implies that I have (and have always had) an isolated cognitive system that receives its inputs from

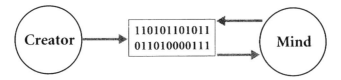

The Matrix Hypothesis

and sends its outputs to processes in physical space-time. In conjunction with the Computational Hypothesis, this implies that my cognitive system receives inputs from and sends outputs to the computational processes that constitute physical space-time. The Creation Hypothesis (along with the rest of the Metaphysical Hypothesis) implies that these processes were artificially designed to simulate a world. It follows that I have (and have always had) an isolated cognitive system that receives its inputs from and sends its outputs to an artificially designed computer simulation of a world. This is just the Matrix Hypothesis. So the Metaphysical Hypothesis implies the Matrix Hypothesis.

The other direction is closely related. To put it informally: if I accept the Matrix Hypothesis, I accept that what underlies apparent reality is just as the Metaphysical Hypothesis specifies. There is a domain containing my cognitive system, which is causally interacting with a computer simulation of physical space-time, which was created by other beings in that domain. This is just what has to obtain in order for the Metaphysical Hypothesis to obtain. If one accepts this, one should accept the Creation Hypothesis, the Computational Hypothesis, the Mind-Body Hypothesis, and the relevant relations among these.

This may be a little clearer through a picture. Here is the shape of the world according to the Matrix Hypothesis.

At the fundamental level, this picture of the shape of the world is exactly the same as the picture of the Metaphysical Hypothesis given earlier. So if one accepts that the world is as it is according to the Matrix Hypothesis, one should accept that it is as it is according to the Metaphysical Hypothesis.

One might make various objections. For example, one might object that the Matrix Hypothesis implies that a computer simulation of physical processes exists, but (unlike the Metaphysical Hypothesis) it does not imply that the physical processes themselves exist. I discuss this objection in section 6 and other objections in section 7. For now, though, I take it that there is a strong case that the Matrix Hypothesis implies the Metaphysical Hypothesis and vice versa.

5. Life in the Matrix

If this is right, it follows that the Matrix Hypothesis is not a skeptical hypothesis. If I accept it, I should not infer that the external world does not exist, that I have no body, that there are no tables and chairs, or that I am not in Tucson. Rather, I should infer that the physical world is constituted by computations beneath the microphysical level. There are still tables, chairs, and bodies. These are made up fundamentally of bits and of whatever constitutes these bits. This world was created by other beings but is still perfectly real. My mind is separate from physical processes and interacts with them. My mind may not have been created by these beings, and it may not be made up of bits, but it still interacts with these bits.

The result is a complex picture of the fundamental nature of reality. The picture is strange and surprising, perhaps, but it is a picture of a full-blooded external world. If we are in a matrix, this is simply the way that the world is.

We can think of the Matrix Hypothesis as a creation myth for the information age. If it is correct, then the physical world was created, although it was not necessarily created by gods. Underlying the physical world is a giant computation, and creators created this world by implementing this computation. Our minds lie outside this physical structure, with an independent nature that interacts with this structure.

Many of the same issues that arise with standard creation myths arise here. When was the world created? Strictly speaking, it was not created within *our* time at all. When did history begin? The creators might have started the simulation in 4004 BC (or in 1999) with the fossil record intact, but it would have been much easier for them to start the simulation at the big bang and let things run their course from there.

(In *The Matrix*, of course, the creators are machines. This gives an interesting twist to common theological readings of the movie. It is often held that Neo is the Christ figure in the movie, with Morpheus corresponding to John the Baptist, Cypher to Judas Iscariot, and so on. But on the reading I have given, the gods of *The Matrix* are the machines. Who, then, is the Christ figure? Agent Smith, of course! After all, he is the gods' offspring, sent down to save the Matrix world from those who wish to destroy it. And in the second movie, he is even resurrected.)

Many of the same issues that arise on the standard Mind-Body Hypothesis also arise here. When do our nonphysical minds start to exist? It depends on just when new envatted cognitive systems are attached to the simulation (perhaps at the time of conception within the matrix or perhaps at the time of birth?). Is there life after death? It depends on just what happens to the envatted systems once their simulated bodies die. How do mind and body interact? By causal links that are outside physical space and time.

Even if we are not in a matrix, we can extend a version of this reasoning to other beings who are in a matrix. If they discover their situation and come to accept that they are in a matrix, they should not reject their ordinary beliefs about the external world. At most, they should come to revise their beliefs about the underlying nature of their world. They should come to accept that external objects are made of bits and so on. These beings are not massively deluded: most of their ordinary beliefs about their world are correct.

There are a few qualifications here. One may worry about beliefs about other people's minds. I believe that my friends are conscious. If I am in a matrix, is this correct? In the Matrix depicted in the movie, these beliefs are mostly fine. This is a multivat matrix: for each of my perceived friends, there is an envatted being in the external reality who is presumably conscious like me. The exception might be beings such as Agent Smith, who are not envatted but are entirely computational. Whether these beings are conscious depends on whether computation is enough for consciousness. I remain neutral on that issue here. We could circumvent this issue by building into the Matrix Hypothesis the requirement that all of the beings we perceive are envatted. However, even if we do not build in this requirement, we are not much worse off than in the actual world, where there is a legitimate issue about whether other beings are conscious, quite independent of whether we are in a matrix.

One might also worry about beliefs about the distant past and about the far future. These will be unthreatened as long as the computer simulation covers all of space-time from the big bang until the end of the universe. This is built into the Metaphysical Hypothesis, and we can stipulate that it is built into the Matrix Hypothesis, too, by requiring that the computer simulation be a simulation of an entire world. There may be other simulations that start in the recent past (perhaps the Matrix in the movie is like this), and there may be others that last for only a short while. In these cases, the envatted beings will have false beliefs about the past or the future in their worlds. But as long as the simulation covers the lifespan of these beings, it is plausible that they will have mostly correct beliefs about the current state of their environment.

There may be some respects in which the beings in a matrix are deceived. It may be that the creators of the matrix control and interfere with much of what happens in the simulated world. (The Matrix in the movie may be like this, though the extent of the creators' control is not quite clear.) If so, then these beings may have much less control over what happens than they think. But the same goes if there is an interfering god in a nonmatrix world. Moreover, the Matrix Hypothesis does not imply that the creators interfere with the world, though it leaves the possibility open. At worst, the Matrix Hypothesis is no more skeptical in this respect than is the Creation Hypothesis in a nonmatrix world.

The inhabitants of a matrix may also be deceived in that reality is much bigger than they think. They might think their physical universe is all there is, when in fact there is much more in the world, including beings and objects that they can never see. Again, however, this sort of worry can arise equally in a nonmatrix world. For example, cosmologists seriously entertain the hypothesis that our universe may stem from a black hole in the "next universe up" and that in reality there may be a whole tree of universes. If so, the world is also much bigger than we think, and there may be beings and objects that we can never see. But either way, the world that we see is perfectly real.

Importantly, none of these sources of skepticism—about other minds, the past and the future, our control over the world, and the extent of the world—casts doubt on our belief in the reality of the world that we perceive. None of them leads us to doubt the existence of external objects such as tables and chairs in the way that the vat hypothesis is supposed to do. Furthermore, none of these worries is especially tied to the matrix scenario. One can raise doubts about whether other minds exist, whether the past and the future exist, and whether we have control over our world quite independently of whether we are in a matrix. If this is right, then the Matrix Hypothesis does not raise the distinctive skeptical issues that it is often taken to raise.

I suggested before that it is not out of the question that we really are in a matrix. One might have thought that this would be a worrying conclusion. But if I am right, it is not nearly as worrying as one might have feared. Even if we are in such a matrix, our world is no less real than we thought it was. It just has a surprising fundamental nature.

6. Objection: Simulation Is Not Reality

(This slightly technical section can be skipped without too much loss.)

A common objection is that a simulation is not the same as reality. The Matrix Hypothesis implies only that a simulation of physical processes exists. By contrast, the Metaphysical Hypothesis implies that physical processes really exist (they are explicitly mentioned in the Computational Hypothesis and elsewhere). If so, then the Matrix Hypothesis cannot imply the Metaphysical Hypothesis. On this view, if I am in a matrix, then physical processes do not really exist.

In response: my argument does not require the general assumption that simulation is the same as reality. The argument works quite differently. However, the objection helps us to flesh out the informal argument that the Matrix Hypothesis implies the Metaphysical Hypothesis.

Because the Computational Hypothesis is coherent, it is clearly *possible* that a computational level underlies real physical processes, and it is possible that the computations here are implemented by further processes in turn. So there is *some* sort of computational system that could yield reality here. But here, the objector will hold that not all computational systems are created equal. To say that some computational systems will yield real physical processes in this role is not to say that they all do. Perhaps some of them are merely simulations. If so, then the Matrix Hypothesis may not yield reality.

To rebut this objection, we can appeal to two principles. First: any abstract computation that could be used to simulate physical space-time is such that it *could* turn out to underlie real physical processes. Second: given an abstract computation that *could* underlie physical processes, the precise way in which it is implemented is irrelevant to whether it *does* underlie physical processes. In particular, the fact that the implementation was designed as a simulation is irrelevant. The conclusion then follows directly.

On the first principle: let us think of abstract computations in purely formal terms, abstracting away from their manner of implementation. For an abstract computation to qualify as a simulation of physical reality, it must have computational elements that correspond to every particle in reality (likewise for fields, waves, or whatever is fundamental), dynamically evolving in a way that corresponds to each particle's evolution. But then, it is guaranteed that the computation will have a rich enough causal structure that it *could* in principle underlie physics in our world. Any computation will do as long as it has enough detail to correspond to the fine details of physical processes.

On the second principle: given an abstract computation that could underlie physical reality, it does not matter how the computation is implemented. We can imagine discovering that some computational level underlies the level of atoms and electrons. Once we have discovered this, it is possible that this computational level is implemented by more basic processes. There are many hypotheses about what the underlying processes could be, but none of them is especially privileged, and none of them would lead us to reject the hypothesis that the computational level constitutes physical processes. That is, the Computational Hypothesis is *implementation-independent*. As long as we have the right sort of abstract computation, the manner of implementation does not matter.

In particular, it is irrelevant whether or not these implementing processes were artificially created, and it is irrelevant whether they were intended as a simulation. What matters is the intrinsic nature of the processes, not their origin. And what matters about this intrinsic nature is simply that they are arranged in such a way as to implement the right sort of computation. If so, the fact that the implementation originated as a simulation is irrelevant to whether it can constitute physical reality.

There is one further constraint on the implementing processes: they must be connected to our experiences in the right sort of way. That is, when we have an experience of an object, the processes underlying the simulation of that object must be causally connected in the right sort of way to our experiences. If this is not the case, then there will be no reason to think that these computational processes underlie the physical processes that we perceive. If there is an isolated computer simulation to which nobody is connected in this way, we should say that it is simply a simulation. However, an appropriate hookup to our perceptual experiences is built into the Matrix Hypothesis on the most natural understanding of that hypothesis, so the Matrix Hypothesis has no problems here.

Overall, then, we have seen that computational processes *could* underlie physical reality, that any abstract computation that qualifies as a simulation of physical reality could play this role, and that any implementation of this computation could constitute physical reality as long as it is hooked up to our experiences in the relevant way. The Matrix Hypothesis guarantees that we have an abstract computation of the right sort, and it guarantees that it is hooked up to our experiences in the relevant ways. So the Matrix Hypothesis implies that the Computational Hypothesis is correct and that the computer simulation constitutes genuine physical processes.

7. Other Objections

When we look at a brain in a vat from the outside, it is hard to avoid the sense that it is deluded. This sense manifests itself in a number of related objections. These are not direct objections to the main argument I have given, but they are objections to its conclusion.

Objection 1: A brain in a vat may think it is outside walking in the sun, when in fact it is alone in a dark room. Surely it is deluded.

Response: The *brain* is alone in a dark room. But this does not imply that the *person* is alone in a dark room. By analogy, just say Descartes is right that we have disembodied minds outside space-time and made of ectoplasm. When I think, "I am outside in the sun," an angel might look at my ectoplasmic mind and note that in fact it is not exposed to any sun at all. Does it follow that my thought is incorrect? Presumably not: I can be outside in the sun even if my ectoplasmic mind is not. The angel would be wrong to infer that I have an incorrect belief. Likewise, we should not infer that the envatted being has an incorrect belief. At least, it is no more deluded than a Cartesian mind.

The moral is that the immediate surroundings of our minds may well be irrelevant to the truth of most of our beliefs. What matters is the processes that our minds are connected to by perceptual inputs and motor outputs. Once we recognize this, the objection falls away.

Objection 2: An envatted being may believe that it is in Tucson when in fact it is in New York and has never been anywhere near Tucson. Surely this belief is deluded.

Response: The envatted being's word "Tucson" does not refer to what we call Tucson. Rather, it refers to something else entirely: call this "Tucson*" or "virtual Tucson." We might think of this as a virtual location (more on this in a moment). When the being says to itself, 'I am in Tucson,' it really is thinking that it is in Tucson*, and it may well be in Tucson*. Because Tucson is not Tucson*, the fact that the being has never been in Tucson is irrelevant to whether its belief is true.

A rough analogy is this: I look at my colleague Terry and say to myself, 'That's Terry'. Elsewhere in the world, a duplicate of me looks at a duplicate of Terry. He says to himself, 'That's Terry,' but he is not looking at the real Terry. Is his belief false? It seems not: my duplicate's word 'Terry' refers not to Terry but to his duplicate, Terry*. My duplicate really is looking at Terry*, so his belief is true. The same sort of thing is happening in the case above.

Objection 3: Before he leaves the Matrix, Neo believes that he has hair. But in reality he has no hair (the body in the vat is bald). Surely this belief is deluded.

Response: This case is like the last one. Neo's word 'hair' does not refer to real hair but to something else that we might call hair* (virtual hair). So the fact that Neo does not have real hair is irrelevant to whether his belief is true. Neo really does have virtual hair, so he is correct. Likewise, when a child in the movie tells Neo, 'There is no spoon,' his concept refers to a virtual spoon, and there really is a virtual spoon. So the child is wrong.

Objection 4: What *sort* of objects does an envatted being refer to? What *are* virtual hair, virtual Tucson, and so on?

Response: These are all entities constituted by computational processes. If I am envatted, then the objects to which I refer (hair, Tucson, and so on) are all made of bits. If I am not envatted but another being is envatted, the objects that it refers to (hair*, Tucson*, and so on) are likewise made of bits. If the envatted being is hooked up to a simulation in my computer, then the objects to which it refers are constituted by patterns of bits inside my computer. We might call these things *virtual objects*. Virtual hands are not hands (assuming I am not envatted), but they exist inside the computer all the same. Virtual Tucson is not Tucson, but it exists inside the computer all the same.

Objection 5: You just said that virtual hands are not real hands. Does this mean that if we are in a matrix, we do not have real hands?

Response: No. If we are *not* in a matrix, but other beings are, we should say that their term 'hand' refers to virtual hands, but our term does not. So in this case, our hands are not virtual hands. However, if we *are* in a matrix, then our term 'hand' refers to something that is made of bits: virtual hands, or at least something that would be regarded as virtual hands by people in the next world up. That is, if we *are* in a matrix, real hands are made of bits. Things look quite different, and our words refer to different things, depending on whether our perspective is from inside or outside the matrix.

This sort of perspective shift is common in thinking about the matrix scenario. From the first-person perspective, we suppose that *we* are in a matrix. Here, real things in our world are made of bits, though the next world up might not be made of bits. From the third-person perspective we suppose that someone *else* is in a matrix but that we are not. Here, real things in our world are not made of bits, but the next world down is made of bits. On the first way of doing things, our words refer to computational entities. On the second way of doing things, the envatted beings' words refer to computational entities, but our words do not.

Objection 6: Just which pattern of bits is a given virtual object? Surely it will be impossible to pick out a precise set.

Response: This question is like asking the following: just which part of the quantum wave function is this chair, and which part is the University of Arizona? These objects are all ultimately constituted by an underlying quantum wave function, but there may be no precise part of the microlevel wave function that we can say "is" the chair or the university. The chair and the university exist at a higher level. Likewise, if we are envatted, there may be no precise set of bits in the microlevel computational process that is the chair or the university. These exist at a higher level. Furthermore, if someone else is envatted, there may be no precise sets of bits in the computer simulation that "are" the objects to which they refer. However, just as a chair exists without being any precise part of the wave function, a virtual chair may exist without being any precise set of bits.

Objection 7: An envatted being thinks it performs actions, and it thinks it has friends. Are these beliefs correct?

Response: One might try to say that the being performs actions* and that it has friends*. However, for various reasons I think it is not plausible that words like 'action' and 'friend' can shift their meanings as easily as words like 'Tucson' and 'hair.' Instead, one can say truthfully (in our own language) that the envatted being performs actions and that it has friends. To be sure, it performs actions in *its* environment, and its environment is not our environment but the virtual environment. Moreover, its friends likewise inhabit the virtual environment (assuming that we have a multivat matrix or that computation suffices for consciousness). But the envatted being is not incorrect in this respect.

Objection 8: Set these technical points aside. Surely, if we are in a matrix, the world is nothing like we think it is.

Response: I deny this. Even if we are in a matrix, there are still people, football games, and particles, arranged in space-time just as we think they are. It is just that the world has a *further* nature that goes beyond our initial conception. In particular, things in the world are realized computationally in a way that we might not have originally imagined. Still, this does not contradict any of our ordinary beliefs. At most, it will contradict a few of our more abstract metaphysical beliefs. But exactly the same goes for quantum mechanics, relativity theory, and so on.

If we are in a matrix, we may not have many false beliefs, but there is much knowledge that we lack. For example, we do not know that the universe is realized computationally. But this is just what one should expect. Even if we are not in a matrix, there may well be much about the fundamental nature of reality that we do not know. We are not omniscient creatures, and our knowledge of the world is at best partial. This is simply the condition of a creature living in a world.

8. Other Skeptical Hypotheses

The Matrix Hypothesis is one example of a traditional "skeptical" hypothesis, but it is not the only example. Other skeptical hypotheses are not quite as straightforward as the Matrix Hypothesis. Still, for many of them, a similar line of reasoning applies. In particular, one can argue that

most of these are not global skeptical hypotheses: that is, their truth
would not undercut all of our empirical beliefs about the physical world.
At worst, most of them are *partial* skeptical hypotheses that undercut
some of our empirical beliefs but leave many other beliefs intact.

New Matrix Hypothesis: I was recently created, along with all of my
memories, and was put in a newly created matrix.

What if both the matrix and I have existed for only a short time? This
hypothesis is a computational version of Bertrand Russell's Recent Creation Hypothesis: the physical world was created only recently (with fossil
record intact), and so was I (with memories intact). On that hypothesis,
the external world that I perceive really exists, and most of my beliefs about
its current state are plausibly true, but I have many false beliefs about the
past. The same should be said of the New Matrix Hypothesis. One can
argue, along the lines presented earlier, that the New Matrix Hypothesis is
equivalent to a combination of the Metaphysical Hypothesis with the
Recent Creation Hypothesis. This combination is not a global skeptical
hypothesis (though it is a partial skeptical hypothesis, where beliefs about
the past are concerned). The same goes for the New Matrix Hypothesis.

Recent Matrix Hypothesis: For most of my life I have not been
envatted, but I was recently hooked up to a matrix.

If I was recently put in a matrix without realizing it, it seems that many
of my beliefs about my current environment are false. Let us say that just
yesterday someone put me into a simulation in which I fly to Las Vegas
and gamble at a casino. Then I may believe that I am in Las Vegas now and
that I am in a casino, but these beliefs are false. I am really in a laboratory
in Tucson.

This result is quite different from the long-term matrix. The difference lies
in the fact that my conception of external reality is anchored to the reality in
which I have lived most of my life. If I have been envatted all of my life, my
conception is anchored to the computationally constituted reality. But if I
were just envatted yesterday, my conception is anchored to the external reality. So when I think that I am in Las Vegas, I am thinking that I am in the
external Las Vegas, and this thought is false.

Still, this does not undercut all of my beliefs about the external world. I
believe that I was born in Sydney, that there is water in the oceans, and so
on, and all of these beliefs are correct. It is only my recently acquired
beliefs, stemming from my perception of the simulated environment, that

will be false. So this is only a partially skeptical hypothesis: its possibility casts doubt on a subset of our empirical beliefs, but it does not cast doubt on all of them.

Interestingly, the Recent Matrix Hypothesis and the New Matrix Hypothesis give opposite results despite their similar nature. The Recent Matrix Hypothesis yields true beliefs about the past but false beliefs about the present, whereas the New Matrix Hypothesis yields false beliefs about the past and true beliefs about the present. The differences are tied to the fact that in the Recent Matrix Hypothesis, I really have a past existence for my beliefs to be about, and that past reality has played a role in anchoring the contents of my thoughts, which has no parallel under the new Matrix Hypothesis.

Local Matrix Hypothesis: I am hooked up to a computer simulation of a fixed local environment in a world.

On one way of doing this, a computer simulates a small fixed environment in a world, and the subjects in the simulation encounter some sort of barrier when they try to leave that area. For example, in the movie *The Thirteenth Floor*, just California is simulated, and when the subject tries to drive to Nevada, a road sign says "Closed for Repair" (with faint green electronic mountains in the distance). Of course, this is not the best way to create a matrix, as subjects are likely to discover the limits to their world.

This hypothesis is analogous to a Local Creation Hypothesis, on which creators create just a local part of the physical world. Under this hypothesis, we will have true beliefs about nearby matters but false beliefs about matters farther from home. By the usual sort of reasoning, the Local Matrix Hypothesis can be seen as a combination of the Metaphysical Hypothesis with the Local Creation Hypothesis so we should say the same thing about it as about the Local Creation Hypothesis.

Extendible Local Matrix Hypothesis: I am hooked up to a computer simulation of a local environment in a world, which is extended when necessary depending on my movements.

This hypothesis avoids the obvious difficulties with a fixed local matrix. Here, the creators simulate a local environment and extend it when necessary. For example, they might right now be concentrating on simulating a room in my house in Tucson. If I walk into another room or fly to another city, they will simulate those. Of course, they need to make sure that when

I go to these places, they match my memories and beliefs reasonably well, with allowance for evolution in the meantime. The same goes for when I encounter familiar people or people I have only heard about. Presumably, the simulators keep up a database of the information about the world that has been settled so far, updating this information whenever necessary as time goes along and making up new details when they need them.

This sort of simulation is quite unlike simulation in an ordinary matrix. In a matrix, the whole world is simulated at once. There are high start-up costs, but once the simulation is up and running, it will take care of itself. By contrast, the extendible local matrix involves "just-in-time" simulation. This has much lower start-up costs, but it requires much more work and creativity as the simulation evolves.

This hypothesis is analogous to an Extendible Local Creation Hypothesis about ordinary reality, under which creators create just a local physical environment and extend it when necessary. Here, external reality exists, and many local beliefs are true, but again beliefs about matters farther from home are false. If we combine that hypothesis with the Metaphysical Hypothesis, the result is the extendible local Matrix Hypothesis. So if we are in an extendible local matrix, external reality still exists, but there is not as much of it as we thought. Of course, if I travel in the right direction, more of it may come into existence.

The situation is reminiscent of the film *The Truman Show*. Truman lives in an artificial environment made up of actors and props that behave appropriately when he is around but may be completely different when he is absent. Truman has many true beliefs about his current environment. There really are tables and chairs in front of him and so on. But he is deeply mistaken about things outside his current environment and farther from home.

It is common to think that while *The Truman Show* poses a disturbing skeptical scenario, *The Matrix* is much worse. But if I am right, things are reversed. If I am in a matrix, then most of my beliefs about the external world are true. If I am in something like *The Truman Show*, then a great number of my beliefs are false. On reflection, it seems to me that this is the right conclusion. If we were to discover that we were (and always had been) in a matrix, this would be surprising, but we would quickly get used to it. If we were to discover that we were (and always had been) in a televised "Truman Show," we might well go insane.

Macroscopic Matrix Hypothesis: I am hooked up to a computer simulation of macroscopic physical processes without microphysical detail.

One can imagine that, for ease of simulation, the makers of a matrix might not bother to simulate low-level physics. Instead, they might just represent macroscopic objects in the world and their properties: for example, that there is a table with such-and-such a shape, position, and color, with a book on top of it with certain properties, and so on. They will need to make some effort to make sure that these objects behave in physically reasonable ways, and they will have to make special provisions for handling microphysical measurements, but one can imagine that at least a reasonable simulation could be created this way.

This hypothesis is analogous to a Macroscopic World Hypothesis: there are no microphysical processes, and instead macroscopic physical objects exist as fundamental objects in the world, with properties of shape, color, position, and so on. This is a coherent way that our world could be, and it is not a global skeptical hypothesis, though it may lead to false scientific beliefs about lower levels of reality. The Macroscopic Matrix Hypothesis can be seen as a combination of this hypothesis with a version of the Metaphysical Hypothesis. As such, it is not a global skeptical hypothesis, either.

One can also combine these various hypotheses in various ways, yielding hypotheses such as a New Local Macroscopic Matrix Hypothesis. For the usual reasons, all of these can be seen as analogs of corresponding hypotheses about the physical world. So all of them are compatible with the existence of physical reality, and none is a global skeptical hypothesis.

God Hypothesis: Physical reality is represented in the mind of God, and our own thoughts and perceptions depend on God's mind.

A hypothesis like this was put forward by Berkeley as a view about how our world might really be. Berkeley intended this as a sort of metaphysical hypothesis about the nature of reality. Most other philosophers have differed from Berkeley in regarding this as a sort of skeptical hypothesis. If I am right, Berkeley is closer to the truth. The God hypothesis can be seen as a version of the Matrix Hypothesis, on which the simulation of the world is implemented in the mind of God. If this is right, we should say that physical processes really exist. It is just that at the most fundamental level, they are constituted by processes in the mind of God.

Evil Genius Hypothesis: I have a disembodied mind, and an evil genius is feeding me sensory inputs to give the appearance of an external world.

This is René Descartes' classical skeptical hypothesis. What should we say about it? This depends on just how the evil genius works. If the evil genius simulates an entire world in his head in order to determine what inputs I should receive, then we have a version of the God hypothesis. Here we should say that physical reality exists and is constituted by processes within the mind of the evil genius. If the evil genius is simulating only a small part of the physical world, just enough to give me reasonably consistent inputs, then we have an analog of the Local Matrix Hypothesis (in either its fixed or flexible versions). Here we should say that just a local part of external reality exists. If the evil genius is not bothering to simulate the microphysical level but just the macroscopic level, then we have an analog of the Macroscopic Matrix Hypothesis. Here we should say that local external macroscopic objects exist, but our beliefs about their microphysical nature are incorrect.

The Evil Genius Hypothesis is often taken to be a global skeptical hypothesis, but if the foregoing reasoning is right, this is incorrect. Even if the Evil Genius Hypothesis is correct, some of the external reality that we apparently perceive really exists, though we may have some false beliefs about it depending on details. It is just that this external reality has an underlying nature that is quite different from what we may have thought.

Dream Hypothesis: I am now and have always been dreaming.

Descartes raised the question: how do you know that you are not currently dreaming? Morpheus raises a similar question:

> Have you ever had a dream, Neo, that you were so sure was real? What if you were unable to wake from that dream? How would you know the difference between the dream world and the real world?

The hypothesis that I am *currently* dreaming is analogous to a version of the Recent Matrix Hypothesis. I cannot rule it out conclusively, and if it is correct, then many of my beliefs about my current environment are incorrect. But presumably I still have many true beliefs about the external world that are anchored in the past.

What if I have always been dreaming? That is, what if all of my apparent perceptual inputs have been generated by my own cognitive system without my realizing this? This case is analogous to the Evil Genius Hypothesis: it is just that the role of the "evil genius" is played by a part of my own cognitive system! If my dream-generating system simulates all of space-time, we have something like the original Matrix Hypothesis. If it models just my local environment or just some macroscopic processes, we have analogs of the more local versions of the Evil Genius Hypothesis. In any of these cases, we should say that the objects that I am currently perceiving really exist (although objects farther from home may not). It is just that some of them are constituted by my own cognitive processes.

> **Chaos Hypothesis:** I do not receive inputs from anywhere in the world. Instead, I have random, uncaused experiences. Through a huge coincidence, they are exactly the sort of regular, structured experiences with which I am familiar.

The Chaos Hypothesis is an extraordinarily unlikely hypothesis, much more unlikely than anything considered earlier. But it is still one that could in principle obtain, even if it has minuscule probability. If I am chaotically envatted, do physical processes in the external world exist? I think we should say that they do not. My experiences of external objects are caused by nothing, and the set of experiences associated with my conception of a given object will have no common source. Indeed, my experiences are not caused by any reality external to them at all. So this is a genuine skeptical hypothesis. If accepted, it would cause us to reject most of our beliefs about the external world.

So far, the only clear case of a global skeptical hypothesis is the Chaos Hypothesis. Unlike the previous hypotheses, accepting this hypothesis would undercut all of our substantive beliefs about the external world. Where does the difference come from?

Arguably, what is crucial is that on the Chaos Hypothesis, there is no causal explanation of our experiences at all, and there is no explanation for the regularities in our experience. In all of the previous cases, there is some explanation for these regularities, though perhaps not the explanation that we expect. One might suggest that as long as a hypothesis involves *some* reasonable explanation for the regularities in our experience, then it will not be a global skeptical hypothesis.

If so, then if we are granted the assumption that there is some explanation for the regularities in our experience, then it is safe to say that some of our beliefs about the external world are correct. This is not much, but it is something.

Afterword: Philosophical Notes

This chapter was written to be accessible to a wide audience, so it deliberately omits technical philosophical details, connections to the literature, and so on. In this afterword I remedy this omission. Readers without a background in philosophy may choose to skip or skim this section.

Note 1: Putnam's Antiskeptical Argument

Hilary Putnam (1981) has argued that the hypothesis that I am (and have always been) a brain in a vat can be ruled out a priori. In effect, this is because my word 'brain' refers to objects in my perceived world, and it cannot refer to objects in an "outer" world in which the vat would have to exist. For my sentence 'I am a brain in a vat' to be true, I would have to be a brain of the sort that exists in the perceived world, but that cannot be the case. So the sentence must be false.

An analogy: I can arguably rule out the hypothesis that I am in the Matrix (capital M). My term 'the Matrix' refers to a specific system that I have seen in a movie in my perceived world. I could not be in that very system, as the system exists within the world that I perceive, so my hypothesis 'I am in the Matrix' must be false.

This conclusion about the Matrix seems reasonable, but there is a natural response. Perhaps this argument rules out the hypothesis that I am in the Matrix, but I cannot rule out the hypothesis that I am in a matrix, where a matrix is a generic term for a computer simulation of a world. The term 'Matrix' may be anchored to the specific system in the movie, but the generic term 'matrix' is not.

Likewise, it is arguable that I can rule out the hypothesis that I am a brain in a vat (if 'brain' is anchored to a specific sort of biological system in my perceived world). But I cannot rule out the hypothesis that I am envatted, where this simply says that I have a cognitive system that receives input from and sends outputs to a computer simulation of a world. The term 'envatted' (and the terms used in its definition) are generic terms, not anchored to specific systems in perceived reality. By using this slightly different language, we can restate the skeptical hypothesis in a way that is invulnerable to Putnam's reasoning.

More technically, Putnam's argument may work for 'brain' and 'Matrix' because one is a natural kind term and the other is a name. These terms are subject to "Twin Earth" thought experiments (Putnam 1975), where duplicates can use corresponding terms with different referents. On Earth, Oscar's term 'water' refers to H_2O, but on Twin Earth (which contains the superficially identical XYZ in its oceans and lakes), Twin Oscar's term 'water' refers to XYZ. Likewise, perhaps my term 'brain' refers to biological brains, while an envatted being's term 'brain' refers to virtual brains. If so, when an envatted being says, 'I am a brain in a vat,' it is not referring to its biological brain, and its claim is false.

However, not all terms are subject to Twin Earth thought experiments. In particular, semantically neutral terms are not (at least when used without semantic deference). Such terms plausibly include 'philosopher,' 'friend,' and many others. Other such terms include 'matrix' and 'envatted,' as defined earlier. If we work with hypotheses such as 'I am in a matrix' and 'I am envatted' rather than 'I am in the Matrix' or 'I am a brain in a vat,' then Putnam's argument does not apply. Even if a brain in a vat could not truly think, 'I am a brain in a vat,' it could truly think, 'I am envatted.' So I think that Putnam's line of reasoning is ultimately a red herring.

Note 2: The Causal Theory of Reference

Despite this disagreement, my main conclusion is closely related to another suggestion of Putnam's. This is the suggestion that a brain in a vat may have true beliefs because it will refer to chemical processes or processes inside a computer. However, I reach this conclusion by a quite different route. Putnam argues by an appeal to the causal theory of reference: thoughts refer to what they are causally connected to, and the thoughts of an envatted being are causally connected to processes in a computer. This argument is clearly inconclusive because the causal theory of reference is so unconstrained. To say that a causal connection is required for reference is not to say what sort of causal connection suffices. There are many cases (like 'phlogiston') where terms fail to refer despite rich causal connections. Intuitively, it is natural to think that the brain in a vat is a case like this, so an appeal to the causal theory of reference does not seem to help.

The argument I have given presupposes nothing about the theory of reference. Instead, it proceeds directly by considering first-order hypotheses about the world, the connections among these, and what we should say if they are true. In answering objections, I have made some claims about reference, and these claims are broadly compatible with a causal theory of reference. But importantly, these claims are very much consequences of the first-order argument rather than presuppositions of it. In general, I think that claims in the theory of reference are beholden to first-order judgments about cases rather than vice versa.

Note 3: Skeptical Hypotheses

I use 'skeptical hypothesis' in a certain technical sense. A skeptical hypothesis (relative to a belief that p) is a hypothesis such that (i) we cannot rule it out with certainty, and (ii) were we to accept it, we would reject the belief that p. A skeptical hypothesis with respect to a class of beliefs is one that is a skeptical hypothesis with respect to most or all of the beliefs in that class. A global skeptical hypothesis is a skeptical hypothesis with respect to all of our empirical beliefs.

The existence of a skeptical hypothesis (with respect to a belief) casts doubt on the relevant belief in the following sense. Because we cannot rule out the hypothesis with certainty and because the hypothesis implies the negation of these beliefs, it seems (given a plausible closure principle about certainty) that our knowledge of these beliefs is not certain. If it is also the case that we do not *know* that the skeptical hypothesis does not obtain (as I think is the case for most of the hypotheses in this chapter), then it follows from an analogous closure principle that the beliefs in the class do not constitute knowledge.

Some use 'skeptical hypothesis' in a broader sense to apply to any hypothesis such that if it obtains, I do not know that p. (A hypothesis under which I have accidentally true beliefs is a skeptical hypothesis in this sense but not in the previous sense.) I have not argued here that the Matrix Hypothesis is not a skeptical hypothesis in this sense. I have argued that if the hypothesis obtains, our beliefs are true, but I have not argued that if it obtains, our beliefs constitute knowledge. Nevertheless, I am inclined to think that if we have knowledge in an ordinary, nonmatrix world, we would also have knowledge in a matrix.

Note 4: Empirical Beliefs

What is the relevant class of beliefs? Of course, there are some beliefs that even a no-external-world skeptical hypothesis might not undercut: the belief that I exist, the belief that $2 + 2 = 4$, or the belief that there are no unicorns. Because of this, it is best to restrict attention to beliefs that (i) are about the external world, (ii) are not justifiable a priori, and (iii) make a positive claim about the world (they could not be true in an empty world). For the purposes of this chapter we can think of these beliefs as our "empirical beliefs." Claims about skeptical hypotheses undercutting beliefs should generally be understood as restricted to beliefs in this class.

Note 5: The Computational Level

Considering the Computational Hypothesis, it is coherent to suppose that there is a computational level underneath physics, but it is not clear whether it is coherent to suppose that this level is fundamental. This last supposition in effect describes a world of "pure bits." Such a world would be a world of pure differences: there would be two basic states that differ from one another without this difference being a difference in some deeper nature. Whether one thinks this is coherent or not is connected to whether one thinks that all differences must be grounded in some basic intrinsic nature, whether one thinks that all dispositions must have a categorical basis, and so on. For the purposes of this chapter, however, the issue can be set aside. Under the Matrix Hypothesis, the computation itself is *implemented* by processes in the world of the creator. As such, there will be a more basic level of intrinsic properties that serves as the basis for the differences between bits.

Note 6: Cartesian Dualism

On the Mind-Body Hypothesis: it is interesting to note that the Matrix Hypothesis shows a concrete way in which Cartesian substance dualism might have turned out to be true. It is sometimes held that the idea of physical processes interacting with a nonphysical mind is not just implausible but also incoherent. The Matrix Hypothesis suggests fairly straightforwardly that this is wrong. Under this hypothesis, our cognitive system involves processes quite distinct from the processes in the physical world, but there is a straightforward causal story about how they interact.

Some questions arise. For example, if the envatted cognitive system is producing a body's motor outputs, what role does the simulated brain play? Perhaps one could do without it, but this will cause all sorts of awkward results, not least when doctors in the matrix open the skull. It is more natural to think that the envatted brain and the simulated brain will always be in isomorphic states, receiving the same inputs and producing the same outputs. If the two systems start in isomorphic states and always receive the same inputs, then (setting aside indeterminism) they will always stay in isomorphic states. As a bonus, this may explain why death in the Matrix leads to death in the outer world!

Which of these actually controls the body? This depends on how things are set up. Things might be set up so the envatted system's outputs are not fed back to the simulation; in this case a version of epiphenomenalism will be true. Things might be set up so that motor impulses in the simulated body depend on the envatted system's outputs with the simulated brain's outputs being ignored; in this case a version of interactionism will be true. Interestingly, this last might be a version of interactionism that is compatible with causal closure of the physical. A third possibility is that the mechanism takes both sets of outputs into account (perhaps averaging the two?). This could yield a sort of redundancy in the causation. Perhaps the controllers of the matrix might even sometimes switch between the two. In any of these cases, as long as the two systems stay in isomorphic states, the behavioral results will be the same.

One might worry that there will be two conscious minds here in a fashion reminiscent of Daniel Dennett's story "Where Am I?" This depends on whether computation in the matrix is enough to support a mind. If anticomputationalists about the mind (such as John Searle) are right, there will be just one mind. If computationalists about the mind are right, there may well be two synchronized minds (which then raises the question: if I am in a matrix, which of the two minds is mine?). The one-mind view is certainly closer to the ordinary conception of reality, but the two-mind view is not out of the question.

One bonus of the computationalist view is that it allows us to entertain the hypothesis that we are in a computer simulation *without* a separate cognitive system attached. Instead, the creators just run the simulation, including a simulation of brains, and minds emerge within it. This is presumably much easier for the creators since it removes any worries tied to the creation and upkeep of the attached cognitive systems. Because of this, it seems quite plausible that there will be many simulations of this sort in the future, whereas it is unclear that there will be many of the more cumbersome Matrix-style simulations. (Because of this, Bostrom's 2003 argument that we may well be in a simulation applies more directly to this sort of simulation than to Matrix-style simulations.) The hypothesis that we are in this sort of computer simulation corresponds to a slimmed-down version of the Metaphysical Hypothesis on which the Mind-Body Hypothesis is unnecessary. As before, this is a nonskeptical hypothesis: if we are in such a simulation (and if computationalism about the mind is true), then most of our beliefs about the external world are still correct.

There are also other possibilities. One intriguing possibility (discussed in Chalmers 1990) is suggested by contemporary work in artificial life, which involves relatively simple simulated environments and complex rules by which simulated creatures interact with these environments. Here the algorithms responsible for the creatures' "mental" processes are quite distinct from those governing the "physics" of the environment. In this sort of simulation, creatures will presumably never find underpinnings for their cognitive processes in their perceived world. If these creatures become scientists, they will be Cartesian dualists, holding (correctly) that their cognitive processes lie outside their physical world. It seems that this is another coherent way that Cartesian dualism might have turned out to be true.

Note 7: Implication and Entailment

I have argued that the Matrix Hypothesis implies the Metaphysical Hypothesis and vice versa. Here, "implies" is an epistemic relation: if one accepts the first, one should accept the second. I do not claim that the Matrix Hypothesis *entails* the Metaphysical Hypothesis in the sense that in any counterfactual world in which the Matrix Hypothesis holds, the Metaphysical Hypothesis holds. That claim seems to be false. For example, there are counterfactual worlds in which physical space-time is created by nobody (so the Metaphysical Hypothesis is false) and in which I am hooked up to an artificially designed computer simulation located within physical space-time (so the Matrix Hypothesis is true). Furthermore, if physics is not computational in the actual world, then physics in this world is not computational, either. One might say that the two hypothesis are a priori equivalent but not necessarily equivalent. (Of course, the term 'physics' as used by my envatted self in the counterfactual world will refer to something that is both computational and created. But 'physics' as used by my current, nonenvatted self picks out the outer noncomputational physics of that world, not the computational processes.)

The difference arises from two different ways of considering the Matrix Hypothesis: as a hypothesis about what might actually be the case or as a hypothesis about what might have been the case but is not. The first hypothesis is reflected in indicative conditionals: if I am actually in a matrix, then I have hands, atoms are made of bits, and the Metaphysical Hypothesis is true. The second version is reflected in subjunctive conditionals: if I had been in a matrix, I would not have had hands, atoms would not have been made of bits, and the Metaphysical Hypothesis would not have been true.

This is analogous to the different ways of thinking about Putnam's Twin Earth scenario, common in discussions of two-dimensional semantics (see the appendix). If I am actually in the XYZ world, then XYZ is water, but if I had been in the XYZ world, XYZ would not have been water (water would still have been H_2O). On the first way of doing things, we consider a Twin Earth world as *actual*. On the second way of doing things, we consider a Twin Earth world as *counterfactual*. We can say that the Twin Earth world *verifies* 'water is XYZ' but that it *satisfies* 'water is not XYZ,' where verification and satisfaction correspond to considering something as actual and as counterfactual.

Likewise, we can say that a matrix world verifies the Metaphysical Hypothesis, but it does not satisfy the Metaphysical Hypothesis. The reason is that the Metaphysical Hypothesis makes claims about physics and the physical world. Moreover, what counts as "physics" differs depending on whether the matrix world is considered as actual or counterfactual. If I am in a matrix, physics is computational, but if I *had been* in a matrix, physics would not have been computational. (The matrix would have been computational, but the computer and my brain would all have been made from computation-independent physics.) In this way, claims about physics and physical processes in a matrix world are analogous to claims about 'water' in the Twin Earth world.

Note 8: Meaning and Reference

The responses to the first few objections in section 7 are clearly congenial to a causal account of reference. There I say that the truth of an envatted being's thoughts depends not on its immediate environment but on what it is causally connected to, that is, on the computational processes to which it is hooked up. As noted earlier, I did not need to assume the causal theory of reference to get to this conclusion but instead got there through a first-order argument. However, once the conclusion is reached, there are many interesting points of contact.

For example, the idea that my term 'hair' refers to hair while my envatted counterpart's term refers to virtual hair has a familiar structure. The case is structurally analogous to a Twin Earth case, in which Oscar (on Earth) refers to water (H_2O), while his counterpart Twin Oscar (on Twin Earth) refers to twin water (XYZ). In both cases, the terms refer to what they are causally connected to. These natural-kind terms function by picking out a certain kind in the subject's environment, and the precise nature of that kind depends on the nature of the environment. Something similar applies to names for specific entities such as 'Tucson.'

The behavior of these terms can be modeled using the two-dimensional semantic framework. As before, when we consider a Twin Earth world as actual, it verifies 'water is XYZ,' and when we consider it as counterfactual, it satisfies 'water is not XYZ.' Likewise, when we consider a matrix world as actual, it verifies 'hair is made of bits,' and when we consider it as counterfactual, it satisfies 'hair is not made of bits.'

The difference between considering something as actual or as counterfactual yields a perspective shift like the one in the response to objection 5.

If the matrix world is considered as merely counterfactual, we should say that the beings in the matrix do not have hair (they have only virtual hair). However, if the matrix world is considered as actual (that is, if we hypothetically accept that we are in a matrix), we should say that the beings in the matrix have hair and that hair is itself a sort of virtual hair.

The Twin Earth analogy may suggest that a wholly externalist view on which the meanings of our terms such as 'hair' and the contents of our corresponding thoughts depend on our environment. But the two-dimensional approach also suggests that there is an internal aspect of content that is shared between twins and does not depend on the environment. The *primary intension* of a sentence is true at a world if the world verifies the sentence, while its *secondary intension* is true at a world if the world satisfies the sentence. Then Oscar and Twin Oscar's sentences 'water is wet' have different secondary intensions (roughly, true when H_2O is wet or when XYZ is wet, respectively), but they have the same primary intension (roughly, true at worlds where the watery-looking stuff is wet). Likewise, utterances of 'I have hair' by me and my envatted counterpart have different secondary intensions (roughly, true at worlds where we have biological hair or computational hair, respectively), but they have the same primary intension (roughly, true at worlds where we have hairlike stuff). The primary intensions of our thought and our language represent a significant shared dimension of content.

Note 9: Semantically Neutral Terms

Why the different response to objection 7, on 'action' and 'friend'? I noted earlier (note 1) that not all terms function like 'water' and 'hair.' There are numerous *semantically neutral* terms that are not subject to Twin Earth thought experiments: any two twins using these terms in different environments will use them with the same meaning (at least if they are using the terms without semantic deference). These terms arguably include 'and,' 'friend,' 'philosopher,' 'action,' 'experience,' and 'envatted.' So while an envatted being's term 'hand' or 'hair' or 'Tucson' may mean something different from our corresponding term, an envatted being's term 'friend' or 'philosopher' or 'action' will arguably mean the same as ours.

It follows that if we are concerned with an envatted being's belief *I have friends* or *I perform actions*, we cannot use the Twin Earth response. These beliefs will be true if and only if the envatted being has friends and performs actions. Fortunately, it seems quite reasonable to say that the envatted being *does* have friends (in its environment, not in ours) and that it does perform actions (in its environment, not in ours). The same goes for other semantically neutral terms: it is for precisely this class of expressions that this response is reasonable.

Note 10: The Ontology of Virtual Objects

What is the ontology of virtual objects? This is a hard question, but it is no harder than the question of the ontology of ordinary macroscopic objects in a quantum-mechanical world. The response to objection 6 suggests that in both cases we should reject claims of token identity between microscopic and macroscopic levels. Tables are not identical to any object characterized purely in terms of quantum mechanics; likewise, virtual tables are not identical to any objects characterized purely in terms of bits. Nevertheless, facts about tables supervene on quantum-mechanical facts, and facts about virtual tables supervene on computational facts. So it seems reasonable to say that tables are constituted by quantum processes and that virtual tables are constituted by computational processes. Further specificity in either case depends on delicate questions of metaphysics.

Reflecting on the third-person case, in which we are looking at a brain in a vat in our world, one might protest that virtual objects do not really exist: there are not real *objects* corresponding to tables anywhere inside a computer. If one says this, though, one may be forced by parity into the view that tables do not truly exist in our quantum-mechanical world. If one adopts a restricted ontology of objects in one case, one should adopt it in the other; if one adopts a liberal ontology in one case, one should adopt it in the other. The only reasonable way to treat the cases differently is to adopt a sort of contextualism about what counts as an "object" (or about what falls within the domain of a quantifier such as 'everything'), depending on the context of the speaker. However, this will just reflect a parochial fact about our language rather than any deep fact about the world. In the deep respects, virtual objects are no less real than ordinary objects.[1]

Note 11: The Intrinsic Nature of Matter

The response to objection 8 is reminiscent of the familiar point, associated with Russell and Kant, that we do not know the intrinsic nature of entities in the external world (see the discussion of type-F monism in chapter 5). When it comes to physical entities, perception and science

---

1. *See my "Ontological Anti-realism" (2009) for more on these issues.

may tell us how these entities affect us and how they relate to each other, but these methods tell us little about what the fundamental physical entities are like in themselves. That is, these methods reveal the causal structure of the external world, but they leave its intrinsic nature open.

The Metaphysical Hypothesis is in part a hypothesis about what underlies this microphysical causal structure: microphysical entities are made of bits. The same goes for the Matrix Hypothesis. One might say that if we are in a matrix, the Kantian Ding-an-sich (thing in itself) is part of a computer-an-sich. This hypothesis supplements our ordinary conception of the external world, but it does not really contradict it, as this ordinary conception is silent on the world's intrinsic nature.[2]

Note 12: The Robustness of the Manifest Image

One general moral is that the "manifest image" is *robust*. Our ordinary conception of the macroscopic world is not easily falsified by discoveries in science and metaphysics. As long as the physical world contains processes with the right sort of causal and counterfactual structure, then it will be compatible with the manifest image. Even a computer simulation has the relevant causal and counterfactual structure, as does a process in the mind of God. This is why they can support a robust external reality despite their surprising nature.

This sort of flexibility in our conception of the world is closely tied to the semantic nonneutrality of many of our concepts. Those concepts such as *water*, *hair*, and *electron*, leave some flexibility in what their referent might turn out to be. We conceive of their referents roughly as whatever actual entity plays a certain causal role or has a certain appearance, while leaving open their intrinsic nature. One can likewise argue that the strongest constraints imposed by our conception of the world are plausibly those associated with semantically neutral concepts, which do not yield this sort of flexibility. These concepts plausibly include many of our causal and nomic concepts, as well as many of our mental concepts. In these cases, we have a sort of "direct" grasp of how the world must be in order to satisfy the concepts. If so, then our causal and mental beliefs impose strong constraints on the way the actual world must be.

One can argue that our most fundamental semantically neutral concepts are mental concepts (*experience*, *belief*), causal concepts (*cause*, *law*),

---

2. * *The Matrix* has been read as illustrating many philosophical ideas: Plato's cave, Descartes' skepticism, Berkeley's idealism, and so on. If I am correct, it might be seen more fundamentally as an illustration of Kantian humility.

logical and mathematical concepts (*and*, *two*), and categorical concepts (*object*, *property*). There are also many semantically neutral concepts that involve more than one of these elements: *friend*, *action*, and *computer* are examples. If this is right, then the fundamental constraints that our beliefs impose on the external world are that it contains relevant mental states (in ourselves and in others) and that it contains objects and properties that stand in relevant causal relations to each other and to the mental states. This sort of conception is weak enough that it can be satisfied by a matrix (at least if it is a multivat matrix or if computationalism about the mind is true).

In my opinion, this issue about the fundamental constraints that our beliefs impose on the world is the deepest philosophical issue that arises from thinking about the matrix. If what I have said in this chapter is right, it is precisely because these constraints are relatively weak that many hypotheses that one might have thought of as "skeptical" turn out to be compatible with our beliefs. In addition, it is this that enables us to produce some sort of response to the skeptical challenge. A little paradoxically, one might say that it is because we demand so little that we know so much.[3]

Note 13: Computation and Causal Structure

Why does a computer simulation of a world satisfy these constraints? The reason is tied to the nature of computation and implementation. Any formal computation can be regarded as giving a specification of (abstract) *causal structure*, specifying the precise manner of interaction between some set of formal states. To implement such a formal computation, the implementation must have concrete states that map directly onto these formal states, where the pattern of (causal and counterfactual) interaction between these states precisely mirrors the pattern of interaction between the formal states (see Chalmers 1994). So any two implementations of the computation will share a certain specific causal structure. A computational description of the physical world will be required to mirror its causal structure down to the level of

---

3. *These remarks about the manifest image need to be supplemented by what I say in the previous chapter. There are some demanding, semantically neutral concepts of the manifest image: the Edenic concepts of color, space, and so on. A matrix world does not meet the standard of these concepts, but neither, it seems likely, does our own post-Fall world. As I argue in the previous chapter, we do not hold the world to the demanding standard of these concepts in our ordinary thought and talk. Edenic concepts are demanding, but everyday non-Edenic concepts are robust.

fundamental objects and properties. So any implementation of this computation will embody this causal structure (in transitions between implementing states, whether these be voltages, circuits, or something quite different). So insofar as our conception of the external world imposes constraints on causal structure that a real physical world can satisfy, these constraints will also be satisfied by a computer simulation.

(This relates to a point made by Hubert Dreyfus and Stephen Dreyfus [2005]. Like me, the Dreyfuses take the view that most of the beliefs of the inhabitants of a matrix will be true, not false. However, the Dreyfuses suggest that many of their causal beliefs will be false: for example, their general belief that "a physical universe with causal powers makes things happen in our world," and perhaps their specific beliefs that germs cause disease, that the sun causes things to get warm, and so on. On my view, this suggestion is incorrect. On my view, the world of someone living in a matrix has real causation going on everywhere within it, grounded in the real causation going on in the computer. Virtual germs in the computer really do cause virtual disease in the computer, so when matrix inhabitants say, 'Germs cause disease,' what they say is true.)

Of course, the mental constraints also need to be satisfied. In particular, it is important that the causal structure stand in the right sort of relation to our experiences, but this constraint will also be satisfied when we are hooked up to a matrix. Constraints regarding other minds will be satisfied as long as we are in a multivat matrix or if computationalism about the mind is true. In this way, a matrix has everything that is required to satisfy the crucial causal and mental constraints on our conception of the world.

Note 14: Spatial Constraints

Perhaps the most important line of objection to the argument in this chapter argues that there are further constraints that our beliefs impose on the world that the Matrix Hypothesis does not satisfy.[4] One could argue that a mere match in mental and causal structure is not enough. Most obviously,

---

4. *Many further objections can be made to the claim that if we are in a Matrix, our beliefs are true. In my experience, the great majority can be handled by observing that analogous objections arise concerning either (i) a creation scenario, (ii) a Cartesian dualist scenario, (iii) a radical-physics scenario (e.g., involving quantum mechanics or cellular automata), or (iv) a Twin Earth scenario. An opponent could embrace the conclusion that the relevant scenario of types (i)–(iv) is itself a skeptical scenario, but this conclusion is usually unattractive and implausible.

one might argue that the world needs to have the right *spatial* properties, where we have some sort of direct grip on what spatial properties are (perhaps because spatial concepts are semantically neutral). In addition, one could suggest that the problem with the matrix is that its spatial properties are all wrong. We believe that external entities are arranged in a certain spatial pattern, but no such spatial pattern exists inside the computer.

In response, one can argue that these further constraints do not exist. It can be argued that spatial concepts are not semantically neutral but instead are subject to Twin Earth thought experiments. Here, as in the previous chapter, one can invoke Brad Thompson's thought experiments (2003) involving a Doubled Earth where 'one meter' refers to (what we call) two meters, an El Greco World where 'square' refers to (what we call) rectangles, and so on. On this view, our spatial concepts pick out whatever manifold of properties and relations in the external world is causally responsible for our corresponding manifold of spatial experiences. In this respect, spatial concepts are analogous to color concepts. Here we do not have any "direct" grip on the basic nature of spatial properties.[5] Instead, once again, the basic constraints are mental and causal.

This line of objection is tacitly engaged in section 6 of this chapter, where I suggest that if there is a computational level underlying physics, then any implementation of the relevant formal computation could serve in principle as a realization of that level without compromising physical reality. Perhaps opponents might deny that there could be a computational level underlying physics or at least might hold that there are constraints on what sort of implementation can serve. For example, they might hold that the implementing level itself must have an appropriate spatial arrangement.

This line of response runs counter to the spirit of contemporary physics, however. Physicists have seriously entertained the idea that space as we understand it is not fundamental and that there is an underlying level, not described in terms of ordinary spatial notions, from which space emerges. The cellular automaton hypothesis is just one such proposal. Here, what is crucial is simply a pattern of causal interaction. If physicists discover that this pattern is realized in turn by an entirely different sort of level with very different properties, they will not conclude that ordinary physical space does not exist. Rather, they will conclude that space is itself constituted by something nonspatial. This sort of discovery might be surprising and revisionary, but again it will be no

---

5. *As in the last chapter, one might suggest that we have a direct (semantically neutral) grip on Edenic spatial properties, but we do not have a direct grip on the ordinary spatial properties instantiated in our world. The same goes for temporal properties.

more so than quantum mechanics. Furthermore, as with quantum mechanics, we would almost certainly not regard it as a skeptical hypothesis about the macroscopic external world. If this is right, then our conception of the macroscopic world does not impose essentially spatial constraints on the fundamental level of reality.

Similar issues arise with respect to time. In one respect, time poses fewer problems than space, as the computer simulation in a matrix unfolds in time in the same temporal order as time in the simulated world. So one cannot object that the relevant temporal arrangements are not present in the matrix in the way that one could object that the relevant spatial arrangements are not present. So even if temporal concepts were semantically neutral, the Matrix Hypothesis could still vindicate our temporal beliefs. Still, one can make a case that our concept of external time is not semantically neutral (it is notable that physicists have entertained hypotheses on which temporal notions play no role at the fundamental level). Rather, it picks out the external manifold of properties and relations that is responsible for our corresponding manifold of temporal experiences. If so, then any computer simulation with the right causal structure and the right relation to our experience will vindicate our temporal beliefs regardless of its intrinsic temporal nature.

Note 15: Whither Skepticism?

The reasoning in this chapter does not offer a knockdown refutation of skepticism, because several skeptical hypotheses are left open. Still, it significantly strengthens one of the standard responses to skepticism. It is often held that although various skeptical hypotheses are compatible with our experiences, the hypothesis that there is a real physical world provides a simpler or better explanation of the regularities in our experiences than these skeptical hypotheses. If so, then, by an inference to the best explanation, we may be justified in believing in the real physical world.

At this point, it is often objected that some skeptical hypotheses seem just as simple as the standard explanation, for example, the hypothesis that all of our experiences are caused by a computer simulation or by God. If so, this response to skepticism fails. If I am right, however, these "equally simple" hypotheses are not skeptical hypotheses at all. If so, then inference to the best explanation may work after all, because all of these simple hypotheses yield mostly true beliefs about an external world.

The residual issue concerns the various remaining skeptical hypotheses on the table, such as the Recent Matrix Hypothesis, the Local

Matrix Hypothesis, and so on. It seems reasonable to hold that these hypotheses are significantly less simple than the earlier hypotheses, however. All of them involve a nonuniform explanation of the regularities in our experiences. In the Recent Matrix Hypothesis, present regularities and past regularities have very different explanations. In the Local Matrix Hypothesis, beliefs about matters close to home and about those far from home have very different explanations. These hypotheses as a whole have a sort of dual-mechanism structure that seems considerably more complex than the earlier uniform-mechanism structures. If this is right, one can argue that inference to the best explanation justifies us in ruling out these hypotheses and in accepting the earlier nonskeptical hypotheses.

Even if one thinks that some of these skeptical hypotheses offer reasonably good explanations of our experience, there is still a promising argument against global external-world skepticism in the vicinity. If I am right, all of these skeptical hypotheses are at worst *partial* skeptical hypotheses: if they are correct, then a good many of our empirical beliefs will still be true, and there will still be an external world. To obtain a *global* skeptical hypothesis, we have to go all the way to the Chaos Hypothesis, but this is a hypothesis on which the regularities in our experience have no explanation at all. Even an extremely weak version of inference to the best explanation justifies us in ruling out this sort of hypothesis. If so, then this sort of reasoning may justify our belief in the existence of the external world.[6]

6. *One might think of the antiskeptical strategy here as a combination of what is sometimes called the "abductive" response to skepticism (the scenarios that best explain our experiences are ones in which our beliefs are true) with the "externalist" response to skepticism (brains in vats have true beliefs because they refer to chemical/computational properties in their environments). For the reasons outlined in note 2, however, my arguments do not require any externalist presuppositions about reference and content. I think of the view more fundamentally as a "structuralist" response to skepticism: one according to which our relevant conception of the external world involves causal structure that is present even in the most putatively skeptical scenarios. I hope to develop this structuralism further in future work.

Part VI

THE UNITY OF CONSCIOUSNESS

14

WHAT IS THE UNITY OF CONSCIOUSNESS?

[with Tim Bayne]

1. Introduction

At any given time, a subject has a multiplicity of conscious experiences. A subject might simultaneously have visual experiences of a red book and a green tree, auditory experiences of birds singing, bodily sensations of a faint hunger and a sharp pain in the shoulder, the emotional experience of a certain melancholy, while having a stream of conscious thoughts about the nature of reality. These experiences are distinct from each other: a subject could experience the red book without the singing birds and the singing birds without the red book. But at the same time, the experiences seem to be tied together in a deep way. They seem to be *unified*, by being aspects of a single, encompassing state of consciousness.

This is a rough characterization of the unity of consciousness. There is some intuitive appeal to the idea that consciousness is unified and to the idea that it must be unified. But as soon as the issue is raised, a number of questions immediately arise.

(1) *What is the unity of consciousness?* What does it mean to say that different states of consciousness are unified with each other, or that they are part of a single, encompassing state? The idea of unity is multifaceted and has been understood in many different ways by different thinkers. In some senses of "unity," the claim that consciousness is unified may be obvious or trivial. In other senses, the claim may be obviously false. So the first project in this area is to distinguish between varieties of unity and to isolate those varieties that pose the most important questions.

(2) *Is consciousness necessarily unified?* Some thinkers (Descartes and Kant, for example) have argued that some sort of unity is a deep and essential feature of consciousness. On this view, the conscious states of a subject are necessarily unified: it is impossible for there to be a subject whose conscious states are disunified. On the other side, some thinkers (e.g., Nagel 1971) have argued that the unity of consciousness can break down. On this view, there are cases (especially neuropsychological cases, such as those involving patients with split brains) in which a subject's states of consciousness are disunified. Some (e.g., Dennett 1992) hold more strongly that consciousness is often or usually disunified and that much of the apparent unity of consciousness is an illusion.

(3) *How can the unity of consciousness be explained?* If consciousness really is unified and especially if it is necessarily unified, then it is natural to look for an explanation of this fact. What is it about consciousness that yields this unity? Is unity a primitive feature of consciousness, or is it explained by something deeper? Further, the unity of consciousness may put strong constraints on a theory of consciousness. If consciousness is necessarily unified, then a correct theory of consciousness should at least be compatible with this unity, and we can hope that it will explain it.

We can see these three questions as clustering around the status of what we can call the unity thesis (UT):

Unity thesis: Necessarily, any set of conscious states of a subject at a time is unified.

The first question raises the issue of how the notion of unity in the unity thesis is to be understood: what is it for a set of conscious states to be unified? The second question raises the issue of whether the unity thesis is true. The third question raises the issue of how, if the unity thesis is true, its truth might be explained.

In this chapter we address all three of these questions. Our central project is to isolate a notion of unity on which the unity thesis is both substantive and plausible. That is, we aim to find a more precise version of the unity thesis that is neither trivially true nor obviously false. With such a thesis in hand, we look at certain arguments that have been made *against* the unity of consciousness to determine whether they are good arguments against the unity thesis as we understand it. Finally, after fleshing out the unity thesis further, we apply the thesis to certain currently popular philosophical theories of consciousness, arguing that the thesis is incompatible with these theories: if the unity thesis is true, then these theories are false.

We do not aim to conclusively prove the unity thesis in this chapter, and indeed we are not certain that it is true. But we suggest at least that the thesis is plausible, that it captures a strong intuition about the nature of consciousness, and that there are no knockdown arguments against it. If the thesis is true, it is likely to have important consequences for a theory of consciousness.

2. Varieties of Unity

To start with, we need to distinguish different notions of unity. In particular, we will distinguish various ways in which different states of consciousness might be said to be unified.

Objectual unity. We can say that two states of consciousness are *objectually unified* when they are directed at the same object. For example, when I look at a red book, I have an experience of redness and an experience of rectangularity. The color experience and the shape experience here are unified in a particularly strong way. They are present in my consciousness as directed at a single entity: the book. The same goes for my experience of a blue car moving down the street. Here I experience color, shape, and motion, all of which are unified by being directed at the same object. I might even have an auditory experience of the car's engine and also experience this as directed at the same object. So there can be objectual unity across different sensory domains.

For two experiences to be objectually unified, their object need not actually exist. If I hallucinate a red book, then my experiences of redness and of rectangularity will be objectually unified despite the book's nonexistence. On the other side of the coin, two experiences can be experiences of the same object without being objectually unified. I might see a car's shape and hear its noise without anything in my conscious state tying the noise to the car (perhaps I perceive the noise as behind me due to an odd environmental effect). If so, the experiences are not objectually unified. For objectual unity, what matters is that two states are experienced *as* being directed at a common object.

The notion of objectual unity is closely tied to a central issue in cognitive psychology and neurophysiology. When I look at a red square, the color and the shape may be represented in different parts of my visual system, but somehow these separate pieces of information are brought together so that I experience a single red square, so that I can identify and report a red square and so on. This phenomenon is often referred to as *binding*, and the question of how it is achieved is often referred to as the *binding problem*.

The binding problem is in large part the problem of how objectual unity is possible. As we will see, this divides into two problems in turn.

Objectual unity is an important phenomenon, but it will not be central for our purposes. Where objectual unity is concerned, the corresponding unity thesis is almost certainly false. While some sets of experiences are objectually unified with each other, it seems that most sets are not. For example, my experience of the color of the book and of the shape of the car are not objectually unified: they are experienced as being directed at *different* objects. My experiences of a bird singing and of a sharp pain do not seem to be directed at the same object at all. If so, then objectual unity cannot unify all of a subject's conscious states. For such a notion of unity, we must look elsewhere.

Spatial unity. A related notion of unity is that of *spatial unity.* We can say that two conscious states are *spatially unified* when they represent objects as being part of the same space. For example, my experiences of a book and of a car are not directed at a common object, but they represent both objects as part of the same visual space. More generally, all of my visual experiences seem to be spatially unified in this way: every visual experience represents something spatially, and everything that is represented is represented as part of a common space. Auditory experiences usually represent objects as part of the same space; such auditory experiences are spatially unified with visual experiences.

The notion of being "represented as part of the same space" can be fleshed out in various ways, but the crucial idea will be something like the following. A set of experiences is spatially unified if (i) each experience has spatial representational content and (ii) the representational content of each is *comparable* in the sense that the objects represented are represented as being in spatial relations to each other. So visual experience might represent a car as being near a tree, behind a truck, or to the left of a building. Auditory experience might represent exhaust noise as coming from the same area as the car, or it might represent a siren as being much farther away. This sort of comparability is endemic to much perceptual experience, and makes for a deep spatial unity in perception.

Like objectual unity, however, spatial unity does not yield a plausible version of the unity thesis. Some experiences seem to have no spatial representational content at all. An emotional experience such as that of melancholy does not obviously represent anything as located within space. A conscious thought about philosophy might have no spatial content at all. If so, these conscious states are not spatially unified with other conscious states. As before, to find a notion of unity that unifies all of a subject's conscious states, we must look elsewhere.

Subject unity. Let us say that two conscious states are *subject unified* when they are had by the same subject at the same time. So all of my current experiences—my perceptual experiences, my bodily sensations, my emotional experiences and conscious thoughts—are subject unified simply because they are all *my* experiences.

If we construe the unity thesis as involving subject unity, the thesis is certainly plausible. If a set of conscious states is had by a subject at a time, then the states will be subject unified by definition. The trouble with this version of the unity thesis is that it is *trivial*. It is true by definition and tells us nothing substantive about consciousness. As such, it cannot capture the intuition that there is some nontrivial way in which consciousness is unified. So subject unity will not be our central focus here.

Still, the notion of subject unity is at least useful in articulating the unity thesis. As it was characterized earlier, the unity thesis holds that if a set of experiences of a subject at a time is subject unified, then that set is unified. So in effect, the unity thesis states that subject unity entails unity. Now we simply need to find a notion of unity for which this entailment is both plausible and nontrivial.

Subsumptive unity. We started the chapter by invoking the intuition that there is some substantial sense in which *all* of a subject's experiences—including at least perceptual, bodily, emotional, and cognitive experiences—are unified. This sense is not object or spatial unity since these notions do not apply to all of the relevant experiences. And this sense is not subject unity since the resulting unity holds trivially. Rather, it involves the idea that these experiences are somehow subsumed within a single state of consciousness.

We can say that two conscious states are *subsumptively unified* when they are both subsumed by a single state of consciousness. The notion of one state being subsumed by another should be taken as intuitive for now; we will spell it out shortly. To take an example, it seems plausible that all of my visual experiences are subsumed by a single encompassing state of consciousness corresponding to my visual field. More generally, my visual and auditory experiences might all be subsumed by a single encompassing state of perceptual consciousness. And it does not seem unreasonable to suppose that there is a single encompassing state of consciousness that subsumes all of my experiences: perceptual, bodily, emotional, cognitive, and any others.

We can think of this last encompassing state of consciousness for a given subject as the subject's *total* conscious state. When it exists, a subject's total conscious state might be thought of as the subject's conscious *field*. It can be thought of as involving at least a conjunction of each of many more specific conscious states: states of perceptual experience, bodily experience, emotional experience, and so on. However, what is important, on the unity thesis, is that this total state is not *just* a conjunction of conscious states but also a conscious state in its own right. If such a total conscious state exists, it can serve as the "singularity behind the multiplicity"—the single state of consciousness in which all of a subject's states of consciousness are subsumed.[1]

It is worth pointing out certain sorts of unity with which subsumptive unity should not be confused. We are not talking about *gestalt unity*, where the conscious experiences of two different objects are deeply related in a way that transforms each of the experiences and produces a "gestalt" experience with a novel content. We are also not talking about *normative* unity, which requires some special coherence or consistency among multiple contents of consciousness. As we have characterized subsumptive unity, two conscious states might be subsumptively unified whether or not their contents stand in a special gestalt relation to each other and whether or not they are especially consistent or coherent with one another. We are also not dealing with *neurophysiological unity*, which requires that conscious states involve a single area or mechanism in the brain. Finally, we are not dealing with *diachronic unity*, or the unity of consciousness across time. It might turn out that one or more of these notions is deeply related to the issues at hand, but none of them is our primary object of discussion.

To spell out the notion of subsumptive unity, we need to go into more detail about just what consciousness involves and just what is involved in the idea of one conscious state being subsumed by another. This requires making some further distinctions.

3. Access Unity and Phenomenal Unity

What is it for a mental state to be a conscious state? There is no single answer to this question. As many have pointed out, the notion of "consciousness" is

---

1. *Since this chapter was first published, Michael Tye (2003b) has put forward a view on which the only experiences are total experiences and on which there are no nontotal experiences. This seemingly radical claim appears to turn either on a verbal issue about what counts as an experience or on a hard-to-motivate metaphysical thesis. Certainly, if experiences are understood as phenomenal states (that is, instances of phenomenal properties), as in the next section, there is little objection to nontotal experiences. I think that any explanatory work done by Tye's view can be done better by the view (discussed late in this chapter) that total states are the *fundamental* phenomenal states and that nontotal states derive from these. This view stands to Tye's view roughly as "priority monism" (the view in metaphysics that the universe as a whole is more fundamental than its parts; see Schaffer 2010) stands to "existence monism" (the view that only the universe exists).

ambiguous and is understood in different ways by different people, so to make progress we have to draw distinctions. For our purposes, the most useful distinction is Ned Block's distinction between access consciousness and phenomenal consciousness (Block 1995).

A mental state is *access conscious* when a subject has a certain sort of access to the content of the state. More precisely, a state is access conscious if, by virtue of having the state, the content of the state is available for verbal report, for rational inference, and for the deliberate control of behavior. When I look at a red book, I can report the presence of the book ("there's a red book"), I can reason about it (e.g., concluding that I must have put it there when reading yesterday), and I can use its presence in deliberately directing my behavior (e.g., picking up the book and putting it back on the shelf). So my perception of the red book gives me the relevant sort of access to information about the red book. My perceptual state here is access conscious One can also say that in such a case, the subject is access conscious of the relevant object. So here, I am access conscious of the red book.

In a similar way, many of my perceptual states are access conscious, and so are many of my emotional and cognitive states. Not all mental states are access conscious, however. In some cases, such as those involving subliminal perception, blindsight, or unconscious belief, a mental state represents information without that information being reportable or usable in reasoning and in rational control of behavior. The exact definition of access consciousness is somewhat flexible and can be varied for different purposes. The most important point is that a state's being access conscious is defined in terms of the causal role that the state plays within the cognitive system and in particular in terms of the role that the state plays in making information available to other parts of the system.

A mental state is *phenomenally conscious* when there is something it is like to be in that state. When a state is phenomenally conscious, being in that state involves some sort of subjective experience. There is something it is like for me to see the red book—I have a visual experience of the book—so my perception of the book is phenomenally conscious. There is something it is like to hear the bird singing and to feel the pain in my shoulder, so these states are phenomenally conscious. There is something it is like to feel melancholy, and there is arguably something it is like when I think about philosophy. If so, then these states are phenomenally conscious. Phenomenal consciousness is often taken to be the most important sort of consciousness and to be the sort of consciousness that poses the most difficulty for scientific explanation.

There is a close empirical connection between phenomenal consciousness and access consciousness. It is arguable that the two almost always go together empirically: when a state is phenomenally conscious, it is access conscious, and vice versa. That is, when there is something it is like to be in a state, a subject can usually report the contents of the state and use it to directly guide reasoning and behavior. And when a subject can report the contents of a state and use it to directly guide reasoning and behavior, there is usually something it is like to be in that state. So when I am phenomenally conscious of the red book, I am access conscious of it, and vice versa.

Despite this empirical connection, there is plausibly a *conceptual* distinction between access consciousness and phenomenal consciousness. Access consciousness is defined in terms of the causal role that a state plays, whereas phenomenal consciousness is defined in terms of the way the state feels. It is arguable that we can at least *imagine* states that are access conscious without corresponding states of phenomenal consciousness (the philosophers' zombie, which is functionally like a normal human being but without any conscious experience, is one such imaginary case). And it seems that we can know about another being's states of access consciousness without knowing about their states of phenomenal consciousness: one might know what information is available for report and for behavioral control in a cognitive system without being in a position to know what it is like to be that system.

When there is something it is like to have a mental state, we can say that the mental state has a phenomenology, or a phenomenal character. Slightly more formally, we can say that such mental states have *phenomenal properties*, or *qualia*, which characterize what it is like to be in them. We can also say that *subjects* have phenomenal properties, characterizing aspects of what it is like to be a subject at a given time. We can then say that a phenomenal state is an instantiation of such a property. For example, the state of experiencing a certain sort of reddish quality is a phenomenal state.

When a subject is in a phenomenally conscious mental state, the subject will thereby be in a phenomenal state that reflects the phenomenology of being in the mental state. For example, if there is something it is like for a given subject to believe that Paris is in France, the subject will be in a corresponding phenomenal state. But the phenomenally conscious mental state (the state of believing that Paris is in France) and the phenomenal state may be distinct states, in that it may be possible to believe that Paris is in France while having a different phenomenology or no phenomenology at all. If so, the belief state is a phenomenally conscious mental state, but it is not a phenomenal state. There is a special class of phenomenally conscious mental states such that the mental state and the corresponding phenomenal states are identical: phenomenal states themselves. Phenomenal states are at the core of phenomenal consciousness.

We can use the distinction between access consciousness and phenomenal consciousness to make a distinction between two corresponding notions of unity: access unity and phenomenal unity. Broadly speaking, two conscious states are *access unified* when they are jointly accessible: that is, when the subject has access to the contents of both states at once. Two conscious states are *phenomenally unified* when they are jointly experienced: when there is something it is like to be in both states at once.

We can construct more precise versions of phenomenal and access unity by combining these distinctions with the distinctions outlined earlier between objectual unity, spatial unity, and field unity. These distinctions cross-classify each other, so that one can isolate notions of objectual phenomenal unity, objectual access unity, spatial access unity, subsumptive phenomenal unity, and so on. The distinction between phenomenal and access unity applies less clearly to the notion of subject unity, so we set that notion aside here.

We can say that two conscious states are *objectually access unified* when their contents involve attributing properties to a single object of representation and these contents are jointly accessible within the system. The contents will be jointly accessible when their *conjunction* is available for report, reasoning, and the rational control of behavior. When I am conscious of a red square, I can report the presence of red and the presence of a square, but I can also report the presence of a red square. Similarly, the presence of a red square can be used in guiding my reasoning and my behavior. So my perception of red and my perception of a square are not just individually access conscious: they are also access unified.

We can say that two conscious states are *objectually phenomenally unified* when they are experienced as representing a single object. When I am conscious of a red square, I experience the presence of red and I experience the presence of a square, but I also experience the presence of a red square. There is a distinctive sort of unity involved in what it is like to experience the redness and the squareness simultaneously here. The two states are unified by being experienced as aspects of a single object.

Objectual access unity and objectual phenomenal unity correspond to two distinct aspects of the binding problem. It has often been pointed out that there are actually two binding problems (see e.g., Revonsuo 1999). The first is that of how a system such as the brain manages to bring together two separately represented pieces of information (e.g., representations of color and shape in different areas of the visual cortex), so that these can play a joint role in the control of behavior (e.g., so that we can report the presence of a red square and a blue circle rather than a red circle and a blue square). This is a sort of engineering problem concerning the design of the cognitive system; one can think of it as the neurophysiological or cognitive binding problem. This binding problem is the problem of explaining objectual access unity. The second binding problem is that of explaining how it is that we perceptually experience separate pieces of information as bound together in pertaining to the same object. This is the problem of explaining objectual phenomenal unity. On the face of it, these two problems are distinct. One could solve the neurophysiological binding problem, giving an explanation of how two pieces of information are brought together in the brain to be jointly accessible while still having no explanation of why the jointly accessible information should be experienced. So objectual phenomenal unity and objectual access unity are at least conceptually distinct.

One can make a similar distinction between spatial phenomenal unity and spatial access unity. We can say that two conscious states are spatially access unified when they have spatial representational contents that can be jointly accessed by the cognitive system, so that they can be spatially compared and the results of the comparison can be made available for report, reasoning, and behavioral control. For example, when I see a car and a tree, I do not just have access to their spatial locations individually; I also have access to the spatial locations jointly, in that I can report that the car is to the left of the tree. So these two perceptual states are spatially access unified. Two conscious states are spatially phenomenally unified when they involve experiencing entities as part of the same space—as part of the same phenomenal space, one might say. I experience the car as being in the same space as the tree and to the left of it, so these two states are spatially phenomenally unified.

The most important distinction is that between subsumptive phenomenal unity and subsumptive access unity. These notions apply to two arbitrary conscious states as long as they are phenomenally conscious in the first instance and access conscious in the second. Because these are the most important versions of unity, we henceforth usually speak simply of "phenomenal unity" and "access unity," where it is understood that we are referring to subsumptive phenomenal unity and subsumptive access unity, respectively.

Two conscious states are *subsumptively access unified* (or simply *access unified*) if the *conjunction* of their contents is available for verbal report, reasoning, and the deliberate control of behavior. So if mental state A has content p and mental state B has content q, these states will be individually access conscious if the information that p is available for report and control and the information that q is available for report and control. They will be *jointly* access conscious, or they will be access unified, if the information that $p\&q$ is available for report and control. More briefly, two states A and B are access unified if and only if the subject is access conscious of the conjunction of their contents. In this case, there is an access-conscious mental state with the conjunctive content. This conjunctive mental state can be seen as subsuming the original states A and B.

For example, when I see a book and feel a pain, I can report the presence of the book and the pain individually, but I can do more than that: I can report them jointly. I can also reason about the book and the pain jointly and use information about both to jointly control my behavior (e.g., looking in the book for a remedy for the pain or ceasing to read the book to help alleviate the pain). Because of the accessibility of this conjunctive content, the two states are (subsumptively) access unified. Similarly, I can often jointly report or reason about an emotion and a sound: if so, the emotional state and the auditory state are access unified.

It is worth noting that for a state to be access conscious, it is not required that the content of the state is actually *accessed* in the sense that it is directly used for report or control. What matters is that it is *accessible* in a certain direct sense: that it be "poised" for use, as Block puts it. The same goes for access unity. For two states to be access unified, they need not be jointly accessed at any given moment. What matters is that they are jointly accessible in that it would be possible for a subject to jointly report them and to use them jointly in reasoning and behavior control. Typically, our conscious states are not jointly accessed, but they are much more often jointly accessible. It is joint accessibility that matters for our notion of unity.

We can use the notion of access unity to put forward a version of the unity thesis:

Access unity thesis: Necessarily, any set of access conscious states of a subject at a time is access unified.

This thesis appeals to the notion of a set of states being access unified. This is a natural generalization of the notion of two states being access unified. We can say that a set of states is access unified if the contents of all of the states are jointly accessible.

It might be objected that in requiring that *any* set of a subject's access-conscious states be access unified, the thesis is highly implausible. A subject might have a large (possibly infinite) number of access conscious states, and the conjunction of the contents of these states might be so complex that it is implausible that a subject could have access to this conjunction. The full conjunction would not be reportable or directly available to guide reasoning and behavior. To get around this, we could put forward a slightly weakened version of the thesis:

Pairwise access unity thesis: Necessarily, any two access conscious states of a subject at a time are access unified.

One might argue that the pairwise version is too weak to count as a full unity thesis (which requires unity of all states at a time) or that it suffers from the same problems as the full unity thesis (since it entails that conjunctions of conjunctions will be access conscious and so on). However, none of this matters here since as we argue in the next section, even a weak version of the access unity thesis, limited to pairwise unity of relatively simple access conscious states, is straightforwardly false.

We can say that two conscious states are *subsumptively phenomenally unified* (or simply *phenomenally unified*) if there is something it is like for a subject to be in both states simultaneously. That is, two states are phenomenally unified when they have a *conjoint phenomenology*: a phenomenology of having both states at once that subsumes the phenomenology of the individual states. When A and B are phenomenally conscious states, there is something it is like for a subject to have A, and there is something it is like for a subject to have B. When A and B are phenomenally unified, there is not just something it is like to have each state individually: there is something it is like to have A and B together. Here the phenomenology of being in A and B together will carry with it the phenomenology of being in A and the phenomenology of being in B.

For example, when I look at a book while feeling a pain, there is something it is like to see the book (yielding a phenomenal state A), and there is something it is like to feel the pain (yielding a phenomenal state B), but there is more than this: there is something it is like to see the book while feeling the pain. Here there is a sort of conjoint phenomenology that carries with it the phenomenology of seeing the book and the phenomenology of feeling the pain. As in the discussion of field unity, we can think of the conjoint state here as involving at least the conjunction $A\&B$ of the original phenomenal states A and B. But importantly, the conjoint state is itself a phenomenal state: a single complex state of consciousness that subsumes the individual states of consciousness A and B. It is this encompassing state of consciousness that unifies A and B.

More generally, a *set* of conscious states is phenomenally unified if there is something it is like for a subject to have all the members of the set at once and if this phenomenology subsumes that of the individual states. As a special case, we can say that the set consisting of all of a subject's conscious states at a given time is phenomenally unified if there is something it is like for the subject to have all of these states at once, where this phenomenology subsumes the phenomenology of the individual states. If so, then the subject has a *total phenomenal state* that encompasses all of the subject's phenomenal states. One can think of a total phenomenal state as capturing what it is like to be a subject at a time. If a subject has a total phenomenal state, there is a clear sense in which all of a subject's phenomenal states are unified within it.

We can put forward a phenomenal version of the unity thesis as follows:

> **Phenomenal unity thesis:** Necessarily, any set of phenomenal states of a subject at a time is phenomenally unified.

This is not quite the same as the thesis that any set of *phenomenally conscious mental states* of a subject at a time is phenomenally unified, but the two theses are clearly equivalent. The first version (regarding phenomenally conscious mental states) entails the second version (regarding phenomenal states) as a special case. In reverse, the second version entails that for any set of phenomenally conscious mental states, their associated phenomenal states will be phenomenally unified. So there will be a phenomenal state that subsumes each of the original phenomenal states. So there will be something it is like to be in all the original mental states simultaneously that subsumes what it is like to be in them individually. It follows that the original mental states will be phenomenally unified.

One can also put forward slightly weaker versions of the phenomenal unity thesis:

> **Pairwise phenomenal unity thesis:** Necessarily, any two phenomenal states of a subject at a time are phenomenally unified.

> **Total phenomenal unity thesis:** Necessarily, the set of all phenomenal states of a subject at a time is phenomenally unified.

The original phenomenal unity thesis clearly entails the pairwise unity thesis and the total unity thesis. The pairwise thesis does not obviously entail the first version. It is plausible that subsumption is transitive, so that, necessarily, if A subsumes B and B subsumes C, then A subsumes C. If so, the pairwise unity thesis will entail the phenomenal unity thesis for any finite set of phenomenal states, as any pair of these will be subsumed by a single phenomenal state, and any pair of those in turn will be subsumed by a single phenomenal state, and so on. But the pairwise thesis does not obviously entail the original thesis where infinite sets of phenomenal states are concerned. The total unity thesis entails the original phenomenal unity thesis, however.

If there is a state that subsumes each phenomenal state of the subject, that state will also subsume each member of an arbitrary set of phenomenal states of the subject, so that set will be phenomenally unified. So the total unity thesis and the original phenomenal unity thesis are equivalent.[2]

The total unity thesis arguably captures the central intuition behind the unity of consciousness. This thesis suggests that there is always a single phenomenal state that subsumes all of the phenomenal states of a subject at a time. That is, it suggests that any conscious subject at any time has a total phenomenal state. If a subject has a total phenomenal state, subsuming every specific phenomenal state of the subject, then the subject's consciousness will be unified in a deep way.

It might be objected that when a subject experiences a number of phenomenal states at once, the original phenomenal states will be transformed. For example, it might be phenomenally different to see a red book in the context of a moving car than to see a red book on its own, and the phenomenal state that was present when one saw the book on its own might not be present at all. This may be so, but it is no objection to the unity thesis. The unity thesis says that the phenomenal states had by a subject *at a time* are subsumed by a complex phenomenal state. So the experience of a red book and a moving car at a given time should subsume the experience of the red book at that time and the experience of the moving car at that time. It is not required that the complex experience should subsume the experience of a red book as the subject might have it at a different time and in a different context. If the experience of the book is itself transformed by the context of the car, then it is the transformed experience that will be subsumed by the complex state.

It might also be objected that these unity theses are *trivial.* If a subject has a set of phenomenal states, there will automatically be a phenomenal state that subsumes them: the conjunction of the original states. But this is not a trivial claim. It is trivial that if a subject is in a number of phenomenal states, the subject will be in the conjunction of those states. However, it is nontrivial that this conjunction will itself be, or be subsumed by, a phenomenal state. That is, it is nontrivial that there will be *something it is like* to be in the conjunctive state. This can be seen from the fact that some philosophers deny the total unity thesis, or at least entertain its denial. For example, when Hurley (1998) discusses the possibility that the unity of consciousness could break down and that consciousness could be "partially

---

2. *Strictly speaking, the total phenomenal unity thesis entails that every set of phenomenal states is subsumed by some state, but (for reasons discussed on pp. 519 and 526) it does not entail that there is a phenomenal state corresponding precisely to their conjoint phenomenology, as the original phenomenal unity thesis arguably requires. Thanks to Ole Koksvik for discussion here.

unified" (so that two phenomenal states are each unified with a third state but not with each other), she says:

> Therefore, we cannot imagine what it is like for there to be partial unity. That doesn't show [that] partial unity is unintelligible, because being partially unified isn't the sort of thing there *could be* anything it is like to be. We shouldn't expect to be able to imagine what it is like. (Hurley 1998, 165)

In general, it seems that a case in which the unity of consciousness breaks down would be precisely a case in which there is no total phenomenal state of the subject. That is, there is nothing it is like to be the subject at that time, or at least there is no single something-it-is-like that captures all the phenomenal states of the subject. Such a subject would have states with a local phenomenal character, but there would be no global phenomenal character involved in having these states. It is certainly very hard to see how this could be the case. Indeed, one might suspect (as we do) that such a scenario is impossible and perhaps incoherent. But to say this is not to say that the unity thesis is trivial: it is a substantive thesis about the nature of consciousness. This is reflected by the fact that (as we discuss later in the chapter) certain theories of consciousness entail that the unity thesis is false. If so, then the thesis puts substantive constraints on a theory of consciousness.

4. When Access Unity Breaks Down

The access unity thesis holds that necessarily, any two access-conscious states are access unified. This entails that whenever a subject is access conscious of p and is access conscious of q, the subject will be access conscious of $p\&q$. This thesis is clearly false.

To see that the thesis is false, we need a case in which a subject is access conscious of p and access conscious of q without being access conscious of $p\&q$. For this to happen, it should be the case that p is reportable and available for guiding reasoning and behavior and that q is reportable and available for guiding reasoning and behavior but that $p\&q$ is not reportable and not available for guiding reasoning and behavior. This can happen in a quite straightforward way. All that is required is that there be an *access bottleneck*. This will be a pathway of information access through which only a limited amount of information can pass at one time. If p and q are both accessible only through the bottleneck, and if each carries an amount of information that is near the capacity of the bottleneck, then p and q will be individually accessible, but the conjunctive content $p\&q$ will not.

This is not merely a description of an imaginary case. Such access bottlenecks can occur in real cognitive systems and are revealed by a number of experiments in the psychological literature. Perhaps the clearest example of such a bottleneck is given by a famous experiment by George Sperling (1960). In Sperling's experiment, a subject is presented with a matrix consisting of three rows with four letters each. The matrix is flashed only briefly, for 250 milliseconds. After the matrix vanishes, a tone sounds, indicating whether the subject is to report the contents of the first, second, or third row. When subjects are required to report the contents of the top row, on average they correctly report 3.3 of the four letters in that row. The same occurs when they are required to report the contents of the middle or the bottom row. But when subjects are asked to report the contents of the entire matrix, on average they correctly report 4.5 of the twelve letters. So, to simplify a little, it seems that the subject has access to the information in any single row, but the subject does not have joint access to the information in all three rows.

In this case, it is natural to hold that the subject (just after the matrix disappears, before the tone sounds) is access conscious of the contents of any individual row. Recalling that access consciousness requires accessibility for report and for reasoning and behavior, the contents of each row are available for report (individually) and could presumably be used to guide both reasoning about those contents and behavior. But it also seems that the subject is not access conscious of the conjunctive contents of the whole matrix or of any two rows. The conjunctive contents of more than one row are not available for verbal report and presumably are not available to guide reasoning and behavior. If so, then a subject can be access conscious of p (one row) and of q (another row) without being access conscious of $p\&q$ (both rows). So two access-conscious states of a subject at a time can fail to be access unified, and the access unity thesis is false.

We do not claim that the Sperling experiment alone *proves* that the access unity thesis is false. There are other possible interpretations of the experiment. For example, one could hold that the subject has some sort of internal access to the conjunctive content but that the process of report destroys this access. However, the interpretation we have suggested is a natural one. On the face of it, the conjunctive content does not seem to be available for any sort of reasoning or control, although the individual contents are available taken singly. And importantly, whether or not this interpretation is correct of the actual case, it seems to be a perfectly coherent interpretation that describes a perfectly reasonable way for a cognitive system to function.

Indeed, given a natural design for cognitive systems with limited resources, we would expect certain restrictions on the flow of information in access and control, and we would expect access bottlenecks to arise in some cases. It may be that most of the time, when a subject has access to p and to q, the subject has access to $p\&q$. But this sort of joint access clearly cannot hold *necessarily.* So even if there is a reasonably high degree of access unity in ordinary conscious states, this sort of access unity cannot hold across the board.

This breakdown of access unity does not entail a breakdown of phenomenal unity. This can be seen by examining the Sperling case. It is difficult to know exactly what is going on in the phenomenology of the subject who is undergoing the Sperling experiment before being asked about the contents of a row. Perhaps the details of all nine letters are present in the subject's phenomenology (as some subjects report); perhaps these details are not present, and there is merely an indeterminate patch in each cell of the matrix; or perhaps there is something in between. Still, whatever the exact phenomenology here, there is little reason to suppose that phenomenal unity breaks down.

No matter what it is like for a subject to experience each individual cell of the matrix in the Sperling case, it is plausible that there will be something it is like for the subject to see the entire matrix. It is also plausible that the phenomenology of seeing the matrix will subsume the phenomenology of seeing the individual cells. If the phenomenology of seeing a cell involves just a hazy patch, then the phenomenology of seeing the matrix will plausibly involve nine hazy patches. If the phenomenology of seeing a cell involves a detailed shape, then the phenomenology of seeing the matrix will plausibly involve nine detailed shapes. Either way, the individual phenomenal states are subsumed by the overall phenomenal state, so there is no reason to deny phenomenal unity here.

At most, this sort of case suggests that a subject does not always have simultaneous access to the contents of all of the subject's phenomenal states. If the subject is indeed experiencing the details of all nine letters, then the subject is in a position where the contents of these experiences can be accessed and reported only a few at a time and not all at the same time. There is nothing paradoxical or contradictory about this. It simply suggests that a subject's access to a total phenomenal state is sometimes piecemeal. But this is just what we might expect.

One consequence of this is that access consciousness and phenomenal consciousness can come apart. We have seen that the subject is access conscious of the individual letters but not of their conjunction. It is also natural to hold that either (i) the subject is phenomenally conscious of neither the individual letters nor their conjunctions, or (ii) the subject is phenomenally conscious of both the individual letters and their conjunction. In case (i), a subject is access conscious of an individual letter but not phenomenally conscious of it. In case (ii), a subject is phenomenally conscious of the conjunction but not access conscious of it. Either way, access consciousness and phenomenal consciousness of a given content can come apart. Our own view is that description (ii) is somewhat more plausible. If this is so, we can still hold that access consciousness and phenomenal consciousness are correlated with each other for *simple* contents. But access consciousness and phenomenal consciousness will not always be correlated for *complex* contents.

The moral of all this is that a breakdown of access unity does not entail a breakdown in phenomenal unity. There is a sense in which a breakdown of access unity is a "disunity" in consciousness, but it is a relatively shallow sense. Such a breakdown is quite compatible with an underlying phenomenal unity. Of course, we have not demonstrated that no breakdowns of access unity involve a breakdown of phenomenal unity, but this discussion does strongly suggest that one cannot *infer* a breakdown of phenomenal unity from a breakdown in access unity. To accept a breakdown of phenomenal unity, one would need a quite distinct reason.

An opponent might try to argue that the Sperling case is a case where phenomenal unity breaks down. For example, the opponent might argue that the phenomenology of seeing each individual cell involves a detailed letter but that the phenomenology of seeing the whole matrix does not and that any "global" phenomenology here involves only hazy patches. Such a response would seem unmotivated and implausible on the face of it, at least in the absence of much supporting argument. If the phenomenology of each letter is detailed, then there seems to be good reason to hold that this phenomenology is present in a global phenomenal state. And even if it is *coherent* for an opponent to hold this, it is equally coherent (and seemingly more plausible) to deny this and to hold that the experience of the letters is phenomenally unified. The mere coherence of the denial is enough to show that one cannot *infer* a breakdown in phenomenal unity from a breakdown of access unity.

5. Can Phenomenal Unity Break Down?

We think that there is a strong prima facie case that the unity thesis is true. This prima facie case is brought out by the fact that there seems to be something *inconceivable* about phenomenal disunity. It is difficult or impossible to imagine a subject having two phenomenal states simultaneously without there being a conjoint phenomenology for both states. And there is a sense that something about the suggestion is incoherent. This prima facie inconceivability—whether it takes the form of unimaginability or apparent incoherence—gives at least some reason to believe that cases in which phenomenal unity break down are impossible, so that the unity thesis is true.

But this is only a prima facie case. There are some possible scenarios that humans cannot imagine, and there are arguably some possible scenarios that no being could imagine. In addition, the judgment of incoherence in this case is not so strong that it could not be incorrect. So the prima facie case for the unity thesis needs to be balanced with the case *against* the unity thesis. A number of philosophers and scientists have argued that the unity of consciousness can break down. So to assess the unity thesis, one needs to examine these arguments in order to see what force they have against the unity thesis as we have understood it.

By far the most common reason for holding that the unity of consciousness can break down is grounded in neuropsychology. It is widely held that patients in various unusual neuropsychological states have a disunified consciousness. The paradigm case here is that of a *split-brain* patient, whose corpus callosum has been severed for medical purposes, preventing the left and right hemispheres of the cerebral cortex from communicating directly (although there is still some connection through lower areas of the brain). Such patients behaves in a surprisingly normal fashion much of the time, but in certain circumstances they behave quite unusually. For example, when presented with different pictures in different halves of their visual field (e.g., a cat on the left and a dog on the right) and asked to report the contents, the patient will report seeing only a dog, since the left hemisphere, which dominates speech, receives input from the right visual field. When asked to write down what she sees with her left hand (is controlled by the right hemisphere), such a patient may slowly write "CAT"; with the right hand, she may write "DOG." If patient writes with her left hand on a paper visible in her right visual field, a conflict may occur when she sees what is written. In some cases, the right hand scratches out what the left hand has written.

It is often held that in cases like this, consciousness is disunified. On one interpretation (e.g., Puccetti 1981), there are two distinct subjects of consciousness, one corresponding to each hemisphere. Such an interpretation is actually compatible with the unity thesis, since the unity thesis requires only that every subject have a unified consciousness. More threatening to the unity thesis are interpretations on which there is a single subject with a disunified consciousness. Some (e.g., Marks 1980) hold that the subject has two separate streams of consciousness, at least under experimental conditions. Others (e.g., Lockwood 1989) hold that the subject has a fragmented consciousness with nontransitive unity between the states: for example, the experiences of "CAT" and of "DOG" might each be unified with some background emotional state but not with each other. Others (e.g., Nagel 1971) hold that our conceptual framework in speaking of subjects may simply break down in this area.

Adjudicating this question requires a very detailed examination of both the empirical details and the philosophical analysis of these phenomena, which we cannot provide here. Here, we will simply note that given what we have said so far in this chapter, the advocate of the phenomenal unity thesis has a natural line of response.

It is plausible that in split-brain cases, there is some sort of breakdown of *access* unity. If we assume that there is a single subject, then it seems that the subject in the preceding case has at least a weak sort of access both to the presence of a cat and to the presence of a dog and can use each in reasoning and in the control of behavior. But it seems that the subject has no access to a conjunctive content involving both the cat and the dog. The conjunctive content is not reported and plays no apparent role in reasoning and in the control of behavior. So this may well be a case in which access unity fails. In this case, it seems that two accessed contents are not jointly accessible because of a disconnection between the relevant access mechanisms.

But as we have seen, a breakdown of access unity does not entail a breakdown of phenomenal unity. So the possibility remains open that split-brain subjects have a unified phenomenal field, with some sort of conjoint phenomenology subsuming each of the separate contents. It is just that the subject has pathologies of access, so that the contents of the field are accessible only singly and not jointly. If so, the subject in the experiment described has a phenomenal field that includes experiences of both a cat and a dog. The subject simply has no conjoint access to these contents. Of course, this implies that the subject has highly imperfect knowledge of her conscious states. She will believe (in both "halves" of the brain) that she is experiencing only one image of an animal when in fact she is experiencing two. Still, it is plausible for many other reasons that knowledge of consciousness is fallible, and it is not unreasonable to suppose that in cases of brain damage, this fallibility might be quite striking.

Nothing here proves that this interpretation is correct. It does suggest, however, that we should not be too quick to conclude that these cases involve a breakdown of phenomenal unity. Most of those who have discussed these cases have not carefully distinguished the relevant notions of unity and consciousness (an exception is Marcel 1994, who distinguishes "reflexive consciousness" from "phenomenal experience" and argues that the disunity concerns the former) and have often discussed things in terms of access and related functional notions. Once we distinguish access unity from phenomenal unity, it becomes clear that the direct evidence concerns access disunity, not phenomenal disunity. To establish phenomenal disunity requires substantial further argument. It may be that such arguments can be given, but the case is far from clear.

One might say something similar about other disorders of consciousness, such as dissociative identity disorder (multiple personality disorder). In this case, it seems that there are pathologies of access between different parts of a cognitive system. But it seems quite tenable to hold that there is nevertheless a single field of consciousness at any given time, subsuming the conscious states of the subject, even if they are in certain respects mutually inaccessible. Of course, as in the split-brain case, subjects may well have various false beliefs about their own consciousness (e.g., that the various states belong to different subjects), but again this is not unexpected.

To completely assess this thesis requires much further analysis. But for now, we conclude that the empirical case against the phenomenal unity thesis is at best inconclusive. Given the strong prima facie positive case for accepting the phenomenal unity thesis, this suggests that the unity thesis remains quite plausible.

6. Formalizing the Unity Thesis

(This section is philosophically technical and can be skipped.)

6.1. More on Subsumption and Entailment

For further analysis, we need to clarify the phenomenal unity thesis and the corresponding notion of phenomenal unity. We have said that a set of states is phenomenally unified when there is something it is like to be in all those states at once. When this is the case, the subject will have a phenomenal state (corresponding to the conjoint what-it-is-like) that *subsumes* each of the states in the original set. So phenomenal unity can be seen as a sort of subsumptive unity, and the phenomenal unity thesis on the table is a sort of subsumptive unity thesis.

Subsumptive unity thesis: For any set of phenomenal states of a subject at a time, the subject has a phenomenal state that subsumes each of the states in that set.

There are also closely related total and pairwise subsumptive unity theses that require subsumptive unity only for pairs of phenomenal states or only for the complete set of a subject's phenomenal states at a time, but we can focus on the preceding thesis for now.

As it stands, the notion of subsumption is something of an intuitive primitive. There are some things we can say about it. It is a relation among token phenomenal states. It is plausibly reflexive (a state subsumes itself), antisymmetric (if A subsumes B and B subsumes A, then $A = B$) and transitive (if A subsumes B and B subsumes C, then A subsumes C). Note that reflexivity eliminates any apparent problem of regress in the unity thesis (if A and B are subsumed by C, there is no need for a further state to subsume A and C, since C subsumes itself).

The paradigm case of subsumption is the relation between a complex phenomenal state and a simpler state that is intuitively one of its "components." One might think of subsumption as analogous to a sort of mereological part/whole relation among phenomenal states, although this should be taken as an aid to intuition rather than as a serious ontological proposal, at least at this point. It is also useful to stipulate that subsumption holds between a phenomenal state and less specific states that intuitively correspond to the same experience: for example, that the state of experiencing a sharp pain subsumes the corresponding state of experiencing a pain. This sort of subsumption is required in order for a highly specific total phenomenal state to be able to subsume all of a subject's phenomenal states, including unspecific states.

It should be noted that there are alternatives to analyzing phenomenal unity in terms of subsumption. Often phenomenal unity is analyzed in terms of an intuitive relation of coconsciousness, where this relation is taken as primitive. We think that the analysis in terms of subsumption runs deeper in certain respects than a primitive analysis in terms of coconsciousness and offers the promise of further analytic tools, as discussed later. But the exact relation between these notions is an open question. (Dainton 2000 gives a thorough and insightful analysis of the unity of consciousness in terms of a primitive coconsciousness relation; Bayne 2001b discusses the relationship between the different accounts.[3])

The notion of subsumption is connected to the notion of "what it is like" in at least the following sense: when A subsumes B, what it is like to have B is an aspect of what it is like to have A. Of course, this appeals to the unexplained notion of an "aspect." One might try to go further by *defining* subsumption wholly in terms of the notion of "what it is like" as

---

3. *See also the appendix to the second edition of Dainton (2000) for an interesting discussion of the relation between the accounts.

follows: a phenomenal state A subsumes phenomenal state B when what it is like to have A and B simultaneously is the same as what it is like to have A. This seems to capture the connection articulated earlier, and it also can ground the connection between subsumptive unity and the original definition of phenomenal unity. If there is something it is like to be in a set of states (as the original definition requires), then this phenomenology will correspond to a phenomenal state A of the subject, and it is clear that this state will subsume the states in the original set in the sense defined earlier. It is arguable that the defined notion of subsumption goes beyond the intuitive notion in certain respects (someone might hold that the "what it is like" locution can be read such that what it is like to have A and B differs from what it is like to have A even when A subsumes B), and we will not rely on it in what follows. Nevertheless, it can serve as a useful aid to the understanding.

(Extending this line of thought, one could say that a state A *precisely subsumes* a set of states S when what it is like to be in A is the same as what it is like to simultaneously be in the members of S. Then if A precisely subsumes S, A subsumes each of the members of S, but the reverse entailment does not hold. For example, a subject's total state of consciousness subsumes each of the subject's visual experiences, but it does not precisely subsume the set of them. One could then articulate a *correspondence thesis* that holds that for any set of phenomenal states of a subject at a time, there is a corresponding phenomenal state that precisely subsumes that set. The correspondence thesis is formally stronger than the original subsumptive unity thesis: the existence of a total phenomenal state suffices for the truth of the original thesis, but it does not suffice for the truth of the correspondence thesis. The correspondence thesis nevertheless has some intuitive plausibility, and one could argue that this thesis, rather than the subsumptive unity thesis, best captures the idea articulated in the original phenomenal unity thesis. The difference between these theses will not be important for our purposes, however.)

6.2. Subsumption, Entailment, and Gestalt Unity

There is a close relation between subsumption and *entailment*. Let us say that a state P entails a state Q when it is impossible (logically or metaphysically impossible) for a subject to instantiate P without instantiating Q. Then it seems clear that when a phenomenal state P subsumes a phenomenal state Q, P will entail Q. For example, if P involves the phenomenal character as of seeing a red book and hearing a bird singing, and if Q involves the phenomenal character as of seeing a red book, then it is impossible to have P without having Q. The same goes with any case of subsumption. By its nature, the subsuming state carries with it the subsumed state.

Note that strictly speaking, entailment is a relation among state types, while subsumption is a relation among state tokens. For present purposes, we can regard entailment as derivatively a relation among state tokens, so that one state token entails another when there is entailment between the corresponding state types (although see the discussion later). We will generally pass over this nicety in discussion, acknowledging it where it is relevant. Note also that a phenomenal state A entails a phenomenal state B iff, necessarily, a subject in A is also in B—*not* if the content of A entails the content of B.[4]

The close relation between entailment and subsumption raises an interesting possibility: perhaps we can simply *define* subsumption in terms of entailment. That is, perhaps we can hold that phenomenal state A subsumes B when A entails B. If this were possible, instead of relying on a novel primitive relation, we could analyze unity in terms of a well-understood relation that allows the use of standard logical tools. To help assess this possibility, we can define a corresponding notion of unity and a corresponding unity thesis. Let us say that a set of phenomenal states of a subject at a time is *logically unified* when the subject has a phenomenal state that entails each of the phenomenal states in that set.

Logical unity thesis: For any set of phenomenal states of a subject at a time, the subject has a phenomenal state that entails each of the states in the set.

This gives an attractively simple formulation of the unity thesis that has some intuitive force. Unfortunately, there is an obstacle to replacing subsumption by entailment. We know that when A subsumes B, A entails B, but the reverse is not obviously the case. In fact, there are two ways in which it may seem that A could entail B without subsuming B.

First, A and B might correspond to intuitively distinct experiences that share a type. For example, a subject might have two pains at the same time or two experiences of red and so will have two distinct phenomenal states of the same type. In this case, one state type will entail the other (as the types are identical), so if entailment among tokens is derivative on

4. *Only under certain highly constrained assumptions will a phenomenal state A entail a phenomenal state B iff the content of A entails the content of B. Most obviously, this will follow from (i) a pure representationalist view on which to have a phenomenal state is just to represent a certain content or a semipure representationalist view on which to have a phenomenal state is just to phenomenally represent a certain content, conjoined with (ii) the view that whenever one (phenomenally) represents a content, one (phenomenally) represents any content that the first content entails.

entailment among types, one state token will entail the other. Here it is not plausible to hold that one state subsumes the other. (What it is like to have A and B simultaneously is quite different from what it is like to have A.) One might instead refine the definition of entailment among state tokens, requiring that it is impossible for one token to exist without the other, in addition to the requirement that one type cannot exist without the other, but one can also deal with this case by a strategy discussed below.

Second, A and B could be intuitively distinct phenomenal states that do not share any simple type but are nevertheless necessarily connected. This would involve a sort of *gestalt unity* that involves constraints on the co-occurrence of distinct phenomenal states. For example, perhaps there are cases where feeling a pain in one's shoulder while also experiencing a splitting headache produces a unique sort of pain that could not be experienced in the absence of the headache. Or perhaps seeing a certain person in the middle of a crowd produces a unique sort of visual experience of that person that could not be had in the absence of the experience of the crowd. Or perhaps (to use an example from Dainton 2000) the experience of the boundaries of a Kanizsa triangle is of a special sort that could not be had in the absence of the circles in which the triangle is embedded. In this sort of case, we can say that the pain is gestalt unified with the headache; the experience of the person is gestalt unified with the experience of the rest of the crowd; and the experience of the boundaries is gestalt unified with the experience of the circles.

Whether there are really any cases of gestalt unity is arguable. One could argue that in the cases in question, it would be possible (perhaps in some very different context) to experience the pain without the headache or to have the visual experience of the person without that of the crowd or to have that of the boundaries without that of the circles. Nonetheless, it is not implausible that at least some experiences put *some* constraints on concurrent experiences and that one cannot mix and match experiences arbitrarily. If this is so, then there is at least a weak sort of gestalt unity since the presence of one phenomenal state puts constraints on the nature of concurrent phenomenal states. In this case one can even say that the presence of one phenomenal state entails the existence of another phenomenal state, where the second is understood as an instantiation of a sufficiently unspecific phenomenal property.

If there is gestalt unity, then there will be cases in which one phenomenal state entails another phenomenal state without the first subsuming the second in any intuitive sense. For example, the experience of the boundary of a Kanizsa triangle might entail something about the experience of the nearby objects, but the experience of the nearby objects does not intuitively subsume that of the boundary of the triangle. Similarly, the experience of the shoulder pain might entail the experience of the headache, but it does not intuitively subsume the experience of the headache. Intuitively, what it is like to have the pain and the headache goes beyond what it is like to have the pain, even if the former is entailed by the latter.

6.3. Logical Unity and Subsumptive Unity

If there is gestalt unity, then subsumption cannot be understood in terms of entailment. But this does not mean that we must give up on the logical unity thesis. Even if subsumption cannot be understood in terms of entailment, one can make a case that the logical unity thesis entails the subsumptive unity thesis.

To see this, we can first note that not *all* phenomenal states are gestalt unified. Even if some pairs of phenomenal states are gestalt unified, it seems very unlikely that all pairs are, and it seems much more plausible that most pairs are not. Given a typical pair of phenomenal states had by a subject such that neither subsumes the other, it usually seems to be straightforwardly possible that a subject could have an instance of the first state without the second. When I see the red book and hear the bird singing, there seems to be no good reason to deny that I could have a visually identical experience without hearing the bird singing and so on. (Dainton 2000 gives a more extended argument for the conclusion that gestalt unity is not universal and is in fact rare.)

If there can be pairs of states that are not gestalt unified, it also seems that there can be subjects none of whose states are gestalt unified. One simply needs a subject all of whose basic phenomenal states are independent in the way described above: each of them could occur without any of the others. There seems to be no obstacle in principle to such a subject, and one could even argue that our own phenomenal states are often like this. Let us say that such a subject is gestalt free. In gestalt-free subjects, the gestalt cases of entailment without subsumption will not arise. So (setting aside for a moment any other cases of entailment without subsumption), we can say that if the logical unity thesis holds, the subsumptive unity thesis holds at least when restricted to gestalt-free subjects.

Now let us assume that the subsumptive unity thesis holds for gestalt-free subjects: for any set of phenomenal states of a gestalt-free subject, there is a subsuming phenomenal state. If so, it is very plausible that the subsumptive unity thesis holds for all subjects. If there is always a subsuming state in gestalt-free cases, there will plausibly always be a subsuming state in gestalt cases. There is nothing about gestalt unity that makes the existence of a subsuming state in such cases *less* likely. If anything, the situation is the reverse. In a case of gestalt unity, the experiences will be connected in such a way that the existence of a subsuming state will be more likely, not less. So if there are cases in which gestalt unified states are not phenomenally unified, there should equally be cases in which gestalt-free states are not phenomenally unified. So the subsumptive unity thesis for gestalt-free subjects plausibly leads to the subsumptive unity thesis for all subjects.

We are close to establishing a connection between the logical unity thesis and the subsumptive unity thesis in general. But we still need to deal with the other case of entailment without subsumption, in which a subject has distinct simultaneous experiences that share a type. We can deal with this in an analogous way. Let us say that a subject has *duplicate* experiences when the subject has two intuitively distinct experiences that share a maximally specific phenomenal type (two pains or two color experiences with exactly the same quality, say). It is not entirely obvious that duplicate experiences are possible, but in any case, let us say that a *duplicate-free* subject is a subject without duplicate experiences. It is plausible that *if* the subsumptive unity thesis is true when restricted to duplicate-free subjects, it is true also of subjects with duplication. If it is possible for duplicate experiences not to be subsumed by a common experience, it will be equally possible for nonduplicate experiences not to be so subsumed. As with gestalt phenomena, there is nothing about duplication per se that contributes to a breakdown of phenomenal unity. So the subsumptive unity thesis for duplication-free subjects plausibly leads to the subsumptive unity thesis for all subjects.

Combining the last two cases, we can say that the subsumptive unity thesis restricted to gestalt-free, duplication-free subjects plausibly entails the subsumptive unity thesis for all subjects. But it is also clear that the logical unity thesis entails the subsumptive unity thesis for gestalt-free, duplication-free subjects. In such subjects, a phenomenal state T that entails all phenomenal states will also subsume all phenomenal states since we have removed the relevant gaps between subsumption and entailment. One might worry that one gap remains. By ruling out duplication, we have ruled out the possibility of entailment without subsumption for maximally specific phenomenal states, but it remains open that two sufficiently nonspecific states of the same type might entail each other without subsuming each other. Nevertheless, since T entails maximally specific versions of each of these nonspecific states, T will subsume these maximally specific states, and so T will subsume the nonspecific states. So T subsumes all of the subject's phenomenal states.

We have established that the logical unity thesis entails the subsumptive unity thesis for gestalt-free, duplication-free subjects, and we have established that the latter thesis plausibly entails the subsumptive unity thesis for all subjects. So the logical unity thesis plausibly entails the subsumptive unity thesis. In reverse, the subsumptive unity thesis clearly entails the logical unity thesis. So it is plausible that the subsumptive unity thesis holds if and only if the logical unity thesis holds. The only obstacle to this equivalence will arise if there are breakdowns of phenomenal unity that are solely due to gestalt unity or to duplication, but there seems to be little reason to take that possibility seriously.

If this is correct, we can assess the truth of the subsumptive unity thesis by assessing the truth of the logical unity thesis. This latter task is in some respects more straightforward, since we no longer have to deal directly with the primitive notion of subsumption. This also allows the possibility of using familiar logical tools to formulate and assess versions of the unity thesis. We will look more closely at some versions of the thesis in the following section.

6.4. Logical Unity and Conjunctive Closure

There are three versions of the subsumptive unity thesis: the pairwise version, the general version, and the total version. There are correspondingly three versions of the logical unity thesis, holding that there is logical unity among either any two states of a subject at a time, any set of states, or the complete set of states. We can state this more directly as follows:

Pairwise logical unity thesis: Necessarily, for any two phenomenal states had by a subject at a time, the subject has a phenomenal state that entails both original states.

General logical unity thesis: Necessarily, for any set of phenomenal states of a subject at a time, the subject has a phenomenal state that entails each state in the set.

Total logical unity thesis: Necessarily, for any conscious subject at a time, the subject has a phenomenal state T such that for any phenomenal state A of the subject at that time, T entails A.

As before, it is clear that the general thesis entails the pairwise thesis and the total thesis as special cases. The total thesis also entails the general thesis and the pairwise thesis since a state that entails all of the phenomenal states of a subject will also entail any pair or any set of states. Arguably the pairwise thesis does not entail the other two theses because of the formal possibility that there might be entailing states for any finite set of states but not for infinite subsets.

We can start by focusing on the total logical unity thesis since this corresponds most closely to the total phenomenal unity thesis, which arguably captures the central intuition behind the unity of consciousness. Intuitively, we can think of T, the entailing state in the thesis, as the subject's total phenomenal state, capturing what it is like to be the subject at that time. If such a state exists, it will fulfill the requirement of the total logical unity thesis.

One can also approach the matter in logical terms. Let us say that the *conjunction* of a set of states is a state C such that necessarily, a subject is in C if and only the subject is in each of the states in that set. (Like entailment, conjunction is fundamentally a relation among state types and derivatively a relation among state tokens. Note also that the conjunction of states is quite different from the conjunction of the *contents* of states.[5]) This identifies C at least up to mutual entailment. For present purposes, it is useful to assume that when two states A and B mutually entail each other (i.e., necessarily, a subject is in A if and only if the subject is in B), then the two states are identical. If so, then C is identified uniquely. Nothing that follows rests essentially on this assumption—one could rephrase things in terms of equivalence classes of states—but this makes the discussion easier.

We can then propose a natural candidate for T: the conjunction C of all of a subject's phenomenal states at a time. It is clear that if T exists, T entails C (since T entails each of the conjuncts of C). And it is clear that if T exists, C entails T (since T is itself a phenomenal state). So if T exists, then T is identical to C (and C is therefore a phenomenal state) by the earlier criterion for state identity. It is also clear that if C is a phenomenal state, then C will satisfy the total logical unity thesis with $T=C$. We can therefore say that an appropriate T exists if and only if C is a phenomenal state.

Let us say that a set of states is *conjunctively unified* when the conjunction of the members of that set is itself a phenomenal state. Then from the discussion here, it follows that the total logical unity thesis is equivalent to the claim that the set of a subject's phenomenal states is conjunctively unified:

---

*5. On some (but only some) representationalist views, the conjunction of a set of phenomenal states will be a phenomenal state whose content is a conjunction of the contents of the original states. For reasons discussed in the next section, this claim is unlikely to hold in general on functionalist versions of representationalism. It is also unlikely to hold on impure versions of representationalism, on which different phenomenal states may involve different manners of representation. The claim is better suited to pure or semipure versions of representationalism, on which phenomenal states are just states of (phenomenally) representing certain contents.

Total conjunctive unity thesis: If C is the conjunction of all of a subject's phenomenal states at a time, then C is itself a phenomenal state.

As before, someone might think that a thesis of this sort is trivially true, but this would be incorrect. It is trivial that for any set of phenomenal states of a subject at a time, there will be a conjunctive state C that entails each of the original states, but it is nontrivial that C will itself be a phenomenal state. That is, it is nontrivial (although very plausible) that there will be something it is like to be in C: some global phenomenal character that a subject will have if and only if the subject is in C. Those who deny the original unity thesis will deny the existence of such a phenomenal character and so will deny that C is itself a phenomenal state.

In effect, we have seen that the original phenomenal unity thesis is equivalent to a thesis about the *conjunctive closure* of coinstantiated phenomenal states (where coinstantiated states are states had by the same subject at the same time): certain conjunctions of states in this class must also be states in this class. This is very useful since conjunctive closure is amenable to relatively straightforward analysis.

One can also formulate conjunctive closure theses that are closely related to the other versions of the logical unity thesis. There is a pairwise version and a general version:

Pairwise conjunctive unity thesis: For any two phenomenal states of a subject at a time, their conjunction is a phenomenal state.

General conjunctive unity thesis: For any set of phenomenal states of a subject at a time, their conjunction is a phenomenal state.

These theses are not quite formally equivalent to the corresponding versions of the logical unity thesis. To see this, note that it is at least a formal possibility that two states might be logically unified but not conjunctively unified. For example, it is at least formally possible that the conjunction of *all* of a subject's phenomenal states might be a phenomenal state but that the conjunctions of certain pairs and subsets might not be. If so, then these pairs and subsets will be logically unified but not conjunctively unified. In this case the pairwise and general conjunctive unity theses will be false, but the pairwise and general logical unity theses will be true.

However, it is clear that these conjunctive unity theses *entail* the corresponding versions of the logical unity thesis. They are also interesting and plausible theses in their own right. The first says that for any two phenomenal states A and B of a subject at a time, there will be something distinctive that it is like to be in A and B: that is, a distinctive conjoint phenomenal character that a subject will have if and only if the subject is in both A and B. The second says the same thing for arbitrary sets of coinstantiated phenomenal states. These theses are not formally trivial, but they are highly plausible theses about phenomenal consciousness. (These theses are closely related to the correspondence thesis discussed in the previous section.)

All three theses are simple and elegant. The pairwise conjunctive unity thesis says that the class of phenomenal states is closed under pairwise coinstantiated conjunction: the conjunction of two coinstantiated phenomenal states is a phenomenal state. The general conjunctive unity thesis says that the class of phenomenal states is closed under general coinstantiated conjunction: the conjunction of any set of coinstantiated phenomenal states is a phenomenal state. The total conjunctive unity thesis says that the class of phenomenal states is closed under maximal coinstantiated conjunction: the conjunction of a maximal set of coinstantiated phenomenal states is a phenomenal state.

The total conjunctive unity thesis remains the core version of the unity thesis, but all of these theses are plausible and useful. Each of them can be used as a tool in assessing the status of the unity of consciousness, its consequences, and its compatibility with various theories of consciousness.

6.5. Hurley, Shoemaker, and What It Is Like

All of the conjunctive unity theses are stated simply in terms of the notions of phenomenal state, coinstantiation, and conjunction. In addition, the notion of a phenomenal state is tied constitutively to the notion of there being something it is like to be a given subject or to be in a given state. So we have an account of unity that requires little more than the existing "what it is like" conception of phenomenal states.

This stands in tension with a claim in a very interesting analysis by Hurley (1998, 165–66) who argues that the unity of consciousness cannot be characterized "subjectively" and that suppositions about the structure of consciousness are not captured by the "what it is like" test, so that we need to appeal to further "objective" properties to give an account of unity. This claim is grounded in the claim that in a case where unity breaks down, there is no "what it is like" that captures the structure of a subject's consciousness. Hurley backs up this claim by considering two cases: (i) two subjects, one experiencing red and hot, the other experiencing red and dizzy; and (ii) a partially unified single subject, in whom red and hot are unified, red and dizzy are unified, but hot and dizzy are not. Hurley argues that no "what it is like" facts can distinguish these two cases.

From the claim that there is no what-it-is-like that characterizes a disunified subject, however, it does not follow that one cannot characterize unity in what-it-is-like terms. Indeed, following Hurley's own claim, one can hold that unity breaks down precisely when there is nothing it is like to have all of a subject's conscious states simultaneously. We can distinguish case (i) from case (ii) by noting that in case (ii), both subjects have a phenomenal state that subsumes all of their phenomenal states, whereas in case (i), the subject has no such phenomenal state. Of course, our characterization of unity appeals to something more than phenomenal states themselves: it also appeals to subsumption and to coinstantiation in a subject. Perhaps Hurley would count these notions as in some sense "objective." There is no point in arguing over terminology here, but we can at least note that subsumption is a phenomenal relation, fixed by phenomenology alone: if A subsumes B, then the phenomenology of A guarantees that it subsumes B. In addition, subjects are simply the bearers of phenomenal states, so we are staying quite close to home in characterizing unity this way.

Hurley might extend her argument by suggesting case (iii): a bifurcated subject with two different (but indistinguishable) tokens of red in separate streams. In this subject, red_1 is unified with hot, red_2 is unified with dizzy, and no state in either pair is unified with a state in the other pair (Hurley [1998, 166] seems to point toward such a case). If (iii) is possible, one could argue that it could not be distinguished from (ii) by talk of subjects and their phenomenal states alone. We would need to appeal to the identity of phenomenal states: a single "red" experience is involved in both complex experiences in (ii) but not in (iii).

There are a number of things one could say in response. One might concede that "what it is like" talk cannot distinguish the two different cases of disunity (ii) and (iii) but hold that it can nevertheless distinguish unity from disunity, which is the most important work we need it to do. If the unity thesis is true, then cases of disunity will be impossible, and distinctions among impossible cases will not matter for characterizing the structure of consciousness. More deeply, one can suggest that Hurley's argument shows at best that one cannot distinguish the cases in terms of the distribution of phenomenal state *types*. If we appeal to facts about the distribution of phenomenal state *tokens*, things are straightforward: there is a token experience that is subsumed by two different complex experiences in (ii) but not in (iii). It may be that (ii) and (iii) will be introspectively indistinguishable, so that the structure of consciousness is not *transparent* to a subject. Nevertheless, a characterization of the structure of consciousness in terms of phenomenal relations among phenomenal state tokens is still, in a deep sense, a characterization in subjective terms.

Our characterization of unity in phenomenal terms also stands in tension with a claim by Shoemaker (2003). Shoemaker suggests that if a conscious state is understood as one with a phenomenal property (i.e., one such that there is something it is like to be in it), this leads to "consciousness atomism": the view that the factors that make a state conscious are independent of the factors that make two states unified. Our discussion here suggests that this is false. What it is for two conscious states to be unified can be understood in terms of the existence of a more complex conscious state, where both the simple state and the complex states are characterized by what it is like to be in them. So the factors that enter into unifying conscious states are the same sort as those that enter into those states being conscious in the first place.

At one point, Shoemaker characterizes "consciousness atomism" differently, as the view that "whether a state is conscious will be independent of whether there are other conscious states with which it is co-conscious." The account here is neutral on this claim. For all we have said here, it may be possible for there to be a subject with a single conscious state. This claim does not seem to us to be obviously objectionable, and it is compatible with the more important view that the factors that enter into consciousness are the same as those that enter into coconsciousness.

In fact, the definitions of unity that we have given here suggest that any account of what it is to be a phenomenal state will automatically yield a theory of what it is for two such states to be unified. We need simply to apply the theory to the relevant conjunctive states in order to determine whether they are phenomenal states. In this way, any substantive theory of phenomenal consciousness can yield unified definitions of consciousness and coconsciousness. It is precisely because of this that the unity thesis (if it is true) puts strong constraints on a theory of phenomenal consciousness, as we will see.

7. Applications of the Unity Thesis

We have already mentioned the objection that the conjunctive versions of the unity thesis are trivial: that is, that it is trivial that the conjunction of a set of coinstantiated phenomenal states is itself a phenomenal state.

It is clear that the thesis is not *formally* trivial in that there are many classes of states that are not closed under coinstantiated conjunction. For example, states of the sort "talking with X" where X is an individual are not closed under co-instantiated conjunction. Closer to home, there are also many classes of *mental* states that are not closed under coinstantiated conjunction.

For example, the class of belief states does not seem to be closed under conjunction. Let us say that a belief state is the state of believing some proposition. Then it is not the case that the conjunction of any set of belief states is a belief state. For example, if A is the state of believing that p, and if B is the state of believing that q, there is plausibly no belief state that a subject will be in precisely when they are in A and B. The only tenable candidate for such a belief state is the state of believing that $p\&q$, but there are well-known reasons to believe that a subject can believe p and believe q without believing the conjunction $p\&q$. For example, p and q might be believed in different "compartments" of a compartmentalized mind. It may even be that, for some p, a subject can believe that p and separately believe that $\sim p$ without believing the contradiction $p\&\sim p$. It also seems quite possible that a subject can have many different beliefs without accepting the massive conjunction of the contents of all of those beliefs. If this is right, then the conjunction of coinstantiated belief states will not in general be a belief state. So the class of belief states is not closed under coinstantiated conjunction

It may seem plausible or even obvious that the class of *phenomenal* states is closed under conjunction. But if so, this is a substantive thesis about the class of phenomenal states and its difference from other classes of mental states. It may even be a *conceptual* truth, in some sense, that the class of phenomenal states is closed under coinstantiated conjunction. But if so, this is again a substantive thesis about the *concept* of a phenomenal state and a way in which it differs from the concept of a belief state and other sorts of states.

The substantive nature of the thesis is also revealed by the fact that it puts strong constraints on theories of consciousness. We have seen that the unity thesis is prima facie plausible, and there seem to be no strong arguments against it. If this is right, then the unity thesis puts a prima facie constraint on theories of consciousness: they must be compatible with the unity thesis. In particular, any account of phenomenal states must be compatible with the total conjunctive unity thesis. Whatever phenomenal states are, according to a given account, the class of phenomenal states must be closed under total coinstantiated conjunction. A number of prominent theories of consciousness appear to be incompatible with this constraint.

7.1. The Higher-Order Thought Theory

One example is the higher-order thought theory of consciousness put forward by Rosenthal (1997) and others. Not all higher-order thought theorists intend the theory as an account of phenomenal consciousness (e.g., Lycan 2000 explicitly rejects the idea), but we are concerned only with versions of the theory that are aimed at phenomenal consciousness. The central idea of these theories is the following:

Higher-order thought thesis: A mental state M is phenomenally conscious if and only if a subject has a higher-order thought about M.

Here, a higher-order thought about M should be understood as a thought by the subject with the content "I am in M." The thesis will usually be modified and qualified in some ways. For example, Rosenthal holds that for M to be conscious, the higher-order thought must be brought about in the right sort of way and in particular must be a noninferential thought. Rosenthal also holds that only sensory states can be phenomenally conscious, so that we would have to insert a qualification to that effect in the preceding definition. This is arguably a mere verbal difference, however, since Rosenthal holds that there will be something it is like to be in a state whenever it is the object of the right sort of higher-order thought, whether the state is sensory or not. In any case, for our purposes we will take the thesis in the simple form above. Our arguments should apply straightforwardly to most modified versions.

Is the higher-order thought thesis compatible with the unity thesis? It is easiest to approach this question by considering the conjunctive versions of the unity thesis. The conjunctive versions say that the class of phenomenal states is closed under conjunction. So we can ask: on the higher-order thought theory, is the class of phenomenal states closed under conjunction?

We can start by thinking about phenomenally conscious mental states. If A and B are phenomenally conscious mental states, is $A\&B$ necessarily a phenomenally conscious mental state? Assuming the higher-order thought thesis, this translates into the following: if a subject has a higher-order thought about A and a higher-order thought about B, does the subject necessarily have a higher-order thought about $A\&B$? That is, if the subject has a thought "I am in A" and a thought "I am in B," does it follow necessarily that the subject has a thought "I am in A and B"?

It seems not. It is surely possible for a subject to think "I am in A" and "I am in B" without connecting these into a thought "I am in A and B." We can take a case like those discussed earlier, in which a subject has contradictory beliefs, knows that she has each belief, but never puts the two together. She might have the thought "I believe p" and the thought "I believe $\sim p$" without ever putting these two together into a thought "I believe both p and $\sim p$." This might be strange or unusual, but there is nothing contradictory about it. There would only be something contradictory here if the beliefs of a subject are necessarily closed under logical consequence, but of course no subject's beliefs are closed under logical consequence.

The same is even clearer where total conjunctivity is concerned. On the higher-order thought theory, if a subject has a number of phenomenally conscious mental states, is their conjunction a phenomenally conscious mental state? That is, if a subject has mental states $A_1, \ldots, A_n$ and has the thoughts *I am in A_1, ..., I am in A_n*, does the subject necessarily have the thought *I am in $A_1 \& A_2 \& \ldots A_n$*? Again, it seems not. One might reasonably argue that this entailment does not even hold *typically*, let alone necessarily. That is, it is arguable that a *typical* subject with these higher-order beliefs would not have the complex conjunctive belief. Whatever one says here, it is hard to dispute that it is *possible* for a subject to have the individual higher-order beliefs without the complex conjunctive belief.

So it appears that if the higher-order thought view is true, the class of phenomenally conscious mental states is not closed under coinstantiated conjunction. This already contradicts the central intuition behind the unity thesis: that necessarily, if there is something it is like to be in each of a set of states, there is something it is like to be in all the states at once. On the higher-order thought view, this thesis will clearly be false.

The official version of the unity thesis is stated in terms of phenomenal states, not phenomenally conscious mental states. The analysis of phenomenal states is slightly trickier since advocates of the higher-order thought view have not usually talked about phenomenal states and phenomenal properties directly. But given that higher-order thought theorists hold that there is something it is like to be in a mental state when the subject has a higher-order thought about it, they presumably hold that what it is like to be in that state is determined by the content of the higher-order thought. If so, it seems that phenomenal properties will be the properties of having higher-order thoughts with certain contents and that phenomenal states will be the states of having such higher-order thoughts.

Do phenomenal states, understood this way, satisfy the unity thesis? It seems not, for much the same reason as before. Here it is useful to take the entailment version of the unity thesis: that necessarily, when a subject has a set of phenomenal states, the subject has a phenomenal state that entails each of the individual states. When a subject has a set of higher-order thoughts $H_1, \ldots, H_n$, does the subject necessarily have a higher-order thought H_H such that being in H_H entails being in $H_1, \ldots, H_n$? It seems not, for the usual reasons. A subject might think *I am in A* and *I am in B* without any higher-order thought (e.g., *I am in A&B*) such that having that thought entails having the original thoughts.

The problem is not that the higher-order thought theory provides no way to understand phenomenal unity. It can do so in a natural way. Two phenomenally conscious mental states *A* and *B* are unified when the subject has a higher-order thought about them not just singly but jointly. And two phenomenal states, the states of having higher-order thoughts *I am in A* and *I am in B* are phenomenally unified when there is a complex phenomenal state that entails them: that is, if there is a complex higher-order thought such that having the complex thought entails having the specific thoughts. This requirement will arguably be satisfied when the subject has a complex higher-order thought such as *I am in A&B*.

The problem is rather that on this account, there is no reason to believe that phenomenal states or phenomenally conscious mental states will always be unified. Certainly it will not be necessary that they be unified, and it seems plausible that in a typical case they will not be unified. So the higher-order thought thesis is incompatible with the unity thesis. It is clearly incompatible with the conjunctive and logical versions of the unity thesis. It is therefore also incompatible with the subsumptive versions since any failure of logical unity automatically entails a failure of subsumptive unity. So if the higher-order thought thesis is true, the unity thesis is false. And if the unity thesis is true, the higher-order thought thesis is false.

Proponents of the higher-order thought thesis might reply in a number of ways. Most straightforwardly, they might reply by denying the unity thesis. This is a tenable response since the truth of the unity thesis cannot be taken for granted. Still, there is a strong intuition that the unity thesis is true, so the incompatibility is at least a cost of the higher-order thought thesis. Proponents might also embrace a more limited version of the unity thesis, arguing, for example, that unity holds typically but not necessarily, or that it holds given contingent facts of human psychology but not for all possible beings. Here there would still be the cost of denying the intuition of necessary unity, and there would be the added difficulty of defending the claim that unity holds in the relevant range of cases when there seems to be no obvious reason why complex conjunctive thoughts about all the objects of our higher-order thoughts should typically exist.

Higher-order thought theorists might also respond by finding fault with the argument for incompatibility. They might hold, for example, that it is necessary that the class of mental states that are objects of higher-order thoughts is closed under conjunction. This would be a difficult case to make in face of the apparent possibility of the failure of this principle, and in face of the general phenomenon that beliefs are not closed under logical consequence.

Finally, proponents might modify the higher-order thought thesis to make it compatible with the unity thesis. To do so, they must modify the definition of a phenomenally conscious mental state. It could be held, for example, that a mental state is phenomenally conscious when either (i) it is the object of a higher-order thought or (ii) it is the conjunction of states that are the objects of higher-order thoughts. This sort of disjunctive account would be contrary to both the letter and the spirit of existing higher-order thought views (which hold that a conscious state is one that the subject is conscious of). One could also raise questions about whether this thesis delivers any *substantive* unity of consciousness or merely a stipulated sort of unity of consciousness that holds trivially. Insofar as the unity of consciousness seems to be a substantive fact about consciousness, one could argue that this modified version of the higher-order thesis does not really account for it.

Of course, all of this is debatable and could lead to fruitful further discussion. But the prima facie incompatibility between the two theses is at least interesting. The incompatibility extends straightforwardly to other "higher-order" views of consciousness, including views on which a conscious state is an object of a higher-order perceptual state or the object of some other sort of higher-order representational state. The existence of a set of higher-order perceptual states does not entail the existence of a complex conjunctive higher-order perceptual state, and the same goes for other sorts of representational states. So if the unity thesis is true, these theses are false, and vice versa.

7.2. Representationalism

The unity thesis is also incompatible with many *representationalist* views of consciousness. According to representationalist views (e.g., Dretske 1995; Tye 1995), all phenomenally conscious mental states are representational states (that is, states with representational content). This is commonly allied with a further functional criterion to yield the following:

Representationalist thesis: A mental state is phenomenally conscious if and only if it is a representational state that plays an appropriate functional role.

We will focus on this broadly functionalist variety of representionalism. The details of the relevant functional role differ among representationalists, but it is typically held to involve some sort of access and control. One can then say that what it is like to be in a mental state is determined by the content of the representional state, on the condition that it plays the relevant functional role. On this sort of view, then, a phenomenal state is a state of having a certain sort of representational state play the appropriate functional role, where distinct phenomenal states are individuated by distinct representational contents.

Two phenomenal states P_1 and P_2 are conjunctively unified when there is a phenomenal state P that entails each of the original states. On the representationalist account, two phenomenal states P_1 and P_2, corresponding to representational states A_1 and A_2 (with contents C_1 and C_2) playing the relevant functional role, will be conjunctively unified when there is a phenomenal state P corresponding to representational state A (with content C) playing the relevant functional role, such that P entails P_1 and P_2. This will occur if and only if the existence of A playing the role entails the existence of both A_1 and A_2 playing the role. The only reasonable way to satisfy this is for the content of A to entail the content of A_1 and the content of A_2: that is, for C to entail both C_1 and C_2, or for C to entail $C_1 \& C_2$. For example, if A_1 has content "red to the left," and A_2 has content "green to the right," P_1 and P_2 will be conjunctively unified if there is a state A (playing the role) whose content entails "red to the left and green to the right." So two phenomenal states, corresponding to two representational states, will be conjunctively unified if and only if there is a conjunctive representational state (playing the appropriate role) whose content entails the conjunction of the contents of the original representational states.

The unity thesis is true if and only if necessarily, every set of phenomenal states is conjunctively unified. On the representationalist view, is this the case? It seems not. It seems at least possible to have a state with content C_1 and a state with content C_2, each playing a certain role, without having a state with content $C_1 \& C_2$ that plays the role. We saw this earlier in the case where the relevant role involves accessibility: it is possible that C_1 is accessible and C_2 is accessible without $C_1 \& C_2$ being accessible. Something similar will hold for any functional role involving access and control. If this is so, then representationalist theses in the relevant class are incompatible with the unity thesis.

As before, representationalists could respond in a number of ways. They could deny the unity thesis, at the cost of denying a strong intuition. They could modify it to apply to a more limited range of cases, at the cost of some intuition and perhaps some empirical constraint. (For example, in the Sperling case, this representationalist may have to deny that the subject has a phenomenally unified visual field.) They could modify the representationalist thesis to allow a disjunctive definition that stipulates that conjunctions of phenomenal states are phenomenal states, at the cost of endangering the substantive status of the unity thesis. Alternatively, they could move to a different sort of representationalism (the sort discussed in chapter 11) that is not so closely tied to functionalism. For example, it might be held that phenomenally conscious states are representational states whose content is represented *phenomenally* or that they are representational states with some other property that is not functionally defined. The resulting version of representationalism might be compatible with the unity thesis (as well as being independently more plausible than the previous versions), at the cost of giving up the reductive aspirations of many representationalist views.

One might also argue that other nonrepresentationalist forms of functionalism are incompatible with the unity thesis on the general grounds that there will not be the relevant conjunctive property among states playing the functional role. The details will depend on the details of the functionalist theory and in particular on the account that is given of phenomenal states and properties. These accounts can vary between functionalist theories and are often not clearly articulated, so it is difficult to give a general analysis of such theories with respect to the unity thesis. Nonetheless, it is clear that it will be at least highly nontrivial for a functionalist account to satisfy the unity thesis.

If the foregoing is correct, then the unity thesis is incompatible with higher-order thought (and other higher-order representation) views of consciousness, with many representationalist views of consciousness, and with many functionalist views of consciousness. So the unity thesis is clearly nontrivial. Nevertheless, it has strong independent plausibility as a thesis about phenomenal states. So the incompatibility of the unity thesis with these views of consciousness should be seen as at least prima facie evidence against these views.

8. Explaining the Unity Thesis

If the unity thesis is true, how is its truth to be explained? We do not know the answer to this question, but in this concluding section, we explore some possibilities.

One common strategy is to try to explain unity in functional terms. For example, one might try to explain unity in terms of some sort of informational integration or in terms of serial processing in the brain. One obvious problem with this sort of strategy is that it is not clear why this sort of functioning should yield phenomenal unity, as opposed to something like access unity. An equally deep problem is that, for reasons similar to those discussed in the previous section, it seems inevitable that this sort of functioning will be present *contingently* and that it will be possible for conscious states to exist that do not stand in the relevant functional relations. If so, unity (on these analyses) will obtain only contingently, and the unity thesis will be false. If unity is to obtain necessarily, as the unity thesis suggests, we must look elsewhere.

Much of the reason for accepting the truth of the unity thesis comes from the fact that its denial seems to be inconceivable and perhaps incoherent. This suggests that the unity thesis may be at some level a *conceptual* truth, although perhaps a deep conceptual truth, whose roots are revealed only by a deep analysis of our concepts. The central concepts involved in the unity thesis are that of a phenomenal state and that of a subject, along with various additional notions such as subsumption, entailment, conjunction, and so on. So one might hope that some light could be shed by attention to the concept of a subject or by attention to the concept of consciousness.

One natural suggestion is that our concept of a subject of experience is somehow premised on unity. For example, one could suggest that ascriptions of subjecthood require as a precondition that subjects correspond to unified phenomenal fields. In the spirit of a sort of bundle theory of the subject, one could argue that we have a prior notion of a phenomenal field and that we then associate subjects with phenomenal fields. If this is the case, we would expect that every subject would have a unified consciousness. A subject with two distinct phenomenal fields, for example, would be ruled out as a conceptual impossibility. Where there are two phenomenal fields, there will automatically be two subjects.

How might this work? Our articulation of the notion of a phenomenal field in this chapter appeals to subjects and coinstantiation, but one might argue that these can be bypassed. For example, one might appeal to a primitive relation of subsumption (or of coconsciousness) among phenomenal states that makes no presuppositions about subjects of those states and then define a phenomenal field as a maximal phenomenal state: a phenomenal state that is not subsumed by any other phenomenal state. But even if something like this works, there is a deeper problem. This strategy might explain why distinct phenomenal fields correspond to distinct subjects, but it cannot explain why states of consciousness come packaged into unified phenomenal fields in the first place. For example, nothing in this strategy explains why a phenomenal state cannot be subsumed by two different phenomenal states such that no further phenomenal state subsumes both of these in turn. More generally, nothing here explains why the subsumption relation does not hold in an unsystematic and fragmented manner. It is possible that an analysis of subsumption itself could do some work. For example, one could argue that subsumption is conceptually akin to a mereological part-whole relation and so must hold reflexively, antisymmetrically, and transitively, perhaps in a way that allows no overlap. Still, this conceptual stipulation does not really make the problem go away. It simply raises the question of why conscious states come packaged as parts and wholes.

One might then take a different approach. Instead of focusing on the concept of a subject, one could focus on the concept of consciousness itself. It could be argued that our *basic* concept of consciousness is not the notion of a simple phenomenal state—what it is like to experience such-and-such at a time. Rather, our basic notion of consciousness is that of a total phenomenal state: what it is like to be a subject at a time. This yields a holistic rather than an atomistic view of consciousness. On this approach, we do not start with basic atomic states of consciousness and somehow glue them together into complex states. Rather, we start with a basic *total* state of consciousness and then differentiate it into simpler states and ultimately into atomic states.

If this were truly our basic notion of consciousness, then it might explain why the unity thesis is true. On this view, any nontotal phenomenal state is *derivative* on a total phenomenal state that subsumes it. It is then to be expected that any phenomenal states of a subject at a time are all simply aspects of what it is like to be that subject at that time. As such, it is to be expected that for any set of coinstantiated phenomenal states, there will be a subsuming state. On this view, the most basic problem with the theories of consciousness discussed in the last section is that they are atomistic rather than holistic, starting with simple states rather than total states. If this view is right, then any such analysis of consciousness will be a misanalysis from the start.

It is not obvious that this sort of conceptual claim on its own yields a substantive unity thesis. But one might naturally tie this analysis to a corresponding substantive view of the metaphysics of consciousness. In nature, it may be that the most basic sort of conscious state is the total phenomenal state, the phenomenal field, or even the phenomenal world.[6] These total

---

6. *As noted earlier, this view is analogous in some respects to Schaffer's priority monism (2010), which holds that the universe as a whole is fundamental and its parts are derivative.

states are basic, but they are not featureless. They come with a complex structure from which one can differentiate many aspects. (As an analogy, one can think of a quantum wave function, which is a basic state in physics but which nevertheless has a complex structure.) So metaphysically, simple conscious states might be derivative on total conscious states. If so, we would have a clean explanation of why a substantive unity thesis is true.

This sort of suggestion is highly speculative and much needs to be worked out. For example, it is far from obvious that our basic concept of consciousness is that of a total state of consciousness, and one needs to make a direct case for this. In addition, the corresponding metaphysics needs to be worked out in much more depth. But there is at least some plausibility in the idea that the concepts of consciousness and states of consciousness are fundamentally holistic rather than atomistic. This squares well with our intuition that consciousness is necessarily unified.

In any case, whether the substantive claims that we have made in this chapter are correct or incorrect, we hope to have pinned down some of the crucial issues. It is clear that there is much need for further work in analyzing the notion of unity, in assessing the truth of the unity thesis, and in seeking an explanation of its truth. It is likely that such work will be philosophically fruitful.

1. Introduction

Two-dimensional approaches to semantics, broadly understood, recognize two "dimensions" of the meaning or content of linguistic items. On these approaches, expressions and their utterances are associated with two different sorts of semantic values that play different explanatory roles. Typically, one semantic value is closely associated with an expression's referent, while the other is associated with the way that reference depends on the external world. Two-dimensional semantics is usually understood as a version of possible-world semantics, so that each dimension is understood in terms of possible worlds and related modal notions.

In possible-world semantics, linguistic expressions and/or their utterances are first associated with an *extension*. The extension of a sentence is its truth value: for example, the extension of 'Plato was a philosopher' is true. The extension of a singular term is its referent: for example, the extension of 'Don Bradman' is Bradman. The extension of a general term is the class of individuals that fall under the term: for example, the extension of 'cat' is the class of cats. Other expressions work similarly.

One can then associate expressions with an *intension*, which is a function from possible worlds to extensions. The intension of a sentence is a function that is true at a possible world if and only if the sentence is true there: the intension of 'Plato was a philosopher' is true at all worlds where Plato was a philosopher. The intension of a singular term maps a possible world to the referent of the term in that possible world: the intension of 'Don Bradman' picks out whoever is Bradman in a world. The intension of a general term maps a possible world to the class of individuals that fall under the term in that world: the intension of 'cat' maps a possible world to the class of cats in that world.

It can easily happen that two expressions have the same extension but different intensions. For example, Quine's terms 'cordate' (creature with a heart) and 'renate' (creature with a kidney) pick out the same class of individuals in the actual world, so they have the same extension. However, there are many possible worlds where they pick out different classes (any possible world in which there are creatures with hearts but no kidneys, for example), so they have different intensions. When two expressions have the same extension and a different intension in this way, the difference in intension usually corresponds to an intuitive difference in meaning. So it is natural to suggest that an expression's intension is at least an aspect of its meaning.

Carnap (1947) suggested that an intension behaves in many respects like a Fregean sense, the aspect of an expression's meaning that corresponds to its cognitive significance. For example, it is cognitively significant that all renates are cordates and vice versa (this was a nontrivial empirical discovery about the world), so that 'renate' and 'cordate' should have different Fregean senses. One might naturally suggest that this difference in sense is captured more concretely by a difference in intension and that this pattern generalizes. For example, one might suppose that when two singular terms are cognitively equivalent (so that '$a = b$' is trivial or at least knowable a priori, for example), then their extension will coincide in all possible worlds, so they will have the same intension. One might also suppose that when two such terms are cognitively distinct (so that '$a = b$' is knowable only empirically, for example), then their extensions will differ in some possible world, so they will have different intensions. If this were the case, the distinction between intension and extension could be seen as a sort of vindication of a Fregean distinction between sense and reference.

However, the work of Kripke (1980) is widely taken to show that no such vindication is possible. According to Kripke, there are many statements that are knowable only empirically but are true in all possible worlds. For example, it is an empirical discovery that Hesperus is Phosphorus, but there is no possible world in which Hesperus is not Phosphorus (or vice versa), as both Hesperus and Phosphorus are identical to the planet Venus in all possible worlds. If so, then 'Hesperus' and 'Phosphorus' have the same intension (one that picks out the planet Venus in all possible worlds), even though the two terms are cognitively distinct. The same goes for pairs of terms such as 'water' and 'H_2O'. It is an empirical discovery that water is H_2O, but according to Kripke, both 'water' and 'H_2O' have the same intension (picking out H_2O in all possible worlds). Something similar even applies to terms such as 'I' and 'David Chalmers,' at least as used by me on a specific occasion: 'I am David Chalmers' expresses nontrivial empirical knowledge, but Kripke's analysis entails that I am David Chalmers in all worlds, so my utterances of these expressions have the same intension. If this is correct, then intensions are strongly dissociated from cognitive significance.

Still, there is a strong intuition that the members of these pairs ('Hesperus' and 'Phosphorus,' 'water' and 'H_2O,' 'I' and 'David Chalmers') differ in some aspect of meaning. Further, there remains a strong intuition that there is *some* way the world could turn out so that these terms would refer to different things. For example, it seems to be at least *epistemically* possible (in some broad sense) that these terms might fail to corefer. On the face of it, cognitive differences between the terms are connected in some fashion to the existence of these possibilities. So it is natural to continue to use an analysis in terms of possibility and necessity to capture aspects of these cognitive differences. This is perhaps the guiding idea behind two-dimensional semantics.

Two-dimensional approaches to semantics start from the observation that the extension and even the intension of many of our expressions depend in some fashion on the external world. As things have turned out, my terms 'water' and 'H_2O' have the same extension and the same (Kripkean) intension. But there are ways things could have turned out so that the two terms could have had different extensions and different Kripkean intensions. So there is a sense in which for a term like 'water,' the term's extension and its Kripkean intension depend on the character of our world. Given that *this* world is actual, it turns out that water is H_2O, and its Kripkean intension picks out H_2O in all possible worlds. However, if another world had been actual (e.g., Putnam's Twin Earth world, in which XYZ is the clear liquid in the oceans), 'water' might have referred to something quite different (e.g., XYZ), and it might have had an entirely different Kripkean intension (e.g., one that picks out XYZ in all worlds).

This suggests a natural formalization. If an expression's (Kripkean) intension itself depends on the character of the world, then we can represent this dependence by a function from worlds to intensions. As intensions are themselves functions from worlds to extensions, this naturally suggests a two-dimensional structure. We can represent this structure diagramatically as follows:

	H_2O world	XYZ world	. . .
H_2O world	H_2O	H_2O	. . .
XYZ world	XYZ	XYZ	. . .
. . .	. . .	. . .	. . .

This diagram expresses an aspect of the two-dimensional structure associated with the term 'water.' It is intended to express the intuitive idea that if the H_2O world turns out to be actual (as it has), then 'water' will have a Kripkean intension that picks out H_2O in all worlds, but if the XYZ world turns out to be actual (as it has not), then 'water' will have a Kripkean intension that picks out XYZ in all worlds. Intuitively, the worlds in the column on the left represent ways the actual world can turn out (these are sometimes thought of more precisely as possible contexts of utterances and sometimes as epistemic possibilities), while the worlds across the top reflect counterfactual ways that a world could have been (these are sometimes thought of more precisely as possible circumstances of evaluation and sometimes as metaphysical possibilities). It is sometimes said that worlds on the left column (one world per row), making up the "first dimension" of the matrix, correspond to different worlds *considered as actual*, while the worlds in the top row (one world per column), making up the "second dimension" of the matrix, correspond to different worlds *considered as counterfactual*.

This two-dimensional matrix can be seen as a *two-dimensional intension*: a function from ordered pairs of worlds to extensions. Such a function is equivalent to a function from worlds to intensions and, seen this way, can be regarded as capturing the intuitive idea that a term's intension depends on the character of the actual world. One can also recover the intuitive idea that a term's *extension* depends on the character of the actual world by examining the "diagonal" of this matrix: the cells that correspond to the same world considered as actual and as counterfactual. In the earlier example, where the H_2O world is considered as actual and as counterfactual, then 'water' picks out H_2O, while if the XYZ world is considered as actual and as counterfactual, then 'water' picks out XYZ. We can say that an expression's *primary intension* is a function mapping a world w to the term's extension when w is taken as both actual and as counterfactual. So the primary intension of 'water' maps the H_2O world to H_2O, the XYZ world to XYZ, and so on.

We can then see how pairs of terms with the same extension and the same Kripkean intension might nevertheless have different two-dimensional intensions and different diagonal intensions. For example, 'water' and 'H_2O' have the same Kripkean intension, but it is plausible that if the XYZ world had turned out to be actual, they would have had different Kripkean intensions. 'Water' would have had an intension that picked out XYZ in all worlds, while 'H_2O' would still have had an intension that picked out H_2O in all worlds. If so, then these terms have different two-dimensional intensions and different diagonal intensions.

One can make a case that something similar applies with 'Hesperus' and 'Phosphorus' and with 'I' and 'David Chalmers': the members of each pair have a different two-dimensional intension and a different primary intension. If so, then this begins to suggest that there is some sort of connection between an expression's two-dimensional intension (or perhaps its diagonal intension) and its cognitive significance. One might even speculate that an expression's diagonal intension behaves in some respects like a Fregean sense, so that a version of Carnap's project might be vindicated.

A number of different two-dimensional approaches to semantics have been developed in the literature by Kaplan (1979, 1989), Stalnaker (1978), Chalmers (1996, 2002a, 2004a), and Jackson (1998), among others, and closely related two-dimensional analyses of modal notions have been put forward by Evans (1979) and by Davies and Humberstone (1981). These approaches differ greatly in the way that they make the foregoing intuitive ideas precise. They differ, for example, in just what they take the "worlds" in the left column to be, and they differ in their analysis of how a term's intension and/or extension depends on the character of the actual world. As a result, different approaches associate these terms with quite different sorts of two-dimensional semantic values, and these semantic values have quite different connections to cognitive significance. In many cases, the connection is limited in scope, applying to indexicals (Kaplan), to descriptive names (Evans), and to expressions that involve 'actually' (Davies and Humberstone), while Stalnaker's later work rejects a connection to apriority altogether.[1]

2. Two-Dimensionalism

In recent years, a number of philosophers (e.g., Chalmers 1996, 2002a, 2004a; Jackson 1998, 2004; see also Braddon-Mitchell 2004; Lewis 1994; Wong 1996) have advocated a two-dimensional approach on which first-dimensional semantic values are connected to apriority and cognitive significance in a much stronger and more general way. On this approach, the framework applies not just to indexicals and descriptive names but also to expressions of all sorts. Proponents hold that any expression (or at least any expression token of the sort that is a candidate for having an extension) can be associated with an intension that is strongly tied to the role of the expression in reasoning and thought. The term *two-dimensionalism* is often used for views of this sort.

Five core claims of two-dimensionalism are as follows:

---

1. *I have omitted a section of the original version of this chapter that discusses these four alternative two-dimensional frameworks in more detail. This material can be found at http://consc.net/papers/twodim.pdf. A more extensive discussion of alternative two-dimensional frameworks can be found in Chalmers (2006).

(T1) Every expression token (of the sort that is a candidate to have an extension) is associated with a primary intension, a secondary intension, and a two-dimensional intension. A primary intension is a function from scenarios to extensions. A secondary intension is a function from possible worlds to extensions. A two-dimensional intension is a function from ordered pairs of scenarios and worlds to extensions.

(T2) When the extension of a complex expression token depends compositionally on the extensions of its part, the value of each of its intensions at an index (world, scenario, or ordered pair) depends in the same way on the values of the corresponding intensions of its parts at that index.

(T3) The extension of an expression token coincides with the value of its primary intension at the scenario of utterance and with the value of the secondary intension at the world of utterance.

(T4) A sentence token S is metaphysically necessary iff the secondary intension of S is true at all worlds.

(T5) A sentence token S is a priori (epistemically necessary) iff the primary intension of S is true at all scenarios.

In what follows I first clarify and motivate these principles without precisely defining all of the key notions or making a case for their truth. In later sections, I discuss how the relevant notions (especially the notion of a primary intension) can be defined in such a way that the principles might be true. These principles should not be taken to provide an exhaustive characterization of two-dimensionalism, but they lie at the core of the view.

Start with claim (T1). Here, a scenario is something akin to a possible world, but it need not be a possible world. In the most common two-dimensionalist treatments, a scenario is a *centered world*: an ordered triple of a possible world along with an individual and a time in that world. Other treatments of scenarios are possible (see Chalmers 2004), but I will use this understanding here.

An expression's secondary intension (or what Jackson calls its C-intension) is just its familiar post-Kripkean intension, picking out the extension of the expression in counterfactual worlds. For example, the secondary intension of a token of 'I' as used by speaker A picks out A in all worlds. The secondary intension of 'water' picks out H_2O in all worlds. The secondary intension of 'Julius' (Evans' term that rigidly designates whoever invented the zip) picks out William C. Whitworth in all worlds. More generally, any rigid designator picks out the same object in all worlds (or at least in all worlds where the object exists).

An expression's primary intension works quite differently. I defer a full characterization, but some examples give a rough idea. The primary intension of a token of 'I,' evaluated at a centered world, picks out the designated individual at the "center" of that world. (So the primary intension of my use of 'I,' evaluated at a world centered on Napoleon, picks out Napoleon rather than David Chalmers.) The primary intension of a token of 'water,' very roughly, picks out the clear, drinkable liquid with which the individual at the center is acquainted. (So the primary intension of my use of 'water,' evaluated at a "Twin Earth" world centered on a subject surrounded by XYZ in the oceans and lakes, picks out XYZ rather than H_2O.) The primary intension of a token of 'Julius' picks out whoever invented the zip in a given world. (So the primary intension of 'Julius,' evaluated at a world where Tiny Tim invented the zip, picks out Tiny Tim rather than William C. Whitworth.) And so on.

Thesis (T1) also holds that expression tokens can be associated with a *two-dimensional intension*: roughly, a function from <scenario, world> pairs to extensions. We can then say that at least on the understanding of scenarios as centered worlds, the primary intension coincides with the "diagonal" of the two-dimensional intension (i.e., the value of S's primary intension in a centered world w coincides with the value of S's two-dimensional intension at the pair $<w, w^*>$, where w^* is the possible-world element of w). Likewise, the secondary intension coincides with the "row" of the two-dimensional intension determined by the scenario of an utterance (i.e., the value of S's secondary intension at a world w coincides with the value of S's two-dimensional intension at $<a, w>$, where a is the scenario of utterance). However, for most purposes the two-dimensional intension of an expression is somewhat less important than its primary and secondary intensions, and the two-dimensionalist need not hold that an expression's primary and secondary intensions are derivative from its two-dimensional intension.

Thesis (T2) says that the primary and secondary intensions of a complex expression depend on the primary and secondary intensions of its parts according to the natural compositional semantics. For example, the primary intension of 'I am Julius' will be true at a scenario if the individual at the center of that scenario is the inventor of the zip in that scenario.

Thesis (T3) states a natural connection between the intensions and the extension of an expression token. This thesis requires that for every utterance, just as there is one world that is the world of the utterance, there is also one scenario that is the scenario of the utterance. If scenarios are understood as centered worlds, this will be a world centered on the speaker and the time of the utterance. When evaluated at the scenario and world of utterance, the primary and secondary intensions (respectively) of an expression token will coincide with the extension of the expression token. At other worlds and scenarios, however, the values of these intensions may diverge from the original extension and from each other.

Turning to claims (T4) and (T5): here, we can say that S is a priori when it expresses a thought that can be justified independently of experiences. S is metaphysically necessary when it is true with respect to all counterfactual worlds (under the standard Kripkean evaluation). Thesis (T4) is a consequence of the standard understanding of metaphysical necessity and the corresponding intensions. Thesis (T5) is intended to be an analog of thesis (T4) in the epistemic domain.

Thesis (T5) is the distinctive claim of two-dimensionalism. It asserts a very strong and general connection between primary intensions and apriority, one much stronger than obtains with the other two-dimensional frameworks discussed earlier. It is possible that a two-dimensionalist might grant some limited exceptions to thesis (T5) (say, for certain complex mathematical statements that are true but unknowable) while still remaining recognizably two dimensionalist. However, it is crucial to the two-dimensionalist position that typical a posteriori identities involving proper names or natural kind terms, such as 'Mark Twain is Samuel Clemens' or 'water is H_2O,' have a primary intension that is false in some scenario.

Consequences of the previous theses include the following:

(T6) A sentence token S is necessary a posteriori iff the secondary intension of S is true at all worlds but the primary intension of S is false at some scenario.

(T7) A sentence token S is contingent a priori iff the primary intension of S is true at all scenarios but the secondary intension of S is false at some world.

So two-dimensionalism proposes a unified analysis of the necessary a posteriori: all such sentences have a necessary secondary intension but a contingent primary intension. Likewise, it proposes a unified analysis of the contingent a priori: all such sentences have a contingent primary intension but a necessary secondary intension.

From the previous theses, one can also draw the following conclusions about the primary and secondary intensions of both sentential and subsentential expressions. Here A and B are arbitrary expressions of the same type, and '$A\equiv B$' is a sentence that is true iff A and B have the same extension. For example, if A and B are singular terms, '$A\equiv B$' is just the identity statement '$A=B$,' while if A and B are sentences, '$A\equiv B$' is the biconditional 'A iff B.'

(T8) '$A\equiv B$' is metaphysically necessary iff A and B have the same secondary intension.

(T9) '$A\equiv B$' is a priori (epistemically necessary) iff A and B have the same primary intension.

It follows that for a posteriori necessary identities involving proper names, such as 'Mark Twain is Samuel Clemens,' the two names involved will have the same secondary intensions but different primary intensions. Something similar applies to kind identities such as 'water is H_2O.' If this is correct, then primary intensions behave in these cases in a manner somewhat reminiscent of a Fregean sense.

3. Epistemic Two-Dimensionalism

For these claims, especially claim (T5), to be grounded, we need to have a better idea of what primary intensions are. Clearly, they must differ from the two-dimensional notions such as Kaplan's characters and Stalnaker's diagonal propositions, at least as these are understood by their proponents. Here, I outline one approach (the approach I favor) to understanding primary intensions. This approach, which we might call *epistemic two-dimensionalism*, is elaborated in much greater detail in other works (Chalmers 2002a, 2004a, 2006).

According to epistemic two-dimensionalism, the connection between primary intension and epistemic notions such as apriority requires that primary intensions be characterized in epistemic terms from the start. On this approach, the scenarios that are in the domain of a primary intension do not represent contexts of utterance. Rather, they represent *epistemic possibilities*: highly specific hypotheses about the character of our world that are not ruled out a priori. The value of an expression's primary intension at a scenario reflects a speaker's rational judgments involving the expression under the hypothesis that the epistemic possibility in question actually obtains.

For example, 'water is not H_2O' is epistemically possible in the sense that its truth is not ruled out a priori. Correspondingly, it is epistemically possible that our world is the XYZ world (or at least that it is qualitatively just like the XYZ world). If we suppose that our world is the XYZ world (that is, that the liquid in the oceans and lakes is XYZ and so on), then we should rationally endorse the claim 'water is XYZ,' and we should rationally reject the claim 'water is H_2O.' So the primary intension of 'water is H_2O' is false at the XYZ world, and the primary intension of 'water is XYZ' is true there.

Likewise, 'Mark Twain is not Samuel Clemens' is epistemically possible in the sense that it is not ruled out a priori. Correspondingly, it is epistemically possible that our world is a world w where one person wrote the books such as *Tom Sawyer* that we associate with the name 'Mark Twain' and a quite distinct person is causally connected to our use of the term 'Samuel Clemens.' If we suppose that w is our world, then we should rationally endorse the claim 'Mark Twain is not Samuel Clemens.' So the primary intension of 'Mark Twain is Samuel Clemens' is false at w.

According to two-dimensionalism, something similar applies to any Kripkean a posteriori necessity. For any such sentence S, $\sim S$ is epistemically possible. It is also plausible that for any such S, there is a world w such that if we suppose that our world is qualitatively like w, we should rationally reject S. If so, then the primary intension of S is false at w. If this pattern generalizes to all a posteriori necessary sentences, then any such sentence has a primary intension that is false at some scenario, as thesis (T6) suggests.

Here, primary intensions are characterized in thoroughly epistemic terms. The preceding claims are not in tension with the Kripkean claims that 'water is H_2O' is metaphysically necessary or that 'water' picks out H_2O in all worlds. Even Kripke allows that 'water is not H_2O' is *epistemically* possible. As chapter 7 notes, it is a familiar Kripkean point that there can be an epistemic necessitation between two statements A and B even when there is no metaphysical necessitation between them (witness 'X is the source of heat sensations' and 'X is heat'). We simply have to strongly distinguish this sort of epistemic evaluation of sentences in worlds (which turns on epistemic necessitation) from the usual sort of counterfactual evaluation (which turns on metaphysical necessitation). Primary intensions are grounded in the former; secondary intensions are grounded in the latter.

4. Defining Primary Intensions

It remains to define primary intensions more precisely. To generalize from the foregoing, we might suggest that the primary intension of a sentence S

is true at a scenario w iff the hypothesis that w is actual should lead us to rationally endorse S. Somewhat more carefully, we can say that the primary intension of S is true at a scenario w iff D epistemically necessitates S, where D is a canonical specification of w. It remains to clarify the notion of a scenario, a canonical specification, and epistemic necessitation.

Scenarios are highly specific epistemic possibilities. In the centered-worlds version of epistemic two-dimensionalism, scenarios are identified with centered worlds.

For any possible world w, it is epistemically possible that w is actual, or at least it is epistemically possible that a world qualitatively identical to w is actual. (More precisely, it is epistemically possible that D is the case, where D is a canonical specification of w, in a sense I will discuss shortly.) However, epistemic possibilities are more fine grained than possible worlds. For example, the information that the actual world is qualitatively like a possible world w is epistemically consistent with various different epistemic possible claims about one's self-location. For example, it is consistent with the claims 'It is now 2004' and 'It is now 2005.'

To handle these claims about self-location, we model epistemic possibilities using centered worlds. The individual and the time marked at the "center" of a centered world serve as a "you are here" marker, which serves to settle these claims about self-location. For a given thinker, the hypothesis that a given centered world w is actual can be seen as the following hypothesis: 'D is the case, I am F, and the current time is G,' where D is a canonical specification of the uncentered world corresponding to w and F and G are semantically neutral descriptions that pick out the individual and the time at the center of w. We can think of this conjunctive claim as a canonical specification of the centered world w.

A canonical specification of an uncentered world w is a complete specification of w in semantically neutral vocabulary. To a first approximation, a semantically neutral vocabulary is one that is free of terms (such as names and natural kind terms) that give rise to Kripkean a posteriori necessities and a priori contingencies. (Restricting world specifications to a vocabulary of this sort avoids obvious problems that would arise if we allowed, for example, 'water is H_2O' into the specification of the XYZ world. For more on the characterization of semantic neutrality, see Chalmers 2006.) A complete specification of w is a sentence D such that (i) D is true of w, and (ii) if E is a semantically neutral sentence that is true of w, then D epistemically necessitates E.

We also need to define epistemic necessitation. To a first approximation, we can say that D epistemically necessitates S iff accepting D should lead one to rationally endorse S (without needing further empirical information, given idealized reflection). On a refined definition, we can say that D epistemically necessitates S iff a conditional of the form '$D \supset S$' is a priori. The refined definition is arguably better in some difficult cases, but for many purposes, the first approximation will suffice.

Because they are defined in epistemic terms, there is an in-built connection between primary intensions and the epistemic domain. In particular, there will be a strong connection to apriority. When a sentence token S is a priori, then it will be epistemically necessitated by any sentence whatsoever (this is especially clear for the second understanding of epistemic necessitation given earlier), so its primary intension will be true in all scenarios. When a sentence token S is not a priori, then its negation will be epistemically possible, and S will be false relative to some highly specific epistemic possibility. As long as there is a scenario for every epistemic possibility, then the primary intension of S will be false in some scenario. If so, then thesis (T5) will be correct.

Still, on the centered-world understanding of scenarios, thesis (T5) is nontrivial and is denied by some philosophers for reasons discussed in chapter 6 (sections 6–8). Some hold that there are more conceivable scenarios than centered metaphysically possible worlds. For example, some hold that 'There is an omniscient being' is conceivably false (it is not a priori) but is true at all centered worlds. If so, then sentences like these are counterexamples to (T5). Similar potential counterexamples arise from conceivable situations involving zombies, according to the type-B materialist. I argue in chapter 6 that there are no such counterexamples and that a conceivability-possibility thesis (CP– in the language of chapter 6) equivalent to (T5) is true, but the issue is controversial.

Alternatively, there is a version of epistemic two-dimensionalism in which scenarios are more strongly dissociated from ordinary possible worlds. On this approach, scenarios are understood in more purely epistemic terms as maximally specific epistemic possibilities. They can be constructed as maximal a priori consistent sets of sentences in an ideal language. On this construction, thesis (T5) is all but guaranteed to be true. For example, even if it is necessary that there is an omniscient being, as long as it is not a priori that there is an omniscient being, there will be scenarios in which 'There is no omniscient being' is true. Likewise, if it is not ruled out a priori that there are zombies, there will be scenarios in which 'There are zombies' is true.

The epistemic construction of scenarios allows many of the semantic and epistemological benefits of two-dimensionalism even for those who are skeptical about associated metaphysical claims. So for the semantic and epistemological purposes of chapters 8, 9, 11, and 12, this construction is at least as useful as the centered-world construction. For the metaphysical purposes of chapter 6, the centered-world construction is crucial. In what follows, I largely use the centered-world construction for reasons of familiarity and concreteness, but most of what I say can easily be translated to the epistemic construction.

One can define the secondary intension of a sentence in a similar, if more familiar, way. The secondary intension of S is true at a world w iff D metaphysically necessitates S, where D is a canonical specification of w. Here a canonical specification can be characterized much as before, although it is not necessary to impose the restriction to semantically neutral vocabulary. Metaphysical necessitation could be taken as basic, or perhaps better, we can define it in terms of subjunctive conditionals: D metaphysically necessitates S when a subjunctive conditional of the form 'if D had been the case, S would have been the case' is true.

One can likewise define the two-dimensional intension of a sentence. The two-dimensional intension of S is true at $<v, w>$ iff D epistemically necessitates that D' metaphysically necessitates S, where D is a canonical specification of the scenario v and D' is a canonical specification of the world w. If we understand epistemic necessitation in terms of a priori material conditionals and metaphysical necessitation in terms of subjunctive conditionals, this will be the case iff '$D \supset (D' \Rightarrow S)$' is a priori, where the outer conditional is material and the inner conditional is subjunctive.

This discussion of the intensions of sentences can be extended to the intensions of subsentential expressions in a reasonably straightforward way. For details, see Chalmers 2006.

5. The Roots of Epistemic Two-Dimensionalism

The epistemic two-dimensional framework is grounded in a thesis about the *scrutability* of reference and truth. This is a version of the thesis discussed in section 3 of chapter 7: once subjects are given enough information about the character of the actual world, then they are in a position to make rational judgments about what their expressions refer to and whether their utterances are true. For example, once we are given enough information about the appearance, behavior, composition, and distribution of various substances in our environment, as well as about their relations to us, then we are in a position to conclude (without needing further empirical information) that water is H_2O. And if instead we are given quite different information, characterizing our environment as a "Twin Earth" environment, then we will be in a position to conclude that water is XYZ.

Of course, if we allow the "enough information" to include arbitrary truths, such as 'water is H_2O,' the scrutability claim will be trivial. But we can impose significant restrictions on the information without compromising the plausibility of the thesis. For example, one can argue that even if we restrict ourselves to truths that do not use the term 'water' or cognates, it remains the case that given enough truths of this kind, we are in a position to know the truth of 'water is H_2O' (see chapter 6). The same goes for many or most other terms, plausibly including most names or natural kind terms.

The upshot is that there is some reasonably restricted vocabulary V, such that for arbitrary statements T, then once we know enough V-truths, we will be in a position to know (without needing further empirical information) the truth value of T. Just how restricted such a vocabulary can be is an open question. Chapter 7 argues that $PQTI$, a conjunction of microphysical, phenomenal, and indexical truths along with a "that's all" truth, can serve as a basis, but this claim is not required here. All that is required for present purposes is that some semantically neutral vocabulary, conjoined with indexical terms such as 'I' and 'now,' is sufficient.[2]

This suggests that for any true sentence token S, there is a V-truth D such that D epistemically necessitates S, in that a subject given the information that D will be in a position to rationally endorse S (given ideal rational reflection). Furthermore, it appears that in principle, no further empirical information is needed to make this judgment; if such information were required, we could simply include it (or equivalent qualitative information) in D to start with. This strongly suggests that there is a nonempirical warrant for the transition from D to S. In particular, one can make the case that in these cases, the material conditional '$D \supset S$' will be a priori. (This case is made at length in chapter 7.) If this is correct, then D epistemically necessitates S in the second, stronger sense given earlier.

---

2. As before, a semantically neutral vocabulary is one that excludes terms, such as names and natural kind terms, that give rise to Kripkean a posteriori necessities. A qualitative vocabulary may include all sorts of high-level expressions: 'friend,' 'philosopher,' 'action,' 'believe,' and 'square,' for example. It will not designate individuals by using names: instead it will make existential claims of the form 'there exist such-and-such individuals with such-and-such qualitative properties.' Some theoretical terms (perhaps including microphysical terms) may be excluded, but information conveyed using these terms can instead be conveyed by the familiar Ramsey-sentence method, characterizing a network of entities and properties with appropriate causal/nomic connections to each other and to the observational and the phenomenal. For familiar reasons, no important information is lost by doing this.

The scrutability claim does not apply only to the actual world. It is plausible that for all sorts of scenarios, if we are given the information that the scenario is actual, then we are in a position to make a rational judgment about the truth value of arbitrary sentences. For example, if we are given a complete qualitative characterization of the bodies visible in the sky at various times, with the feature that no body is visible both in the morning sky and the evening sky, then we should rationally reject the claim 'Hesperus is Phosphorus.' This sort of judgment is part of the *inferential role* associated with our use of the terms 'Hesperus' and 'Phosphorus.' The point is general: for any expression we use, then given sufficient information about the actual world, certain judgments using the expression will be irrational, and certain other judgments using the expression will be rational. It is arguable that the expressions of any language user will have this sort of normative inferential role. This is just part of what being a language user involves.

It is this sort of inferential role that grounds the primary intension of an arbitrary expression (as used by an arbitrary speaker). A given sentence token will be associated with a raft of conditional rational judgments across a wide variety of scenarios. This raft of conditional judgments corresponds to the sentence's primary intension. Something very similar applies to subsentential expressions. For a singular term, for example, there will be a raft of conditional rational judgments using the expression across a wide variety of scenarios, and these can be used to define the extension of the expression relative to those scenarios (see Chalmers 2006), so we will have substantial primary intensions for a wide range of sentential and subsentential expression tokens.

For reasons discussed in chapter 6, nothing here requires that the expressions in question be definable in simpler terms (such as in semantically neutral terms) or that they be equivalent to descriptions (even to rigidified descriptions or descriptions involving "actually"). The inferential roles in question will exist whether or not the term is definable and whether or not it is equivalent to a description.

These claims are quite compatible with Kripke's epistemological argument that terms such as 'Gödel' are not equivalent to descriptions. In effect, Kripke describes a scenario w, where someone called 'Schmidt' proved the incompleteness of arithmetic, and then it was stolen by someone called 'Gödel,' who moved to Princeton, and so on. Kripke's argument might be put by saying that (i) w is not ruled out a priori, and (ii) if we accept that w obtains, we should reject the claim 'Gödel proved the incompleteness of arithmetic,' so (iii) 'Gödel proved the incompleteness of arithmetic' is not a priori. A two-dimensionalist will put this by saying that the primary intension of 'Gödel proved the incompleteness of arithmetic' is false at w, so that the primary intension of 'Gödel' differs from that of 'the prover of the incompleteness of arithmetic.' If Kripke's argument generalizes to other descriptions, it will follow that the primary intension of Gödel is not equivalent to the primary intension of any such description. But nothing here begins to suggest that 'Gödel' lacks a primary intension.

Although the primary intension of an expression may not be equivalent to that of a description, one can often at least approximately characterize an expression's primary intension by using a description. For example, one might roughly characterize the primary intension of a typical use of 'water' by saying that in a centered world w, it picks out the dominant clear, drinkable liquid with which the individual at the center of w is acquainted. One might also roughly characterize the primary intension of 'Gödel' by saying that it picks out that individual who was called 'Gödel' by those from whom the individual at the center acquired the name. However, these characterizations will usually be imperfect, and it will be possible to find Kripke-style counterexamples to them. Ultimately, a primary intension is not grounded in any description but rather is grounded in an expression's inferential role.

6. Two-Dimensionalism and Semantic Pluralism

Two-dimensionalism is naturally combined with a *semantic pluralism*, according to which expressions and utterances can be associated with many different semantic (or quasi-semantic) values by many different semantic (or quasi-semantic) relations.[3] On this view, there should be no question about whether the primary intension of the secondary intension is *the* content of an utterance. Both can be systematically associated with utterances, and both can play some of the roles that we want contents to play. Furthermore, there will certainly be explanatory roles that neither one plays, so two-dimensionalism should not be seen as offering an exhaustive account of the content of an utterance. Rather, it is characterizing some aspects of utterance content that can play a useful role in the epistemic and modal domains.

Likewise, there should be no question about which of the two-dimensional frameworks that have been developed by various theorists is the "correct" framework. Each framework offers a different quasi-semantic relation that associates expressions with two-dimensional semantic values,

---

3. *Semantic pluralism is closely akin to the content pluralism discussed in chapter 12, except that it applies to linguistic expressions rather than to mental states.

and each of these may play an explanatory role in different domains. Each
has different properties. Most importantly, primary intensions have a
stronger connection to apriority and cognitive significance than the semantic values described earlier. These differences arise from the differences in
the way the semantic relations are defined. Kaplan and Stalnaker define
their two-dimensional notions in terms of certain sorts of context-
dependence, while Evans defines his notions in terms of a prior notion of
content and Davies and Humberstone define theirs in terms of the behavior of an 'actually' operator. Primary intensions are not defined in any of
these ways but instead are defined in epistemic terms. Because they are
defined in epistemic terms, primary intensions can often vary between
tokens of an expression type. This will happen most obviously for context-
dependent terms such as 'tall,' for which tokens in different contexts will
be associated with different inferential roles. Primary intensions may also
vary among different tokens of the same name (especially by different
speakers), for different tokens of the same demonstrative (e.g., 'this' or
'that'), and perhaps also for different tokens of the same natural kind term.
It follows that, in these cases, a primary intension does not constitute an
expression's linguistic meaning, where this is understood as what is common
to all tokens of an expression type or as what is required for any competent
use of the expression. Instead, a primary intension can be seen as a kind of
utterance content.

Even if they are not always part of linguistic meaning, primary intensions are nevertheless a sort of truth-conditional content. The primary intension of an utterance yields a condition under which the utterance will
be true. For example, the primary intension of 'there is water in the glass'
will be true at some scenarios and false at others, and the utterance will be
true iff the primary intension is true at the scenario of the utterance (roughly,
if the glass picked out by the individual at the center of the scenario contains the dominant watery stuff in the environment around the center).
This can be seen as an *epistemic* truth condition for the utterance, specifying
how the truth of the utterance depends (epistemically) on which epistemically possible scenario turns out to be actual. This contrasts with the "metaphysical" truth condition corresponding to the secondary intension, which
might be seen as specifying how the truth of the utterance depends (metaphysically) on which metaphysically possible world is actual. Again, there is
no need to decide the question of which of these is *the* truth condition
associated with an utterance.

Are primary intensions a sort of semantic content? This depends on how
we understand the notion of semantic content. If we stipulate that the
semantic content of an utterance is truth-conditional content, then

primary intensions are a variety of semantic content. On the other hand, if we stipulate that semantic content is linguistic meaning in the sense just discussed or that semantic content is always associated with expression types and not tokens, then primary intensions are not in general part of semantic content (though they may be part of semantic content for some expressions, such as some indexicals and qualitative expressions). In any case, once we are clear on the various properties of these intensions, nothing important to the framework turns on the terminological question of whether they count as "semantic."

A semantic pluralist can allow that for some explanatory purposes it may be useful to modify two-dimensionalist semantic values in some respects. For example, one might define the *structured* primary intension of a complex expression as a structured entity involving the primary intensions of the simple expressions involved in the expression's logical form. One might likewise define structured secondary and two-dimensional intensions. Given compositionality, a structured primary intension will determine an unstructured primary intension (and likewise for the other intensions), but the reverse need not be the case. This means that structured primary intensions are finer grained than unstructured primary intensions. For example, all a priori truths will have the same unstructured primary intension (one that is true at all scenarios), but they will have different structured primary intensions. The fine-grainedness of structured intensions makes a difference for certain purposes, described later.

What are *propositions*, according to two-dimensionalism? Some two-dimensionalists (e.g., Jackson 1998) hold that propositions are sets of possible worlds, in which case a given utterance expresses two propositions (a primary proposition and a secondary proposition). This view is naturally combined with the view that there are no necessary a posteriori propositions: necessary a posteriori sentences have both a primary proposition that is contingent and knowable only a posteriori and a secondary proposition that is necessary and knowable a priori. Other two-dimensionalists may hold that propositions have more structure than this. For example, one could hold that propositions are structured entities involving both the primary and the secondary intensions (and/or perhaps the two-dimensional intension) of the simple expressions involved. A two-dimensionalist of this sort may allow that there are necessary a posteriori propositions.

A semantic pluralist view tends to suggest that there are numerous entities that can play some of the explanatory roles that propositions are supposed to play and that there is no need to settle which of these best deserves the label 'proposition.' My own view (see Chalmers forthcoming) is that if one has to identify propositions with one sort of entity that can be modeled in the framework, there is a good case for choosing structured two-dimensional entities of some sort and in particular those discussed as candidates for Fregean senses in the following section. However, one might also allow that, at least for some purposes, propositions should be seen as entities that are finer grained than any two-dimensional objects, so that propositions can be associated with intensions without themselves being intensions. In any case, core two-dimensionalism as characterized earlier is compatible with a wide range of views here.

7. Applications of Two-Dimensionalism

I will briefly sketch some applications of the two-dimensionalism outlined in the previous section.

(i) *Fregean sense* (Chalmers 2002b, forthcoming). Thesis (T9) says that two expressions A and B have the same primary intensions iff '$A{\equiv}B$' is epistemically necessary. This is reminiscent of the Fregean claim that two singular terms a and b have the same sense iff '$a{=}b$' is cognitively insignificant. It suggests that primary intensions can play at least some of the roles of a Fregean sense, individuating expressions by their epistemic role. Of course, there are some differences. For example, primary intensions are not as fine grained as Fregean senses: a priori equivalent expressions (such as '7+3' and '10') will have different Fregean senses, but they have the same primary intension (though they will usually have different structured primary intensions). Further, there are differences between primary intensions and Fregean senses in the case of indexicals. For example, uses of 'I' by different speakers have the same primary intension, whereas Frege held that they have different senses. Relatedly, where Frege held that sense determines reference, primary intensions do not determine extensions in a strong sense (although they may still determine extension relative to context), as two expressions may have the same primary intensions and different extensions. Still, one may nevertheless think of primary intensions as a broadly Fregean aspect of an expression's content.

One can also use the two-dimensional framework to define semantic values that behave more like Frege's own senses. We might stipulate that the sense of a simple expression token is an ordered pair of its primary intension and its extension (that is, an ordered pair of its Fregean and Russellian content, as explicated in chapter 11) and that the sense of a complex expression token is a structured complex made up of the senses of its parts. Now, most pairs of a priori equivalent expressions, such as

'7+3' and '10,' will have different senses. (The only potential exceptions will arise if there are a priori equivalent but cognitively distinct simple expressions, which is not obvious.) Furthermore, uses of 'I' by different speakers will have different senses. And now, sense determines reference in the strong sense. So entities of this sort might be seen as very much akin to Fregean senses, and we might think of the structured entity associated with a sentence token as akin to a Fregean thought. See Chalmers (forthcoming) for much more on this.

(ii) *Contents of thoughts* (Chalmers 2002a). One can extend the earlier framework so that primary and secondary intensions are not just associated with sentences but also with thoughts, where these are understood as occurrent mental states. For example, my thought *water is H_2O* will have a contingent primary intension (false in the XYZ scenario) but a necessary secondary intension. One can then argue that a thought's primary intension is a sort of *narrow content*: content that is shared between intrinsically identical thinkers. For example, when Oscar on Earth and Twin Oscar on Twin Earth say 'water is wet,' the thoughts they express will have different secondary intensions (so secondary intensions are a sort of "wide content"), but they will have the same primary intension.

(iii) *Conceivability and possibility* (chapter 6). If thesis (T5) is correct, it licenses a certain sort of move from conceivability to possibility. Let us say that S is conceivable when it is epistemically possible: that is, when S is not ruled out a priori. If (T5) is correct, then when S is conceivable, the primary intension of S will be true in some scenario. If scenarios are centered worlds, then there will be some centered (metaphysically possible) world w satisfying the primary intension of S. This does not entail that S is metaphysically possible, but it nevertheless allows us to draw conclusions about metaphysically possible worlds from premises about conceivability. As discussed in chapter 6, reasoning of this sort is central to some uses of conceivability arguments in the philosophy of mind.

8. Objections to Two-Dimensionalism

A number of objections to two-dimensionalism have been made in the literature. Some objections (the first eight considered here) rest on the attribution of views to which two-dimensionalism is not committed. They might be considered objections to certain versions of two-dimensionalism, but they do not apply to the epistemic two-dimensionalism that I have outlined. Other objections (the next two considered here) show that the claims of two-dimensionalism must be restricted in certain respects. Still others (the last three considered here) raise substantive issues whose adjudication is an ongoing project.

What is held constant? (Block and Stalnaker 1999). Evaluation of primary intensions turns on claims about what a term such as 'water' would have picked out in counterfactual circumstances. This raises the question of what is held constant across worlds in counting an expression as a token of 'water.' If only orthography is held constant, then many tokens of 'water is watery' will be false; if reference is held constant, then no token of 'water is H_2O' will be false. So to yield the desired results, a two-dimensionalist must hold constant some intermediate sort of content, such as Fregean or descriptive or narrow content. But it is question-begging for a two-dimensionalist to presuppose such a notion of content.

Response: Evaluation of primary intensions does not turn on metalinguistic claims about what a term would have picked out in counterfactual circumstances. One could define an expression's *contextual intension* as a mapping from worlds containing a token of the expression to the extension of that token in that world. The question of what is held constant would then become relevant: one would obtain different sorts of contextual intensions depending on just what one counts as a relevant token. But primary intensions are not defined like this. They simply turn on the epistemic properties of an expression in the actual world. For example, it is epistemically possible (not ruled out a priori) that there are no utterances, and so the primary intension of 'There are no utterances' will be true in an utterance-free world (whereas the contextual intension of 'There are no utterances' will not be defined there). Because properties of counterfactual tokens are irrelevant to the evaluation of primary intensions (except in some special cases), the problem of "what is held constant" does not arise.

Twin Earth intuitions are irrelevant (Soames 2004). Intuitions about the reference of 'water' as used on Twin Earth are irrelevant to the meaning of our term 'water,' as the term 'water' on Twin Earth has a different meaning.

Response: Again, evaluation of primary intensions does not depend on the referents of homonymous terms in counterfactual worlds. Rather, it depends on certain epistemic properties associated with uses of 'water' in our world. For example, if we are given the information that the liquid in the oceans and lakes is and has always been XYZ, we should conclude that water is XYZ. This is a fact about the inferential role associated with uses of *our* term 'water.' Epistemic two-dimensionalism uses this inferential role to analyze an aspect of the content of these uses of the term.

Names and natural-kind terms are not indexicals (Nimtz 2004; Soames 2005): Two-dimensionalism entails that terms such as 'water' are really disguised indexicals that can pick out different referents in different contexts. But such terms are not indexicals. Any utterance of the English term 'water' in any context picks out H_2O.

Response: Epistemic two-dimensionalism does not entail that names and natural kind terms are disguised indexicals, and it is consistent with the claim that any utterance of the English term 'water' refers to H_2O. If primary intensions were Kaplanian characters or contextual intensions, then the claim that 'water' refers to H_2O in any context would be inconsistent with the two-dimensionalist claim that the primary intension of 'water' picks out XYZ in the Twin Earth world. However, primary intensions are not Kaplanian characters or contextual intensions. To ground the desired behavior of primary intensions, the two-dimensionalist simply requires the plausible claim that it is *epistemically* possible (i.e., not ruled out a priori) that water is XYZ. This claim is consistent with the claim that (given that 'water' actually refers to H_2O) all metaphysically possible tokens of the English term 'water' refer to H_2O.

Names are not rigidified descriptions (Soames 2005). Two-dimensionalism entails that names and natural kind terms are disguised rigidified descriptions (of the form 'the actual ϕ' for some ϕ). However, Kripke's epistemic arguments show that names are not rigidified descriptions, as do considerations concerning the way that names and descriptions behave in belief ascriptions.

Response: Two-dimensionalism does not entail that names and natural kind terms are rigidified descriptions. I have noted already that Kripke's epistemic arguments are accommodated by the observation that primary intensions cannot always be encapsulated into a description. Furthermore, as noted earlier, it is consistent with two-dimensionalism to hold that names and natural kind terms, unlike rigidified descriptions, have the same referent in any context of utterance. It is also consistent with two-dimensionalism to hold that the primary intension of a name or natural kind term may vary between speakers. The account of belief ascriptions given in Chalmers (2002a) does not entail that names will behave like rigidified descriptions in belief contexts and handles the relevant data straightforwardly.

Speakers lack identifying knowledge (Byrne and Pryor 2005; Schiffer 2003). Two-dimensionalism requires that every name N (at least as used by a speaker) be associated with a "uniqueness property" ϕ (such that at most one individual has ϕ) and also requires that the speaker have a priori "identifying knowledge" of the form 'N is ϕ,' but speakers in general lack this sort of knowledge.

Response: Two-dimensionalism does not require that speakers possess identifying knowledge. It is true that primary intensions can be associated with uniqueness properties (or better, uniqueness relations, because of the role of centering), but speakers need not have beliefs about these uniqueness properties (e.g., of the form '*N* is ϕ'). Epistemic two-dimensionalism simply requires that speakers have a *conditional ability* (of the sort discussed in chapter 7) to determine the referent of *N* (or better, to determine the truth value of claims using *N*), given relevant information about the character of the actual world and given idealized rational reflection. This conditional ability need not be grounded in the possession of identifying knowledge. Furthermore, the invocation of rational reflection makes this a normative claim that idealizes away from the speaker's cognitive limitations. For example, even if children cannot actually identify a referent across all circumstances, there may still be idealized inferential norms on how they should update their relevant beliefs given relevant information about the world. These norms are all that the framework requires.

Ordinary expressions are not ambiguous (Bealer 2002; Marconi 2005). Two-dimensionalism explains the difference in truth value between

1. It is metaphysically necessary that water is H_2O.
2. It is epistemically necessary that water is H_2O.

by saying that 'water' expresses its primary intension in the first context and its secondary intension in the second context, but this entails implausibly that 'water' is ambiguous. Further, this view cannot handle combined contexts such as 'It is metaphysically necessary but not epistemically necessary that water is H_2O.'

Response: Two-dimensionalism does not hold that ordinary expressions are ambiguous. 'Water' has exactly the same content in both 1 and 2. In both contexts (and in all contexts) it has both a primary intension and a secondary intension (or equivalently, it has a complex semantic value involving both a primary and a secondary intension). This does not entail that 'water' is ambiguous any more than the distinction between character and content entails that indexicals are ambiguous. The distinction between 1 and 2 is handled is handled instead by the difference between the modal operators. The semantics of these operators are such that 'It is metaphysically necessary that *S*' is true when *S* has a necessary secondary intension, while 'It is epistemically necessary that *S*' is true when *S* has a necessary primary intension. Combined contexts are handled in the obvious combined way.

Two-dimensionalism cannot handle belief ascriptions (Soames 2005). It is natural for two-dimensionalists to hold that '*x* believes that *S*' is true when the subject has a belief whose primary intension is the primary intension of *S*, but this view gives the wrong result in a number of cases, and no better two-dimensionalist treatment of belief ascriptions is available.

Response: The view of belief ascriptions mentioned here is considered and rejected in Chalmers (2002a), and to the best of my knowledge no two-dimensionalist endorses the view. The account of belief ascriptions developed in Chalmers (2002a, forthcoming) straightforwardly handles most of the puzzle cases developed by Soames.

Two-dimensionalism requires global descriptivism (Stalnaker 2003, 2004). Two-dimensionalism holds that the primary intension of an utterance or a belief is determined by the internal state of the speaker or believer. This requires an internalist "metasemantic" theory, showing how intentional content is determined by internal state. The main candidate for such a theory is the "global descriptivism" of Lewis (1984), which holds that the content of our utterances and beliefs is determined by whatever assignment of content yields the "best fit" between the beliefs and the world. But global descriptivism is false.

Response: Two-dimensionalism does not require global descriptivism. Of course, there is not yet any satisfactory theory of the basis of intentionality, but there are many possible internalist alternatives. For example, one might hold that the primary intension of a mental state is determined in part by its internal functional role and in part by associated phenomenal states (where the latter may be especially relevant for phenomenal and perceptual concepts).

The wrong sentences are a priori: Two-dimensionalism requires the claim that sentences such as 'Hesperus (if it exists) is Phosphorus' are not a priori, while sentences such as 'Julius (if he exists) invented the zip' are a priori. However, these claims are incorrect. The former sentence expresses a trivial singular proposition that can be justified a priori, while the latter sentence expresses a nontrivial singular proposition that cannot be justified a priori.

Response: If one stipulated that apriority of a name-involving sentence is to be understood in terms of the a priori knowability of an associated singular proposition, these (controversial and counterintuitive) claims would be correct. However, the two-dimensionalist takes this as good reason to reject the stipulation or at least stipulates a different understanding of apriority for the purposes of the framework. For these purposes, an utterance can be said to be a priori when it expresses a belief (or at least an occurrent thought) that can be justified nonempirically, yielding a priori knowledge. There is an obvious epistemic difference between beliefs expressed by typical occurrences of 'Hesperus is Hesperus' and 'Hesperus is Phosphorus.' No amount of nonempirical reasoning can convert the latter belief into a priori knowledge, but the former is easily justified a priori. (Note that on this definition of apriority, two different beliefs might be related to the same singular propositional content while differing in their epistemic status: the epistemic status attaches primarily to belief tokens, not to belief types or to propositional contents.) This epistemic difference at the level of thought can be used to ground the relevant claims about the apriority of utterances. More generally, the primary intensions of utterances are grounded in the (normative) cognitive role of associated thoughts.

Primary intensions are not linguistic meaning. Different speakers can use the same name ('Fred') or natural kind term ('water') with quite different cognitive roles and with distinct patterns of epistemic evaluation. If so, the same expression will have different primary intensions for different speakers. So an expression's primary intension is not part of its linguistic meaning, where this is understood as meaning that is associated with an expression type simply by virtue of the conventions of a language.

Response: This point is correct. Primary intensions are not always part of linguistic meaning. For example, it can happen that an identity statement (e.g., 'Bill Smith is William Smith') can be cognitively insignificant for one speaker (e.g., his wife, who uses the two names interchangeably) but not for another (e.g., a colleague who uses the names in quite different domains without knowing that they are coextensive). If so, then the primary intensions of the names will coincide for one speaker but not for another, so that the primary intension of at least one of them must vary across speakers. Primary intensions can also vary for context-dependent terms such as 'tall' and 'heavy.' The moral is that for maximal generality, primary intensions should be associated with expression tokens (or with utterances of expression types) rather than with expression types.

Primary intensions are insufficiently fine grained. Cognitively distinct expressions may have the same primary intensions. When expressions are equivalent a priori, their primary intensions will coincide. For example, logical and mathematical truths all have the same primary intension (true in all scenarios) and have the same secondary intension, too. But these truths clearly differ in meaning and in cognitive significance. So two-dimensional semantic values do not exhaust meaning (or utterance content) and are not as fine-grained as Fregean senses.

Response: A two-dimensionalist can accommodate many of the relevant cases here by invoking structured intensions. This will distinguish between different logical and mathematical truths, for example. The only residual problem will arise if there are pairs of simple expressions that are equivalent a priori but are cognitively distinct. It is not obvious that there are such pairs, but if there are, there is more to meaning than primary intensions. We might say that primary intensions individuate expressions by their *idealized* cognitive significance and so do not capture differences in *nonidealized* cognitive significance. One might try to capture these differences by moving to intensions that are defined over a space of finer-grained epistemic possibilities. Alternatively, a two-dimensionalist might simply allow that, in addition to intensions, expressions are associated with finer-grained semantic values (such as the structured semantic values discussed earlier) that lie behind and determine these intensions. In any case, this point is no threat to the two-dimensionalist who is a semantic pluralist. Primary and secondary intensions are not all there is to meaning, but utterances can nevertheless be associated with primary and secondary intensions in a way that can play the various explanatory roles described earlier.

There are epistemic possibilities that correspond to no centered world (Yablo 1999, 2002). A key two-dimensionalist claim holds that when S is not ruled out a priori, then there is some centered world at which the primary intension of S is true. This may be so for typical Kripkean a posteriori necessities such as 'water is not H_2O,' but there are other sentences for which the claim is false. For example, it may be that the existence (or nonexistence) of a god is necessary without being a priori. If so, 'There is no god' (or 'There is a god') is not ruled out a priori, but it is necessarily false. There appears to be no relevant difference between primary and secondary intensions here, so the primary intension is true in no possible world. Something similar applies if the laws of nature in our world are the laws of all possible worlds. If these views are correct, then the space of epistemic possibilities outstrips the space of metaphysical possibilities in a way that falsifies the two-dimensionalist claim.

Response: All of these purported counterexamples rest on controversial claims about modality or apriority, and I argue in chapter 6 that none of them succeed. I also argue there that the concept of metaphysical modality itself has roots in the epistemic domain, so that there cannot be "strong necessities" that exhibit this sort of disconnect between epistemic and metaphysical modalities. Still, the existence or nonexistence of strong necessities is a delicate and controversial issue. A two-dimensionalist can remain neutral on this issue by understanding scenarios not as centered metaphysically possible worlds but instead as maximal epistemic possibilities. Then even if no metaphysically possible world verifies 'There is no god,' some maximal epistemic possibility will verify 'There is no god,' so there will be a scenario at which the primary intension of this sentence will be true. Understood in this neutral way, two-dimensionalism does not ground inferences from conceivability to metaphysical possibility (those inferences will turn on a further claim about the relationship between scenarios and metaphysically possible worlds), but it can still play much the same role as before in the epistemic and semantic domains. (This version of the framework suffices for the purposes of chapters 8, 9, 11, and 12, although not for the purposes of chapter 6.)

Complete canonical specifications are not available (Schroeter 2004). Epistemic two-dimensionalism requires that there be semantically neutral specifications of a given scenario that are complete in that they epistemically determine the truth value of arbitrary judgments. However, there may be some features of the world, such as intrinsic physical features, that cannot be captured in a semantically neutral specification.

Response: It is not clear whether there are intrinsic properties that cannot be captured in a semantically neutral specification, but if there are, this will be irrelevant to epistemically determining the truth value of any of our sentences. When information about these features is needed to epistemically determine the truth value of a sentence in a scenario, a semantically neutral characterization of the features (e.g., an existential or a Ramsey-sentence characterization) will suffice. (Such a characterization may not suffice for metaphysical determination and for evaluating truth values of sentences in counterfactual worlds according to their secondary intensions, but semantically neutral specifications are needed only for primary intensions.) The minimal size of a vocabulary that can epistemically determine the truth of all sentences is an important open question (which I address in forthcoming work), but there is good reason to believe that some semantically neutral (and indexical) vocabulary suffices. It should also be noted that if we take the purely epistemic approach to scenarios described in the previous response, a restriction to semantically neutral vocabulary is not needed, and so the issue here does not arise.

Objections to the role of apriority (Block and Stalnaker 1999; Yablo 2002). It is true that there is an epistemic relation between information about the world and claims about reference. For example, given the information that we are in the H_2O world (appropriately characterized), we should conclude that water is H_2O, and given the information that we are in the XYZ world, we should conclude that water is XYZ. It is also true that we can make these conditional inferences from the armchair without needing to perform further investigation of the environment. Nevertheless, these inferences are not justified a priori. The inferences are justified in part by background empirical knowledge of the world (Block and Stalnaker 1999) or by "peeking" at our own judgments (Yablo 2002). As a result, primary intensions are not connected to apriority as strongly as the two-dimensionalist supposes.

Response: In chapter 7, Jackson and I argue that these connections are in fact a priori. Although empirical facts about the world can play a causal role in determining the relevant patterns of inference, there is good reason to believe that they do not play a justifying role. (Chalmers 2002b responds to Yablo.) It is also worth noting that even a skeptic about apriority can use the epistemic two-dimensional framework. Even if the relevant inferential connections are not a priori, one can still use them to define primary intensions, and the resulting primary intensions will still behave much as they are supposed to (assigning a necessary intension to 'Hesperus is Hesperus' but not to 'Hesperus is Phosphorus,' for example). The connection between primary intensions and apriority will be lost, but primary intensions will still be strongly connected to the epistemic domain.

BIBLIOGRAPHY

Akins, K. 1993. What Is It Like to Be Boring and Myopic? In B. Dahlbom, ed., *Dennett and His Critics*. Oxford: Blackwell.

Albert, D. Z. 1993. *Quantum Mechanics and Experience*. Cambridge, Mass.: Harvard University Press.

Allport, A. 1988. What Concept of Consciousness? In A. Marcel and E. Bisiach, eds., *Consciousness in Contemporary Science*. New York: Oxford University Press.

Alter, T. 2006. On the Conditional Analysis of Phenomenal Concepts. *Philosophical Studies* 131(3): 777–78.

Andersen, R. 1997. Neural Mechanisms in Visual Motion Perception in Primates. *Neuron* 18: 865–72.

Ashwell, L. 2003. Conceivability and Modal Error. Master's thesis, University of Auckland.

Austin, D. F. 1990. *What's the Meaning of "This"?* Ithaca: Cornell University Press.

Aydede, M., and G. Güzeldere. 2005. Cognitive Architecture, Concepts, and Introspection: An Information-theoretic Solution to the Problem of Phenomenal Consciousness. *Nous* 39: 197–255.

Baars, B. J. 1988. *A Cognitive Theory of Consciousness*. New York: Cambridge University Press.

———, ed. 1996. Mental Imagery. Special issue, *Consciousness and Cognition* 5(3).

Bailey, A. Forthcoming. The Unsoundness of Arguments from Conceivability. http://www.uoguelph.ca/~abailey/.

Balog, K. 1999. Conceivability, Possibility, and the Mind-body Problem. *Philosophical Review* 108: 497–528.

———. Forthcoming. In defense of the phenomenal concept strategy. *Philosophy and Phenomenological Research*.

Bateson, G. 1972. *Steps to an Ecology of Mind*. San Francisco: Chandler.

Bayne, T. 2001a. Chalmers on Acquaintance and Phenomenal Judgment. *Philosophy and Phenomenological Research* 62: 407–19.

———. 2001b. Co-consciousness: Review of Barry Dainton's *Stream of Consciousness*. *Journal of Consciousness Studies* 8: 79–92.

———, A. Cleeremans, and P. Wilken. 2009. *The Oxford Companion to Consciousness*. New York: Oxford University Press.

Bealer, G. 1994. Mental Properties. *Journal of Philosophy* 91: 185–208.

———. 2002. Modal Epistemology and the Rationalist Renaissance. In T. Gendler and J. Hawthorne, eds., *Conceivability and Possibility*. New York: Oxford University Press.

————. 2007. Mental Causation. *Philosophical Perspectives* 21: 23–54.

Biggs, S. 2009. The Scrambler: An Argument Against Representationalism. *Canadian Journal of Philosophy* 39: 215–36.

Block, N. 1978. Troubles with Functionalism. In C. W. Savage, ed., *Perception and Cognition: Issues in the Foundation of Psychology.* Minneapolis: University of Minnesota Press.

————. 1990. Inverted Earth. *Philosophical Perspectives* 4: 53–79.

————. 1995. On a Confusion about a Function of Consciousness. *Behavioral and Brain Sciences* 18: 227–47.

————. 2006a. Max Black's Objection to Mind-body Identity. *Oxford Studies in Metaphysics* 2:3–78. Also in T. Alter and S. Walter, eds., *Phenomenal Concepts and Phenomenal Knowledge: New Essays on Consciousness and Physicalism.* New York: Oxford University Press.

————. 2006b. Two Neural Correlates of Consciousness. *Trends in Cognitive Science* 9: 46–52.

————. 2007. Consciousness, Accessibility, and the Mesh between Psychology and Neuroscience. *Behavioral and Brain Sciences* 30: 481–548.

————, O. Flanagan, and G. Güzeldere, eds. 1997. *The Nature of Consciousness: Philosophical Debates.* Cambridge, Mass.: MIT Press.

Block, N., and R. Stalnaker. 1999. Conceptual Analysis, Dualism, and the Explanatory Gap. *Philosophical Review* 108: 1–46.

Bogen, J. E. 1995a. On the Neurophysiology of Consciousness, Part I: An Overview. *Consciousness and Cognition* 4(1): 52–62.

————. 1995b. On the Neurophysiology of Consciousness, Part II: Constraining the Semantic Problem. *Consciousness and Cognition* 4(2): 137–58.

Boghossian, P., and J. D. Velleman. 1989. Color as a Secondary Quality. *Mind* 98: 81–103.

BonJour, L. 1969. Knowledge, Justification, and Truth: A Sellarsian Approach to Epistemology. PhD diss., Princeton University. http://www.ditext.com/bonjour/bonjour0.html.

————. 1978. Can Empirical Knowledge Have a Foundation? *American Philosophical Quarterly* 15: 1–13.

————, and Sosa, E. 2003. *Epistemic Justification.* Malden, MA: Blackwell.

Boring, E. G. 1929. *A History of Experimental Psychology.* New York: Century.

Bostrom, N. 2003. Are You Living in a Computer Simulation? *Philosophical Quarterly* 53: 243–55.

Braddon-Mitchell, D. 2003. Qualia and Analytic Conditionals. *Journal of Philosophy* 100: 111–35.

————. 2004. Masters of our Meanings. *Philosophical Studies* 188: 133–52.

Bradley, D. C., G. C. Chang, and R. A. Andersen. 1998. Encoding of Three-dimensional Structure-from-Motion by Primate Area MT Neurons. *Nature* 392: 714–17.

Broad, C. D. 1925. *The Mind and Its Place in Nature.* London: Routledge and Kegan Paul.

Brogaard, B. Forthcoming. Centered Worlds and the Content of Perception. In S. Hales, ed., *The Blackwell Companion to Relativism.* Oxford: Blackwell.

Brown, R. 2010. Deprioritizing the a priori arguments against physicalism. *Journal of Consciousness Studies* 17: 47–69.

Burge, T. 1979. Individualism and the Mental. *Midwest Studies in Philosophy* 4: 73–122.

————. 1991. Vision and Intentional Content. In E. Lepore and R. van Gulick, eds., *John Searle and His Critics.* Oxford: Blackwell.

Byrne, A. 1999. Cosmic Hermeneutics. *Philosophical Perspectives* 13: 347–83.

———. 2001. Intentionalism Defended. *Philosophical Review* 110: 199–240.

———. 2006. Color and the Mind-body Problem. *Dialectica* 60: 223–44.

———. 2007. Color Primitivism. *Erkenntnis* 66: 73–105.

———, and D. R. Hilbert. 2003. Color Realism and Color Science. *Behavioral and Brain Sciences* 26: 3–21.

Campbell, J. 1993. A Simple View of Color. In J. Haldane and C. Wright, eds., *Reality, Representation, and Projection.* New York: Oxford University Press.

———. 2002. *Reference and Consciousness.* New York: Oxford University Press.

Campbell, K. K. 1970. *Body and Mind.* London: Doubleday.

Carnap, R. 1947. *Meaning and Necessity.* University of Chicago Press.

Carruthers, P. 2000. *Phenomenal Consciousness: A Naturalistic Theory.* New York: Cambridge University Press.

———. 2004. Phenomenal Concepts and Higher-order Experiences. *Philosophy and Phenomenological Research* 68(2): 316–36.

———, and B. Veillet. 2007. The Phenomenal Concept Strategy. *Journal of Consciousness Studies* 14: 212–36.

Cauller, L. J., and A. T. Kulics. 1991. The Neural Basis of the Behaviorally Relevant N1 Component of the Somatosensory Evoked Potential in Awake Monkeys: Evidence that Backward Cortical Projections Signal Conscious Touch Sensation. *Experimental Brain Research* 84: 607–19.

Chalmers, D. J. 1990. How Cartesian Dualism Might Have Been True. http://consc.net/notes/dualism.html.

———. 1994. A Computational Foundation for the Study of Cognition. http://consc.net/papers/computation.html.

———. 1996. *The Conscious Mind: In Search of a Fundamental Theory.* New York: Oxford University Press.

———. 1997a. Availability: The Cognitive Basis of Experience? *Behavioral and Brain Sciences* 20: 148–9. Also in N. Block, O. Flanagan, and G. Güzeldere, eds., *The Nature of Consciousness: Philosophical Debates*, 421. Cambridge, Mass.: MIT Press, 1997. http://consc.net/papers/availability.html.

———. 1997b. Moving Forward on the Problem of Consciousness. *Journal of Consciousness Studies* 4: 3–46. Reprinted in J. Shear, ed., *Explaining Consciousness: The Hard Problem* (Cambridge, Mass.: MIT Press, 1997). http://consc.net/papers/moving.html.

———. 1999. Materialism and the Metaphysics of Modality. *Philosophy and Phenomenological Research* 59: 473–93. http://consc.net/papers/modality.html.

———. 2002a. The Components of Content. In D. J. Chalmers, ed., *Philosophy of Mind: Classical and Contemporary Readings.* New York: Oxford University Press. http://consc.net/papers/content.html.

———. 2002b. Does Conceivability Entail Possibility? In T. Gendler and J. Hawthorne, eds., *Conceivability and Possibility.* New York: Oxford University Press. http://consc.net/papers/conceivability.html.

———. 2004a. Epistemic Two-dimensional Semantics. *Philosophical Studies* 118: 153–226.

———. 2004b. Imagination, Indexicality, and Intensions. *Philosophy and Phenomenological Research* 68: 182–90. http://consc.net/papers/perry.html.

————. 2005. Phenomenal Concepts and the Knowledge Argument. In P. Ludlow, Y. Nagasawa, and D. Stoljar, eds., *There's Something about Mary.* Cambridge, Mass.: MIT Press. http://consc.net/papers/knowledge.html.

————. 2006. The Foundations of Two-dimensional Semantics. In M. Garcia-Carpintero and J. Macia, eds., *Two-dimensional Semantics: Foundations and Applications.* New York: Oxford University Press. http://consc.net/papers/foundations.pdf.

————. 2009. Ontological Anti-realism. In D. Chalmers, D. Manley, and R. Wasserman, eds., *Metametaphysics: New Essays on the Foundations of Ontology.* New York: Oxford University Press. http://consc.net/papers/ontology.pdf.

————. 2011. The Nature of Epistemic Space. In A. Egan and B. Weatherson, eds., *Epistemic Modality.* New York: Oxford University Press. http://consc.net/papers/espace.pdf.

————. Forthcoming. Propositions and Attitude Ascriptions: A Two-dimensional Account. *Nous.* http://consc.net/papers/propositions.pdf.

Chappell, R. 2006. Modal Rationalism. Honours thesis, Australian National University. http://www.princeton.edu/~chappell/ModalRationalism.pdf

Chisholm, R. 1942. The Problem of the Speckled Hen. *Mind* 204: 368–73.

————. 1957. *Perceiving: A Philosophical Study.* Ithaca: Cornell University Press.

Churchland, Patricia S. 1997. The Hornswoggle Problem. In J. Shear, ed., *Explaining Consciousness: The Hard Problem.* Cambridge, Mass.: MIT Press.

Churchland, Paul M. 1995. *The Engine of Reason, the Seat of the Soul: A Philosophical Journey into the Brain.* Cambridge, Mass.: MIT Press.

————. 1996. The Rediscovery of Light. *Journal of Philosophy* 93: 211–28.

Clark, Andy. 2000. A Case Where Access Implies Qualia? *Analysis* 60: 30–38.

Clark, Austen. 1992. *Sensory Qualities.* New York: Oxford University Press.

————. 2000. *A Theory of Sentience.* New York: Oxford University Press.

Conee, E. 1985. The Possibility of Absent Qualia. *Philosophical Review* 94: 345–66.

Cotterill, R. 1994. On the Unity of Conscious Experience. *Journal of Consciousness Studies* 2: 290–311.

Cowey, A., and P. Stoerig. 1995. Blindsight in Monkeys. *Nature* 373: 247–49.

Crane, T. 2003. The Intentional Structure of Consciousness. In Q. Smith and A. Jokic, eds., *Consciousness: New Philosophical Perspectives.* New York: Oxford University Press.

Crick, F. 1994. *The Astonishing Hypothesis: The Scientific Search for the Soul.* New York: Scribner.

————, and C. Koch. 1990. Toward a Neurobiological Theory of Consciousness. *Seminars in the Neurosciences* 2: 263–75.

————. 1995. Are We Aware of Neural Activity in Primary Visual Cortex? *Nature* 375: 121–23.

————. 1998. Consciousness and Neuroscience. *Cerebral Cortex* 375: 121–23.

————. 2004. A Framework for Consciousness. In M. Gazzaniga ed., *The Cognitive Neurosciences III*, 3rd ed. Cambridge, Mass.: MIT Press.

Dainton, B. 2000. *Stream of Consciousness: Unity and Continuity in Conscious Experience.* London: Routledge.

Davidson, D. 1986. A Coherence Theory of Truth and Knowledge. In E. Lepore, ed., *Truth and Interpretation: Perspectives on the Philosophy of Donald Davidson.* Oxford: Blackwell.

Davies, M. & Humberstone, I.L. 1981. Two Notions of Necessity. *Philosophical Studies* 58: 1–30.

Dehaene, S. 2001. *The Cognitive Neuroscience of Consciousness*. Cambridge, MA: MIT Press.

———, and J. Changeux. 2004. Neural Mechanisms for Access to Consciousness. In M. Gazzaniga, ed., *The Cognitive Neurosciences III*, 3rd ed. Cambridge, Mass.: MIT Press.

Dennett, D. C. 1968. *Content and Consciousness*. London: Routledge.

———. 1978. Where Am I? In D. C. Dennett, *Brainstorms: Philosophical Essays on Mind and Psychology*. Cambridge, Mass.: MIT Press.

———. 1979. On the absence of phenomenology. In D. F. Gustafson & B. L. Tapscott, eds., *Body, Mind, and Method*. Dordrecht: Kluwer.

———. 1991. *Consciousness Explained*. Boston: Little, Brown.

———. 1992. The Self as a Center of Narrative Gravity. In F. Kessel, P. Cole, and D. Johnson, eds., *Self and Consciousness: Multiple Perspectives*. Hillsdale, N.J.: Erlbaum.

———. 1996. Facing Backward on the Problem of Consciousness. *Journal of Consciousness Studies* 3: 4–6.

———. 2001. The Fantasy of First-person Science. http://ase.tufts.edu/cogstud/papers/chalmersdeb3dft.htm. Revised in *Sweet Dreams: Obstacles to a Science of Consciousness* (Cambridge, Mass.: MIT Press, 2005).

Descartes, R. 1641/1996. *Meditations on First Philosophy*. Trans. and ed. J. Cottingham. New York: Cambridge University Press.

Diaz Leon, E. Forthcoming a. Can Phenomenal Concepts Explain the Explanatory Gap. *Mind*.

———. Forthcoming b. Reductive Explanation, Concepts, and A Priori Entailment. *Philosophical Studies*.

Dretske, F. 1995. *Naturalizing the Mind*. Cambridge, Mass.: MIT Press.

Dreyfus, H. & Dreyfus, S. 2005. Existential Phenomenology and the Brave New World of the Matrix. In C. Grau, ed., *Philosophers Explore the Matrix*. New York: Oxford University Press.

Droege, P. 2003. *Caging the Beast: A Theory of Sensory Consciousness*. Amsterdam: Benjamins.

Eccles, J. C. 1994. *How the Self Controls Its Brain*. New York: Springer.

Eckhorn, R., Bauer, R., Jordan, W., Brosch, M., Kruse, W., Munk, M., and Reitboeck, H. J. 1988. Coherent oscillations: A mechanism of feature linking in the visual cortex? *Biological Cybernetics* 60: 121–130.

Edelman, G. M. 1989. *The Remembered Present: A Biological Theory of Consciousness*. New York: Basic Books.

Edwards, J. 1998. The Simple Theory of Colour and the Transparency of Sensory Experience. In C. MacDonald, B. Smith, and C. Wright, eds., *Knowing Our Own Minds: Essays on Self-knowledge*. New York: Oxford University Press.

Egan, A. 2006. Appearance Properties? *Nous* 40: 495–521.

Engel, S., X. Zhang, and B. Wandell. 1997. Colour Tuning in Human Visual Cortex Measured with Functional Magnetic Resonance Imaging. *Nature* 388(6637): 68–71.

Evans, G. 1979. Reference and Contingency. *Monist* 62: 161–89.

Farah, M. J. 1994. Visual Perception and Visual Awareness after Brain Damage: A Tutorial Overview. In C. Umilta and M. Moscovitch, eds., *Consciousness and Unconscious Information Processing: Attention and Performance 15*. Cambridge, Mass.: MIT Press.

Feigl, H. 1958. The "Mental" and the "Physical." *Minnesota Studies in the Philosophy of Science* 2: 370–497. Reprinted (with a postscript) as *The "Mental" and the "Physical": The Essay and a Postscript* (Minneapolis: University of Minnesota Press, 1967).

Fine, K. 2002. The Varieties of Necessity. In T. Gendler and J. Hawthorne, eds., *Conceivability and Possibility*. New York: Oxford University Press.

Flohr, H. 1992. Qualia and Brain Processes. In A. Beckermann, H. Flohr, and J. Kim, eds., *Emergence or Reduction?: Prospects for Nonreductive Physicalism*. Berlin: de Gruyter.

———. 1995. Sensations and Brain Processes. *Behavioral Brain Research* 71: 157–61.

Foster, J. 1991. *The Immaterial Self: A Defence of the Cartesian Dualist Conception of the Mind*. London: Routledge.

Francescotti, R. M. 1994. Qualitative Beliefs, Wide Content, and Wide Behavior. *Nous* 28: 396–404.

Frankish, K. 2007. The Anti-Zombie Argument. *Philosophical Quarterly* 57(229): 650–66.

Fredkin, E. 1990. Digital Mechanics: An Informational Process Based on Reversible Universal Cellular Automata. *Physica D* 45: 254.

Fumerton, R. 1995. *Metaepistemology and Skepticism*. Lanham, Md.: Rowman and Littlefield.

Garrett, B. J. 2006. What the History of Vitalism Teaches Us about Consciousness and the "Hard Problem." *Philosophy and Phenomenological Research* 72(3): 576–88.

Gazzaniga, M. S., ed. 2004. *The Cognitive Neurosciences III*, 3rd ed. Cambridge, Mass.: MIT Press.

Gertler, B. 2001. Introspecting Phenomenal States. *Philosophy and Phenomenological Research* 63: 305–28.

Goodale, M. A. 2004. Perceiving the World and Grasping It: Dissociations between Conscious and Unconscious Visual Processing. In M. Gazzaniga, ed., *The Cognitive Neurosciences III*, 3rd ed. Cambridge, Mass.: MIT Press.

Gray, J. A. 1995. The Contents of Consciousness: A Neuropsychological Conjecture. *Behavioral and Brain Sciences* 18: 659–722.

Greenfield, S. 1995. *Journey to the Centers of the Mind*. New York: Freeman.

Greenwald, A. G. 1992. New Look 3: Reclaiming Unconscious Cognition. *American Psychologist* 47: 766–79.

Griffin, D. R. 1998. *Unsnarling the World-knot: Consciousness, Freedom, and the Mind-body Problem*. Berkeley: University of California Press.

Gur, M., and D. M. Snodderly. 1997. A Dissociation between Brain Activity and Perception: Chromatically Active Cortical Neurons Signal Chromatic Activity That Is Not Perceived. *Vision Research* 37: 377–82.

Güzeldere, G. 1999. There Is No Neural Correlate of Consciousness. Paper presented at Toward a Science of Consciousness: Fundamental Approaches, Tokyo, May 25–28, 1999.

Hameroff, S. R. 1994. Quantum Coherence in Microtubules: A Neural Basis for Emergent Consciousness. *Journal of Consciousness Studies* 1: 91–118.

———, and Penrose, R. 1996. Conscious Events as Orchestrated Space-time Selections. *Journal of Consciousness Studies* 3: 36–53.

Hardin, C. L. 1987. *Color for Philosophers*. Indianapolis: Hackett.

———. 1992. Physiology, Phenomenology, and Spinoza's True Colors. In A. Beckermann, H. Flohr, and J. Kim, eds., *Emergence or Reduction?: Prospects for Nonreductive Physicalism*. Berlin: de Gruyter.

Harman, G. 1990. The Intrinsic Quality of Experience. *Philosophical Perspectives* 4: 31–52.

Hawthorne, J. 2002a. Advice to Physicalists. *Philosophical Studies* 101: 17–52.

———. 2002b. Deeply Contingent A Priori. *Philosophy and Phenomenological Research* 65: 247–69.

———. 2006. Dancing Qualia and Direct Reference. In T. Alter and S. Walter, eds., *Phenomenal Concepts and Phenomenal Knowledge: New Essays on Consciousness and Physicalism*. New York: Oxford University Press.

He, S., P. Cavanagh, and J. Intriligator. 1996. Attentional Resolution and the Locus of Visual Awareness. *Nature* 384: 334–37.

Heck, R. 2000. Nonconceptual Content and the Space of Reasons. *Philosophical Review* 109: 483–523.

Hill, C. S. 1991. *Sensations: A Defense of Type Materialism*. New York: Cambridge University Press.

———. 1997. Imaginability, Conceivability, Possibility, and the Mind-body Problem. *Philosophical Studies* 87: 61–85.

———, and B. P. McLaughlin. 1999. There Are Fewer Things in Reality Than Are Dreamt of in Chalmers's Philosophy. *Philosophy and Phenomenological Research* 59: 445–54.

Hobson, J. A. 1997. Consciousness as a State-dependent Phenomenon. In J. Cohen and J. Schooler, eds., *Scientific Approaches to Consciousness*. Mahweh, N.J.: Erlbaum.

Hodgson, D. 1991. *The Mind Matters: Consciousness and Choice in a Quantum World*. New York: Oxford University Press.

Holman, E. 2002. Color Eliminativism and Color Experience. *Pacific Philosophical Quarterly* 83: 8–56.

Horgan, T. 1984. Supervenience and Cosmic Hermeneutics. *Southern Journal of Philosophy* Supplement 22: 19–38.

———, and J. Tienson. 2002. The Intentionality of Phenomenology and the Phenomenology of Intentionality. In D. J. Chalmers, ed., *Philosophy of Mind: Classical and Contemporary Readings*. New York: Oxford University Press.

Howell, R. 2008. The Two-dimensionalist Reductio. *Pacific Philosophical Quarterly* 89: 348–58.

Humphrey, N. 1992. *A History of the Mind*. New York: Simon and Schuster.

Hurlburt, R. T. 1990. *Sampling Normal and Schizophrenic Inner Experience*. New York: Plenum.

Hurley, S. 1998. Unity, Neuropsychology, and Action. In *Consciousness in Action*. Cambridge, Mass.: Harvard University Press.

———. 2002. Action, the Unity of Consciousness, and Vehicle Externalism. In A. Cleeremans, ed., *The Unity of Consciousness: Binding, Integration, Dissociation*. New York: Oxford University Press.

Huxley, T. 1874. On the Hypothesis That Animals Are Automata, and Its History. *Fortnightly Review* 95: 555–80. Reprinted in *Collected Essays* (London: Macmillan, 1893).

Ismael, J. 1999. Science and the Phenomenal. *Philosophy of Science* 66: 351–69.

Jackendoff, R. 1987. *Consciousness and the Computational Mind.* Cambridge, Mass.: MIT Press.

Jackson, F. 1979. A Note on Physicalism and Heat. *Australasian Journal of Philosophy* 58: 26–34.

———. 1982. Epiphenomenal Qualia. *Philosophical Quarterly* 32: 127–36.

———. 1994a. Armchair Metaphysics. In J. O'Leary-Hawthorne and M. Michael, eds., *Philosophy in Mind.* Dordrecht: Kluwer.

———. 1994b. Finding the Mind in the Natural World. In R. Casati, B. Smith, and S. White, eds., *Philosophy and the Cognitive Sciences.* Vienna: Hölder-Pichler-Tempsky.

———. 1996. The Primary Quality of Color. *Philosophical Perspectives* 10: 199–219.

———. 1998. *From Metaphysics to Ethics: A Defence of Conceptual Analysis.* New York: Oxford University Press.

———. 2003. Mind and Illusion. In A. O'Hear, ed., *Minds and Persons.* New York: Cambridge University Press.

———. 2004. Why We Still Need A-Intensions. *Philosophical Studies* 118: 257–277.

———, P. Pettit, and M. Smith. 2000. Ethical Particularism and Patterns. In B. Hooker and M. Little, eds., *Moral Particularism.* New York: Oxford University Press.

Jacoby, L. L., D. S. Lindsay, and J. P. Toth. 1992. Unconscious Influences Revealed: Attention, Awareness, and Control. *American Psychologist* 47: 802–809.

Jakab, Z. 2003. Phenomenal Projection. *Psyche* 9 (4).

James, W. 1890. *The Principles of Psychology. New York:* Henry Holt and Co.

Johnston, M. 1992. How to Speak of the Colors. *Philosophical Studies* 68: 221–63.

———. 2004. The Obscure Object of Hallucination. *Philosophical Studies* 120: 113–83.

———. Forthcoming. *The Manifest.*

Kallestrup, J. 2006. Physicalism, Conceivability, and Strong Necessities. *Synthese* 151: 273–95.

Kaplan, D. 1979. Dthat. In P. Cole, ed., *Syntax and Semantics.* New York: Academic Press.

Kaplan, D. 1989. Demonstratives. In J. Almog, J. Perry, and H. Wettstein, eds., *Themes from Kaplan.* New York: Oxford University Press.

Kaszniak, A., ed. 1998. *Emotions, Qualia, and Consciousness.* Singapore: World Scientific.

Kirk, R. 1974. Zombies vs. Materialists. *Proceedings of the Aristotelian Society* (suppl. vol.) 48: 135–52.

———. 1994. *Raw Feeling: A Philosophical Account of the Essence of Consciousness.* New York: Oxford University Press.

———. 1999. Why There Couldn't Be Zombies. *Aristotelian Society Supplement* 73: 1–16.

Koch, C. 2004. *The Quest for Consciousness: A Neuroscientific Approach.* Englewood, Colo.: Roberts.

Kouider, S. 2009. Neurobiological Theories of Consciousness. In W. Banks, ed., *Encyclopedia of Consciousness.* Boston: Elsevier.

Kreiman, G., I. Fried, and C. Koch. 2002. Single Neuron Correlates of Subjective Vision in the Human Medial Temporal Lobe. *Proceedings of the National Academy of Sciences USA* 99: 8378–83.

Kriegel, U. 2002a. PANIC Theory and the Prospects for a Representational Theory of Phenomenal Consciousness. *Philosophical Psychology* 15: 55–64.

———. 2002b. Phenomenal Content. *Erkenntnis* 57: 175–98.

———. 2009. *Subjective Consciousness: A Self-representational Theory.* New York: Oxford University Press.

Kripke, S. A. 1980. *Naming and Necessity.* Cambridge, Mass.: Harvard University Press.

———. 1981. *Wittgenstein on Rules and Private Language.* Cambridge, Mass.: Harvard University Press.

Lamme, V. 2006. Toward a True Neural Stance on Consciousness. *Trends in Cognitive Sciences* 10: 494–501.

Leopold, D. A., and N. K. Logothetis. 1996. Activity Changes in Early Visual Cortex Reflect Monkeys' Percepts during Binocular Rivalry. *Nature* 379: 549–53.

Leopold, D. A., A. Maier, and N. K. Logothetis. 2003. Measuring Subjective Visual Perception in the Nonhuman Primate. *Journal of Consciousness Studies* 10: 115–30.

Leuenberger, S. 2008. *Ceteris Absentibus* Physicalism. *Oxford Studies in Metaphysics* 4: 145–70.

Levin, J. 2007. What Is a Phenomenal Concept? In T. Alter and S. Walter, eds., *Phenomenal Concepts and Phenomenal Knowledge: Essays on Consciousness and Physicalism.* New York: Oxford University Press.

Levine, J. 1983. Materialism and Qualia: The Explanatory Gap. *Pacific Philosophical Quarterly* 64: 354–61.

———. 1993. On Leaving Out What It's Like. In M. Davies and G. Humphreys, eds., *Consciousness: Psychological and Philosophical Essays.* Oxford: Blackwell.

———. 1998. Conceivability and the Metaphysics of Mind. *Nous* 32: 449–80.

———. 2001. *Purple Haze: The Puzzle of Consciousness.* New York: Oxford University Press.

———. 2003. Experience and Representation. In Q. Smith and A. Jokic, eds., *Consciousness: New Philosophical Perspectives.* New York: Oxford University Press.

———. 2007. Phenomenal Concepts and the Materialist Constraint. In T. Alter and S. Walter, eds., *Phenomenal Concepts and Phenomenal Knowledge: Essays on Consciousness and Physicalism.* New York: Oxford University Press.

———. Forthcoming. The Q-Factor: Modal Rationalism and Modal Autonomism. *Philosophical Review.*

Lewis, D. 1984. Putnam's paradox. *Australasian Journal of Philosophy* 62: 221–237.

———. 1986. *On the Plurality of Worlds.* Oxford: Blackwell.

———. 1988. What Experience Teaches. *Proceedings of the Russellian Society.* Sydney: University of Sydney. Reprinted in W. G. Lycan, ed., *Mind and Cognition: A Reader* (London: Blackwell, 1989).

———. 1994. Reduction of Mind. In S. Guttenplan, ed., *A Companion to the Philosophy of Mind.* Oxford: Blackwell.

Libet, B. 1982. Brain Stimulation in the Study of Neuronal Functions for Conscious Sensory Experiences. *Human Neurobiology* 1: 235–42.

———. 1993. The Neural Time Factor in Conscious and Unconscious Events. In *Experimental and Theoretical Studies of Consciousness* (Ciba Foundation Symposium 174), pp. 123–37. New York: John Wiley and Sons.

Llinas, R. R., U. Ribary, M. Joliot, and X.-J Wang. 1994. Content and Context in Temporal Thalamocortical Binding. In G. Buzsaki, R. R. Llinas, and W. Singer, eds., *Temporal Coding in the Brain.* Berlin: Springer.

Lloyd, D. 1991. Leaping to Conclusions: Connectionism, Consciousness, and the Computational Mind. In T. Horgan and J. Tienson, eds., *Connectionism and the Philosophy of Mind.* London: Kluwer.

Loar, B. 1990/1997. Phenomenal States. *Philosophical Perspectives* 4: 81–108. Revised in N. Block, O. Flanagan, and G. Güzeldere, eds., *The Nature of Consciousness* (Cambridge, Mass.: MIT Press, 1997).

———. 1999. David Chalmers's *The Conscious Mind. Philosophy and Phenomenological Research* 59: 464–71.

———. 2003. Phenomenal Intentionality as the Basis of Mental Content. In M. Hahn and B. Ramberg, eds., *Reflections and Replies.* Cambridge, Mass.: MIT Press.

Lockwood, M. 1989. *Mind, Brain, and the Quantum.* New York: Oxford University Press.

———. 1993. The Grain Problem. In H. Robinson, ed., *Objections to Physicalism.* New York: Oxford University Press.

Logothetis, N. K. 1998. Single Units and Conscious Vision. *Philosophical Transactions of the Royal Society of London, Series B, Biological Sciences* 353: 1801–18.

———, and J. Schall. 1989. Neuronal Correlates of Subjective Visual Perception. *Science* 245: 761–63.

Lowe, E. J. 1996. *Subjects of Experience.* New York: Cambridge University Press.

Lutz, A., J. Lachaux, J. Matrinerie, and F. Varela. 2002. Guiding the Study of Brain Dynamics by Using First-person Data: Synchrony Patterns Correlate with Ongoing Conscious States during a Simple Visual Task. *Proceedings of the National Academy of Science USA* 99: 1586–91.

Lycan, W. G. 1996. *Consciousness and Experience.* Cambridge, Mass.: MIT Press.

———. 2000. Representational Theories of Consciousness. In E. Zalta, ed., *The Stanford Encyclopedia of Philosophy.* http://plato.stanford.edu/.

———. 2001. The Case for Phenomenal Externalism. *Philosophical Perspectives* 15: 17–35.

Lynch, M. 2006. Zombies and the Case of the Phenomenal Pickpocket. *Synthese* 149: 37–58.

Mack, A., and I. Rock. 1998. *Inattentional Blindness.* Cambridge, Mass.: MIT Press.

Macpherson, F. 2010. A Disjunctive Theory of Introspection. *Philosophical Issues.*

Mandik, P., and J. Weisberg. 2008. Type-Q Materialism. In C. Wrenn, ed., *Naturalism, Reference, and Ontology: Essays in Honor of Roger F. Gibson.* New York: Lang.

Marcel, A. J. 1994. What Is Relevant to the Unity of Consciousness? In C. Peacocke, ed., *Objectivity, Simulation, and the Unity of Consciousness.* New York: Oxford University Press.

Marconi, D. 2005. Two-Dimensional Semantics and the *Articulation Problem. Synthese* 143 (3): 321–49.

Marcus, E. 2004. Why Zombies Are Inconceivable. *Australasian Journal of Philosophy* 82: 477–90.

Marge, E. 1991. Magnetostimulation of Vision: Direct Noninvasive Stimulation of the Retina and the Visual Brain. *Optometry and Vision Science* 68: 427–40.

Marks, C. 1980. *Commissurotomy, Consciousness, and Unity of Mind.* Cambridge, Mass.: MIT Press.

Martin, M. G. F. 2002. Particular Thoughts and Singular Thought. In A. O'Hear, ed., *Logic, Thought, and Language.* New York: Cambridge University Press.

Marton, P. 1998. Zombies vs. Materialists: The Battle for Conceivability. *Southwest Philosophy Review* 14: 131–38.

Maund, J. B. 1995. *Colours: Their Nature and Representation.* New York: Cambridge University Press.

Maxwell, G. 1979. Rigid Designators and Mind-brain Identity. *Minnesota Studies in the Philosophy of Science* 9: 365–403.

Maxwell, N. 1968. Understanding Sensations. *Australasian Journal of Philosophy* 46: 127–45.

McDowell, J. 1994. *Mind and World.* Cambridge, Mass.: Harvard University Press.

McGinn, C. 1988. Consciousness and Content. *Proceedings of the British Academy* 74: 219–39.

———. 1989. Can We Solve the Mind-body Problem? *Mind* 98: 349–66.

———. 1996. Another Look at Color. *Journal of Philosophy* 93: 537–53.

McLaughlin, B. 2003. Color, Consciousness, and Color Consciousness. In Q. Smith and A. Jokic, eds., *Consciousness: New Philosophical Perspectives.* New York: Oxford University Press.

Merikle, P. M., and M. Daneman. 2000. Conscious vs. Unconscious Perception. In M. S. Gazzaniga, ed., *The New Cognitive Neurosciences.* Cambridge, Mass.: MIT Press.

Merikle, P. M., and E. M. Reingold. 1992. Measuring Unconscious Processes. In R. Bornstein and T. Pittman, eds., *Perception without Awareness.* New York: Guilford.

Metzinger, T. 1995. *Conscious Experience.* Lawrence, Kans.: Allen.

———. 2000. *Neural Correlates of Consciousness: Empirical and Conceptual Questions.* Cambridge, Mass.: MIT Press.

Mills, E. 1996. Interactionism and Overdetermination. *American Philosophical Quarterly* 33: 105–15.

Milner, A. D. 1995. Cerebral Correlates of Visual Awareness. *Neuropsychologia* 33: 1117–30.

———, and M. A. Goodale. 1995. *The Visual Brain in Action.* New York: Oxford University Press.

Nagel, T. 1971. Brain Bisection and the Unity of Consciousness. *Synthese* 22: 396–413. Reprinted in T. Nagel, *Mortal Questions* (New York: Cambridge University Press, 1979).

———. 1974. What Is It Like To Be a Bat? *Philosophical Review* 4: 435–50.

Nelkin, N. 1993. What Is Consciousness? *Philosophy of Science* 60: 419–34.

Newell, A. 1990. *Unified Theories of Cognition.* Cambridge, Mass.: Harvard University Press.

Newman, J. B. 1997. Putting the Puzzle Together: Toward a General Theory of the Neural Correlates of Consciousness. *Journal of Consciousness Studies* 4: 47–66; 4: 100–21.

Nida-Rümelin, M. 1995. What Mary Couldn't Know: Belief about Phenomenal States. In T. Metzinger, ed., *Conscious Experience.* Lawrence, Kans.: Allen.

———. 1996. Pseudonormal Vision: An Actual Case of Qualia Inversion? *Philosophical Studies* 82: 145–57.

———. 1997. On Belief about Experiences: An Epistemological Distinction Applied to the knowledge argument. *Philosophy and Phenomenological Research* 58: 51–73.

———. 2007. Grasping Phenomenal Properties. In T. Alter and S. Walter, eds., *Phenomenal Concepts and Phenomenal Knowledge: New Essays on Consciousness and Physicalism.* New York: Oxford University Press.

Nimtz, C. 2004. Two-dimensionalism and Natural Kind Terms. *Synthese* 138: 125–48.

Noë, A., and E. Thompson. 2004. Are There Neural Correlates of Consciousness? *Journal of Consciousness Studies* 11: 3–28.

Nordby, K. 1990. Vision in a Complete Achromat: A Personal Account. In R. Hess, L. Sharpe, and K. Nordby, eds., *Night Vision: Basic, Clinical, and Applied Aspects.* New York: Cambridge University Press.

Nordby, K. 2007. What is this thing you call color? Can a totally color blind person know about color? In T. Alter and S. Walter, eds., *Phenomenal Concepts and Phenomenal Knowledge: New Essays on Consciousness and Physicalism.* New York: Oxford University Press.

O'Dea, J. 2002. The Indexical Nature of Sensory Concepts. *Philosophical Papers* 31: 169–81.

Papineau, D. 1993. Physicalism, Consciousness, and the Antipathetic Fallacy. *Australasian Journal of Philosophy* 71: 169–83.

———. 2002. *Thinking about Consciousness.* New York: Oxford University Press.

———. 2007. Phenomenal and Perceptual Concepts. In T. Alter and S. Walter, eds., *Phenomenal Concepts and Phenomenal Knowledge: New Essays on Consciousness and Physicalism.* New York: Oxford University Press.

Peacocke, C. 1983. *Sense and Content: Experience, Thought, and Their Relations.* New York: Oxford University Press.

———. 1992. *A Study of Concepts.* New York: Oxford University Press.

———. 2001. Does Perception Have a Non-conceptual Content? *Journal of Philosophy* 98: 239–64.

Penfield, W. 1937. The Cerebral Cortex and Consciousness. In *The Harvey Lectures.* Reprinted in R. H. Wilkins, ed., *Neurosurgical Classics* (New York: Johnson Reprint Corp., 1965).

———, and T. Rasmussen. 1950. *The Cerebral Cortex of Man: A Clinical Study of Localization of Function.* New York: Macmillan.

Penrose, R. 1989. *The Emperor's New Mind.* New York: Oxford University Press.

———. 1994. *Shadows of the Mind.* New York: Oxford University Press.

Perry, J. 1979. The Problem of the Essential Indexical. *Nous* 13: 3–21.

———. 2001. *Knowledge, Possibility, and Consciousness.* Cambridge, Mass.: MIT Press.

Pessoa, L., E. Thompson, and A. Noe. 1998. Finding Out about Filling In: A Guide to Perceptual Completion for Visual Science and the Philosophy of Perception. *Behavioral and Brain Sciences* 21: 723–48.

Piccinini, G. 2009. First-Person Data, Publicity, and Self-Measurement. *Philosophers' Imprint* 9.

Pollock, J. 1986. *Contemporary Theories of Knowledge.* Lanham, Md.: Rowman and Littlefield.

Pope, K. S. 1978. *The Stream of Consciousness: Scientific Explorations into the Flow of Human Experience.* New York: Plenum.

Popper, K., and J. Eccles. 1977. *The Self and Its Brain: An Argument for Interactionism.* New York: Springer.

Puccetti, R. 1981. The Case for Mental Duality: Evidence from Split-brain Data and Other Considerations. *Behavioral and Brain Sciences* 4: 93–123.

Putnam, H. 1975. The Meaning of "Meaning." In *Mind, Language, and Reality.* New York: Cambridge University Press.

————. 1981. *Reason, Truth, and History.* New York: Cambridge University Press.

Quine, W. V. 1951. Two Dogmas of Empiricism. *Philosophical Review* 60: 20–43.

Raffman, D. 1995. On the Persistence of Phenomenology. In T. Metzinger, ed., *Conscious Experience.* Lawrence, Kans.: Allen.

Ramachandran, V. S., and E. M. Hubbard. 2001. Psychophysical Investigations into the Neural Basis of Synaesthesia. *Proceedings of the Royal Society London* 268: 979–83.

Reber, A. 1996. *Implicit Learning and Tacit Knowledge: An Essay on the Cognitive Unconscious.* New York: Oxford University Press.

Rees, G. 2004. Neural Correlates of Visual Consciousness in Humans. In M. Gazzaniga, ed., *The Cognitive Neurosciences III,* 3rd ed. Cambridge, Mass.: MIT Press.

Revonsuo, A. 1999. Binding and the Phenomenal Unity of Consciousness. *Consciousness and Cognition* 8: 173–85.

Rey, G. 1995. Toward a Projectivist Account of Conscious Experience. In T. Metzinger, ed., *Conscious Experience.* Lawrence, Kans.: Allen.

————. 1998. A Narrow Representationalist Account of Qualitative Experience. *Philosophical Perspectives* 12: 435–58.

Robinson, W. S. 1988. *Brains and People: An Essay on Mentality and Its Causal Conditions.* Philadelphia: Temple University Press.

Roca-Royes, S. Forthcoming. Conceivability and *De Re* Modal Knowledge. *Nous.*

Rosenthal, D. M. 1997. A Theory of Consciousness. In N. Block, O. Flanagan, and G. Güzeldere, eds., *The Nature of Consciousness.* Cambridge, Mass.: MIT Press.

Russell, B. 1910. Knowledge by Acquaintance and Knowledge by Description. *Proceedings of the Aristotelian Society* 11: 108–28.

————. 1927. *The Analysis of Matter.* London: Kegan Paul.

Ryle, G. 1949. *The Concept of Mind.* London: Hutchinson.

Salmon, N. 1986. *Frege's Puzzle.* Cambridge, Mass.: MIT Press.

————. 1989. The Logic of What Might Have Been. *Philosophical Review* 98: 3–34.

Salzman, C. D., K. H. Britten, and W. T. Newsome. 1990. Cortical Microstimulation Influences Perceptual Judgments of Motion Direction. *Nature* 346: 174–77.

Schacter, D. L., and T. Curran. 2000. Memory without Remembering and Remembering without Memory: Implicit and False Memories. In M. S. Gazzaniga, ed., *The New Cognitive Neurosciences.* Cambridge, Mass.: MIT Press.

Schaffer, J. 2010. Monism: The Priority of the Whole. *Philosophical Review* 119: 31–76.

Schellenberg, S. 2010. The Particularity and Phenomenology of Perceptual Experience. *Philosophical Studies* 149: 19–48.

Schiff, N. D. 2004. The Neurology of Impaired Consciousness. In M. Gazzaniga, ed., *The Cognitive Neurosciences III,* 3rd ed. Cambridge, Mass.: MIT Press.

Schiffer, S. 2003. Two-dimensional Semantics and Propositional Attitude Content. In *The Things We Mean.* New York: Oxford University Press.

Schooler, J. W., and S. M. Fiore. 1997. Consciousness and the Limits of Language. In J. Cohen and J. Schooler, eds., *Scientific Approaches to Consciousness.* Hillsdale, N.J.: Erlbaum.

Schroeder, T., and B. Caplan. 2007. On the Content of Experience. *Philosophy and Phenomenological Research* 75: 590–611.

Schroeter, L. 2004. The Rationalist Foundations of Chalmers' Two-Dimensional Semantics. *Philosophical Studies* 18: 227–55.

Schwitzgebel, E. 2008. The Unreliability of Naïve Introspection. *Philosophical Review* 117: 245–73.

Seager, W. E. 1991. *Metaphysics of Consciousness*. London: Routledge.

———. 1995. Consciousness, Information, and Panpsychism. *Journal of Consciousness Studies* 2: 272–288.

Searle, J. R. 1980. Minds, Brains, and Programs. *Behavioral and Brain Sciences* 3: 417–57.

———. 1983. *Intentionality*. New York: Cambridge University Press.

———. 1984. Can Computers Think? In *Minds, Brains, and Science*. Cambridge, Mass.: Harvard University Press.

———. 1990. Consciousness, Explanatory Inversion, and Cognitive Science. *Behavioral and Brain Sciences* 13: 585–642.

———. 1991. *The Rediscovery of the Mind*. Cambridge, Mass.: MIT Press.

Sellars, W. 1956. Empiricism and the Philosophy of Mind. *Minnesota Studies in the Philosophy of Science* 1: 253–329. Reprinted as *Empiricism and the Philosophy of Mind* (Cambridge, Mass: Harvard University Press, 1997).

———. 1981. Is Consciousness Physical? *Monist* 64: 66–90.

Shallice, T. 1972. Dual Functions of Consciousness. *Psychological Review* 79: 383–93.

———. 1988. Information-processing Models of Consciousness: Possibilities and Problems. In A. Marcel and E. Bisiach, eds., *Consciousness in Contemporary Science*. New York: Oxford University Press.

Shannon, C. E. 1948. A Mathematical Theory of Communication. *Bell Systems Technical Journal* 27: 379–423.

Shear, J., ed. 1997. *Explaining Consciousness: The Hard Problem*. Cambridge, Mass.: MIT Press.

Sheinberg, D. L., and N. K. Logothetis. 1997. The Role of Temporal Cortical Areas in Perceptual Organization. *Proceedings of the National Academy of Sciences USA* 94: 139–41.

Shoemaker, S. 1975. Functionalism and Qualia. *Philosophical Studies* 27: 291–315.

———. 1981. Some Varieties of Functionalism. *Philosophical Topics* 12: 93–119.

———. 1990. Qualities and Qualia: What's in the Mind? *Philosophy and Phenomenological Research* (suppl.) 50: 109–31.

———. 1994. Phenomenal Character. *Nous* 28: 21–38.

———. 1998. Causal and Metaphysical Necessity. *Pacific Philosophical Quarterly* 79: 59–77.

———. 1999. On David Chalmers's *The Conscious Mind*. *Philosophy and Phenomenological Research* 59: 539–44.

———. 2001. Introspection and Phenomenal Character. *Philosophical Topics*. Reprinted in D. Chalmers, ed., *Philosophy of Mind: Classical and Contemporary Readings* (New York: Oxford University Press, 2002).

———. 2002. Consciousness and Co-consciousness. In A. Cleeremans, ed., *The Unity of Consciousness: Binding, Integration, Dissociation*. New York: Oxford University Press.

———. 2006. The Ways Thing Seem. In T. Gendler and J. Hawthorne, eds., *Perceptual Experience*. New York: Oxford University Press.

Sidelle, A. 2002. On the Metaphysical Contingency of Laws of Nature. In T. Gendler and J. Hawthorne, eds., *Conceivability and Possibility*. New York: Oxford University Press.

Siegel, S. 2005. Subject and Object in the Contents of Visual Experience. *Philosophical Review* 115: 335–58.

———. 2006. Which Properties Are Represented in Perception? In T. Gendler and J. Hawthorne, eds., *Perceptual Experience.* New York: Oxford University Press.

Siewert, C. 1998. *The Significance of Consciousness.* Princeton: Princeton University Press.

Smart, J. J. C. 1959. Sensations and Brain Processes. *Philosophical Review* 68: 141–56.

Soames, S. 2004. *Reference and Description: The Case against Two-dimensionalism.* Princeton: Princeton University Press.

Sperling, G. 1960. The Information Available in Brief Visual Presentations. *Psychological Monographs* 498: 1–29.

Stalnaker, R. 1978. Assertion. In P. Cole, ed., *Syntax and Semantics: Pragmatics*, vol. 9. New York: Academic Press.

———. 2001. On Considering a Possible World as Actual. *Proceedings of the Aristotelian Society* (suppl. volume) 75: 141–156.

———. 2002. What Is It Like To Be a Zombie? In T. Gendler and J. Hawthorne, eds., *Conceivability and Possibility.* New York: Oxford University Press.

———. 2003. Conceptual Truth and Metaphysical Necessity. In *Ways a World Might Be: Metaphysical and Anti-Metaphysical Essays.* Oxford University Press.

———. 2004. Assertion Revisited: On the Interpretation of Two-Dimensional Modal Semantics. *Philosophical Studies* 118: 299–322.

Stapp, H. 1993. *Mind, Matter, and Quantum Mechanics.* Berlin: Springer.

Stoljar, D. 2001a. The Conceivability Argument and Two Conceptions of the Physical. *Philosophical Perspectives* 15: 393–413.

———. 2001b. Two Conceptions of the Physical. *Philosophy and Phenomenological Research* 62: 253–81.

———. 2005. Physicalism and Phenomenal Concepts. *Mind and Language* 20: 296–302.

———. 2007. Consequences of Intentionalism. *Erkenntnis* (special issue) 66(1–2): 247–70.

Strawson, G. 1994. *Mental Reality.* Cambridge, Mass.: MIT Press.

———. 2000. Realistic Materialist Monism. In S. Hameroff, A. Kaszniak, and D. Chalmers, eds., *Toward a Science of Consciousness III.* Cambridge, Mass.: MIT Press.

Sturgeon, S. 1994. The Epistemic Basis of Subjectivity. *Journal of Philosophy* 91: 221–35.

———. 2000. Zombies and Ghosts. In *Matters of Mind.* New York: Routledge.

———. 2010. Apriorism about Modality. In B. Hale and A. Hoffman, eds., *Modality: Metaphysics, Logic and Epistemology.* New York: Oxford University Press.

Swinburne, R. 1986. *The Evolution of the Soul.* New York: Oxford University Press.

Taylor, J. G., and F. N. Alavi. 1993. Mathematical Analysis of a Competitive Network for Attention. In J. G. Taylor, ed., *Mathematical Approaches to Neural Networks.* New York: Elsevier.

Teller, D. Y., and E. N. Pugh. 1984. Linking Propositions in Color Vision. In J. D. Mollon and L. T. Sharpe, eds., *Color Vision: Physiology and Psychophysics.* London: Academic Press.

Thau, M. 2002. *Consciousness and Cognition.* New York: Oxford University Press.

Thomas, N. J. T. 1998. Zombie Killer. In S. Hameroff, A. Kaszniak, and A. Scott, eds., *Toward a Science of Consciousness II.* Cambridge, Mass.: MIT Press.

Thompson, B. 2003. The Nature of Phenomenal Content. PhD diss., University of Arizona.

————. Forthcoming. The Spatial Content of Experience. *Philosophy and Phenomenological Research.* http://faculty.smu.edu/bthompso/spatialcontent.html.

Tong, F., K. Nakayama, J. T. Vaughan, and N. Kanwisher. 1998. Binocular Rivalry and Visual Awareness in Human Extrastriate Cortex. *Neuron* 21: 753–59.

Tononi, G. 2004. An Information Integration Theory of Consciousness. *BMC Neuroscience* 5: 42.

Tootell, R. B., J. B. Reppas, A. M. Dale, R. B. Look, M. I. Sereno, R. Malach, J. Brady, and B. R. Rosen. 1995. Visual Motion Aftereffect in Human Cortical Area MT Revealed by Functional Magnetic Resonance Imaging. *Nature* 375: 139–41.

Travis, C. 2004. The Silence of the Senses. *Mind* 113: 57–94.

Treisman, A. 2003. Consciousness and Perceptual Binding. In A. Cleeremans, ed., *The Unity of Consciousness: Binding, Integration, Dissociation.* New York: Oxford University Press.

Tye, M. 1995. *Ten Problems of Consciousness: A Representational Theory of the Phenomenal Mind.* Cambridge, Mass.: MIT Press.

————. 1997. Qualia. In E. Zalta, ed., *Stanford Encyclopedia of Philosophy* (fall 1997 ed.).

————. 2003a. Blurry Images, Double Vision, and Other Oddities: New Problems for Representationalism? In Q. Smith and A. Jokic, eds., *Consciousness: New Philosophical Perspectives.* New York: Oxford University Press.

————. 2003b. *Consciousness and Persons: Unity and Identity.* MIT Press.

————. 2003c. A Theory of Phenomenal Concepts. In A. O'Hear, ed., *Minds and Persons.* New York: Cambridge University Press.

————. 2009. *Consciousness Revisited: Materialism without Phenomenal Concepts.* Cambridge, Mass.: MIT Press.

Vaidya, A. 2008. Modal Rationalism and Modal Monism. *Erkenntnis* 68: 191–212.

Van Gulick, R. 1993. Understanding the Phenomenal Mind: Are We All Just Armadillos? In M. Davies and G. Humphreys, eds., *Consciousness: Philosophical and Psychological Aspects.* Oxford: Blackwell.

————. 1999. Conceiving beyond Our Means: The Limits of Thought Experiments. In S. Hameroff, A. Kaszniak, and D. J. Chalmers, eds., *Toward a Science of Consciousness III.* Cambridge, Mass.: MIT Press.

Varela, F. 1997. Neurophenomenology: A Methodological Remedy for the "Hard Problem." In J. Shear, ed., *Explaining Consciousness: The Hard Problem.* Cambridge, Mass.: MIT Press.

————, and J. Shear. 2001. *The View from Within: First-person Methodologies in the Study of Consciousness.* London: Imprint Academic.

Velmans, M. 1991. Is Human Information-processing Conscious? *Behavioral and Brain Sciences* 14: 651–69.

————. 2007. Heterophenomenology versus Critical Phenomenology. *Phenomenology and the Cognitive Sciences* 6: 221–30.

————, and S. Schneider. 2007. *The Blackwell Companion to Consciousness.* Blackwell.

Vinueza, A. 2000. Sensations and the Language of Thought. *Philosophical Psychology* 13: 373–92.

Warfield, T. 1999. Against Representational Theories of Consciousness. *Journal of Consciousness Studies* 6: 66–69.

Weatherson, B. 2004. Luminous Margins. *Australasian Journal of Philosophy* 82: 373–83.

Wheeler, J. A. 1990. Information, Physics, Quantum: The Search for Links. In W. Zurek, ed., *Complexity, Entropy, and the Physics of Information.* Redwood City, Calif.: Addison-Wesley.

White, S. 1986. Curse of the Qualia. *Synthese* 68: 333–68.

———. 2007. Property Dualism, Phenomenal Concepts, and the Semantic Premise. In T. Alter and S. Walter, eds., *Phenomenal Concepts and Phenomenal Knowledge: New Essays on Consciousness and Physicalism.* New York: Oxford University Press.

Wigner, E. P. 1961. Remarks on the Mind-body Question. In I. J. Good, ed., *The Scientist Speculates.* London: Basic Books.

Wilkes, K. V. 1988. —, Yishi, Duh, Um, and Consciousness. In A. Marcel and E. Bisiach, eds., *Consciousness in Contemporary Science.* New York: Oxford University Press.

Williamson, T. 2000. *Knowledge and Its Limits.* New York: Oxford University Press.

Wittgenstein, L. 1953. *Philosophical Investigations.* Oxford: Blackwell.

Wolfram, S. 2002. *A New Kind of Science.* Champaign, Ill.: Wolfram Media.

Wong, K.-Y. 1996. Sentence-Relativity and the Necessary A Posteriori. *Philosophical Studies* 83: 53–91.

Worley, S. 2003. Conceivability, Possibility, and Physicalism. *Analysis* 63: 15–23.

Wright, W. 2003. Projectivist Representationalism and Color. *Philosophical Psychology* 16: 515–33.

Yablo, S. 1999. Concepts and Consciousness. *Philosophy and Phenomenological Research* 59: 455–63.

———. 2000. Textbook Kripkeanism and the Open Texture of Concepts. *Pacific Philosophical Quarterly* 81: 98–122.

———. 2002. Coulda, Woulda, Shoulda. In T. Gendler and J. Hawthorne, eds., *Conceivability and Possibility.* New York: Oxford University Press.

Zeki, S. 2007. A Theory of Micro-consciousness. In Velmans and Schneider 2007.

SUBJECT INDEX

NAME INDEX

29402980R00344

Printed in Great Britain
by Amazon